I0066322

Gene Therapy: Biomedical Applications

Gene Therapy: Biomedical Applications

Editor: Sylvester Noble

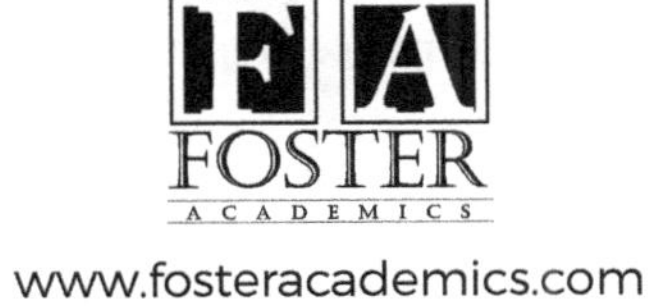

www.fosteracademics.com

www.fosteracademics.com

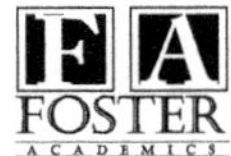

Cataloging-in-Publication Data

Gene therapy : biomedical applications / edited by Sylvester Noble.
p. cm.
Includes bibliographical references and index.
ISBN 978-1-63242-892-9
1. Gene therapy. 2. Medical sciences. 3. Biomedical engineering. 4. Genetic engineering.
5. Therapeutics. I. Noble, Sylvester.
RB155.8 .G46 2020
615.895--dc23

Foster Academics,
118-35 Queens Blvd., Suite 400,
Forest Hills, NY 11375, USA

ISBN 978-1-63242-892-9 (Hardback)

Contents

Preface

The world is advancing at a fast pace like never before. Therefore, the need is to keep up with the latest developments. This book was an idea that came to fruition when the specialists in the area realized the need to coordinate together and document essential themes in the subject. That's when I was requested to be the editor. Editing this book has been an honour as it brings together diverse authors researching on different streams of the field. The book collates essential materials contributed by veterans in the area which can be utilized by students and researchers alike.

In the field of medicine, the emerging frontier of gene therapy holds great potential in the treatment of many human diseases and conditions. It is characterized by the intent of direct therapeutic effect and the precision of the procedure. In this model, nucleic acid is delivered into a patient's cells which results in the replacement or knocking out of genes that cause a disease. Gene therapy can be classified into somatic and germline gene therapy. In somatic cell gene therapy, therapeutic genes are transferred into the somatic cells of the body and the resulting modifications affect the patient only, without being passed on to the offspring. In germline gene therapy, the germline itself is modified due to the introduction of functional genes into the genome of germ cells. Such changes are inherited by generations of individuals. This book covers in detail some existing theories and innovative concepts revolving around gene therapy. Some of the diverse topics covered in this book address the varied biomedical applications of gene therapy. As this field is emerging at a fast pace, this book will help the readers to better understand the advanced concepts of this field.

Each chapter is a sole-standing publication that reflects each author´s interpretation. Thus, the book displays a multi-facetted picture of our current understanding of application, resources and aspects of the field. I would like to thank the contributors of this book and my family for their endless support.

Editor

1

Theranostic Studies of Human Sodium Iodide Symporter Imaging and Therapy using ^{188}Re: A Human Glioma Study in Mice

Rui Guo[1], M Zhang[1], Yun Xi[1], Yufei Ma[2], Sheng Liang[2], Shuo Shi[1], Ying Miao[1], Biao Li[1]*

1 Department of Nuclear Medicine, Rui Jin Hospital, School of medicine, Shanghai JiaoTong University, Shanghai, China, **2** Department of Nuclear Medicine, Xin Hua Hospital, School of medicine, Shanghai JiaoTong University, Shanghai, China

Abstract

Objective: To investigate the role of ^{188}Re in human sodium iodide symporter (hNIS) theranostic gene-mediated human glioma imaging and therapy in model mice.

Methods: The human glioma cell line U87 was transfected with recombinant lentivirus encoding the hNIS gene under the control of cytomegalovirus promoter (U87-hNIS). The uptake and efflux of ^{188}Re were determined after incubating the cells with ^{188}Re. ^{188}Re uptake experiments in the presence of various concentrations of sodium perchlorate were carried out. In vitro cell killing tests with ^{188}Re were performed. U87-hNIS mediated ^{188}Re distribution, imaging and therapy in nude mice were also tested.

Results: U87-hNIS cell line was successfully established. The uptake of ^{188}Re in U87-hNIS cells increased up to 26-fold compared to control cells, but was released rapidly with a half-life of approximately 4 minutes. Sodium perchlorate reduced hNIS-mediated ^{188}Re uptake to levels of control cell lines. U87-hNIS cells were selectively killed following exposure to ^{188}Re, with a survival of 21.4%, while control cells had a survival of 92.1%. Unlike in vitro studies, U87-hNIS tumor showed a markedly increased ^{188}Re retention even 48 hours after ^{188}Re injection. In the therapy study, there was a significant difference in tumor size between U87-hNIS mice (317±67 mm^3) and control mice (861±153 mm^3) treated with ^{188}Re for 4 weeks ($P<0.01$).

Conclusion: The results indicate that inserting the hNIS gene into U87 cells is sufficient to induce specific ^{188}Re uptake, which has a cell killing effect both in vitro and in vivo. Moreover, our study, based on the function of hNIS as a theranostic gene allowing noninvasive imaging of hNIS expression by ^{188}Re scintigraphy, provides detailed characterization of in vivo vector biodistribution and level, localization, essential prerequisites for precise planning and monitoring of clinical gene therapy that aims to individualize gene therapy concept.

Editor: Gabriele Multhoff, Technische Universitaet Muenchen, Germany

Funding: This work was supported by grants from the National Natural Science Foundation of China (Nos. 81101071, 81271610, and 81101066), http://www.nsfc.gov.cn/publish/portal0/default.htm,the Medical Engineering (Science) Cross Foundation of Shanghai Jiaotong University (YG2013MS27), http://en.sjtu.edu.cn/, the Funding Scheme for Training Young Teachers in Colleges and Universities in Shanghai, http://www.studyshanghai.org/controller.asp?action=index_en. The funders had no role in study design, data collection and analysis, decision to publish, or preparation of the manuscript.

Competing Interests: The authors have declared that no competing interests exist.

* Email: lb10363@rjh.com.cn

Introduction

Glioma remains one of the most common cancers and is a leading cause of cancer-related deaths worldwide. Furthermore, glioma carries a poor prognosis and survival rate. Aside from tumor resection, radiotherapy is the major curative therapy for glioma. However, patients often develop normal brain tissue necrosis following external radiation [1]; thus, new therapeutic strategies are required. The theranostic strategy [2,3] using radionuclide-based imaging reporter genes shows great treatment promise for various clinical fields, particularly in the field of cancer gene therapy.

As a theranostic gene, the sodium iodide symporter (NIS) is a plasma membrane glycoprotein, which mediates active iodide uptake in the thyroid and other tissues [4,5]. One of the most exciting current areas of NIS research is radioiodine treatment of extrathyroidal cancers by the ectopic transfer of the NIS gene into otherwise non-NIS-expressing cancers. Many investigators have successfully obtained ectopic NIS expression by gene transfer techniques in prostate cancer [6], melanoma [7], glioma cells [8] and myeloma cells [9].

Our previous studies [10–13] suggest that baculovirus mediate human NIS (hNIS) expression leads to ^{131}I uptake in several types of tumors and presents as a promising target for gene therapy. Although the baculovirus can mediate gene transduction effectively and achieve desirable expression in various tumor cell lines in vitro, there are still some obstacles to overcome concerning the in vivo application of this system in gene therapy. For example, a major concern is the inactivation of baculovirus by the serum complement in baculovirus-based gene therapy in vivo.

In previous studies [14–15], extrathyroidal tissues are generally not able to organify iodide after NIS gene transfer. In the contrast, ^{131}I accumulates and is organified in the thyroid, which exhibits competitive inhibition in extrathyroidal tumor ^{131}I uptake, preventing the delivery of a radiation dose high enough to affect cell viability; therefore, the therapeutic efficacy of ^{131}I is limited [16]. The application of alternative radioisotopes that are also transported by hNIS with a shorter physical half-life and a high energy to ^{131}I may provide a powerful method for enhancing the therapeutic efficacy of hNIS-targeted radionuclide therapy [17,18]. ^{188}Re is a β-emitting radionuclide with a short physical half-life (0.71 day) that has been used in a variety of therapeutic applications in humans, including cancer radioimmunotherapy and palliation of skeletal bone pain [19]. Due to its higher relative energy compared to ^{131}I, administration of ^{188}Re offers the possibility of higher energy deposition over a shorter time period. Compared to ^{131}I (E = 0.192 MeV), ^{188}Re has been proposed as an ideal alternative emitter (E = 0.778 MeV) to ^{131}I for cancer treatment. Kang et al [20] investigated ^{188}Re accumulation of a human hepatocellular carcinoma cell line, SK-Hep1, by transfer of human sodium iodide symporter (hNIS) gene and found it has the potential to be used in hepatocellular carcinoma management. To date, no studies have explored whether lentivirus-mediated hNIS gene expression and ^{188}Re uptake can be used for glioma imaging and therapy. In this study, we investigated the role of ^{188}Re as a potential alternative radionuclide for hNIS-mediated imaging and treatment of human glioma in model mice.

Materials and Methods

Plasmid construction, lentivirus preparation, and U87 cell transfection with Lenti-CMV-hNIS

The human NIS gene was removed from the pcDNA3.1-hNIS vector (kindly provided by Dr. Sissy Jhiang from Ohio University, OH, USA) by restriction enzyme digestion. All plasmid construction and lentivirus (Lenti-CMV-hNIS) production was performed according to Life Technologies (Carlsbad, CA, USA) manufacturing instructions. Lenti-CMV-0 with no hNIS was prepared as a control. U87 human glioma cell line (American Type Culture Collection, AT CC) were maintained in Dulbecco's modified Eagle's medium (DMEM) supplemented with 10% fetal bovine serum, 5% CO_2, 37°C, 100 U/ml penicillin and 100 μg/ml streptomycin. To generate cell lines expressing hNIS controlled by the cytomegalovirus (CMV)-enhancer/promoter, the Lenti-CMV-hNIS vector was transfected into U87 cells and selected for weeks according to the manufacturer's instructions. Established cells (U87-hNIS) were confirmed through ^{188}Re uptake experiments. U87-0 cells transfected with Lenti-CMV-0 (hNIS gene negative) were prepared as controls. Cells were maintained in Dulbecco's modified eagle medium (DMEM; Life Technologies) supplemented with fetal bovine serum (10%), and maintained at 37°C in a humidified atmosphere with 5% CO_2. Cells were seeded in 24-well plates 24 hours before experiments to achieve a density of 10^5 cells/well at the day of study.

In vitro isotope uptake experiments

^{188}Re was eluted from a ^{188}W/^{188}Re generator (LaiTai Company, Suzhou, People's Republic of China) using 0.9% saline. hNIS expression in U87-hNIS cells was tested in vitro by ^{188}Re uptake as Weiss et al. described previously with minor modifications [21]. All activity data were corrected for decay and normalized. U87-hNIS cells were washed with 0.5 mL Hank's balanced salt solution (bHBSS; HBSS supplemented with 10 μM sodium iodide and buffered with Hepes, pH 7.3) once, and incubated for 1, 2, 5, 10, 20, 30, 60, and 120 minutes, respectively, in the presence of 0.5 mL bHBSS containing 3.7 kBq ^{188}Re. The cells were then washed twice with ice-cold bHBSS and incubated with 1 mL of 100% ice-cold dehydrated alcohol for 20 minutes. The radioactivity (counts per minute [cpm]) in cell lysates was measured using a multi-well gamma-counter (Shanghai Institute of Nuclear Research Rihuan Instrument Company, China). All experiments were performed in triplicate. U87-0 transfected cells were prepared as a control.

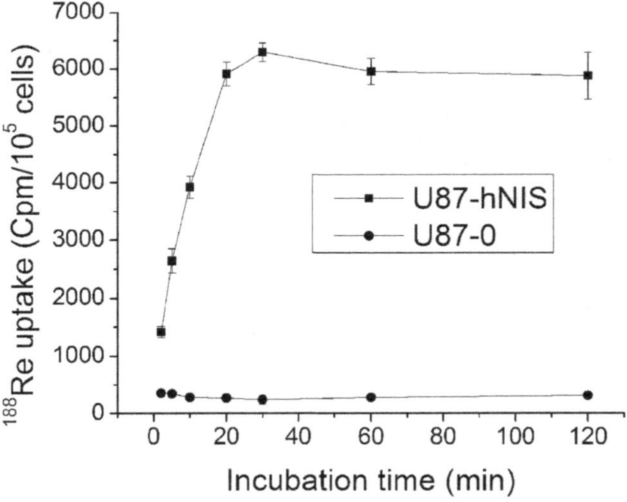

Figure 1. Time dependent ^{188}Re uptake by U87-hNIS cells. ^{188}Re uptake was measured by incubation for various time periods with 3.7 kBq of ^{188}Re in bHBSS. Results are expressed in numbers of counts per minute for 10^5 cells. The upper line represents U87-hNIS cells, while the lower line represents U87-0 cells. Data points are means ± SD (n = 3).

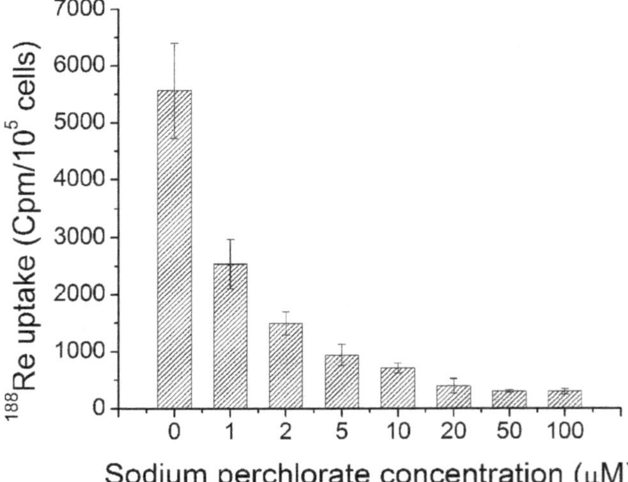

Figure 2. Sodium perchlorate inhibition study. Sodium perchlorate was added at the indicated concentration (0, 1, 2, 5, 10, 20, 50, and 100 μM) and ^{188}Re uptake was measured. Results are expressed in numbers of counts per minute for 10^5 cells. Bars are means ± SD (n = 3).

Sodium perchlorate inhibition study

We used a sodium perchlorate inhibition study to test the specificity of ^{188}Re uptake. U87-hNIS cells were incubated for 30 minutes in 3.7 kBq ^{188}Re medium supplemented with sodium perchlorate (Sigma-Aldrich, St. Louis, MI, USA) at concentrations of 0, 1 μM, 2 μM, 5 μM, 10 μM, 20 μM, 50 μM, and 100 μM. Then the cells were washed, lysed, and counted as described previously.

Isotope efflux study *in vitro*

We evaluated ^{188}Re efflux kinetics in cells expressing hNIS as previously described by Weiss et al [21]. Briefly, U87-hNIS cells were exposed to 3.7 kBq/well ^{188}Re at 37°C for 20 minutes. Cell medium was then replaced with fresh, nonradioactive bHBSS. The cells were incubated for 2, 4, 6, 8, 10, 12, 14, 16, 18 or 20 min and immediately lysed as described previously. After the incubation period, the cells were extracted with 1 mL of dehydrated alcohol, and the residual activity in the cells were measured.

In vitro assessment of isotope toxicity by clonogenic assay

U87-hNIS and U87-0 cells were seeded in 24-well plates 24 hours before the experiment to achieve a density of 10^5 cells/well on the day of study. As shown in Table 1, cells were divided into six groups: Group 1 included U87-hNIS cells washed with bHBSS and allowed to incubate for 7 hours (5% CO_2, 37°C) after the addition of 740 kBq ^{188}Re/mL; Group 2 was processed as Group 1, but without addition of ^{188}Re; Group 3 included U87-0 cells washed with bHBSS and allowed to incubate for 7 hours after the addition of 740 kBq ^{188}Re/mL; Group 4 was processed as Group 3, but without addition of ^{188}Re; Group 5 included non-transfected U87 cells that were washed with bHBSS and allowed to incubate for 7 hours after the addition of 740 kBq ^{188}Re/mL; Group 6 was processed as Group 5, but without addition of ^{188}Re. Groups 2, 3, 4, 5 and 6 all served as controls. The six groups of cells were then washed twice with bHBSS, trypsinized, counted, and plated at a density of 200 cells/well in 6-well plates in triplicate. The cells were placed in 5% CO_2 at 37°C for 7 days. After removing the culture medium, each plate was stained with crystal violet solution (0.1%), and colonies including more than 30 cells were counted. Results are expressed as the percentage of surviving cells, ie, the percentage of colonies obtained after treatment with lentivirus and/or ^{188}Re compared to treatment with bHBSS alone (Group 6).

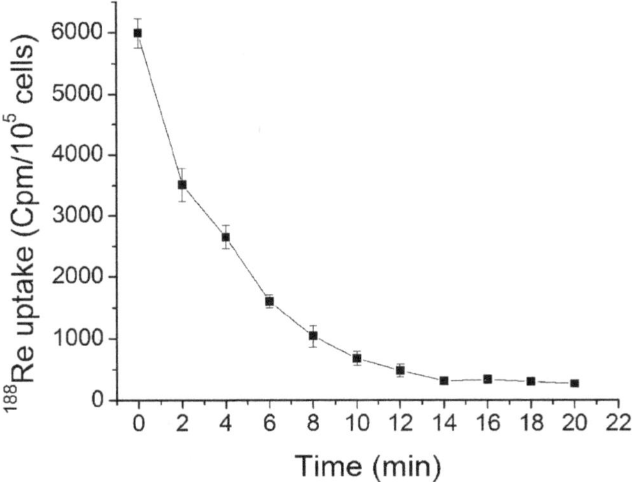

Figure 3. Time dependent ^{188}Re efflux assay in U87-hNIS cells after a 20 minute incubation with 3.7 kBq ^{188}Re in 0.5 mL bHBSS. Results are expressed as counts per minute for 105 cells. Data points are means ± SD (n = 3).

Biodistribution of ^{188}Re in xenografted mice

For biodistribution studies, the U87-hNIS tumor xenografted mice were randomly divided into 4 groups with 6 mice per group. Each animal received a 370 kBq intravenous (i.v.) injection of ^{188}Re to evaluate biodistribution of the tracer in the tumor and major organs. The mice were sacrificed 0.5 h, 2 h, 12 h and 24 h after the radionuclide injection, the main organs and xenografted tumors were removed, weighed, and counted for radioactivity by using a gamma counter. All tissue counts were corrected for background and decay during the time of counting. Results were expressed as a percentage of the injected dose per gram (% ID/g) of tissue. Each value represents the mean and SD of 6 animals. The U87-0 tumor xenografted mice were served as controls and processed as described above.

Tumor imaging and therapy study in a xenograft model

Animal procedures were carried out following the approval of the Ethics Committee and Animal Care Committee of Shanghai Jiaotong University, School of Medicine. Five-week-old female, athymic Balb/c nude mice were used in the following experiments; six mice were used in each group. A xenograft model was generated by subcutaneous injection of U87-hNIS or U87-0 cells (5×10^6 cells suspended in 150 μL phosphate buffered saline) into the right axilla of the mice. Approximately 6 weeks after inoculation when the tumor diameter reached 0.8–1.0 cm, the mice were used for imaging and therapeutic studies.

Xenograft models of U87-hNIS and U87-0 cells were established (n = 6 for each group). ^{188}Re (55.5 MBq) was injected through the caudal vein. Immediately after intravenous injection of ^{188}Re into the mice, the time dependent accumulation of radioactivity in the mice was monitored 15 minutes, 0.5, 1, 2, 4, 24, and 48 hours after injection using a γ-camera (GE Healthcare, Cleveland, OH, USA), equipped with a high-resolution pinhole collimator with a matrix size of 256×256. Elliptical regions of interest (ROI) were placed on the tumor and on the contralateral armpit region, from which tumor-to-nontumor (T/NT) contralateral armpit count ratios of each group were measured and calculated in every time point.

To evaluate the in vivo effects of hNIS-mediated radioiodine therapy, U87-hNIS tumor size of xenograft models were measured before and after the intravenous injection of 18.5 MBq, 55.5 MBq and 111 MBq ^{188}Re respectively (n = 6 for each group). U87-0 tumor xenograft models were treated with 55.5 MBq ^{188}Re and served as controls. All mice were followed for a total of 4 weeks. Tumor volume was estimated using the following formula: $\text{length}\times\text{width}^2\times0.52$.

Statistical analysis

Origin 7.5 (OriginLab Corporation, Northampton, MA, USA) and SPSS 16.0 (IBM Corporation, Armonk, NY, USA) were used for all statistical analyses. Numeric data are expressed as means ± standard deviation (SD). Data comparisons between groups were performed by analysis of variance (ANOVA) test. P values <0.05 were considered statistically significant.

Table 1. The subgroups used in the in vitro ^{188}Re clonogenic assay.

	Group1	Group2	Group3	Group4	Group5	Group6
U87-hNIS	+	+				
U87-0			+	+		
U87					+	+
^{188}Re	+		+		+	

Results

Plasmid construction, lentivirus preparation, and U87 cell transfection with Lenti-CMV-hNIS

We successfully developed a lentivirus-derived vector containing the hNIS gene under the control of the CMV promoter and yielded virus (Lenti-CMV-hNIS) stocks. Lenti-CMV-0 was also prepared as control with the same titer. Approximately 3 weeks later, after infection of U87 cells with the recombinant lentiviruses, stable cell lines U87-hNIS and U87-0 were established. In order to investigate the function of hNIS in the recombinant U87-hNIS cell lines, ^{188}Re uptake experiments were performed.

hNIS-mediated *in vitro* ^{188}Re uptake

^{188}Re uptake in U87-hNIS cells with respect to ^{188}Re incubation time is shown in Figure 1; the initial uptake of ^{188}Re was dependent on incubation time. ^{188}Re influx rapidly increased into U87-hNIS cells, with half-maximal uptake observed at about 5 minutes, reaching a maximum after about 30 minutes. ^{188}Re uptake in U87-hNIS cells was 26-fold higher than in U87-0 cells after incubation with ^{188}Re for 30 minutes. At that time point, ^{188}Re accumulation achieved a peak; therefore, 30 minutes represented the U87-hNIS maximal ^{188}Re uptake and was selected as the incubation time for subsequent experiments. The intracellular radioactivity was calculated to be up to 3.3% of the total radioactivity in cell lysate and media. Assuming that U87-hNIS cells have a mean diameter of 10 μm, we estimated that an up to 328-fold higher concentration of ^{188}Re was observed in cells compared to media. The radioactivity measured 2 hours after ^{188}Re incubation was 93.3% of the maximal uptake. There is a plateau, as Zuckier et al. [22] reported in similar studies, which suggest steady-state uptake.

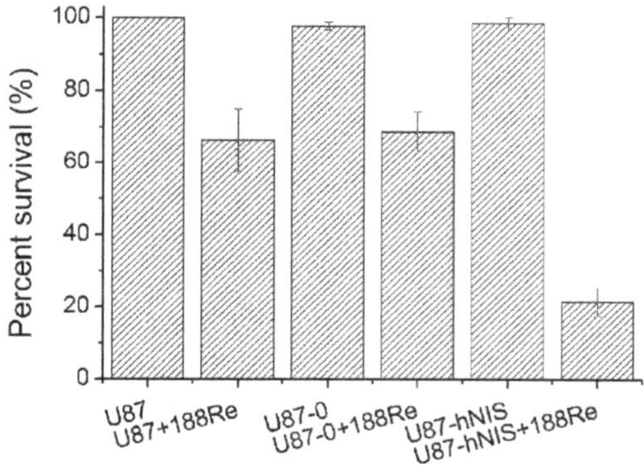

Figure 4. Survival rates of U87-hNIS cells treated with 740 kBq ^{188}Re/mL ^{188}Re. Groups 2, 3, 4, 5, and 6 all served as controls. Bars are means ± SD (n = 3).

Sodium perchlorate inhibition study

To evaluate whether ^{188}Re accumulation was specifically induced by the functional activity of the hNIS gene product, ^{188}Re uptake was determined in U87-hNIS cells in the presence of various concentrations of sodium perchlorate, an established competitive inhibitor. Figure 2 shows the effect of sodium perchlorate on ^{188}Re uptake in U87-hNIS cells. Uptake of ^{188}Re showed dose-dependent inhibition in U87-hNIS cells in experiments performed within a range of 1–50 μM $NaClO_4$; 5 μM $NaClO_4$ decreased ^{188}Re uptake to 16.8%, while at a concentration of 50 μM, sodium perchlorate inhibited ^{188}Re accumulation in U87-hNIS cells by 94.6%. ^{188}Re uptake was blocked and significantly decreased in the presence of sodium perchlorate, indicating that ^{188}Re is uptaken through functional hNIS in U87-hNIS cells.

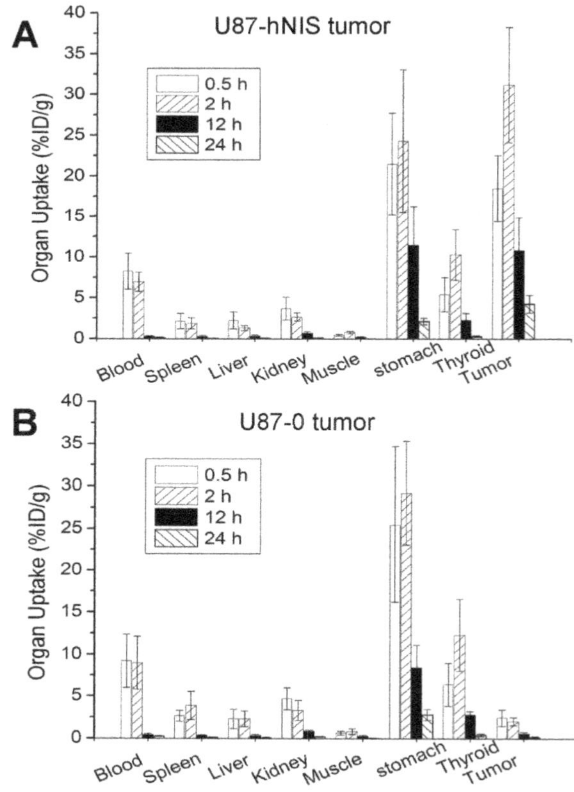

Figure 5. Biodistribution of ^{188}Re in nude mice bearing subcutaneously xenografted U87-hNIS glioma tumors (A) and U87-0 glioma tumors (B). Data are expressed as the % ID/g of tissue. Bars are the mean ± standard deviation (n = 6).

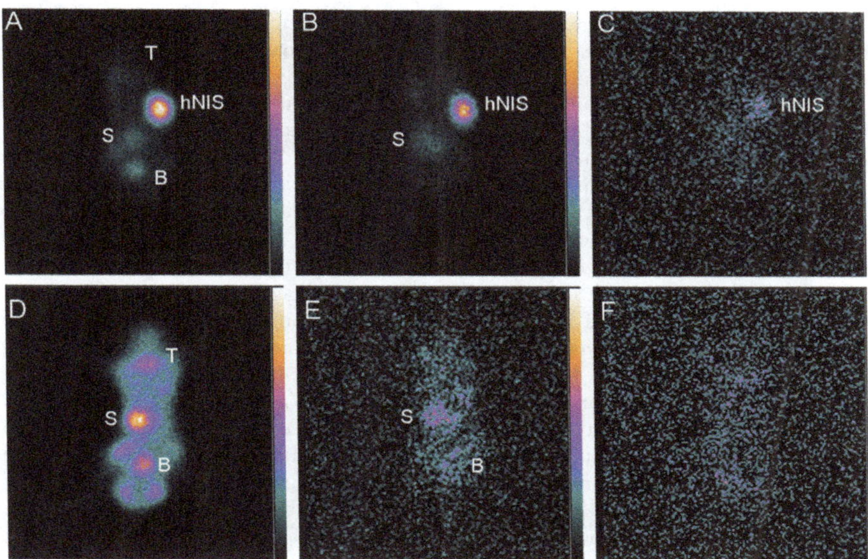

Figure 6. Whole-body scintigraphic images (anterior view) of hNIS-expressing U87-hNIS tumors (the first line, right axilla) or U87-0 tumors (the second line, right axilla) at 1-hour (A, D), 24 hours (B, E), and 48 hours (C, F) after intravenous injection of ^{188}Re. T = thyroid; S = stomach; B = bladder; hNIS = hNIS-expressing tumor.

Radionuclide efflux assay

On reaching maximum ^{188}Re uptake after approximately 30 min, the ^{188}Re efflux assay was continued for 20 min (Figure 1). As shown in Figure 3, the amount of remaining ^{188}Re in U87-hNIS cell lysate was determined as a function of time after replacement of ^{188}Re containing media with nonradioactive media. The cellular radioactivity was rapidly and continuously released into the media, with 55.7% of the total cellular ^{188}Re released within 4 minutes, and 95.5% efflux was observed after 20 minutes, indicating that the radiotracer was rarely trapped in U87-hNIS cells. Accordingly, under in vitro conditions limiting re-uptake, a rapid release of ^{188}Re was observed.

^{188}Re toxicity assessed by colony-forming assay

In vitro ^{188}Re toxicity experiments were performed on U87-hNIS cells to demonstrate whether it was possible to obtain a cell killing effect with ^{188}Re. After ^{188}Re treatment, clonogenic assays were performed, the results of which are shown in Figure 4. The data is expressed as the percentage of surviving cells. In Group 2 and Group 4, U87-hNIS and U87-0 cells treated without ^{188}Re, the numbers of colonies were 98.3% and 97.7% of blank cells (Group 6), respectively, indicating that transfection with the lentivirus did not affect cell survival. In Group 3 and Group 5, after exposure to ^{188}Re, 68.7% and 66.3% of the cells survived, respectively. In Group 1, the number of ^{188}Re treated U87-hNIS colonies that recovered were significantly lower than in the other five groups, with a survival of about 21.3%, demonstrating a selective killing effect of ^{188}Re in hNIS-expressing cells, which is the end goal of this system.

Biodistribution of ^{188}Re in xenografted mice

The biodistribution data of ^{188}Re in U87-hNIS tumor

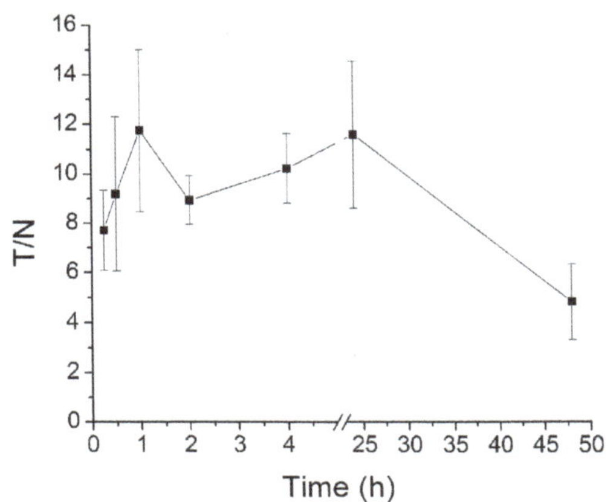

Figure 7. Time dependent tumor/non-tumor (T/NT) ratio of ^{188}Re uptake by U87-hNIS tumor bearing nude mice. Data points are means ± SD (n = 6).

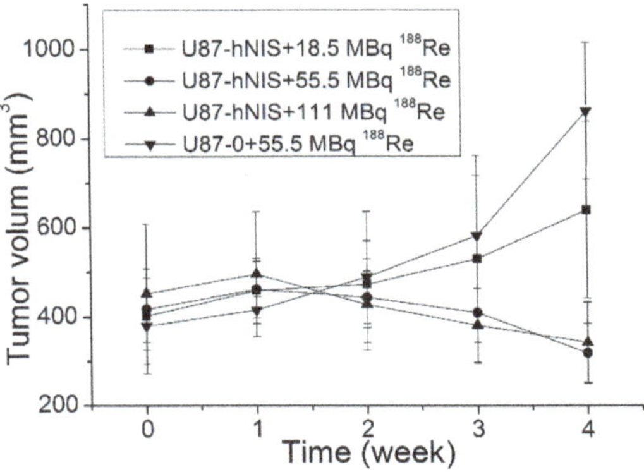

Figure 8. Human NIS induced ^{188}Re therapy in U87-hNIS tumor bearing nude mice; 18.5 MBq, 55.5 MBq and 111 MBq of ^{188}Re were injected intravenously in each mouse. The tumor size was measured before and after ^{188}Re administration. U87-0 tumor bearing nude mice were severd as controls. Data points are means ± SD (n = 6).

xenografted models are illustrated in Fig. 5A. The radiotracer exhibited a rapid decrease in radioactivity over time in blood and most organs. The high activity of stomach was evidently attributable to the excretion of ^{188}Re in the gastric mucosa. The highest tumor uptake of ^{188}Re (31.13±7.09% ID/g) was found 2 h after injection and keeped to 10.72±4.09% ID/g 12 h after injection, even 4.23±1.07% ID/g 24 h after injection, suggesting that the ^{188}Re was present in the U87-hNIS tumor up to at least 24 h after injection. While in U87-0 tumor xenografted mice, the tumor showed little ^{188}Re uptake. The highest tumor uptake of ^{188}Re (2.41±0.97% ID/g) was found 0.5 h after injection and decreased to 0.57±0.19% ID/g 12 h after injection. There is rarely ^{188}Re retention (0.17±0.08% ID/g) 24 h after injection, suggesting that little ^{188}Re was present in the U87-0 tumor.

Tumor imaging and therapy study

^{188}Re uptake and efflux in vivo was not consistent with the data obtained from the in vitro studies. For instance, U87-hNIS tumors showed efficient ^{188}Re uptake in vivo, and ^{188}Re rapidly and significantly accumulated in the right axilla of mice (Figure 6A, B, C), leading to scintigraphic visualization, whereas the U87-0 control tumors were not visible (Figure 6D, E, F). As expected, tissues naturally expressed NIS (in the thyroid and stomach, for example) or in organs involved in ^{188}Re elimination (such as the bladder) were also visualized, but significantly lower relative to tumor uptake. In U87-hNIS tumors, as shown in Figure 7, the tracer accumulation increased to maximum levels 1-hour after administration (T/NT 11.75±3.27), remained steady up to 24 hours (T/NT 11.58±2.96), and ^{188}Re remained in U87-hNIS tumors even 48 hours later (T/NT 4.83±1.55). These are consistent with the results of biodistribution studies in U87-hNIS tumor xenografts. Furthermore, little ^{188}Re is retained in the thyroid gland; the reason for this is that ^{188}Re cannot be organified by the thyroid gland, which alongside with its shorter half-life, should substantially reduce the risk of post-treatment hypothyroidism.

As shown in Figure 8, although U87-hNIS tumors treated with 18.5 MBq ^{188}Re showed no significant shrinkage, the tumor growth was retarded significantly 4 weeks after treatment, whereas the U87-0 tumors treated with 55.5 MBq ^{188}Re rapidly increased in size. A significant difference in tumor size could be observed in U87-hNIS tumors treated with 18.5 MBq ^{188}Re (640±199 mm^3) compared to U87-0 tumors treated with 55.5 MBq ^{188}Re (861±153 mm^3) after 4 weeks of ^{188}Re treatment ($P<0.05$). The difference of tumor volume between U87-hNIS tumors treated with 18.5 MBq ^{188}Re (640±199 mm^3) and 55.5 MBq ^{188}Re (317±67 mm^3) was statistically significant ($P<0.01$). While the difference of tumor volume between U87-hNIS tumors treated with 111 MBq ^{188}Re (342±90 mm^3) and 55.5 MBq ^{188}Re (317±67 mm^3) showed no statistical significance ($P>0.05$).

Discussion

Most gliomas are resistant to currently available chemotherapy regimens. Besides tumor resection, external radiotherapy is a major curative therapy for glioma. However, patients are often either not responsive to or suffer from side effects from these conventional therapies. Radionuclide-based theranostic strategies have been widely used in the diagnosis and treatment of patients with hyperthyroidism or differentiated thyroid cancer, and the sodium iodide symporter gene is the radionuclide-based reporter gene used in theranostics. Theranostics is a promising approach offering the ideal combination of accurate diagnosis and successful therapy in various clinical fields, which is expected to become a key area of personalized medicine in the near future. In order to attain the ultimate goals of personalized medicine, which is to provide the highest therapeutic effect and to avoid adverse effects for each patient, a tailored therapeutic plan should be developed by obtaining accurate, detailed diagnostic information regarding the patient's unique circumstances. Theranostics are an example of rapid advancement in biotechnologies for use with theranostic reporter genes and theranostic radiochemistry, which has led to the development of the concept of using theranostics with radionuclide-based imaging reporter genes [3].

NIS-mediated radionuclide therapy has several features that make it an attractive theranostic approach for the imaging and treatment of gliomas. For instance, complex radiolabeling procedures are not required for NIS-mediated radionuclide therapy. The small sizes of NIS radioactive substrates should result in both increased penetration of the blood-brain barrier and better diffusion capacity within the tumor. Radioisotopes have the potential of a bystander effect, in that tumor cells that do not express NIS can still be destroyed by electrons emitted from the surrounding, transduced tumor cells that express NIS and concentrate the isotope [23].

The traditionally used ^{131}I after NIS gene transfer demonstrates limited therapeutic efficacy due to rapid iodide efflux. A strategy to enhance the therapeutic efficacy of NIS-targeted radionuclide therapies in tumors with rapid iodide efflux might be the application of more potent isotopes, such as ^{188}Re, which are also transported by NIS, but in contrast to ^{131}I offer the possibility of higher energy deposition in the tumor over a shorter period of time due to its shorter physical half-life and higher energy; together, this suggests a superior therapeutic efficacy in medium or large tumors by an enhanced "crossfire effect". In this study, we explored an alternative method of hNIS-mediated therapy using ^{188}Re. As can be seen from our in vivo study results, the degree of uptake and retention is sufficient for delivery of therapeutic doses of radiation to NIS-expressing tumors, considering the average energy of ^{188}Re ($E = 0.778$ MeV vs. 0.192 MeV for ^{131}I, which is 4.05-fold higher than that of ^{131}I) and its considerably shorter physical half-life (0.71 days vs. 8.02 days for ^{131}I) [23]. These properties make ^{188}Re a worthy candidate for investigating its therapeutic efficacy after targeted NIS gene transfer in nonthyroidal cancers.

In our study, we demonstrated that ^{188}Re uptake was very rapid in U87-hNIS cells; the initial kinetic of ^{188}Re uptake was similar to what is observed in other virus transfected cells [24,25], reaching a maximum concentration after about 30 minutes. ^{188}Re accumulation was 26-fold higher compared to U87-0 control cells. There is a plateau phase, as is demonstrated in other studies [24,25], which represents the steady-state of transport processes when influx and efflux are balanced [21]. Similar to other NIS related studies, relatively low radionuclide retention was a problem in our in vitro study; the amount of ^{188}Re retained in U87-hNIS cells decreased significantly. However, U87-hNIS cells were efficiently killed by ^{188}Re, as revealed by clonogenic assays. In our study, the absorbed dose of ^{188}Re was sufficient for a significant selective killing effect of 78.7% using ^{188}Re in an in vitro clonogenic assay, while U87-0 cells showed a non-selective killing effect of approximately 31.3%.

In this context, it is also important to mention that the in vitro monolayer system is an artificial system and does not allow the full assessment of the therapeutic efficacy of a radionuclide due to the lack of a three-dimensional structure, which requires further exploration in in vivo xenotransplant models. Dinglia et al. [26] suggested that therapy depends on adequate retention of the isotope in the tumor. In the absence of iodide organification, isotope trapping is a dynamic process either due to slow efflux or re-uptake of the isotope by cells expressing NIS. With sufficient NIS expression, iodide efflux is a zero-order process and iodide organification is insignificant. In our in vivo imaging study, ^{188}Re remained in the U87-hNIS tumor even 48 hours after administration. In the following therapy study, there was a significant difference in tumor size between U87-hNIS mice (317 ± 67 mm^3) and U87-0 mice (861 ± 153 mm^3) treated with 55.5 MBq ^{188}Re for 4 weeks. Higher dose of ^{188}Re did not increase therapeutic effect. Unlike thyroid cells, U87-hNIS cells are not polarized and therefore should express hNIS over all regions of their plasma membrane. In vivo, U87-hNIS tumors have a three-dimensional structure that places tumor cells in close proximity to each other. This geometry may allow rapid re-uptake of any isotope that leaks from one cell by surrounding cells and serve as a mechanism for isotope trapping by the tumor, which is in part responsible for the observed therapeutic effect of hNIS and ^{188}Re in xenograft models. Therefore, cell arrangement can influence cytotoxicity. Studies [27] with hNIS cDNA transfected human glioma cells also showed increased cytotoxicity of ^{131}I if cells were grouped in a three-dimensional spheroid culture compared to a monolayer culture. This was believed to be due to bystander toxicity, which is maximized in a three-dimensional model. As a corollary, to maximize the therapeutic effect of hNIS, high level transduction and expression are required. Thus, aiming for high level expression of hNIS makes sense not only for maximal radioisotope uptake but also to ensure adequate retention if the isotope is to have its desired effect.

In our study, little ^{188}Re is retained in the thyroid gland, as ^{188}Re cannot be organified by this organ. Studies have demonstrated a similar biodistribution pattern for ^{131}I and ^{188}Re in mice, with the exception of the thyroid gland, in which only ^{131}I is retained by organification. In fact, the absence of organification of ^{188}Re by the thyroid gland may also be considered an advantage for therapy of nonthyroidal hNIS-bearing tissues [18], in that the thyroid will not serve as a sink for radiopharmaceuticals and will sustain less radiation damage, and more ^{188}Re can be uptaken by U87-hNIS cells due to ^{188}Re recirculation.

Considering that in our current study a stably hNIS transfected cell line was used with maximum hNIS expression levels, which is not directly applicable for clinical use in humans, the efficacy of ^{188}Re needs to be evaluated further in future studies after systemic in vivo hNIS gene transfer with the typical limited transduction efficiency and a more heterogeneous hNIS expression pattern. Provided that these studies confirm our findings, ^{188}Re may serve as an attractive alternative to ^{131}I, particular in tumors with short iodide retention time.

Conclusions

Our study is the first in vivo application of ^{188}Re as an alternative radionuclide for the treatment of human glioma after lentivirus transfected sodium iodide symporter gene expression. Transfecting the hNIS gene by a lentiviral vector coupled with ^{188}Re administration appears to be a novel and promising strategy for tumor imaging and therapy. Moreover, our study, based on the function of hNIS as a theranostic gene allowing the noninvasive imaging of hNIS expression by ^{188}Re scintigraphy, provides detailed characterization of in vivo vector biodistribution and level, localization, and duration of transgene expression. These are essential prerequisites for precise planning and monitoring of clinical gene therapies that aim to individualize the hNIS gene therapy concept.

Acknowledgments

We thank Elixigen Corporation (Huntington Beach, California, USA) for helping in proofreading and editing the English of final manuscript.

Author Contributions

Conceived and designed the experiments: RG BL. Performed the experiments: RG MZ Y. Ma SL SS Y. Miao. Analyzed the data: YX. Contributed reagents/materials/analysis tools: BL. Wrote the paper: RG.

References

1. Prados MD, Levin V (2000) Biology and treatment of malignant glioma. Semin Oncol 27: 1–10.
2. Grunwald GK, Vetter A, Klutz K, Willhauck MJ, Schwenk N, et al. (2013) Systemic image-guided liver cancer radiovirotherapy using dendrimer-coated adenovirus encoding the sodium iodide symporter as theranostic gene. J Nucl Med 54: 1450–1457.
3. Ahn BC (2014) Requisites for successful theranostics with radionuclide-based reporter gene imaging. J Drug Target. May 22: 295–303.
4. Tazebay U, Wapnir IL, Levy O, Dohan O, Zuckier LS, et al. (2000) The mammary gland iodide transporter is expressed during lactation and in breast cancer. Nat Med 6: 871–878.
5. Darrouzet E, Lindenthal S, Marcellin D, Pellequer JL, Pourcher T (2014) The sodium/iodide symporter: state of the art of its molecular characterization. Biochim Biophys Acta 1838: 244–253.
6. Gao XF, Zhou T, Chen GH, Xu CL, Ding YL, et al. (2014) Radioiodine therapy for castration-resistant prostate cancer following prostate-specific membrane antigen promoter-mediated transfer of the human sodium iodide symporter. Asian J Androl 16: 120–123.
7. Mandell RB ML, Link CJ (1999) Radioisotope concentrator gene therapy using the sodium/iodide symporter gene. Cancer Res 59: 661–668.
8. Cho JY, Xing S, Liu X, Buckwalter TL, Hwa L, et al. (2000) Expression and activity of human Na+/I− symporter in human glioma cells by adenovirus-mediated gene delivery. Gene Ther 7: 740–749.
9. Dingli D, Diaz RM, Bergert ER, O'Connor MK, Morris JC, et al. (2003) Genetically targeted radiotherapy for multiple myeloma. Blood 102: 489–496.
10. Guo R, Tian L, Han B, Xu H, Zhang M, et al. (2011) Feasibility of a novel positive feedback effect of 131I-promoted Bac-Egr1-hNIS expression in malignant glioma via baculovirus. Nucl Med Biol 38: 599–604.
11. Guo R, Zhang R, Pan Y, Xu H, Zhang M, et al. (2011) Feasibility of a novel positive feedback effect of 131I-promoted Bac-Egr1-hNIS expression in malignant glioma through baculovirus: a comparative study with Bac-CMV-hNIS. Nucl Med Commun 32: 402–409.
12. Guo R, Zhang Y, Liang S, Xu H, Zhang M, et al. (2010) Sodium butyrate enhances the expression of baculovirus-mediated sodium/iodide symporter gene in A549 lung adenocarcinoma cells. Nucl Med Commun 31: 916–921.
13. Yin HY, Zhou X, Wu HF, Li B, Zhang YF (2010) Baculovirus vector-mediated transfer of NIS gene into colon tumor cells for radionuclide therapy. World J Gastroenterol 16: 5367–5374.
14. Boland A, Magnon C, Filetti S, Bidart JM, Schlumberger M, et al. (2002) Transposition of the thyroid iodide uptake and organification system in nonthyroid tumor cells by adenoviral vector-mediated gene transfers. Thyroid 12: 19–26.
15. Dohán O, De la Vieja A, Paroder V, Riedel C, Artani M, et al. (2003) The sodium/iodide Symporter (NIS): characterization, regulation, and medical significance. Endocr Rev 24: 48–77.
16. Mallick UK, Charalambous H (2004) Current issues in the management of differentiated thyroid cancer. Nucl Med Commun 25: 873–881.
17. Nakamoto Y, Saga T, Misaki T, Kobayashi H, Sato N, et al. (2000) Establishment and characterization of a breast cancer cell line expressing Na+/I-symporters for radioiodide concentrator gene therapy. J Nucl Med 41: 1898–1904.
18. Dadachova E, Bouzahzah B, Zuckier LS, Pestell RG (2002) Rhenium-188 as an alternative to Iodine-131 for treatment of breast tumors expressing the sodium/iodide symporter (NIS). Nucl Med Biol 29: 13–18.
19. Lambert B, de Klerk JM (2006) Clinical applications of 188Re-labelled radiopharmaceuticals for radionuclide therapy. Nucl Med Commun 27: 223–229.
20. Kang JH, Chung JK, Lee YJ, Shin JH, Jeong JM, et al. (2004) Establishment of a Human Hepatocellular Carcinoma Cell Line Highly Expressing Sodium Iodide Symporter for Radionuclide Gene Therapy. J Nucl Med 45: 1571–1576.
21. Weiss SJ, Philp NJ, Grollman EF (1984) Iodide transport in a continuous line of cultured cells from rat thyroid. Endocrinology 114: 1090–1098.
22. Zuckier LS, Dohan O, Li Y, Chang CJ, Carrasco N, et al. (2004) Kinetics of perrhenate uptake and comparative biodistribution of perrhenate, pertechnetate,

and iodide by NaI symporter-expressing tissues in vivo. J Nucl Med 45: 500–507.

23. O'Donoghue JA, Bardiès M, Wheldon TE (1995) Relationships between tumor size and curability for uniformly targeted therapy with beta-emitting radionuclides. J Nucl Med 36: 1902–1909.
24. Chen L, Altman A, Mier W, Lu H, Zhu R, et al. (2006) 99mTc-pertechnetate uptake in hepatoma cells due to tissue-specific human sodium iodide symporter gene expression. Nuclear Medicine and Biology 33: 575–580.
25. Boland A, Ricard M, Opolon P, Bidart JM, Yeh P, et al. (2000) Adenovirus-mediated transfer of the thyroid sodium/iodide symporter gene into tumors for a targeted radiotherapy. Cancer Res 60: 3484–3492.
26. Dingli D, Bergert ER, Bajzer Z, O'connor MK, Russell SJ, et al. (2004) Dynamic iodide trapping by tumor cells expressing the thyroidal sodium iodide symporter. Biochemical and Biophysical Research Communications 325: 157–166.
27. Carlin S, Cunningham SH, Boyd M, McCluskey AG, Mairs RJ (2000) Experimental targeted radioiodide therapy following transfection of the sodium iodide symporter gene: effect on clonogenicity in both two- and three-dimensional models. Cancer Gene Ther 7: 1529–1536.

2

AAV-Mediated Cone Rescue in a Naturally Occurring Mouse Model of CNGA3-Achromatopsia

Ji-jing Pang[1,2*◔], Wen-Tao Deng[1◔], Xufeng Dai[1,2], Bo Lei[3], Drew Everhart[4], Yumiko Umino[4], Jie Li[1], Keqing Zhang[3], Song Mao[1], Sanford L. Boye[1], Li Liu[1], Vince A. Chiodo[1], Xuan Liu[1], Wei Shi[1], Ye Tao[1], Bo Chang[5], William W. Hauswirth[1]

1 Department of Ophthalmology, College of Medicine, University of Florida, Gainesville, Florida, United States of America, **2** Eye Hospital, School of Optometry and Ophthalmology, Wenzhou Medical College, Wenzhou, China, **3** Chongqing Key Laboratory of Ophthalmology, Ophthalmology, The First Affiliated Hospital of Chongqing Medical University, Chongqing, China, **4** Ophthalmology, SUNY Upstate Medical University, Syracuse, New York, United States of America, **5** The Jackson Laboratory, Bar Harbor, Maine, United States of America

Abstract

Achromatopsia is a rare autosomal recessive disorder which shows color blindness, severely impaired visual acuity, and extreme sensitivity to bright light. Mutations in the alpha subunits of the cone cyclic nucleotide-gated channels (*CNGA3*) are responsible for about 1/4 of achromatopsia in the U.S. and Europe. Here, we test whether gene replacement therapy using an AAV5 vector could restore cone-mediated function and arrest cone degeneration in the *cpfl5* mouse, a naturally occurring mouse model of achromatopsia with a *CNGA3* mutation. We show that gene therapy leads to significant rescue of cone-mediated ERGs, normal visual acuities and contrast sensitivities. Normal expression and outer segment localization of both M- and S-opsins were maintained in treated retinas. The therapeutic effect of treatment lasted for at least 5 months post-injection. This study is the first demonstration of substantial, relatively long-term restoration of cone-mediated light responsiveness and visual behavior in a naturally occurring mouse model of CNGA3 achromatopsia. The results provide the foundation for development of an AAV5-based gene therapy trial for human *CNGA3* achromatopsia.

Editor: Richard Libby, University of Rochester, United States of America

Funding: This work was funded by National Institutes of Health grants EY018331 (JP), EY021721 (WWH), EY017246 (DE), and by grants from the Macular Vision Research Foundation, Foundation Fighting Blindness, Fight for Sight (DE), Lions of Central NY, Research to Prevent Blindness, Inc., and Juvenile Diabetes Research Foundation. The funders had no role in study design, data collection and analysis, decision to publish, or preparation of the manuscript.

Competing Interests: WWH and the University of Florida have a financial interest in the use of AAV therapies, and own equity in a company (AGTC Inc.) that might, in the future, commercialize some aspects of this work.

* E-mail: jpang@ufl.edu

◔ These authors contributed equally to this work.

Introduction

The human retina contains about 6 million cone photoreceptors, which are responsible for fine resolution, central and color vision. The distribution of cones increases from peripheral retina to central macula or fovea that is comprised nearly 100% of the cones. Achromatopsia is a relatively rare, autosomal recessive congenital retinal disorder that is characterized by cone dysfunction. There are two clinical forms of achromatopsia: incomplete and complete. Patients with incomplete achromatopsia display a milder phenotype and retain residual cone function. Individuals with complete achromatopsia suffer from severely reduced visual acuity, pendular nystagmus, photophobia and color blindness. Since the only functional photoreceptors in complete achromatopsia are rods, which are more sensitive to light, or become saturate at higher levels of illumination, these individuals experience extreme light sensitivity and daylight blindness [1–3].

In humans, four genes that all encode essential components in the cone phototransduction cascade have been identified to cause achromatopsia. Mutations in the two subunits (CNGA3, CNGB3) of cone photoreceptor cyclic nucleotide-gated (CNG) channels account for approximately 75% of all cases of complete achromatopsia [1,4–9]. Some of the remaining cases are caused by mutations in alpha subunit of cone transducin (GNAT2) [10,11] and the catalytic alpha subunit of cone phosphodiesterase (PDE6C) [12,13]. In cone photoreceptors, CNG ion channels are integral tetrameric plasma membrane proteins composed of two A3 and two B3 subunits. Photoreceptors respond to light by closure of the CNG channels induced by hydrolysis of cGMP, resulting in membrane hyperpolarization and decreased synaptic glutamate release [1,14]. A3 and B3 are related proteins composed of six transmembrane helices (S1–S6), a pore-forming region between S5 and S6, a cyclic nucleotide-binding domain (CNBD), and a C-linker region between S6 and CNBD, which mediates channel gating [15,16].

The majority of mutations in the *CNGA3* gene in human patients identified so far are missense mutations, suggesting that CNG channel function has little tolerance for amino acid substitutions [6,9,17]. Missense mutations that ablate CNG channel function typically occur at amino acid residues conserved among the members of the CNG channel family. The majority of these changes are located within structurally and functionally important regions of the CNGA3 polypeptide, i.e., the transmembrane helices, the pore, and the cGMP-binding domain [9].

A new cone photoreceptor function loss 5 (*cpfl5*) mouse strain recently discovered at The Jackson Laboratory exhibits an ocular phenotype similar to complete human achromatopsia. The *cpfl5* mouse carries a missense mutation in exon 5 of the *Cnga3* gene [18]. A single nucleotide A to G change at position 492 in exon 5 results in a substitution of alanine for threonine. The *cpfl5* mouse exhibits selective loss of cone-mediated light responses accompanied by cone cell loss, similar to the phenotype of complete achromatopsia patients with *Cnga3* mutations. Our early study with an AAV5 vector containing a human blue cone promoter (HB570) showed partial restoration of cone function up to 2 months in cpfl5 mouse [18]. Others have shown partial restoration of cone function in a CNGA3$^{-/-}$ knock out mouse model using a capsid mutant AAV5 vector containing a mouse S-opsin promoter [19]. However, in both studies, cone function and cell survival were evaluated in a relatively short-term [18,19]. Moreover, in the later study, photopic b-wave responses were restored only to an average of 1/3 of normal amplitudes at 10 weeks post-injection. Here we report 5-month preservation of cone structure and function in the cpfl5 mouse, a natural missense *Cnga3* mutant, when the therapeutic transgene is driven by a CBA promoter in an AAV5 vector.

Results

AAV-mediated CNGA3 Expression in cpfl5 Mice

Gene therapy in the *cpfl5* mouse was tested by subretinal delivery of the mouse *Cnga3* gene driven by the ubiquitous CBA promoter packaged into an AAV5 vector. Subretinal injection was performed at P14 before significant cone photoreceptor degeneration had initiated. As seen in normal mice (Fig. 1A, 1B), immunostaining showed robust CNGA3 expression in the cone outer segment (OS) layer of treated *cpfl5* retina (Fig. 1D) 5 months following treatment with AAV5-CBA-m*Cnga3* whereas the contralateral uninjected eye lacked detectible CNGA3 labeling (Fig. 1C). Colocalization of CNGA3 and cone-specific lectin peanut agglutinin (PNA) staining suggests that CNGA3 expression is targeted primarily to cone outer segments (Fig. 1E), and a small amount was detected in cone cell bodies.

Cone Opsin Expression and Localization were Restored in *cpfl5* Mice

It has been shown previously that loss of CNGA3 resulted in impaired expression and trafficking of cone opsins as well as cone cell death in the *Cnga3*$^{-/-}$ mouse [20]. Here we documented the retinal morphology and expression patterns of M- and S-cone opsins in *cpfl5* mice (Fig. 2). 5-month-old *cpfl5* mice (Fig. 2B) exhibited photoreceptor outer & inner segment lengths and outer nuclear layer thickness similar to normal C57 BL/6J mice (Fig. 2A). However, retinal wholemounts stained with cone outer segment sheath specific PNA (green) revealed that moderate cone structure loss had occurred at this time point, primarily in the inferior (ventral) and nasal regions of the retina (Fig. 2D). Cone densities in these regions (Fig. 2D) have decreased compared to the dorsal (superior) and temporal regions of the normal retina (Fig. 2C). Expression and localization of cone opsins were then analyzed at different ages in *cpfl5* eyes by immunostaining retinal sections with antibodies to M- or S-opsin. 3-week-old *cpfl5* mice (Fig. 3B) exhibited M-opsin staining intensity and localization to OS consistent with that of wild type controls (Fig. 3A). However, by 10 weeks of age, M-opsin was mislocalized to the inner segment, cone nuclei, and cone pedicles (Fig. 3C). The loss of S-opsin staining proceeded more rapidly than M-opsin. In 3-week-old *cpfl5* mice (Fig. 4B), the intensity of S-opsin immunostaining started to decrease (Fig. 4A), but still localized in the OS. However, by 10 weeks of age, no S-opsin staining was seen in *cpfl5* mice indicating that profound S-cone OS loss had occurred (Fig. 4C).

To evaluate whether AAV5-CBA-m*Cnga3* treatment could arrest cone opsin loss and maintain its normal OS localization following P14 treatment, we analyzed retinal sections from untreated and contralateral treated *cpfl5* eyes with M- and S-opsin antibodies at 5 months after treatment. In untreated eyes, M-opsin can be detected in the superior retinal hemisphere but rarely in the inferior hemisphere (Fig. 3D). This is consistent with PNA staining showing that cones are preserved in the superior region at this age (Fig. 2B). As noted above however, the remaining M-opsin was mislocalized to the inner segments, cone nuclei, cone pedicles (Fig. 3E). In contrast, in vector-treated contralateral eyes, more intense M-opsin staining was detected throughout the retina (Fig. 3G), with an exclusive OS localization pattern (Fig. 3F). In untreated eyes, virtually no S-opsin staining can be detected in any part of the retina (Fig. 4D, 4E) whereas in treated eyes S-opsin was detected throughout the retina and was localized primarily in the cone OS (Fig. 4G, 4F). In summary, AAV5-CBA-Cnga3 P14 treatment prevented cone degeneration and maintained normal M- and S-opsin expression and localization in the *cpfl5* mice for at least 5 months.

Cone Function is Restored in AAV-treated *cpfl5* Mice

We find that *cpfl5* mice treated with AAV5-CBA-m*Cnga3* vector significantly restored cone photoreceptor function as measured by

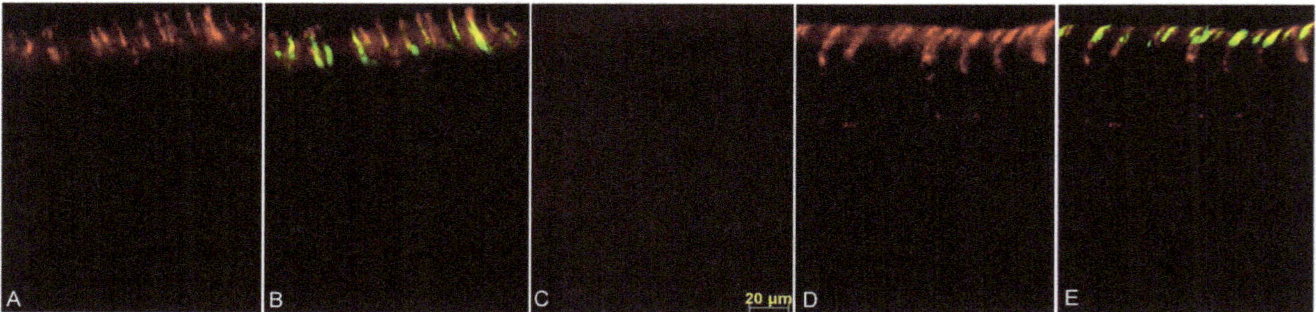

Figure 1. AAV5-CBA-m*Cnga3* leads to CNGA3 expression specifically in cone photoreceptors. A. CNGA3 expression (red) in a normal C57BL/6J mouse. B. Same field as (A) with PNA staining (green) to show CNGA3 expression in cones. C. No CNGA3 expression was found in an untreated *cpfl5* eye. D. AAV-mediated expression of CNGA3 (red) in cone photoreceptors of the partner treated *cpfl5* eye. E. Same field as (D) with PNA staining (green) to show CNGA3 expression in cones. OS, outer segments; IS, inner segments.

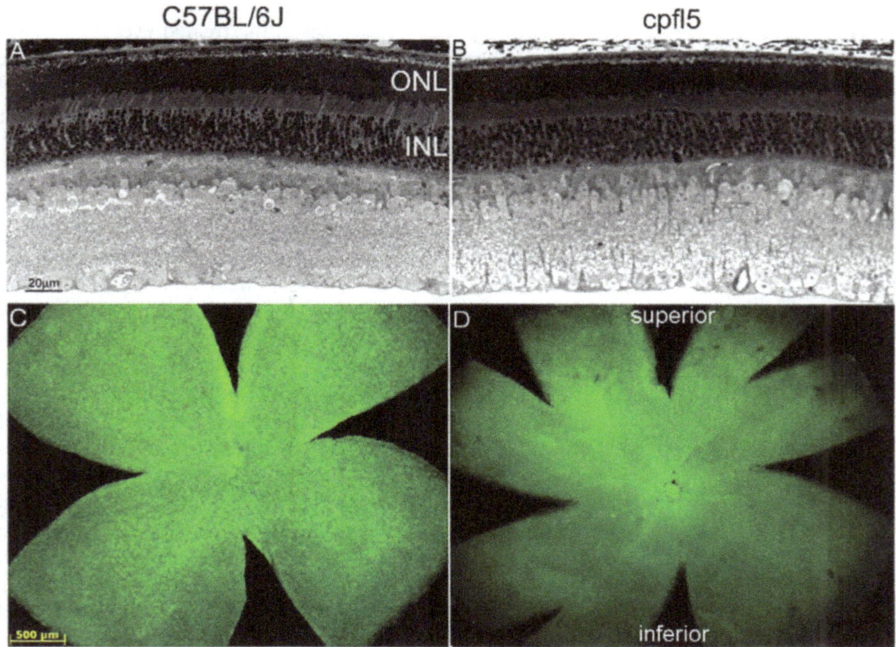

Figure 2. Cone photoreceptors degenerate in *cpfl5* mice. Representative light microscopic images of retinal paraffin sections from the superior hemisphere of a normal 5 month old C57BL/6J (A) and an age matched *cpfl5* mouse (B) showing similar appearing outer and inner nuclear layers. Whole mount PNA staining (green dots) of a 5 month C57BL/6J retina (C, right eye): and a *cpfl5* retina at 5 months (D, left eye) showing that cones outside the superior hemisphere, primarily in the nasal inferior quadrant of the *cpfl5* retina where most of the S-cones are located have degenerated. Panels A and B and Panels C and D are at the same scale.

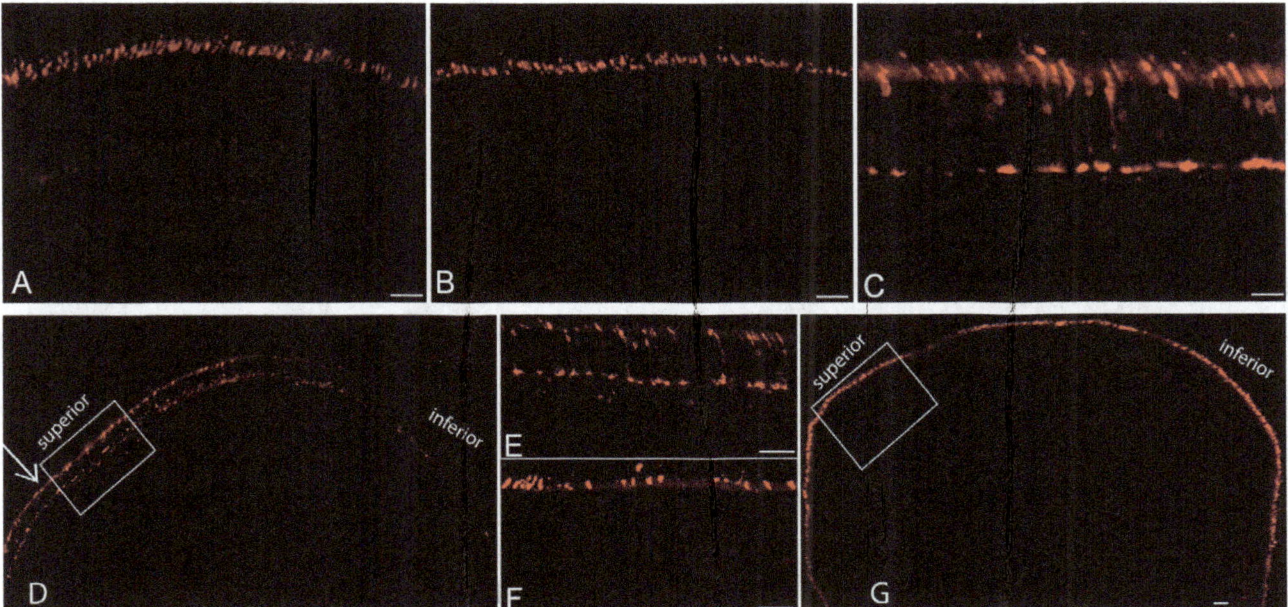

Figure 3. AAV-mediated CNGA3 expression restores expression and localization of M-opsin in *cpfl5* mice. By immunostaining, a 3-week-old C57 BL/6J wild type control retinal section (A) and an age-matched *cpfl5* retina (B) has identical expression and localization of M-opsin in the outer segments. In contrast, a section of a 10-week-old *cpfl5* mouse (C) shows that M-opsin has become mislocalized to cone inner segments, nuclei, and synaptic termini. Upon CNGA3 vector treatment, M-opsin expression and localization is nearly normal (D-G). Retinal sections from untreated (D and E, E is inset of D) and the contralateral treated (F, G, F is an insert of G) *cpfl5* eyes at 5 months post-treatment show that M-opsin can be detected only in the superior region (arrow) of the retina in an untreated 5-month-old *cpfl5* mouse (D); in addition, the remaining M-opsin in superior (dorsal) region is mislocalized (E). In contrast, intense M-opsin staining was detected throughout the entire retina in the contraleteral vector-treated eye (G) and was exclusively localized to the cone outer segments (F). Scale bars are equal to 50 μm.

both single-stimulus ERG and 10 Hz flicker ERG recordings. Dark- and light-adapted single-stimulus ERG analyses were initiated at 3 weeks post-treatment (Fig. 5A, 5B), and repeated regularly until 5 months post-treatment. At 3 weeks post-injection, the average light-adapted b-wave amplitude (Fig. 5C, 5D) was 82 ± 16 μV (n = 3) in treated eyes, about 80% of the wild-type controls (652 ± 55 μV, n = 3, P = 0.09) at a stimulus intensity of 1.08 log cd-s/m^2. No ERG responses were detected in untreated eyes (2 ± 2.6 μV, n = 3). Although the untreated cpfl5 (561 ± 31 μV) and normal C57BL/67 eyes (652 ± 55 μV) had statistically similar dark-adapted b-wave amplitudes (n = 3, P = 0.19), there was a reduction in the average of dark-adapted b-wave amplitude in treated eyes (427 ± 23 μV at 0.43 log cd-s/m^2) vs. in untreated eyes (561 ± 31 μV, n = 3, P< 0.05) (Fig. 5A, 5B. This decreased rod-mediated ERG amplitude upon treatment is likely the consequence of injection-related damage since this difference diminished (P>0.05) when the same mice were similarly analyzed at 5 months post-injection (Fig. 5F, 5H). We have consistently observed that rod-mediated ERG responses in 5.5 months old untreated cpfl5 eyes were lower than the age-matched wild-type controls (P<0.05), and the reason is under investigation.

At 5 months post-injection, the average light-adapted ERG response in treated cpfl5 was 58.40 ± 18.87 μV (n = 3), about 70% of the wild-type controls at a stimulus intensity of 0.65 log cd-s per m^2 (Fig. 5E, 5F). 10 Hz flicker ERG (Fig. 5G, 5H) showed that untreated and treated *cpfl5* eyes at lower stimulus intensities (≤ -1.85 log cd-s per m^2) which reflect pure rod-mediated responses [21], were similar. At high stimulus intensities (> -1.85 log cd-s per m^2), cone-driven responses in treated eyes showed much higher amplitudes than partner untreated eyes. The average b-wave amplitudes plotted against light intensities from untreated, contralateral treated, and wild type control eyes (Fig. 5H) showed a cone peak of 68.29 ± 15.19 μV in the treated eyes at 0.65 log cd-s/m^2 whereas a signal is undetectable in untreated eyes (n = 3, P < 0.01). These cone ERG responses in the treated eyes were about 60% of that recorded in the same session from uninjected wild type controls (113.68 ± 26.61 μV, n = 5). In summary, cone-mediated ERG responses were restored and maintained for at least 5 months in AAV5-CBA-m*Cnga3* treated eyes.

Restoration of Cone-mediated Acuity and Contrast Sensitivity in *cpfl5* mice

We also tested whether maintenance of cone structure, normal cone opsin localization and restoration of cone ERG function translated into improvement in cone-mediated visual behavior by measuring optomotor responses to rotating sine-wave gratings [22,23]. Optomotor behavioral analysis revealed significant improvement in cone-mediated acuity and contrast sensitivity of AAV-treated *cpfl5* eyes. Untreated eyes displayed poor visual acuities of 0.273 ± 0.111 cycles per degree whereas in treated eyes, acuities were 0.457 ± 0.059 cycles per degree (Fig. 6A), a level essentially identical to that in wild type controls (0.477 ± 0.026) and significantly better than untreated cpfl5 eyes (n = 4, P<0.05). In parallel, contrast sensitivities tested at a spatial frequency of 0.256 cycles/degree in treated eyes (9.20 ± 2.30, n = 4) showed similar contrast thresholds as wild type controls (8.49 ± 2.78, n = 4), and were significantly better than untreated eyes (2.34 ± 0.74, P<0.01, n = 4; Fig. 6B). Thus, cone-mediated visual acuity and contrast sensitivity were restored to wild type levels, demonstrating a positive therapeutic effect on visual behavior in treated *cpfl5* mice.

Discussion

We demonstrate here that AAV5-CBA-mCnga3-mediated gene replacement therapy restored cone-specific ERG, cone-mediated visual acuity and visual contrast in the *cpfl5* mouse, a naturally

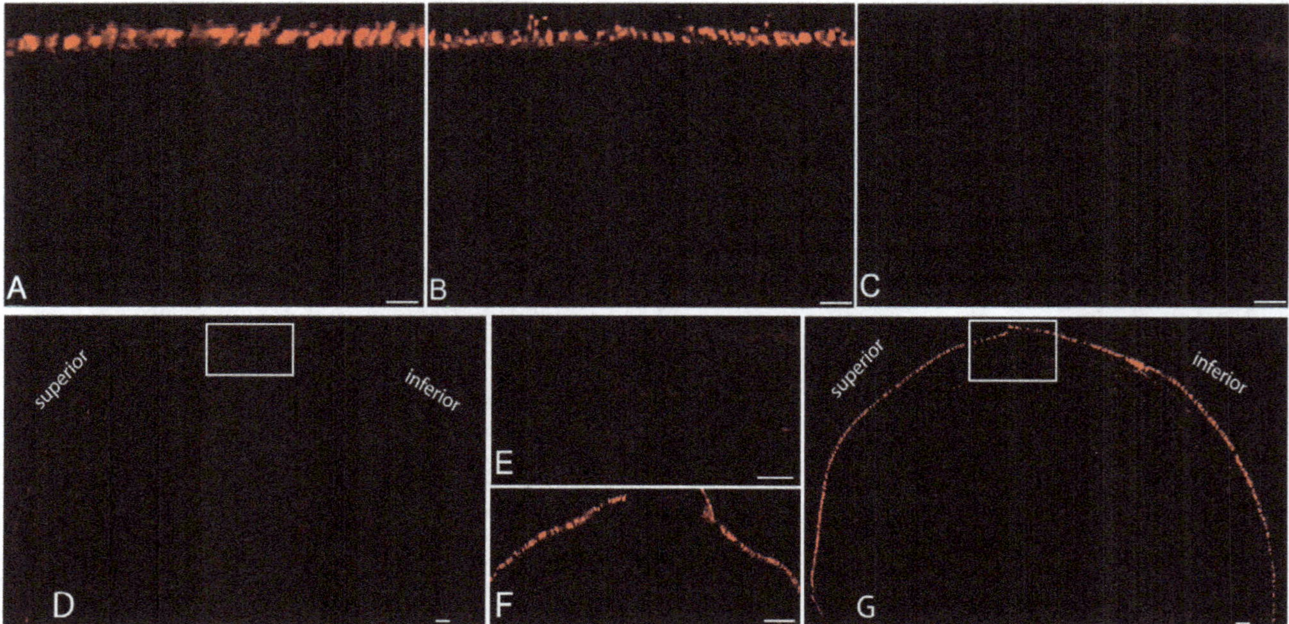

Figure 4. AAV-mediated CNGA3 expression maintains expression and localization of S-opsin in *cpfl5* mice. Retinal sections immunostained with S-opsin antibody from 3-week-old C57 BL/6J wild type control mouse (A) and an age-matched *cpfl5* retina (B) showing robust S-opsin expression in cone outer segments. Section from a 10-week-old *cpfl5* retina (C) showed no S-opsin staining indicating that profound S-cone degeneration had occurred. Five months after vectored CNGA3 expression, a treated *cpfl5* retina maintained normal expression and localization of S-opsin immunostaining (G and inset F) for at least 5 months in contrast to the contralateral untreated retina (D and E). Scale bars equal 50 μm.

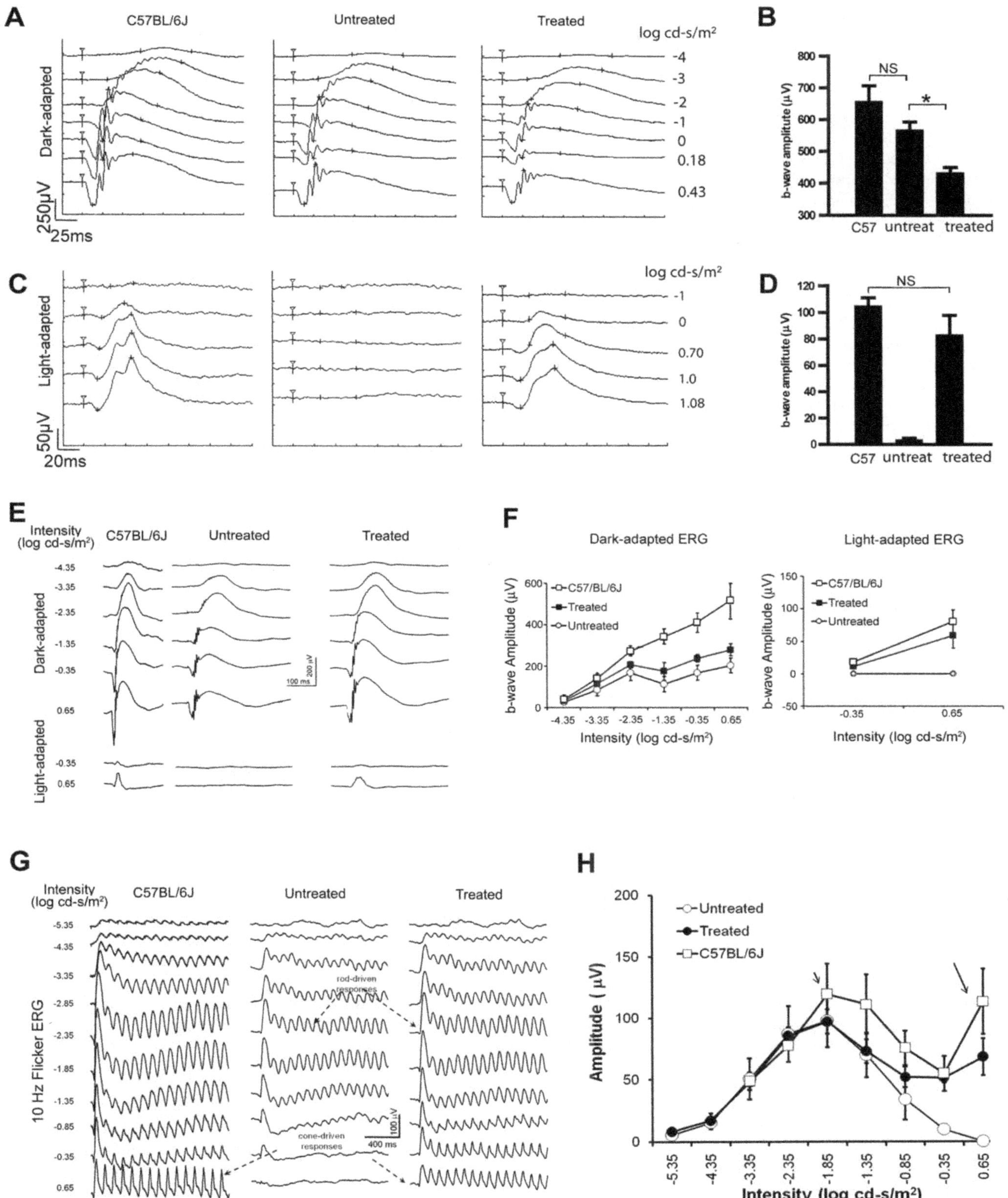

Figure 5. AAV5-CBA-m*Cnga3* treatment restores cone-mediated ERG. A-D. Single-stimulus ERG recordings from *cpfl5* mice 3 weeks post-treatment compared with normal C57BL/6J controls. Representative rod-mediated (A) ERG responses and statistical analysis (B) of b-wave amplitudes at 0.43 log cd-s per m^2. Representative cone-mediated ERG (C) responses and statistical analysis (D) of b-wave amplitudes at 1.08 log cd-s per m^2. n = 3 for each group. G-H. 10 Hz flicker ERG recordings from *cpfl5* mice 5 months post-treatment compared with normal C57BL/6J controls. Representative dark-adapted 10Hz flicker ERG (G) from normal C57 BL/6J, untreated and the contralateral treated *cpfl5* eyes. Statistical analysis (H)

showed that the cone-mediated ERG amplitudes were restored up to 60% of wild type levels for at least 5 months post-treatment; short arrow: pure rod-mediated responses; long arrow: pure cone-mediated responses. NS: No statistical difference; *: $P<0.05$.

occurring mouse model of achromatopsia caused by *Cnga3* deficiency. We also showed that gene therapy restored normal levels and localization of cone opsins. These therapeutic effects were maintained for at least 5 months after treatment.

We previously reported that AAV5-mediated gene therapy using the HB570 human blue cone opsin promoter (HB570) [18,24] or human red/green opsin promoter (PR2.1) (our unpublished work) leads to partial restoration of both S- and M-cone visual function in cpfl5 mice. A recent study using an AAV5 vector with a surface exposed tyrosine to phenylalanine mutation on the capsid (Y719F) containing a mouse S-opsin promoter also demonstrated partial cone functional restoration in a CNGA3$^{-/-}$ mouse model 11 weeks after injection [19]. In that study photopic b wave responses were on average 1/3 the amplitude of matched wild type controls. Compared to both previous studies, our current results using the strong, fast acting CBA promoter showed more robust and longer term restoration of ERG amplitudes, and vision elicited behavior.

Based on immunostaing using a CNGA3-specific antibody, CNGA3 expression driven by CBA promoter was primarily restricted to cone photoreceptors of cpfl5 retina with majority of CNGA3 found in the cone OS where it is normally localized, suggesting that off-target expression is inefficient, likely due to a posttranscriptional process mediating the instability of CNGA3 protein in non-cone cells. This phenomenon is not unexpected, particularly when the treatment is longer than 2–3 months. Similar observations of cell specific expression have also been found when using CBA or a truncated version of CBA (smCBA) to express RPE65 in the RPE cells [25],GC1 [26] and PDEβ proteins [27,28] in photoreceptors. In addition, the *RPE65*-LCA clinical trials have demonstrated the ability of the CBA promoter to support therapeutic transgene expression in the retina and restoration of visual function [29–33]. Although a cone-specific promoter might be preferred if off-target expression from a CBA promoter is a concern, it remains unclear which promoter would be best for transducing all cone subtypes. The human blue cone promoter (HB570) [18] or 2.1 kb human red/green opsin promoter (PR2.1. unpublished work) used in our previous cpfl5 mice studies, or the mouse S-opsin promoter used in the CNGA3 knockout mice study [19] have not been investigated in non-human primates. In fact, when evaluated in dog, the HB570 promoter did not drive expression in S-cones, only in M/L cones. Therefore, the current study using the CBA promoter combined with AAV5 serotype might remain the preferred combination of promoter and AAV serotype.

GFP expression in photoreceptor cells from AAV5-CBA-GFP vector can be detected as early as 7 days after subretinal injection [34]. Early onset AAV5 expression is also supported by the fact that almost half the magnitude of the final cone ERG restoration is obtained one week after P14 injection with AAV5-CBA-*Cnga3* vector (data not shown). It takes about 3 weeks for the AAV5-CBA- *Cnga3* vector to express sufficient CNGA3 protein to restore a stable cone ERG function (Figure 1A &1B). Cone opsins are almost normal in untreated 3-week-old cpfl5 mice (Figure 3 & 4) and cone structure is intact by whole mount PNA staining at P35 (data not shown). That explains why we can maintain most of the cone opsins 5-month after P14 treatment.

The rapid loss of S-opsin labeling in cpfl5 mouse suggests treatment earlier than P14 might lead to even more recovery of cone function, however, it is difficult to detach a significant fraction of the mouse retina prior to eye opening at P14 via trans-cornea subretinal injection without substantial injection-related damage [27,34]. We have noted a close correlation between maximal stable rescue and the extent of retinal coverage by the vector. For example, P14 treatment [27] was more therapeutically robust than P2 treatment in the rapid degenerating rd10 mouse that carries a PDEβ mutation [35]. Unlike the human retina, in which of the density of cones is very high in the central macula (fovea), M- and S-cones in the mouse retina are relatively evenly distributed in fixed topographic patterns across the entire retina. Currently, the most reliable way to evaluate successful cone therapy in mouse would be to limit analysis to eyes where the majority of cone photoreceptors were transduced, i.e. in retinas in which subretinal vector had detached all or nearly all of the retina. We found one microliter of vector sufficient to detach nearly the entire mouse retina, resulting in a homogenous "shallow bleb", which appears to minimize subsequent retinal detachment-related photoreceptor loss. From our previous work on cone therapy in the rd12 (mutant RPE65) mouse, we found that a single subretinal injection of AAV-RPE65 can restore cone ERG amplitudes to about 2/3 of wild type levels [25], similar to that reported here. This approach may therefore, in part, explain the better cone ERG rescue reported here than previously [19], in which subretinal vector detached only 30% of the retina.

It has been shown that AAV vectors with capsid surface exposed tyrosine residues mutated to phenylalanine (Y-F) have increased transgene expression levels and transduction kinetics relative to the corresponding standard wild-type AAV vectors [36]. An AAV8 Y-F capsid mutant vector demonstrated more effective and longer therapeutic effect compared to standard AAV8 and AAV5 in the rd10 mouse model of retinal degeneration [28]. A side by side comparison of AAV5 and the AAV5 (Y719F) utilized in the Michalakis et al. study [19] was not presented, therefore, it is uncertain whether there is any advantage of AAV5 (Y719F) over unmutated AAV5 for achieving cone rescue. In our case, perhaps the robust nature of CBA expression precluded the need for an AAV5 capsid variant. It may also be that the differences in level of rescue are related to the fact that the two studies were performed in different mouse models of CNGA3 deficiency.

Both cpfl5 and CNGA3$^{-/-}$ mice display the essential hallmarks of achromatopsia observed in human patients, in which cone responses are absent whereas rod function is retained [18,20,37]. In both mouse strains, cones gradually degenerated, possibly as a result of the impaired phototranduction cascade or the structural instability of cone outer segments [20]. Both models displayed defective cone opsin transport and failure to target cone opsin to the outer segments. Cones in the dorsal (superior) hemisphere containing mainly M-opsin survived significantly longer than ventral (inferior) cones with primarily S-opsin. Interestingly, the same pattern of S-cone loss preceding M-cone loss has been observed in other mouse models of retinal degeneration [38,39].

In 5-month-old cpfl5 eyes, M-opsin can be only detected in superior region of the retina, and is mislocalized to inner segments and cone cell bodies (Fig. 3D). However, M-cone structure in superior retina is still relatively intact as shown by cone outer segment sheath specific PNA staining (Fig. 2D).It would be interesting to test whether delayed treatment in older cpfl5 mice would still lead to rescue of the remaining M-cones as has been

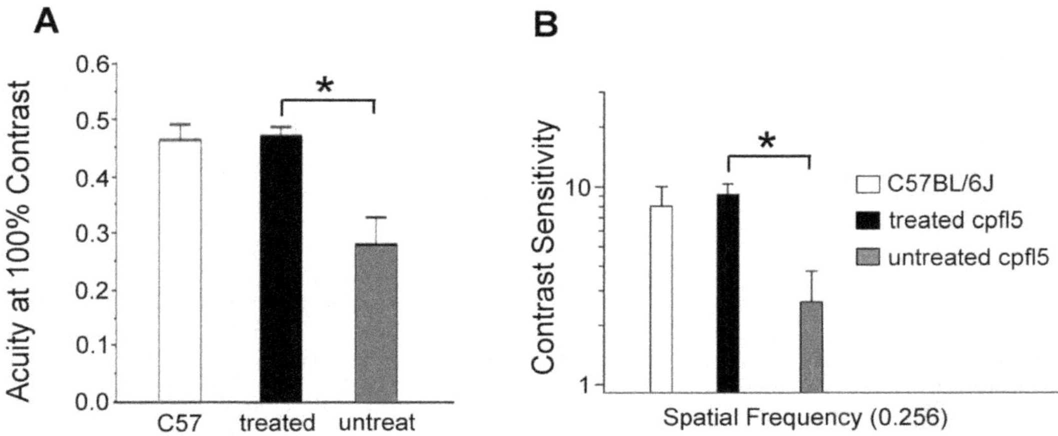

Figure 6. Rescue of visual acuity and contrast sensitivity in *cpfl5* mice. Comparison of average values for photopic acuities (A) and contrast sensitivities (B) from untreated, treated, and wild type mice (n = 4 for each group) 5 months post injection. Values are expressed as the mean ± SD for each group (* $P < 0.05$ for acuity and $P<0.01$ for contrast sensitivity).

seen with delayed treatment of rd12 mice [38]. If so, correct intracellular M-opsin distribution should also be restored since cone cell bodies are still be present although cone functional degeneration has occurred early. This would have important implications for human *Cnga3* achromatopsia which is characterized by a gradual and variable degree of cone loss [9,40].

In summary, we demonstrate restoration of cone function for at least 5 months in a naturally occurring mouse model of *Cnga3* achromatopsia using an AAV5 vector. Both M-cone and S-cone degeneration was prevented and correct trafficking of cones opsins restored. As mutations in CNG channels are the most common cause of human achromatopsia (CNGB3 ≥ 50%, CNGA3 ≥ 25%), the demonstration of successful gene therapies by AAV vectors to rescue cone function in this model [18,41], in CNGB3-mutant dogs [42] and in *Cnga3*$^{-/-}$ mice [19] provides key proof-of-principle for future achromatopsia clinical trials in humans.

Materials and Methods

Animals

Cpfl5 mice and the isogenic wild type strain C57BL/6J mice were obtained from The Jackson Laboratory (Bar Harbor, ME). All mice were bred and maintained in the University of Florida Health Science Center Animal Care Services Facilities under a 12hr/12hr light/dark cycle. All experiment protocols were approved by the University of Florida Institutional Animal Care and Use Committee and conducted in accordance with the Association for Research in Vision and Ophthalmology (ARVO) Statement for the Use of Animals in Ophthalmic and Vision Research and National Institute of Health (NIH) regulations.

Construction of the AAV5-CBA-m*Cnga3* Vector

Serotype 5 AAV vectors were used in this study as they have been demonstrated previously to mediate robust transduction efficiency and relatively rapid expression onset in photoreceptors [43]. A Mammalian Gene Collection (MGC) clone that contains full length mouse *Cnga3* cDNA was purchased from Invitrogen (Carlsbad, CA). NotI restriction enzyme sites were added to both ends of the cDNA by PCR utilizing forward 5′ –TTAGCGGCCGCGCAGAGATGG-CAAAGGTGA- 3′ and reverse 5′ –TTAGCGGCCGCTG-CATTTTCAGTCAGTCTTTGAA-3′ primers. The PCR fragment was then cloned into pCRblunt plasmid (Invitrogen) and sequence verified. Using the AAV vector plasmid pTR-CBA-hGFP, containing the CBA promoter driving expression of GFP, the *hGFP* cDNA was replaced with *mCnga3* via NotI digestion. AAV vectors were packaged and tittered according to previously published methods [44,45].

Subretinal Vector Injection

One microliter of AAV5-CBA-m*Cnga3* vector containing 10^{10} total DNAse resistant vector genomes was injected subretinally into the left eye of each P14 *cpfl5* mouse (n = 30) and the right eyes remained uninjected as controls. Subretinal injections were performed as described previously [27,28,38,39]. Only those mice that had more than 95% retinal detachment and minimal complications following subretinal injections were kept for further evaluation [25]. Eighteen cpfl5 mice (60% of total) met this criterion, which resulted in at least three animals for each experiment.

Electroretinographic Analysis

Initial ERG responses of *cpfl5* mice and isogenic wild type controls were recorded at 3 weeks following injection, and repeated at the 3rd and 5th month post-treatment using a Toennies Multiliner Vision instrument (Höchberg, Germany) according to protocols described previously [26,39,46]. Briefly, mice were dark adapted overnight and anesthetized with a mixture of 100 mg/kg ketamine, 20 mg/kg xylazine and saline at a ratio of 1:1:5. Full field ERGs were recorded using gold wire loop electrodes placed on each cornea and a reference electrode placed subcutaneously between the eyes. Scotopic rod recordings were performed with seven increasing light intensities of white light between 0.01 mcds/m^2 and 5 cds/m^2. Ten responses were recorded and averaged at each light intensity. Photopic cone recordings were done after mice were light adapted to a white background light of 100 cds/m^2 for 5 min. Recordings were performed with five increasing flash intensities between 100 mcds/m^2 and 12 cds/m^2 in the presence of a constant 100 mcds/m^2 rod suppressing background light. Fifty responses were recorded and averaged at each intensity. Photopic b-wave amplitudes from untreated, treated *cpfl5* and wild type eyes at each intensity were averaged and compared by repeated-measures ANOVA with the Bonferroni post hoc test for ANOVA ($P < 0.05$) to compare means at individual flash intensities.

For flicker ERG responses at 5 months after P14 treatment, untreated, treated *cpfl5* and wild type control eyes were analyzed with a custom-designed ERG system with a Ganzfeld illumination using Grass PS22 Xenon visual stimulator (Grass Instrument Inc. West Warwick, RI). Procedures were performed as described previously [39]. ERG data are presented as mean ± standard deviation (mean ± SD). Statistical significance was examined with ANOVA as above. Pairwise comparisons between groups for the ERG were performed by the Bonferroni post hoc test ($P < 0.05$).

Optomotor Testing

Photopic and scotopic visual acuities and contrast sensitivities of treated and untreated mouse eyes were measured using a two-alternative forced choice paradigm as described previously [22,23,26,39] with minor modifications. Acuity was defined as the highest spatial frequency (100% contrast) yielding a threshold response, and contrast sensitivity was defined as 100 divided by the lowest percent contrast yielding a threshold response (sinusoidal pattern at 0.256 cycles/degree). For both photopic and scotopic acuity, the initial stimulus was a 0.200 cycles/degree sinusoidal pattern with a fixed 100% contrast. For photopic contrast sensitivity measurements, the initial pattern was presented at 100% contrast, with a fixed spatial frequency of 0.256 cycles/degree. For scotopic contrast sensitivity measurements, the spatial frequency was fixed at 0.031 cycles/degree, a spatial frequency tuned for rod vision [22]. All patterns were presented at a speed of 12 degrees per second. Photopic vision was measured at a mean luminance of 70 cd/m^2. For scotopic measurements, mice were dark-adapted overnight and light levels were attenuated to 3.5×10^{-5} cd/m^2 through the use of neutral density filters. Visual acuities and contrast sensitivities were measured for both eyes of each mouse four to six times over a period of 1–2 weeks. Wild type control animals were 6 months old at testing time (n = 5), and P14 treated animals were at least 5.5 months old (n = 5). Unpaired t-tests were carried out on acuity and percent contrast values to determine significance of results.

Tissue Preparation and Immunohistochemistry

Eyes were enucleated at 5 months after P14 treatment. Retinal sections were prepared according to previously described methods [34,39]. Briefly, immediately following sacrifice, the limbus of injected and uninjected eyes was marked at "12 o'clock" with a hot needle which facilitated orientation. The eyes were then enucleated and fixed in 4% paraformaldehyde overnight. The cornea and lens were then removed from each eye without disturbing the retina. The remaining eyecup was rinsed with PBS and then cryoprotected by placing it in 30% sucrose in PBS for 4 hours at 4°. Eyecups were then embedded in cryostat compound (Tissue TEK OCT, Sakura Finetek USA, Inc., Torrance, CA) and frozen at - 80°C.

Retinal cryosections were cut at 12μM thickness, then rinsed in PBS and blocked in 2% normal goat serum, 0.3% Triton X-100 in 1% BSA in PBS for 1 hour at room temperature. Lectin PNA conjugated to a Alexa Fluor 488 (1: 200, L21409, Invitrogen), S-cone opsin, M-cone opsin primary antibodies (1:200, Santa Cruz Biotechnology, Santa Cruz, CA), or rabbit polyclonal CNGA3 (generously provided by Dr. Martin Biel (Ludwig-Maximilians-Universität, München) was diluted to 1:400 in 0.1% Triton X-100 and 1% BSA in PBS, and incubated overnight at 4°C. The sections were then washed 3 times with PBS, then incubated with IgG secondary antibody tagged with Alexa-594 (molecular Probes, Eugene OR) diluted 1:500 in PBS at room temperature for 1 hour and washed with PBS. Sections were mounted with Vectashiled Mounting Medium for Fluorescence (H-1000, Vector lab, In. Burlingame, CA) and coverslipped. Sections were analyzed with a Zeiss CD25 microscope fitted with Axiovision Rel. 4.6 software. All fluorescent images were acquired using identical exposure settings.

Acknowledgments

We thank M. Biel at Center for Integrated Protein Science Munich (CIPSM), Department of Pharmacy–Center for Drug Research, Ludwig-Maximilians-Universität München, Munich, Germany for offering the anti-mouse CNGA3 antibody. We also thank Tom Doyle, Min Ding, and Thomas Andresen at the University of Florida for technical support.

Author Contributions

Conceived and designed the experiments: JP WWH. Performed the experiments: JP WTD XD BL DE YU JL KZ SM SLB LL VAC XL WS. Analyzed the data: JP BL DE. Contributed reagents/materials/analysis tools: BC WTD YT. Wrote the paper: JP WTD. Revision: JP WTD WWH.

References

1. Kohl S, Varsanyi B, Antunes GA, Baumann B, Hoyng CB, et al. (2005) CNGB3 mutations account for 50% of all cases with autosomal recessive achromatopsia. Eur J Hum Genet 13: 302–308.
2. Michaelides M, Hunt DM, Moore AT (2004) The cone dysfunction syndromes. Br J Ophthalmol 88: 291–297.
3. Michaelides M, Hardcastle AJ, Hunt DM, Moore AT (2006) Progressive cone and cone-rod dystrophies: phenotypes and underlying molecular genetic basis. Surv Ophthalmol 51: 232–258.
4. Ahuja Y, Kohl S, Traboulsi EI (2008) CNGA3 mutations in two United Arab Emirates families with achromatopsia. Mol Vis 14: 1293–1297.
5. Kaupp UB, Seifert R (2002) Cyclic nucleotide-gated ion channels. Physiol Rev 82: 769–824.
6. Kohl S, Marx T, Giddings I, Jagle H, Jacobson SG, Apfelstedt-Sylla E, et al. (1998) Total colourblindness is caused by mutations in the gene encoding the alpha-subunit of the cone photoreceptor cGMP-gated cation channel. Nat Genet 19: 257–259.
7. Kohl S, Baumann B, Broghammer M, Jagle H, Sieving P, et al. (2000) Mutations in the CNGB3 gene encoding the beta-subunit of the cone photoreceptor cGMP-gated channel are responsible for achromatopsia (ACHM3) linked to chromosome 8q21. Hum Mol Genet 9: 2107–2116.
8. Milunsky A, Huang XL, Milunsky J, DeStefano A, Baldwin CT (1999) A locus for autosomal recessive achromatopsia on human chromosome 8q. Clin Genet 56: 82–85.
9. Wissinger B, Gamer D, Jagle H, Giorda R, Marx T, et al. (2001) CNGA3 mutations in hereditary cone photoreceptor disorders. Am J Hum Genet 69: 722–737.
10. Aligianis IA, Forshew T, Johnson S, Michaelides M, Johnson CA, et al. (2002) Mapping of a novel locus for achromatopsia (ACHM4) to 1p and identification of a germline mutation in the alpha subunit of cone transducin (GNAT2). J Med Genet 39: 656–660.
11. Kohl S, Baumann B, Rosenberg T, Kellner U, Lorenz B, et al. (2002) Mutations in the cone photoreceptor G-protein alpha-subunit gene GNAT2 in patients with achromatopsia. Am J Hum Genet 71: 422–425.
12. Thiadens AA, den Hollander AI, Roosing S, Nabuurs SB, Zekveld-Vroon RC, et al. (2009) Homozygosity mapping reveals PDE6C mutations in patients with early-onset cone photoreceptor disorders. Am J Hum Genet 85: 240–247.
13. Chang B, Grau T, Dangel S, Hurd R, Jurklies B, et al. (2009) A homologous genetic basis of the murine cpfl1 mutant and human achromatopsia linked to mutations in the PDE6C gene. Proc Natl Acad Sci U S A 106: 19581–19586.
14. Burns ME, Arshavsky VY (2005) Beyond counting photons: trials and trends in vertebrate visual transduction. Neuron 48: 387–401.
15. Matveev AV, Quiambao AB, Browning FJ, Ding XQ (2008) Native cone photoreceptor cyclic nucleotide-gated channel is a heterotetrameric complex comprising both CNGA3 and CNGB3: a study using the cone-dominant retina of Nrl-/- mice. J Neurochem 106: 2042–2055.
16. Peng C, Rich ED, Varnum MD (2004) Subunit configuration of heteromeric cone cyclic nucleotide-gated channels. Neuron 42: 401–410.
17. Johnson S, Michaelides M, Aligianis IA, Ainsworth JR, Mollon JD, et al. (2004) Achromatopsia caused by novel mutations in both CNGA3 and CNGB3. J Med Genet 41: e20.
18. Pang JJ, Alexander J, Lei B, Deng W, Zhang K, et al. (2010) Achromatopsia as a potential candidate for gene therapy. Adv Exp Med Biol 664: 639–646.

19. Michalakis S, Muhlfriedel R, Tanimoto N, Krishnamoorthy V, Koch S, et al. (2010) Restoration of Cone Vision in the CNGA3(-/-) Mouse Model of Congenital Complete Lack of Cone Photoreceptor Function. Mol Ther 18: 2057–2063.
20. Michalakis S, Geiger H, Haverkamp S, Hofmann F, Gerstner A, et al. (2005) Impaired opsin targeting and cone photoreceptor migration in the retina of mice lacking the cyclic nucleotide-gated channel CNGA3. Invest Ophthalmol Vis Sci 46: 1516–1524.
21. Seeliger MW, Grimm C, Stahlberg F, Friedburg C, Jaissle G, et al. (2001) New views on RPE65 deficiency: the rod system is the source of vision in a mouse model of Leber congenital amaurosis. Nat Genet 29: 70–74.
22. Umino Y, Solessio E, Barlow RB (2008) Speed, spatial, and temporal tuning of rod and cone vision in mouse. J Neurosci 28: 189–198.
23. Alexander JJ, Umino Y, Everhart D, Chang B, Min SH, et al. (2007) Restoration of cone vision in a mouse model of achromatopsia. Nat Med 13: 685–687.
24. Glushakova LG, Timmers AM, Pang J, Teusner JT, Hauswirth WW (2006) Human blue-opsin promoter preferentially targets reporter gene expression to rat s-cone photoreceptors. Invest Ophthalmol Vis Sci 47: 3505–3513.
25. Pang JJ, Chang B, Kumar A, Nusinowitz S, Noorwez SM, et al. (2006) Gene therapy restores vision-dependent behavior as well as retinal structure and function in a mouse model of RPE65 Leber congenital amaurosis. Mol Ther 13: 565–572.
26. Boye SE, Boye SL, Pang J, Ryals R, Everhart D, et al. (2010) Functional and behavioral restoration of vision by gene therapy in the guanylate cyclase-1 (GC1) knockout mouse. PLoS One 5: e11306.
27. Pang JJ, Boye SL, Kumar A, Dinculescu A, Deng W, et al. (2008) AAV-mediated gene therapy for retinal degeneration in the rd10 mouse containing a recessive PDEbeta mutation. Invest Ophthalmol Vis Sci 49: 4278–4283.
28. Pang JJ, Dai X, Boye SE, Barone I, Boye SL, et al. (2011) Long-term Retinal Function and Structure Rescue Using Capsid Mutant AAV8 Vector in the rd10 Mouse, a Model of Recessive Retinitis Pigmentosa. Mol Ther 19: 234–242.
29. Cideciyan AV, Aleman TS, Boye SL, Schwartz SB, Kaushal S, et al. (2008) Human gene therapy for RPE65 isomerase deficiency activates the retinoid cycle of vision but with slow rod kinetics. Proc Natl Acad Sci U S A 105: 15112–15117.
30. Cideciyan AV, Hauswirth WW, Aleman TS, Kaushal S, Schwartz SB, et al. (2009) Vision 1 year after gene therapy for Leber's congenital amaurosis. N Engl J Med 361: 725–727.
31. Hauswirth WW, Aleman TS, Kaushal S, Cideciyan AV, Schwartz SB, et al. (2008) Treatment of leber congenital amaurosis due to RPE65 mutations by ocular subretinal injection of adeno-associated virus gene vector: short-term results of a phase I trial. Hum Gene Ther 19: 979–990.
32. Jacobson SG, Cideciyan AV, Ratnakaram R, Heon E, Schwartz SB, et al. (2011) Gene Therapy for Leber Congenital Amaurosis Caused by RPE65 Mutations: Safety and Efficacy in 15 Children and Adults Followed Up to 3 Years. Arch Ophthalmol 130: 9–24.
33. Maguire AM, Simonelli F, Pierce EA, Pugh EN Jr., Mingozzi F, et al. (2008) Safety and efficacy of gene transfer for Leber's congenital amaurosis. N Engl J Med 358: 2240–2248.
34. Kong F, Li W, Li X, Zheng Q, Dai X, et al. (2010) Self-complementary AAV5 vector facilitates quicker transgene expression in photoreceptor and retinal pigment epithelial cells of normal mouse. Exp Eye Res 90: 546–554.
35. Allocca M, Manfredi A, Iodice C, Di VU, Auricchio A (2011) AAV-mediated gene replacement either alone or in combination with physical and pharmacological agents results in partial and transient protection from photoreceptor degeneration associated with beta PDE deficiency. Invest Ophthalmol Vis Sci 52: 5713–5719.
36. Petrs-Silva H, Dinculescu A, Li Q, Min SH, Chiodo V, et al. (2009) High-efficiency transduction of the mouse retina by tyrosine-mutant AAV serotype vectors. Mol Ther 17: 463–471.
37. Biel M, Seeliger M, Pfeifer A, Kohler K, Gerstner A, et al. (1999) Selective loss of cone function in mice lacking the cyclic nucleotide-gated channel CNG3. Proc Natl Acad Sci U S A 96: 7553–7557.
38. Li X, Li W, Dai X, Kong F, Zheng Q, et al. (2011) Gene Therapy Rescues Cone Structure and Function in the 3-Month-Old rd12 Mouse: A Model for Midcourse RPE65 Leber Congenital Amaurosis. Invest Ophthalmol Vis Sci 52: 7–15.
39. Pang J, Boye SE, Lei B, Boye SL, Everhart D, et al. (2010) Self-complementary AAV-mediated gene therapy restores cone function and prevents cone degeneration in two models of Rpe65 deficiency. Gene Ther 17: 815–826.
40. Genead MA, Fishman GA, Rha J, Dubis AM, Bonci DM, et al. (2011) Photoreceptor structure and function in patients with congenital achromatopsia. Invest Ophthalmol Vis Sci 52: 7298–7308.
41. Pang J, Lei L, Dai X, Shi W, Liu X, et al. (2012) AAV-mediated gene therapy in mouse models of recessive retinal degeneration. Current Molecular Medicine 12;3): 316–330.
42. Komaromy AM, Alexander JJ, Rowlan JS, Garcia MM, Chiodo VA, et al. (2010) Gene therapy rescues cone function in congenital achromatopsia. Hum Mol Genet 19: 2581–2593.
43. Yang GS, Schmidt M, Yan Z, Lindbloom JD, Harding TC, et al. (2002) Virus-mediated transduction of murine retina with adeno-associated virus: effects of viral capsid and genome size. J Virol 76: 7651–7660.
44. Jacobson SG, Acland GM, Aguirre GD, Aleman TS, Schwartz SB, et al. (2006) Safety of recombinant adeno-associated virus type 2-RPE65 vector delivered by ocular subretinal injection. Mol Ther 13: 1074–1084.
45. Zolotukhin S, Potter M, Zolotukhin I, Sakai Y, Loiler S, et al. (2002) Production and purification of serotype 1, 2, and 5 recombinant adeno-associated viral vectors. Methods 28: 158–167.
46. Deng WT, Sakurai K, Liu J, Dinculescu A, Li J, et al. (2009) Functional interchangeability of rod and cone transducin alpha-subunits. Proc Natl Acad Sci U S A 106: 17681–17686.

3

Efficacious and Safe Tissue-Selective Controlled Gene Therapy Approaches for the Cornea

Rajiv R. Mohan[1,2,3]*, Sunilima Sinha[1,2], Ashish Tandon[1,2], Rangan Gupta[1,2], Jonathan C. K. Tovey[1,2], Ajay Sharma[1,2]

1 Harry S. Truman Veterans Memorial Hospital, Columbia, Missouri, United States of America, **2** Mason Eye Institute, School of Medicine, University of Missouri, Columbia, Missouri, United States of America, **3** College of Veterinary Medicine, University of Missouri, Columbia, Missouri, United States of America

Abstract

Untargeted and uncontrolled gene delivery is a major cause of gene therapy failure. This study aimed to define efficient and safe tissue-selective targeted gene therapy approaches for delivering genes into keratocytes of the cornea *in vivo* using a normal or diseased rabbit model. New Zealand White rabbits, adeno-associated virus serotype 5 (AAV5), and a minimally invasive hair-dryer based vector-delivery technique were used. Fifty microliters of AAV5 titer (6.5×10^{12} vg/ml) expressing green fluorescent protein gene (GFP) was topically applied onto normal or diseased (fibrotic or neovascularized) rabbit corneas for 2-minutes with a custom vector-delivery technique. Corneal fibrosis and neovascularization in rabbit eyes were induced with photorefractive keratectomy using excimer laser and VEGF (630 ng) using micropocket assay, respectively. Slit-lamp biomicroscopy and immunocytochemistry were used to confirm fibrosis and neovascularization in rabbit corneas. The levels, location and duration of delivered-GFP gene expression in the rabbit stroma were measured with immunocytochemistry and/or western blotting. Slot-blot measured delivered-GFP gene copy number. Confocal microscopy performed in whole-mounts of cornea and thick corneal sections determined geometric and spatial localization of delivered-GFP in three-dimensional arrangement. AAV5 toxicity and safety were evaluated with clinical eye exam, stereomicroscopy, slit-lamp biomicroscopy, and H&E staining. A single 2-minute AAV5 topical application via custom delivery-technique efficiently and selectively transduced keratocytes in the anterior stroma of normal and diseased rabbit corneas as evident from immunocytochemistry and confocal microscopy. Transgene expression was first detected at day 3, peaked at day 7, and was maintained up to 16 weeks (longest tested time point). Clinical and slit-lamp eye examination in live rabbits and H&E staining did not reveal any significant changes between AAV5-treated and untreated control corneas. These findings suggest that defined gene therapy approaches are safe for delivering genes into keratocytes *in vivo* and has potential for treating corneal disorders in human patients.

Editor: Neeraj Vij, Johns Hopkins School of Medicine, United States of America

Funding: The work was supported by the RO1EY17294 (RRM) and RO1EY17294S2 (RRM) grants from the National Eye Institute, National Institutes of Health, Bethesda, Maryland, USA, 1I01BX000357-01 (RRM) grant from the Veteran Health Affairs, Washington, DC, USA and an Unrestricted grant from the Research to Prevent Blindness, New York, New York, USA. The funders had no role in study design, data collection and analysis, decision to publish, or preparation of the manuscript.

Competing Interests: The authors have declared that no competing interests exist.

* E-mail: mohanr@health.missouri.edu

Introduction

The success of gene therapy to treat diseases in human patients was first demonstrated over a decade ago [1]. Recent studies reporting significant improvement in vision with gene therapy in adult patients with Leber's congenital amaurosis affirmed the promise of gene therapy to treat eye diseases and prevent blindness in humans [2,3]. In spite of the progress in gene therapy research, many challenges including the severe side effects caused by the vector and untargeted gene transfer remain to be resolved [4–6]. The success in the restoration of vision with gene therapy by curing retinal disorders has encouraged more research for defining gene therapy modalities for other ocular tissues. The potential of gene therapy to treat corneal disease has been investigated using various animal and *in vitro* models [7–13]. The cornea is an attractive organ for gene therapy because of its accessibility, immune-privileged status and ability to be monitored visually. The three major cellular layers of the cornea are: epithelium, stroma and endothelium. Gene therapy reagents can be administered into epithelium and stroma topically, as well as into stroma and endothelium with simple surgical procedures such as microinjection [13].

Major benefits of gene therapy are that it repairs the cause of the problem and not merely suppress symptoms, provides long-term cure, does not require repeated application or clinic visits. Various viral and non-viral vectors have been tested to deliver genes in the cornea [11–13]. Among viral vectors, adenoviruses and retroviruses have been shown to deliver genes into the cornea for short periods of time with moderate-to-severe inflammatory responses [14–20]. However, both of these vectors are of limited use for corneal gene therapy because of their inability to transduce non-dividing cells, low transduction efficiency for corneal cells and induction of immune reactions [12,13]. Adeno-associated virus (AAV) and disabled lentivirus vectors offer better alternatives for delivering genes into the corneal stroma and endothelium because of their ability to transduce non-dividing cells [12,13]. Additionally, these vectors are non-pathogenic and typically drive long-term transgene expression. AAV vectors are preferred over lentivirus because of their superior safety profile and non-pathogenicity to humans. More than 100 serotypes of AAV are known but serotypes 1-9 have been extensively tested for gene therapy [4,11–13,21]. AAV serotypes have shown a varied degree of tissue selective tropism [21–27]. These reports led us to the hypothesis that vector regulates amount of gene delivery in the cornea. Indeed our recent studies supported our hypothesis as AAV serotypes 2, 5, 6, 8, and 9 showed significantly different transduction in the rodent and rabbit cornea *in vitro* and *in vivo* [11,21,27,28]. Our studies also suggested that AAV serotypes 5, 8 and 9 are most efficient for transporting genes in the rodent and rabbit stroma *in vivo* among various tested AAV serotypes [11,21,27]. AAV5-treated rodent corneas continued to express delivered transgene up to 1 year *in vivo* without any apparent side effects (Mohan et al Unpublished data), and thus was selected for this study.

The poor targeted delivery of therapeutic genes into corneal cells *in vivo* is another major challenge that sharply limits clinical application of gene therapy to treat corneal disorders and diseases. Previously, we demonstrated that AAV and plasmid vectors could deliver significant amount of genes into keratocytes of the rabbit stroma *in vivo* if applied on bare stroma employing a lamellar flap technique [28]. This led us to hypothesize that administration of an efficient vector via a custom vector-delivery technique would provide tissue-selective targeted transgene delivery in the cornea with no major side effects. Thus, multiple minimally invasive vector-delivery techniques to administer vector into keratocytes, stroma or endothelium of the rabbit and rodent cornea *in vivo* were optimized. Among many defined vector-delivery techniques, the hair-dryer based technique manipulating corneal hydration, the microinjection techniques using glass needle and Hamilton microsyringes, the topical cloning cylinder based technique employing 20% alcohol and the epithelial scrape technique using #64 surgical blade have provided the most targeted gene delivery into the targeted cells of the cornea *in vivo* [29]. The aim of this study was to define site-selective tissue-targeted gene therapy approaches using a suitable combination of efficacious AAV5 vector and newly-defined vector-delivery techniques to express therapeutic genes selectively in keratocytes or the stroma of the normal and damaged (fibrotic or neovascularized) rabbit cornea *in vivo*.

Results

Characterization of AAV5-mediated gene transfer in rabbit cornea

Figure 1 shows AAV5-mediated delivery of GFP gene in the normal rabbit cornea detected using stereo- (Fig. 1A) and fluorescent- (Fig. 1B–D) microscopy. Rabbits were subjected to fluorescence imaging every 12 h for the first 3 days after AAV5 vector application, and thereafter once a week until euthanasia. All rabbit corneas showed initial appearance of GFP gene expression at day-3 (Fig. 1 C), which reached its maximum level at day-7. Fig. 1D shows a representative image of peak level of GFP expression in rabbit corneal tissue section detected at 2-week time point. No fluorescence was detected in corneas of early tested time points (12 h, 24 h, 48 h or 60 h). Rabbit corneas of later time points (2-week, 4-week and 16-week) showed fluorescence levels similar to the levels of 7-day time point. These observations suggest that AAV5 delivered transgene expression first appeared between 60 h to 72 h after vector application, continued to increase for the next 4 days, peaked at day-7, and maintained high transgene expression up to the longest tested time point of 16-week (4 months) in the rabbit corneas *in vivo*.

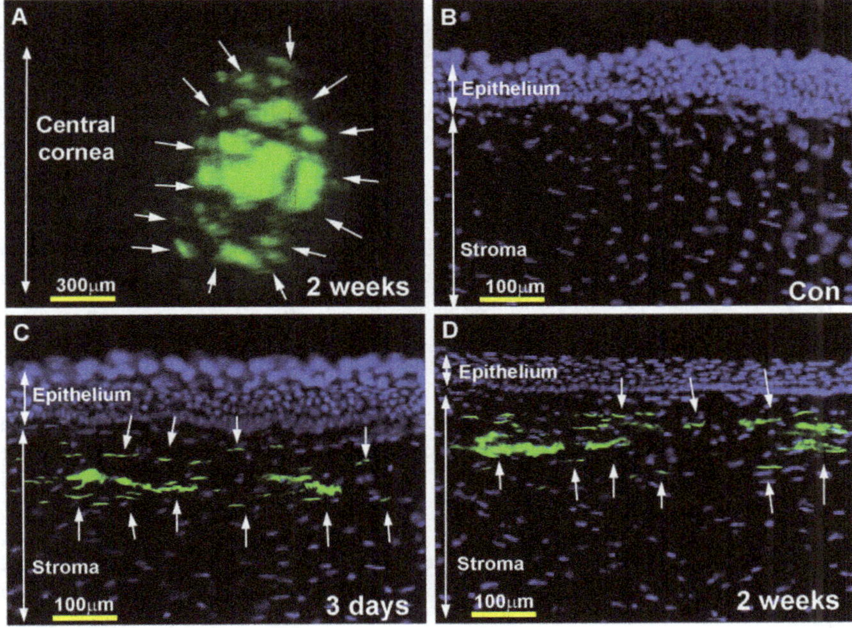

Figure 1. Representative *in vivo* fluorescence stereomicrograph (A) and tissue sections (B–D) of rabbit corneas showing AAV5-mediated GFP gene expression at 3-day and 2-week time points. Topical application of AAV5-GFP vector selectively transduced anterior keratocytes (arrows) located beneath the epithelium (C, D). No transgene expression was detected in control corneas (A). The rabbit corneas collected at 4-week and 16-week showed similar levels of GFP expression with immunostatining (data not shown). Nuclei are stained blue with DAPI. Scale bar denotes 100 μm.

Quantification of AAV5-mediated gene transfer

The level of AAV5 delivered GFP gene expression was quantified using western blot. Figure 2 shows the levels of delivered GFP protein in rabbit corneas at various tested time points (2-day, 3-day, 7-day, 2-week, 4-week and 16-week) after single topical application of AAV5. The digital quantification of the western blot depicting the average pixels of three independent experiments is shown in Figure 2. The first detectable expression was noted at day-3 (4099 pixels±682). The maximum GFP expression was observed at day-7 (7100 pixels±154), which was significantly higher compared to day-3 ($p<0.05$) and balanced salt solution (BSS)-treated controls ($p<0.01$). Also, the GFP expression detected at other tested time points of 2-weeks (7021 pixels±462), 4-weeks (6998 pixels±473) and 16 weeks (6880 pixels±698) was significantly ($p<0.05$) higher than the GFP expression detected at day-3 as well as BSS-treated controls. No GFP expression was detected in BSS-treated control rabbit corneas. Equal loading of protein was confirmed by the detection of similar intensity β-actin bands.

Spatial localization of AAV5-mediated GFP gene transfer

To detect spatial localization of AAV5-mediated gene transfer in the rabbit cornea, we performed confocal microscopy in rabbit corneal tissues collected 3 days and 2 weeks after AAV5 application. The three-dimensional z-stack confocal images presented in Figure 3 reveal localization of GFP in rabbit corneas of 3-day (A) and 2-week (B) time points. As evident from this figure, the delivered-GFP gene expression was detected in the anterior stroma just below the corneal epithelium. No transgene expression was detected either in the corneal epithelium or posterior stroma or corneal endothelium. These observations suggest that AAV5 vector administered to the rabbit cornea with defined vector-delivery technique provided tissue-selective localized gene delivery in the anterior stroma.

Determination of delivered-GFP gene copies with AAV5

To understand the correlation between delivered-GFP gene copy number and expression of delivered-GFP protein, we measured AAV5-delivered GFP gene copy number in rabbit corneas using slot blot. Figure 4 shows the gene copy number delivered in two separate rabbit corneas detected at 2-week time point using slot blot method. Densitometric analysis revealed that 10^8–10^{10} genomic copies of transgene were detected in the rabbit corneas. This data complement the results of immunocytochemistry (Fig. 1) and western blotting (Fig. 2).

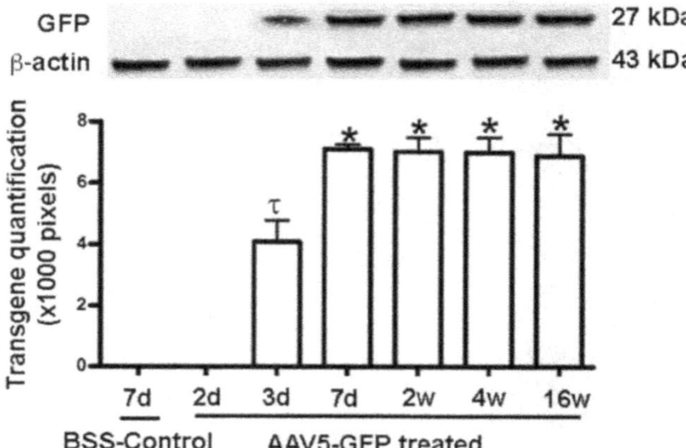

Figure 2. Representative western blot (upper panel) and digital quantification (lower panel) of delivered trangene in rabbit corneas at various time points. The delivered transgene expression first detected at 3-day, peaked at 7-day and maintained up to longest tested 16-week time point. β-actin was used to confirm equal loading of protein in each well and normalization of data. * $p<0.05$ compared to BSS-treated controls and 3-day time point, and τ $p<0.01$ compared to BSS-treated control.

AAV5-mediated gene delivery in diseased rabbit corneas

Diseases affecting the corneas are associated with significant alterations in corneal homeostatic and/or cellular phenotype. Thus, we raised a question "do gene transfer parameters optimized using normal rabbit corneas are applicable for the diseased cornea?" To answer this question we used two most acceptable *in vivo* rabbit disease models; the PRK-based corneal scarring model and the VEGF-induced corneal neovascularization model to test the potential of optimized tissue-targeted gene transfer approaches using AAV5 for treating corneal diseases such as corneal fibrosis and corneal neovascularization. The gene transfer data observed in scarred rabbit cornea is shown in Figure 5. The detection of transdifferentiated keratocytes (myofibroblasts) with αSMA (a fibrosis biomarker) immunostaining (Fig. 5A) shown in red confirmed the scarring in rabbit corneas induced by PRK surgery. AAV5-delivered GFP gene expression (shown in green color) detected at 3-day (Fig. 5B) and 2-week (Fig. 5C) time points is shown in green. As evident from Figure 5B and 5C, AAV5 delivered significant levels of GFP in the anterior stroma of the scarred rabbit cornea. Furthermore, co-localization of GFP and αSMA (detected in yellow) suggests that transgene was also delivered into transdifferentiated keratocytes (myofibroblasts) in addition to keratocytes by this technique. These observations revealed that defined gene transfer parameters are efficient for corneal gene therapy.

Next, we evaluated the efficiency of defined gene transfer parameters using AAV5 for delivering genes into neovascularized rabbit corneas. Figure 6 shows that a single 2 minutes topical application of AAV5-GFP vector on the rabbit stroma delivered significant levels of transgene into neovascularized rabbit corneas further validated suitability of optimized parameters and tested AAV5 vector for delivering therapeutic genes in diseased corneas. The increased GFP expression detected at 7-day (Fig. 6C) compared to 3-day (Fig. 6B) time point suggests that neovascularization did not alter kinetics of AAV5-mediated gene transfer. GFP delivery and blood vessel formation in the rabbit corneal section in Figure 6 is shown with GFP immmunostaining with green and lectin staining in red, respectively.

Safety determinations with slitlamp biomicroscopy and histology of AAV5-treated rabbit corneas

To analyze the effects of AAV5 on corneal health, visual and slit-lamp clinical examinations were performed in the eyes of live rabbits 1-day, 2-day, 3-day, 7-day and 4-week after BSS or AAV5 application. Neither BSS (Fig. 7A) nor AAV5-GFP (Fig. 7B) treated rabbit eyes showed inflammation, unusual discharge, swelling, redness or infection in the eye during clinical examination suggesting that AAV5 vector and used topical delivery technique are safe for the rabbit cornea. The hematoxylin and eosin-staining of BSS-treated control (Fig. 7C) and AAV5-treated rabbit corneas (Fig. 7D) collected at various time points did not exhibit any apparent structural abnormalities or abnormal infiltration of inflammatory cells in the rabbit cornea further confirming the safety of AAV5 vector for corneal gene delivery.

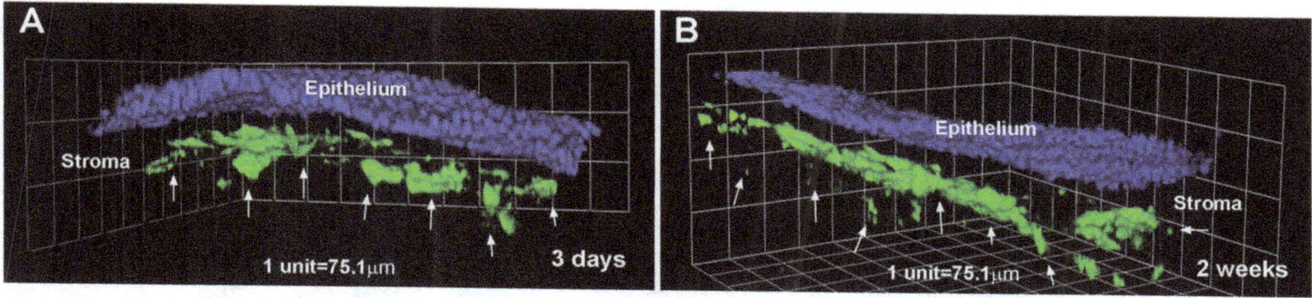

Figure 3. Representative three-dimensional confocal microscopy images showing spatial localization of GFP-expressing keratocytes (arrows) in whole-mount rabbit corneas exposed to AAV5. Corneas collected 3 days (A) and 2 weeks (B) after topical application of AAV5-GFP vector showed GFP-positive keratocytes beneath the epithelium in the anterior stroma. Nuclei are stained blue with DAPI. Scale bar denotes 75 μm.

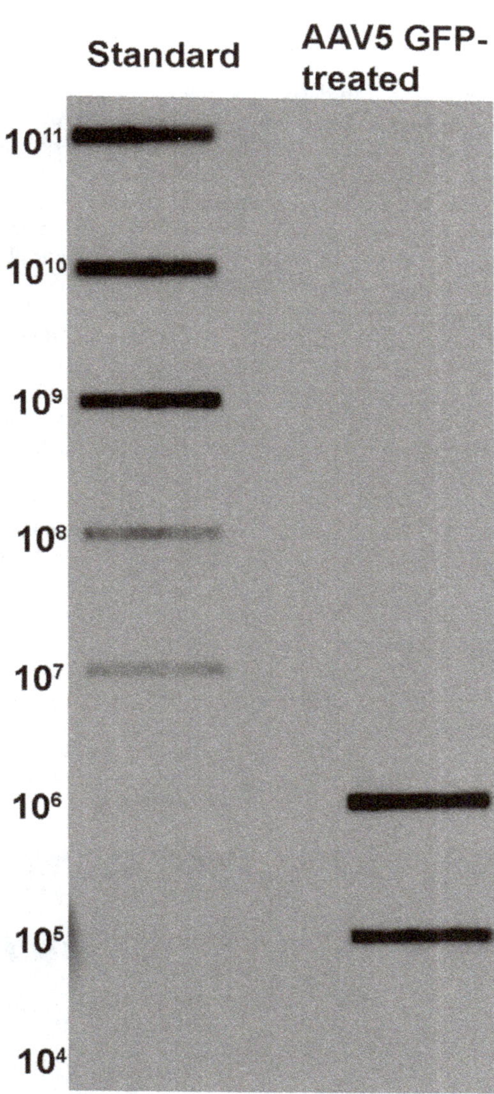

Figure 4. Slot blot showing GFP gene copy number in AAV5-GFP treated rabbit corneas. Densitometric comparison detected 10^8–10^{10} copies of GFP gene in AAV5 GFP-treated rabbit corneas. Left lane shows standard plot of GFP plasmid DNA copies blotted at 10-fold dilution series. The right lane shows delivered GFP DNA copies detected in rabbit corneas collected 2-week after AAV5-GFP application.

Discussion

Gene therapy offers a novel opportunity to cure ocular surface disorders by targeting the underlying cause as opposed to simply treating the symptoms with conventional drug treatment. Safe and successful progression of gene therapy from bench-to-bedside application requires delivery of therapeutic genes into targeted tissue in a selective manner. The major reasons for the failure of gene therapy are the severe side effects because of the uncontrolled and untargeted delivery of therapeutic genes into tissues [5]. This study, for the first time, demonstrates site-selective targeted gene delivery into keratocytes of normal and damaged corneas *in vivo* using a rabbit model, and reports optimal conditions for achieving controlled and targeted expression of therapeutic genes in the cornea for treating blindness due to corneal disorders. Furthermore, our data demonstrate that AAV5 is an efficacious and safe vector for corneal gene therapy as a single two minute topical application of vector provided high levels of delivered-gene starting from day three and lasting over several months without causing significant side effects.

Corneal epithelium spans 5–7 cell layers and acts as a barrier to prevent entry of foreign particles and pathogens into the eye. We previously found that removal of corneal epithelium is a critical step for achieving high levels of transgene delivery in the stroma of mouse and rabbit corneas *in vivo* [21,28,29]. The removal of corneal epithelium via gentle scraping is a common clinical practice in the ophthalmology clinic to treat corneal epithelial defects, and its removal is a standard step in photorefractive keratectomy and laser epithelial keratomileusis surgeries. The healthy corneal epithelium regenerates within 24–72 hours after removal without causing any detrimental effects to the eye. Thus, to test our postulate that direct interaction of AAV to the bare stroma would provide enhanced gene delivery into keratocytes we took advantage of a common clinical practice of removing corneal epithelium, and topically applied AAV5 on de-epitheliazed corneas. Based on the lessons learned from our earlier studies that epithelial injury could lead keratocyte apoptosis in the anterior stroma and affect corneal healing, epithelial removal was carried-out by gentle scarping by advancing the blade from a 45° angle. This minor technique adjustment showed minimal apoptosis and depletion in keratocyte density in anterior stroma of the rabbit cornea. Topical application is the most acceptable method for delivering therapeutics to the eye and was therefore chosen for the study. However, topical dispensing not only renders contact of therapeutics to the cornea but also to other ocular tissues such as conjunctiva, sclera, iris, etc. To limit non-targeted ocular tissue transduction and maximize transgene delivery into

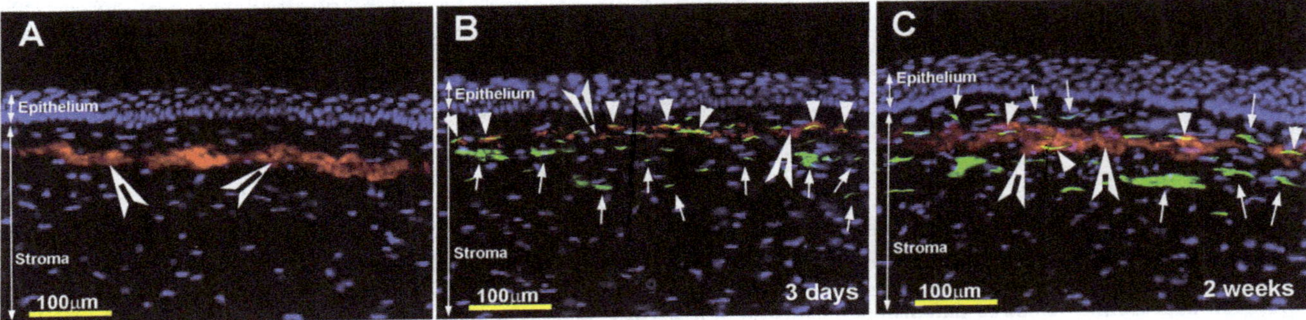

Figure 5. Representative images of corneal sections showing efficacy of AAV5-mediated transgene delivery in fibrotic rabbit corneas. Corneal fibrosis was produced by PRK laser surgery which induces transdifferentiation of keratocytes (myofibroblasts showing red staining for αSMA). Keratocytes expressing delivered GFP are shown in green (arrow), transdifferentiation keratocytes (myofibroblasts) expressing GFP and α-smooth muscle actin are shown in yellow (arrowheads), and transdifferentiation keratocytes (myofibroblasts) expressing α-smooth muscle actin are shown in red (Cut arrowheads). Nuclei are stained blue with DAPI. Scale bar denotes 100 µm.

keratocytes, a custom-cloning cylinder was used [29]. It has been our central hypothesis that localized and controlled administration of vector in the cornea via minimally invasive simple surgical techniques would allow targeted therapeutic gene delivery into desired cells of the cornea, *in vivo*. We used this approach for defining tissue-selective gene therapy approaches for the cornea because it does not require usage of a cornea-tissue specific promoter. At present, keratocan and the aldehyde dehydrogenase 3 cornea-specific promoter are generally used but both have their own limitations including leaky expression [30–32].

Corneal stroma is affected in many clinical disorders including corneal scarring, neovascularization, keratitis, graft rejection, ulcer and genetic dystrophies. Keratocytes residing in the stroma play an important role in maintaining corneal homeostasis, wound healing and clarity [33,34]. Identification of efficacious and safe gene therapy approaches for the stroma has potential to lead to the development of novel therapeutic modalities for treating these corneal diseases and disorders [8,12,13]. It is well documented that during pathologic conditions keratocytes undergo phenotypic changes. This raises a question whether gene therapy methods optimized using normal corneas or healthy keratocytes could also be applicable to diseased conditions. In this study we addressed this issue by evaluating the efficiency of defined tissue targeted gene therapy approaches using two well-established animal disease models; rabbit corneal scarring and rabbit corneal neovascularization. In scarred rabbit corneas, AAV5 efficiently delivered GFP gene in the stroma and transduced a significant population of keratocytes as well as other cell types such as myofibroblasts whereas in neovascularized rabbit cornea transgene delivery was detected predominantly in keratocytes. On one hand, these findings confirmed that defined gene transfer approaches could efficiently deliver therapeutic genes to diseased corneas; on the other hand, the findings prompted us to raise another clinically relevant and important question "what would be a more effective therapeutic strategy: to deliver therapeutic gene into transdifferentiated keratocytes or normal keratocytes?" We postulate that it will largely depend on the selection of the therapeutic gene. For example, corneal scarring treatment with basic fibroblast growth factor (FGF2) gene would require targeted delivery of FGF2 gene into myofibroblasts (transdifferentiated keratocytes) as Maltseva et al. have shown transdifferentiation of myofibroblasts to keratocytes by FGF2 *in vitro* [35]. There is a possibility that FGF2 gene delivery into normal keratocytes could induce neovascularization in the cornea. This assumption is based on the fact that implantation of recombinant FGF2 pellet in the stroma is used to induce angiogenesis in the cornea [36,37]. Our future studies will address such important questions.

Preclinical studies testing gene delivery in cornea have used a wide array of viral vectors. Multiple factors such as tissue tropism, duration of gene expression, vector gene carrying capacity, integrating or non-integrating nature of the vector, toxicity and safety of vector etc. dictate the choice of vector for clinical

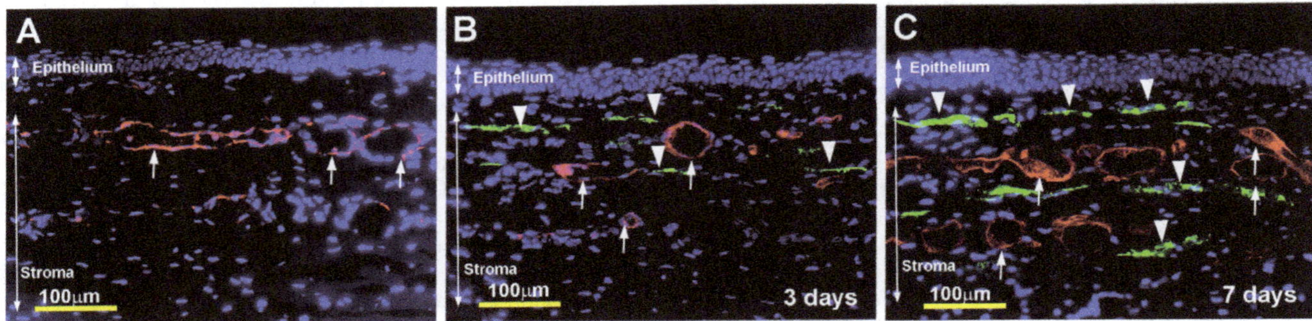

Figure 6. Representative *in vivo* images of corneal tissue sections showing efficacy of AAV5-mediated transgene delivery in neovascularized rabbit cornea. Keratocytes expressing delivered GFP are shown in green (arrowheads). Blood vessels are stained red with lectin (arrows). Nuclei are stained blue with DAPI. Scale bar denotes 100 µm.

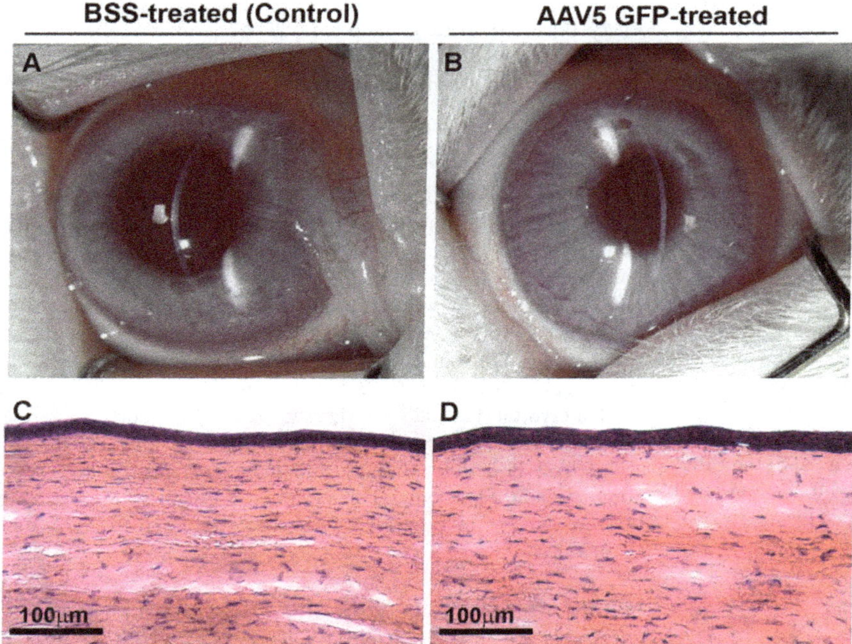

Figure 7. Representative slit lamp microscopy and images demonstrating safety of tested AAV5 to the cornea. No inflammation, redness, water discharge, swelling, etc was observed in BSS-treated control (A) or AAV5-treated corneas (B). Hematoxylin and eosin staining of corneal tissue sections (D) obtained from AAV5-treated rabbit eyes showed corneal morphology comparable to control corneas (C). Panels A–D shows data of 1-day time point. Similar observations were recorded for other tested time points (data not shown). Scale bar denotes 100 μm.

application of gene therapy. The safety and toxicity of vector to the patient and the environment remained a major determinant that enabled AAV to emerge as a vector of choice among viral vectors for ocular gene therapy. AAV is considered the safest viral vector because of its low immunogenic properties and non-pathogenicity to humans. The ocular gene therapy clinical trials carried-out with AAV serotype 2 (AAV2) for the retina have not reported any severe immune or inflammatory reactions among patients with used AAV vectors [38–40]. Like AAV2, AAV5 employed in this study did not show any significant side effects including the immune reaction or corneal damage suggesting that selected AAV5 is safe for corneal gene therapy. Scores of studies have demonstrated that AAV5 has superior transduction efficacy than AAV2 for ocular and non-ocular tissues [8,38,41]. Another factor that favors use of AAV5 for human gene therapy is the presence of AAV2 neutralizing antibodies in humans, which diminishes efficacy of AAV2 [42].

In summary, the site-selective controlled gene therapy approaches for the cornea defined using AAV5 vector and minimally invasive simple surgical technique may be effectively applied clinically to deliver genes in the eye to treat blindness from corneal stromal abnormalities. The AAV5 may potentially be a preferred vector for corneal gene therapy because of higher transduction efficiency and safety profile compared to AAV2.

Materials and Methods

Animals

The Institutional Animal Care and Use Committee of the University of Missouri-Columbia, Missouri USA USA (ID# 4279 and 6487) and Harry S. Truman Memorial Veterans' Hospital Columbia, Missouri USA (ID# 0041 and 0089) approved the study. Animals were treated in adherence to the principles of the ARVO Statement for the Use of Animals in Ophthalmic and Vision Research. New Zealand White rabbits (Myrtle laboratories Inc., Thompson's Station, TN) weighing 2.5–3.0 kg were used in this study. Rabbits were anesthetized by intramuscular injection of ketamine hydrochloride (50 mg/kg) and xylazine hydrochloride (10 mg/kg) for performing PRK, VEGF-implantation, stereo- and slit-lamp biomicroscopy.

AAV5 vector generation

The AAV5 expressing green fluorescent protein gene (AAV5-GFP) titer produced at the Gene Therapy Vector Core Lab, University of Florida, Gainesville, Florida was procured from Prof. Gregory S. Schultz and Dr. Vince A. Chido. Following an earlier reported method the AAV2 plasmid pTRUF11 expressing fluorescent green protein gene under control of a hybrid promoter (cytomegalovirus enhancer and chicken β-actin) and simian virus 40 polyadenylation site was packaged into AAV5 [43]. In brief, AAV5 vector was produced by the 2-plasmid, co-transfection method. One Cell Stack (Corning Inc., Corning, NY, USA) with approximately 1×10^9 HEK 293 cells was cultured in Dulbecco's Modified Eagle's Medium (Hyclone Laboratories, Inc. Logan UT, USA), supplemented with 5% fetal bovine serum and antibiotics. A $CaPO_4$ transfection precipitation was set up by mixing a 1:1 molar ratio of AAV2 plasmid DNA containing GFP and AAV5 rep–cap helper plasmid DNA. This precipitate was applied to the cell monolayer and the transfection was allowed to incubate at 37°C, 7% CO_2 for 60 h. The cells were then harvested and lysed by freeze/thaw cycles and subjected to discontinuous iodixanol gradients centrifugation at 350,000 g for 1 h. This iodixanol fraction was further purified and concentrated by column chromatography on a 5-ml HiTrap Q Sepharose column using a Pharmacia AKTA FPLC system (Amersham Biosciences, Piscataway, NJ, USA). The vector was eluted from the column using 215 mM NaCl buffer, pH 8.0, and the rAAV peak collected. AAV5 GFP vector-containing fraction was then concentrated and buffer exchanged in Alcon BSS with 0.014% Tween 20, using a Biomax 100 K concentrator (Millipore, Billerica, MA, USA). Vector was titered for DNAse-resistant vector genomes by Real-Time PCR relative to a standard.

AAV5 transduction to rabbit cornea

Twenty-eight rabbits ware used for the study. Only one eye of each rabbit selected randomly was used for the experiment. Sixteen rabbits were divided into two groups for the optimization of gene delivery parameters for the cornea. Rabbits of AAV5-treated group (n = 10) received 100 μl titer (6.5×10^{12} vg/ml) of AAV5 expressing green fluorescent protein gene under control of cytomegalovirus enhancer and chicken β-actin promoters topically for 2 minutes on de-epithelialized cornea via a custom hairdryer based vector delivery technique reported recently [29]. The control group (n = 6) received balance salt solution (BSS) topically using similar conditions. Twelve rabbits were used to evaluate the efficiency of optimized gene transfer parameters for delivering genes into diseased corneas namely rabbit corneal scarring model (n = 6) and rabbit neovascularization model (n = 6) were used. The AAV5 vector was topically applied to scarred rabbit cornea 4 weeks after PRK (n = 6) or neovascularized rabbit corneas 5-day after VEGF implantation (n = 6) using similar vector volume, titer, delivery technique, and experimental conditions. The contralateral eyes served as a naive control.

Corneal neovascularization and haze generation

Neovascularization in rabbit cornea was induced by corneal micro-pocket assay [44]. Rabbits were anesthetized with ketamine and xylazine, and 3–4 drops of 0.5% topical proparacaine hydrochloride solution (Alcon, Ft. Worth, TX, USA) was applied to the eye prior to cornea micropocket surgery. Only one eye of each animal was used for surgical procedure. The contralateral eye served as naive control. A wire speculum was positioned in the eye and a sucralfate-hydron pellet containing 650 ng of VEGF (PeproTech, Rocky Hill, NJ) was implanted into the cornea after making a micropocket in the cornea using standard surgical tools. Triple antibiotic ointment (Alcon) was applied to the surface of the cornea after pellet implantation to prevent infection. The ingrowth of blood vessels in the cornea towards the VEGF implant started from day 2, peaked around day 10 and continued to grow progressively up to 15 days before regressing.

Haze in rabbit cornea was produced by performing photo-refractive keratectomy (PRK) surgery in an anaesthetized rabbit [45]. Topical proparacaine hydrochloride 0.5% (Alcon, Ft. Worth, TX, USA) was applied to each eye just before PRK. A wire lid speculum was positioned and a 7 mm-diameter area of epithelium overlying the pupil was removed by scraping with a #64 blade (Beaver; Becton-Dickinson, Franklin Lake, NJ, USA). The −9.0 diopter PRK surgery with a 6 mm ablation zone on the central stroma was performed using the Summit Apex excimer laser (Alcon, Ft. Worth, TX). Only one eye from each animal was used for PRK and the contralateral eye served as naive control. The corneal haze in animals peaked 4 weeks after PRK.

Clinical and slit-lamp biomicroscopy

The health of the cornea in eyes of live rabbits was examined by visual clinical and slit-lamp microscopic (BX 900 Slit Lamp, Haag-Streit-USA, Mason OH) examinations before and after AAV5 application in normal and diseased (hazy or neovascularized) rabbit corneas by two ophthalmologists and a researcher, independently and in a blinded manner while animals were under general anesthesia. Thereafter, corneal health was monitored every third day with a hand-held slit-lamp microscope (SL-15, Kowa Optimed Inc., Torrance, CA). Photographs of the cornea were taken with a digital camera attached to the BX 900 slit-lamp microscope.

Tissue collection

Rabbits were humanely euthanized with pentobarbitone (150 mg/kg) overdose under general anesthesia at selected time points. Rabbit corneas were removed with forceps and sharp Westcott scissors and cut into 2 equal halves. One half was embedded in liquid optimal cutting temperature (OCT) compound (Sakura FineTek, Torrance, CA) within a 24 mm×24 mm×5 mm mold (Fisher, Pittsburgh, PA) and snap frozen. Frozen tissue blocks were maintained at −80°C. Tissue sections were cut 7 μm thick with a cryostat (HM 525 M, Microm GmbH, Walldorf, Germany). Sections were placed on 25 mm×75 mm×1 mm microscope Superfrost Plus slides (Fisher), and maintained frozen at −80°C until staining. The other half of rabbit corneal tissues was snap frozen directly in liquid nitrogen for isolating RNA, DNA or protein.

Immunohistochemistry and hematoxylin and eosin staining

Corneal tissues were stained with hematoxylin and eosin (H & E). Immunofluorescence staining for alpha smooth muscle actin (αSMA), a marker for myofibroblasts, was performed using mouse monoclonal primary αSMA antibody (1:200 dilution, catalog no. M0851, Dako, Carpinteria, CA). Tissue sections were incubated with 2% bovine serum albumin for 30 minutes at room temperature and then with αSMA monoclonal antibody for 90 minutes. For the detection of the primary antibody, Alexa 488 goat anti-mouse IgG secondary antibody (1:1000 dilution; catalog no. A11001, Invitrogen Inc., Carlsbad, CA) for 1 hour was used.

Blood vessel formation was confirmed with tomato lectin staining which entailed the incubation of corneal sections with 20 μg/ml Texas red-conjugated tomato lectin (cat # TL-1176; Vector laboratories, Burlingame, CA) for 90 min. Tissue sections were washed in HEPES buffer and mounted using Vectashield medium containing 4′-6-diamidino-2-phenylindole (DAPI; Vector laboratories). The stained sections were viewed and photographed with a Leica fluorescent microscope (Leica DM 4000B; Leica) equipped with a digital camera (SpotCam RT KE).

Immunoblotting

Protein lysates were prepared by homogenizing corneas in protein lysis buffer containing protease inhibitor cocktail (Roche Applied Sciences, Indianapolis, IN). Total protein was determined with Bradford assay. The same amount of protein of each sample was suspended in Laemmli denaturing sample buffer, vortexed and heated for 10 min at 70°C. The proteins were resolved on 4–20% SDS-PAGE gel and transferred onto 0.45 μm pore size PVDF membrane (Invitrogen, San Diego, CA). The membrane was incubated with GFP (cat # sc-33856; Santa Cruz) or β-actin (cat # sc-69879; Santa Cruz) primary antibody followed by alkaline phosphatase-conjugated anti-goat or anti-mouse secondary antibody (Santa Cruz). The bands were visualized by NBT/BCIP.

Stereo-biomicroscopy and confocal microscopy

Fluorescent stereomicroscope (model MZ16F, Leica) was used to track GFP expression in the eye of live rabbits under general anesthesia. The spatial localization of delivered-GFP gene in whole-mounts of normal cornea and thick tissue sections of damaged corneas was determined with confocal microscope (TCS-SP; Leica or Radiance 2000; Bio-Rad) using corresponding lasers for DAPI and GFP. The paraformaldehyde (4%) fixed corneal whole-mount tissues were stained with DAPI for 3 days to stain nuclei. The 20 μm thick corneal sections of the damaged rabbit corneas were subjected to triple staining (nuclei with DAPI in blue, cells expressing-GFP in green, and cells expressing SMA or lectin with red). The Z-stacks were generated in 0.45 μm increments and 3-D reconstructions were created by computer using Velocity software (Impro Vision Inc., Lexington, MA). The 3-D images were rotated 360° for spatial and perceptual visualization of the corneal regions. The exact location and quantity of the EGFP-positive cells in the cornea were measured with Velocity software (Impro Vision) and NIH Image J software.

Slot blot analysis

The copies of delivered plasmid were determined with slot blot analysis. Frozen corneal tissues were ground in liquid nitrogen and DNA was isolated using the DNA easy kit (Qiagen, cat # 69504). The standards were prepared using 10^4–10^{11} copies of decorin gene cloned into pTRUF11 vector. The DNA probe was prepared by digesting 5 μg of decorin plasmid with Not1 restriction enzyme and labeling 1 μg of isolated decorin fragment with digoxigenin (DIG)-labeled UTP, using DIG starter Kit II (catalog no. 11585614910 Roche Applied Science, Indianapolis, IN). Two microliters of the standard as well as the DNA isolated from corneal tissues was denatured by alkali and heat treatment. Denatured DNA samples were blotted onto nylon membrane using slot blot apparatus (BioRad lab) and were UV-cross linked. The membrane was hybridized with 300 ng of digoxigenin (DIG)-labeled probe overnight at 30°C, followed by incubation in 1:5000 anti-digoxigenin-AP antibody. Chemiluminiscent detection was used following vendor's instructions (catalog no. 11585614910 Roche Applied Science, Indianapolis, IN) and membrane was exposed to X-ray film. Image J 1.38× image analysis software was used to determine delivered gene copies in samples by measuring dot intensities of samples and comparing the data with standards.

Acknowledgments

Authors thank Dr. Frank G. Rieger M.D. and Chuck W. Hamm COT, CRA, OCT-C of Mason Eye Institute, University of Missouri-Columbia Missouri for their help in slitlamp biomicroscopy and undergraduate students (Tyler Cebulko and Yasaman Hemmat) for their assistance in tissue sectioning and immunocytochemistry.

Author Contributions

Conceived and designed the experiments: RRM. Performed the experiments: RRM SS AT RG JCKT AS. Analyzed the data: RRM SS AT RG JCKT AS. Contributed reagents/materials/analysis tools: RRM. Wrote the paper: RRM. Obtained material transfer agreement from University of Florida, Gainesville, Florida: RRM.

References

1. Cavazzana-Calvo M, Hacein-Bey S, de Saint Basile G, Gross F, Yvon E, et al. (2000) Gene therapy of human severe combined immunodeficiency (SCID)-X1 disease. Science 28: 669–672.
2. Bainbridge JW, Smith AJ, Barker SS, Robbie S, Henderson R, et al. (2008) Effect of gene therapy on visual function in Leber's congenital amaurosis. N Engl J Med 358: 2231–2239.
3. Maguire AM, Simonelli F, Pierce EA, Pugh Jr. Mingozzi EN, et al. (2008) Safety and efficacy of gene transfer for Leber's congenital amaurosis. N Engl J Med 358: 2240–2248.
4. Herzog RW, Cao O, Srivastava A (2010) Two decades of clinical gene therapy–success is finally mounting. Discov Med 9: 105–11.
5. Check E (2002) A tragic setback. Nature 420: 116–118.
6. Gura T (2001) Hemophilia. After a setback, gene therapy progresses…gingerly. Science 2 291: 1692–1697.
7. Behrens A, McDonnell PJ (2002) Gene therapy for the prevention of corneal haze after photorefractive/phototherapeutic keratectomy excimer laser surgery. Adv Exp Med Biol 506: 1315–1321.
8. Mohan RR, Sharma A, Netto MV, Sinha S, Wilson SE (2005) Gene therapy in the cornea. Prog Retin Eye Res 24: 537–559.
9. Chen P, Yin H, Wang Y, Mi J, He W, et al. (2010) Multi-gene targeted antiangiogenic therapies for experimental corneal neovascularization. Mol Vis 16: 310–319.
10. Saghizadeh M, Kramerov AA, Yu FS, Castro MG, Ljubimov AV (2010) Normalization of wound healing and diabetic markers in organ cultured human diabetic corneas by adenoviral delivery of c-Met gene. Invest Ophthalmol Vis Sci 51: 1970–1980.
11. Sharma A, Ghosh A, Hansen ET, Newman JM, Mohan RR (2010) Transduction efficiency of AAV 2/6, 2/8 and 2/9 vectors for delivering genes in human corneal fibroblasts. Brain Res Bull 81: 273–278.
12. Williams KA, Coster DJ (2010) Gene therapy for diseases of the cornea - a review. Clin Experiment Ophthalmol 38: 93–103.
13. Sharma A, Ghosh A, Siddapa C, Mohan RR (2010) Ocular Surface: Gene Therapy. In: Besharse J, Dana R, Dartt DA, eds. Encyclopedia of the eye. Elsevier; pp 185–194.
14. Larkin DF, Oral HB, Ring CJ, Lemoine NR, George AJ (1996) Adenovirus-mediated gene delivery to the corneal endothelium. Transplantation 61: 363–370.
15. Klebe S, Sykes PJ, Coster DJ, Krishnan R, Williams KA (2001) Prolongation of sheep corneal allograft survival by ex vivo transfer of the gene encoding interleukin-10. Transplantation 71: 1214–1220.
16. Borras T, Gabelt BT, Klintworth GK, Peterson JC, Kaufman PL (2001) Non-invasive observation of repeated adenoviral GFP gene delivery to the anterior segment of the monkey eye in vivo. J Gene Med 3: 437–449.
17. Carlson EC, Liu CY, Yang X, Gregory M, Ksander B, et al. (2004) In vivo gene delivery and visualization of corneal stromal cells using an adenoviral vector and keratocyte-specific promoter. Invest Ophthalmol Vis Sci 45: 2194–2200.
18. Mohan RR, Possin DE, Mohan RR, Sinha S, Wilson SE (2003) Development of genetically engineered tet HPV16-E6/E7 transduced human corneal epithelial clones having tight regulation of proliferation and normal differentiation. Exp Eye Res 77: 395–407.
19. Seitz B, Moreira L, Baktanian E, Sanchez D, Gray B, et al. (1998) Retroviral vector-mediated gene transfer into keratocytes in vitro and in vivo. Am J Ophthalmol 1998, 126: 630–639.
20. Behrens A, Gordon EM, Li L, Liu PX, Chen Z, et al. (2002) Retroviral gene therapy vectors for prevention of excimer laser-induced corneal haze. Invest Ophthalmol Vis Sci 43: 968–977.
21. Sharma A, Tovey JC, Ghosh A, Mohan RR (2010) AAV serotype influences gene transfer in corneal stroma in vivo. Exp Eye Res 91: 440–448.
22. Ghosh A, Yue Y, Duan D (2006) Viral serotype and the transgene sequence influence overlapping adeno-associated viral (AAV) vector-mediated gene transfer in skeletal muscle. J Gene Med 8: 298–305.
23. Lebherz C, Maguire A, Tang W, Bennett J, Wilson JM (2008) Novel AAV serotypes for improved ocular gene transfer. J Gene Med 10: 375–382.
24. Ghosh A, Yue Y, Duan D (2006) Viral serotype and the transgene sequence influence overlapping adeno-associated viral (AAV) vector-mediated gene transfer in skeletal muscle. J Gene Med 8: 298–305.
25. Klein RL, Dayton RD, Leidenheimer NJ, Jansen K, Golde TE, et al. (2006) Efficient neuronal gene transfer with AAV8 leads to neurotoxic levels of tau or green fluorescent proteins. Mol Ther 13: 517–527.
26. Limberis MP, Vandenberghe LH, Zhang L, Pickles RJ, Wilson JM, et al. (2009) Transduction efficiencies of novel AAV vectors in mouse airway epithelium in vivo and human ciliated airway epithelium in vitro. Mol Ther 17: 294–301.
27. Liu J, Saghizadeh M, Tuli SS, Kramerov AA, Lewin AS, et al. (2008) Different tropism of adenoviruses and adeno-associated viruses to corneal cells: implications for corneal gene therapy. Mol Vis 14: 22087–22096.
28. Mohan RR, Schultz GS, Hong JW, Mohan RR, Wilson SE (2003) Gene transfer into rabbit keratocytes using AAV and lipid-mediated plasmid DNA vectors with a lamellar flap for stromal access. Exp Eye Res 76: 373–383.
29. Mohan RR, Sharma A, Cebulko TC, Tandon A (2010) Vector delivery technique affects gene transfer in the cornea in vivo. Mol Vis 16: 2494–2501.
30. Carlson EC, Liu CY, Chikama T, Hayashi Y, Kao CW, et al. (2005) Keratocan, a cornea-specific keratan sulfate proteoglycan, is regulated by lumican. J Biol Chem 280: 25541–25547.
31. Kays WT, Piatigorsky J (1997) Aldehyde dehydrogenase class 3 expression: identification of a cornea-preferred gene promoter in transgenic mice. Proc Natl Acad Sci U S A 94: 13594–135999.
32. Liu C, Arar H, Kao C, Kao WW (2000) Identification of a 3.2 kb 5′-flanking region of the murine keratocan gene that directs beta-galactosidase expression in the adult corneal stroma of transgenic mice. Gene 250: 85–96.
33. West-Mays JA, Dwivedi DJ (2006) The keratocyte: corneal stromal cell with variable repair phenotypes. Int J Biochem Cell Biol 38: 1625–31.

34. Netto MV, Mohan RR, Ambrósio R, Jr., Hutcheon AE, Zieske JD, et al. (2005) Wound healing in the cornea: a review of refractive surgery complications and new prospects for therapy. Cornea 24: 509–522.
35. Maltseva O, Folger P, Zekaria D, Petridou S, Masur SK (2001) Fibroblast growth factor reversal of the corneal myofibroblast phenotype. Invest Ophthalmol Vis Sci 42: 2490–2495.
36. Oliveira HB, Sakimoto T, Javier JA, Azar DT, Wiegand SJ, et al. (2010) VEGF Trap (R1R2) suppresses experimental corneal angiogenesis. Eur J Ophthalmol 20: 48–54.
37. Azar DT (2006) Corneal angiogenic privilege: angiogenic and antiangiogenic factors in corneal avascularity, vasculogenesis, and wound healing (an American Ophthalmological Society thesis). Trans Am Ophthalmol Soc 104: 264–302.
38. Surace EM, Auricchio A (2008) Versatility of AAV vectors for retinal gene transfer. Vision Res 48: 353–359.
39. Buch PK, Bainbridge JW, Ali RR (2008) AAV-mediated gene therapy for retinal disorders: from mouse to man. Gene Ther 15: 849–857.
40. Bennicelli J, Wright JF, Komaromy A, Jacobs JB, Hauck B, et al. (2008) Reversal of blindness in animal models of leber congenital amaurosis using optimized AAV2-mediated gene transfer. Mol Ther 16: 458–465.
41. Dinculescu A, Glushakova L, Min SH, Hauswirth WW (2005) Adeno-associated virus-vectored gene therapy for retinal disease. Hum Gene Ther 16: 649–663.
42. Calcedo R, Vandenberghe LH, Gao G, Lin J, Wilson JM (2009) Worldwide epidemiology of neutralizing antibodies to adeno-associated viruses. J Infect Dis 199: 381–390.
43. Zolotukhin S, Potter M, Zolotukhin I, Sakai Y, Loiler S, et al. (2002) Production and purification of serotype 1, 2, and 5 recombinant adeno-associated viral vectors. Methods 28: 158–67.
44. Sharma A, Bettis DI, Cowden JW, Mohan RR (2010) Localization of angiotensin converting enzyme in rabbit cornea and its role in controlling corneal angiogenesis in vivo. Mol Vis 16: 720–728.
45. Sharma A, Mehan MM, Sinha S, Cowden JW, Mohan RR (2009) Trichostatin A inhibits corneal haze in vitro and in vivo. Invest Ophthalmol Vis Sci 50: 2695–2701.

4

AAV2-Mediated Subretinal Gene Transfer of hIFN-α Attenuates Experimental Autoimmune Uveoretinitis in Mice

Lichun Tian[1,2], Peizeng Yang[2*], Bo Lei[2], Ju Shao[2], Chaokui Wang[2], Qin Xiang[2], Lin Wei[2], Zhougui Peng[2], Aize Kijlstra[3]

1 Zhongshan Ophthalmic Center, Sun Yat-sen University, Guangzhou, People's Republic of China, **2** The First Affiliated Hospital of Chongqing Medical University, Chongqing Key Laboratory of Ophthalmology and Chongqing Eye Institute, Chongqing, People's Republic of China, **3** Eye Research Institute Maastricht, Department of Ophthalmology, University Hospital Maastricht, Maastricht, The Netherlands

Abstract

Background: Recent reports show that gene therapy may provide a long-term, safe and effective intervention for human diseases. In this study, we investigated the effectiveness of adeno-associated virus 2 (AAV2) based human interferon-alpha (hIFN-α) gene therapy in experimental autoimmune uveoretinitis (EAU), a classic model for human uveitis.

Methodology/Principal Findings: An AAV2 vector harboring the hIFN-α gene (AAV2.hIFN-α) was subretinally injected into B10RIII mice at two doses (1.5×10^6 vg, 1.5×10^8 vg). AAV2 vector encoding green fluorescent protein (AAV2.GFP) was used as a control (5×10^8 vg). The expression of hIFN-α in homogenized eyes and serum was detected by ELISA three weeks after injection. The biodistribution of vector DNA in the injected eyes, contralateral eyes and distant organs was determined by PCR. EAU was induced by immunization with $IRBP_{161-180}$ three weeks following vector injections, and evaluated clinically and pathologically. IRBP-specific proliferation and IL-17 expression of lymphocytes from the spleen and lymph nodes were assayed to test the influence of the subretinal delivery of AAV2.hIFN-α on the systemic immune response. hIFN-α was effectively expressed in the eyes from three weeks to three months following subretinal injection of AAV2.hIFN-α vector. DNA of AAV2.GFP was observed only in the injected eyes, but not in the distant organs or contralateral eyes. Subretinal injection of both doses significantly attenuated EAU activity clinically and histologically. For the lower dose, there was no difference concerning lymphocyte proliferation and IL-17 production among the AAV2.hIFN-α, AAV2.GFP and PBS injected mice. However, the higher dose of AAV2.hIFN-α significantly suppressed lymphocyte proliferation and IL-17 production.

Conclusions/Significance: Subretinal delivery of AAV2.hIFN-α lead to an effective expression within the eye for at least three months and significantly attenuated EAU activity. AAV2.hIFN-α was shown to inhibit the systemic IRBP-specific immune response.

Editor: Alfred Lewin, University of Florida, United States of America

Funding: This work was funded by Natural Science Foundation Major International (Regional) Joint Research Project (30910103912), http://159.226.244.15/portal/Proj_List.asp; Program for the Training of a Hundred Outstanding S&T Leaders of Chongqing Municipality, http://cqkjdj.cstc.gov.cn/View.aspx?id = 1000; PAR-EU Scholars Program, http://www.cqhrss.gov.cn/u/cqhrss/news_37398.shtml; National Basic Research Program of China (973 Program) (2011CB510200), http://www.most.gov.cn/tztg/201010/W020101021511061090978.pdf; Key Project of Natural Science Foundation of Chongqing (CSTC, 2009BA5037) http://www.ctin.ac.cn/Class.aspx?clsId = 226; Chongqing Key Laboratory of Ophthalmology (CSTC, 2008CA5003), http://www.ctin.ac.cn/View.aspx?id = 14380. The funders had no role in study design, data collection and analysis, decision to publish, or preparation of the manuscript.

Competing Interests: The authors have declared that no competing interests exist.

* E-mail: peizengycmu@126.com

Introduction

Uveitis is a common eye disease [1] and is one of the major causes of blindness worldwide [2]. It manifests either as an isolated intraocular inflammation or as a part of systemic autoimmune diseases such as Behcet's disease, systemic sarcoidosis or ankylosing spondylitis. Corticosteroids and immunosuppressive agents are commonly used for the treatment of uveitis. However, long-term application of these drugs frequently leads to numerous side effects. Furthermore, there are still a number of patients who do not respond to immunosuppressive treatment.

The introduction of biologic agents such as tumor necrosis factor-alpha (TNF-α) antibodies and interferon alpha (IFN-α) provides a new intervention regimen for patients with refractory uveitis [3,4,5]. IFN-α has been shown to have multiple immunoregulatory and immunosuppressive effects [6]. It helps to upregulate Tregs and inhibits IL-17-expressing cells in patients with Behcet's disease and other immune-related disorders [7,8,9]. Others found that it could suppress synthesis of IL-17 in both PBMCs and Th17 cells [10]. The capability of IFN-α in blocking IL-17, to some extent, is associated with the upregulation of Tregs and this may be one of the possible pathways in the treatment of autoimmunity diseases. However, potential side effects of these biologic agents have limited their use [3,4]. The improvement of ocular gene transfer techniques and the application of viral vectors allow the therapeutic transgene to target the eye and are considered to overcome these drawbacks.

Currently, gene therapy has achieved remarkable success in human and animal models in various retinal diseases [11,12,13,14]. The eye is a suitable organ for gene therapy [15] because of its following features. The small size and enclosed structure allow low dose administration to achieve a therapeutic effect. The convenient access and various routes of vector delivery can be used to target different layers in the eye [16]. In addition, many eye examination methods are currently available to monitor the treatment. Although recent studies have shown that immune responses can be generated after intraocular administration of AAV vector, this dose not necessarily to inhibit transgene expression nor dose it create retinal toxicity [17,18].

Although AAV-mediated gene therapy of retinal disease caused by single-gene defects has been undergoing clinical trials [19], only few studies have been attempted in the EAU modal [20,21]. We have developed a recombinant AAV2 vector containing the human IFN-α gene. After subretinal injection of the recombinant vectors into B10RIII mice, sufficient marked expression of this therapeutic molecule was associated with an attenuated development of EAU, a classic model for human uveitis.

Materials and Methods

Ethics Statement

This study was carried out according to the ARVO Statement for the Use of Animals in Ophthalmic and Vision Research. The protocol was approved by the Ethics Committee of the First Affiliated Hospital of Chongqing Medical University, Chongqing, China (Permit Number: 2009-201009). All surgery was performed under anesthesia, and all efforts were made to minimize animal suffering.

Animals and Reagents

B10RIII mice were purchased from Jackson Laboratory (Bar Harbor, ME). All animals were housed under standard (specific pathogen free) conditions. Human interphotoreceptor retinoid binding protein peptide spanning amino acid residues 161–180 ($IRBP_{161-180}$, SGIPYIISYLHPGNTILHVD) was synthesized by Shanghai Sangon Biological Engineering Technology & Services Ltd. Co. Complete Freund's adjuvant (CFA) containing 1.0 mg/ml mycobacterium tuberculosis (H37RA, ATCC 25177) was obtained from Sigma-Aldrich (St. Louis, MO).

Vectors

The recombinant adeno-associated virus vector harboring human interferon alpha 2a gene (AAV2.hIFN-α) was prepared as follows. Total mRNA was extracted from freshly isolated human PBMCs using RNeasy Plus Mini Kit (QIAGEN, Valencia, CA) and first-strand cDNA was synthesized with the Superscript III Reverse Transcriptase system (Invitrogen, Carlsbad, CA, USA). The coding sequence of human interferon alpha 2a was obtained from GenBank database (http://www.ncbi.nlm.nih.gov/genbank/, GenBank accession number BC074936) and the specific primers were designed (forward, 5′ GGGGTAC-CATGGCCTTGACCTTTGCTTT 3′ and reverse, 5′ CTG-TCGACTCATTCCTTACTTCTTAAACTTT 3′) to amplify the human IFN-α coding sequence. The PCR product was inserted into T vector (T-hIFN-α) and verified by DNA sequencing on the Applied Biosystems Model 3730 DNA Sequencing System (Invitrogen Biotechnology Co., Shanghai, China). The hIFN-α coding sequence was cut from T-hIFN-α with *Kpn*I and *Sal*I, and subcloned into an AAV2-CMV backbone between the sites of *Kpn*I and *Sal*I. After sequence verification, hIFN-α was driven by a human cytomegalovirus (CMV) intermediate-early promoter and followed by BGH poly A. The expression cassette was flanked by AAV2 inverted terminal repeats (ITRs) (Figure 1). Large-scale production and purification of vectors were performed by Vector Gene Technology Company Ltd. Vector AAV2.GFP served as a control. Titer of vectors batches were 3×10^{11} vg/ml for AAV2.hIFN-α and 1×10^{12} vg/ml for AAV2.GFP, respectively.

Subretinal injection

Subretinal injection was performed according to the method described previously [22]. All procedures were performed under sterile conditions. Under a dissecting microscope, an aperture within the dilated pupil area was made through the cornea with a 30-gauge needle, and a blunt 33-gauge needle was inserted through the corneal opening, avoiding damage to the lens and penetrating the neuroretina. A total amount of 0.5 μl of vector suspension or PBS was slowly delivered into the subretinal space with the aid of a micro-injection system. The successful delivery of vector was confirmed by partial retinal detachment. All animals received antibiotic ointment to the cornea and were observed daily after operation. The retinal detachment resolved spontaneously. The damages occasionally induced by ocular injection included temporal corneal edema, iris-cornea adhesion or iris hemorrhage and cataract formation. The animals with any of these complications were excluded from further study.

Human interferon-α immunoassay

Mice were sacrificed at various time points following subretinal injection of AAV2.hIFN-α. The undiluted serum was collected for assay of hIFN-α. For ocular fluid samples, AAV2.hIFN-α-injected eyes and contralateral eyes were enucleated respectively. The conjunctival tissues were carefully removed and the globes were briefly sonicated with homogenizing solution(20% glycerol, 10 mM KCl, 2 mM $MgCl_2$, 0.1% Triton, 300 mM NaCl, 0.5 mM dithiothreitol, 20 mM HEPES and Anti-protease Complete TM cocktail in H_2O, 10 μl/mg). After centrifugation at $12000\times g$ for 5 min, supernatants from homogenized eyes were collected. All procedures were conducted on ice. hIFN-α concentration was determined using a VeriKine Human IFN Alpha ELISA Kit according to the manufacturer's instructions (PBL Interferon Source, USA) with a detection limit of 12.5 pg/ml.

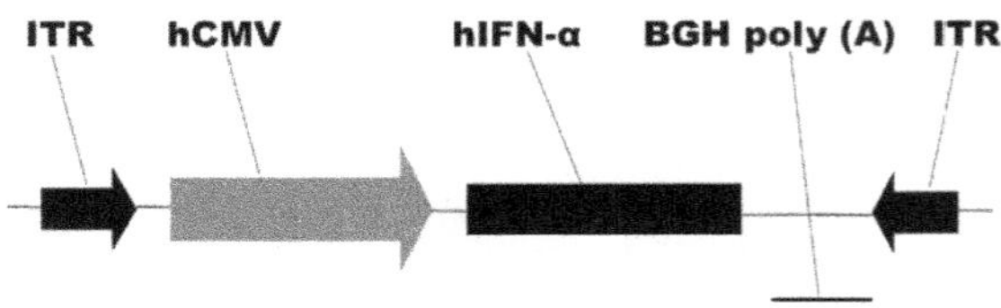

Figure 1. Scheme of the AAV2.hIFN-α construct. The hIFN-α coding sequence is under the control of a CMV promoter and followed by BGH poly (A). The expression cassette is flanked by ITRs. CMV promoter, human cytomegalovirus immediate early promoter; hIFN-α, human interferon-alpha; BGH poly (A), BGH poly-adenylation signal; ITR, AAV2 inverted terminal repeats.

Vector DNA biodistribution

PCR analysis was performed to evaluate the biodistribution of rAAV2 vector DNA. Mice were sacrificed and total DNA was extracted from AAV2.GFP injected eyes, contralateral eyes and distant organs using a Qiagen DNeasy kit. Primers for GFP (forward, 5′ TGGCCCGCCTGGCATTATGC 3′; reverse, 5′ TGGAGACTTGGAAATCCCCGTGAGT 3′) and GAPDH (forward, 5′ TGACGTGCCGCCTGGAGAAA 3′; reverse, 5′AGTGTAGCCCAAGATGCCCTTCAG 3′) were used to amplify 750 bp and 98 bp fragments respectively.

Induction and clinical assessment of EAU

Mice were immunized subcutaneously at the base of the tail and both thighs with 50 μg human $IRBP_{161-180}$ peptide in 100 μl PBS, emulsified 1:1 v/v in complete Freund's adjuvant (CFA) supplemented with 1.0 mg/ml *Mycobacterium tuberculosis* strain (MTB). A total of 200 μl emulsion was given for one mouse. EAU activity was examined clinically by slit lamp microscopy from day 8 to 21 after immunization. The clinical severity of ocular inflammation was assessed by two independent observers in a masked manner, and scored on a scale of 0–5 in half-point increments, according to five separate criteria described previously [23], with some modifications (table 1).

Histopathology

Eyes were enucleated on day 14 following IRBP immunization and were fixed in 4% buffered formaldehyde for 1 hour at room temperature. Tissues were embedded in paraffin. Serial 4–6 μm sections were cut through the papillary-optic nerve axis and stained by haematoxylin and eosin. At least four sections of each eye cut at different levels were prepared and evaluated histologically. The intensity of EAU was graded in a masked fashion on a scale of 0 to 4, as described earlier [24].

Table 1. Criteria of EAU Clinical Scoring in B10RIII mice.

Criteria			
Corneal edema	Mild	+	
	Moderate	++	Total 15 "+"
	Gross	+++	
Conjunctival hyperemia	Mild	+	
	Moderate	++	Grade:
	Gross	+++	0
Ciliary injection of the cornea	Mild	+	1 1~3 "+"
	Moderate	++	2 4~6 "+"
	Gross	+++	3 7~9 "+"
Anterior chamber inflammation	Occasional cells present	+	4 10~12 "+"
	Moderate or heavy cells present	++	5 13~15 "+"
	Hypopyon or exudate in the chamber	+++	
Posterior synechiae	Mild (<1/4 of Posterior synechiae)	+	
	Moderate(1/4~1/2 of Posterior synechiae)	++	
	Total seclusion of the pupil	+++	

IRBP-specific lymphocyte responses

The spleen and draining lymph nodes were removed from immunized mice on day 21. A single cell suspension was prepared by mechanical disruption and followed by a passage through a sterile stainless steel screen. For proliferation and cytokines assay, cells (2×10^6 cells/ml) were cultured in triplicate with RPMI 1640 medium (Gibco, Grand Island, NY, USA) containing 2 mM L-glutamine, 5×10-5 M2-ME, 0.1 Mm nonessential amino acids, 1 mM sodium pyruvate and 10% FBS in the presence of 10 μg/ml $IRBP_{161-180}$, 1 μg/ml Concanavalin A (Sigma) or medium alone for 72 hours. Proliferation was detected by a modified MTT assay using a cell counting kit (Cell Counting Kit-8; Sigma) as described previously [25]. IL-17 concentration in the supernatants was measured using a commercially available ELISA kit according to the manufacturer's directions (R&D System, Minneapolis, MN) with a detection limit of 15 pg/ml.

Statistical analysis

Data are expressed as mean ± standard deviation (SD). Severity of EAU was analyzed using the Kruskal-Wallis test followed by the Mann-Whitney U test with Bonferroni correction. Lymphocyte proliferation and cytokine production was analyzed using ANOVA. $P<0.05$ was considered to be significantly different. All experiments were repeated at least twice.

Results

hIFN-α expression following subretinal injection of AAV2.hIFN-α vector

Different groups of mice were injected subretinally with two doses of AAV2.hIFN-α, 1.5×10^8 vg or 1.5×10^6 vg. The hIFN-α level in supernatants from homogenized eyes was assayed by ELISA. In the eye receiving a subretinal injection of the higher dose of AAV2.hIFN-α (1.5×10^8 vg), expression of hIFN-α was detectable on day 14 (mean 4.41 ng/ml) increasing further on day 21 (mean 7.8 ng/ml). A high level of hIFN-α was observed on day 42 (10.15 ng/ml) and remained detectable until three months after injection (the last detection point). For the lower dose (1.5×10^6 vg), the level of hIFN-α was 0.128 ng/ml on day 14, 0.25 ng/ml on day 21, sharply increased on day 42 (mean 1.067 ng/ml) and day 90 (mean 3.057 ng/ml) following subretinal injection (Figure 2). The hIFN-α expression in the low dose of AAV2.hIFN-α injected group was about thirty fold lower than that from the high dose injected group. For both doses of AAV2.hIFN-α, hIFN-α expression was undetectable in the undiluted serum or contralateral uninjected eyes over time.

Biodistribution of vector DNA

PCR analysis was performed to determine the biodistribution of vector DNA after AAV2.GFP subretinal delivery. Total DNA was extracted from the injected eyes, contralateral eyes and distant organs (liver, spleen, heart, brain, lung and kidney) three weeks after subretinal injection. AAV2 vector DNA was PCR-amplified using GFP-specific primers. A 750 bp GFP-specific product was only detected in the AAV2.GFP treated eyes and no PCR product could be measured in the other tested organs or contralateral eyes (Figure 3).

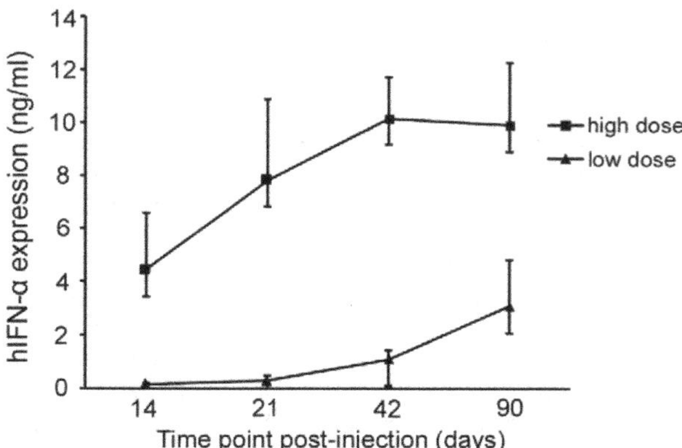

Figure 2. The expression of transgenes following subretinal injection of AAV2.hIFN-α. The ocular hIFN-α levels at various time points show that hIFN-α expression starts before day 14 following injection (the first time point tested). For the higher dose, hIFN-α expression reaches a peak on day 42 and remains high until day 90. In the eyes receiving a lower dose of vector, hIFN-α level shows an unremitting increase from three weeks to three months. Results are expressed as the mean ± standard deviation.

The effect of AAV2.hIFN-α on EAU

All normal B10RIII mice immunized with 50 µg human $IRBP_{161-180}$ peptide emulsified in CFA developed EAU as evidenced by conjunctival hyperemia, ciliary injection, corneal edema, posterior synechiae, aqueous flare and cells. The inflammatory signs appeared on day 8 or 9 after immunization, reached a peak by day 12 and were followed by a gradual regression. There was no inflammation in the control mice which received CFA alone.

To test the effect of AAV2.hIFN-α on EAU, it was subretinally injected into right eyes at two doses, 1.5×10^8 vg and 1.5×10^6 vg. AAV2.GFP (5×10^8 vg) was injected into the contralateral eyes as internal control [20]. Mice were immunized with $IRBP_{161-180}$ peptide emulsified in CFA three weeks after subretinal injection. Mice receiving a subretinal injection of PBS and a subsequent immunization with $IRBP_{161-180}$ peptide emulsified in CFA served as a separate control group.

Clinical signs were monitored after immunization by slit lamp microscopy. In PBS or AAV2.GFP injected eyes, severe uveitis, as evidenced by conjunctival hyperemia, ciliary injection, corneal edema, aqueous cells and posterior synechiae was observed (Figure 4A, B). A minor inflammatory reaction as manifested by conjunctival hyperemia or ciliary injection was found in both doses of AAV2.hIFN-α treated eyes (Figure 4C, D). Severity of inflammation was clinically scored on a scale from 0 to 5. Both doses of AAV2.hIFN-α treated eyes showed a significantly decreased activity of EAU throughout the course of disease as compared with PBS or AAV2.GFP injected controls (Figure 4E). Clinical scoring on day 12 showed that a significantly decreased severity of EAU was observed in AAV2.hIFN-α^{low} and AAV2.hIFN-α^{high} treated groups when compared with PBS and AAV2.GFP injected controls ($p<0.0001$). There was no significant difference between the two groups receiving different doses of AAV2.hIFN-α. Histological examination on day 14 showed severe intraocular inflammation in the AAV2.GFP injected eyes and PBS injected control mice as evidenced by massive infiltration of inflammatory cells into the iris, vitreous cavity, throughout all retinal layers and the choroid, intensive retinal vasculitis, obvious iris thickening, destruction of the retinal architecture with severe retinal folding and detachment, as well as photoreceptor damage (Figure 5A, C). However, in both doses of AAV2.hIFN-α treated eyes, only scattered infiltration of inflammatory cells into the vitreous body and retina was observed (Figure 5E, G). Additionally, the inflammatory changes in the anterior segment in both doses of AAV2.hIFN-α treated groups were less than those in the AAV2.GFP injected eyes and PBS injected mice (Figure 5B, D, F, H). Pathological grading showed that PBS injected eyes (EAU grade, 3.08±0.66) and AAV2.GFP treated eyes (EAU grade, 3.2±0.76) had significantly more intensive inflammation as compared to the AAV2.hIFN-α treated eyes (1.33±0.6 for low dose, 1.4±0.58 for high dose) ($P<0.0001$) (Figure 5I).

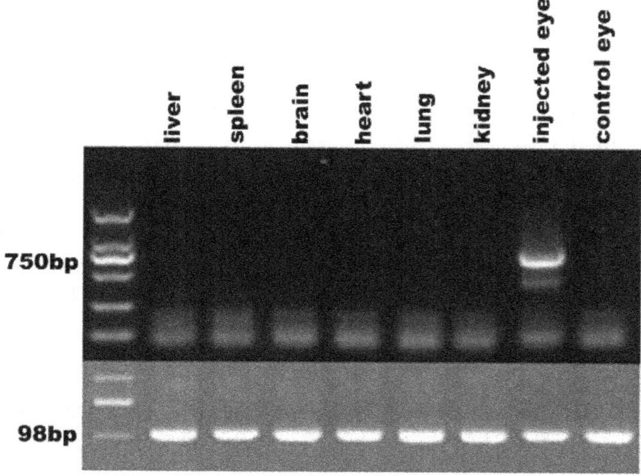

Figure 3. Biodistribution of vector DNA three weeks after the subretinal injection of AAV2.GFP. Vector DNA is detectable only in the injected eye, but not in the contralateral eye and distant tissues including liver, spleen, brain, heart, lung, and kidney.

Effects of subretinal injection of rAAV2.hIFN-α on the IRBP-specific systemic immune response

To determine whether there was an effect of AAV2.hIFN-α on the IRBP-specific immune response, lymphocytes from spleen and lymph nodes were isolated and incubated for 72 hours in vitro with $IRBP_{161-180}$ peptide, ConA (positive control), or medium alone (negative control) respectively. The proliferation and IL-17 production of lymphocytes were assayed. The result showed a similar response in proliferation and IL-17 production of lymphocytes incubated with ConA among the two doses of AAV2.hIFN-α treated mice, AAV2.GFP treated mice and PBS treated mice. A somewhat lower response in IL-17 production and proliferation of lymphocytes was observed in all the tested four groups when exposed to $IRBP_{161-180}$ peptide. There was no difference concerning IRBP-specific lymphocyte proliferation and IL-17 production among lower dose of AAV2.hIFN-α treated mice, AAV2.GFP treated mice and PBS treated mice ($p>0.05$). However, the higher dose of AAV2.hIFN-α treated mice exhibited significantly reduced IRBP-specific lymphocyte proliferation as compared with PBS treated mice ($p=0.012$), AAV2.GFP treated mice ($p=0.019$) and lower dose of AAV2.hIFN-α treated mice ($p=0.027$) (Figure 6A). Also, IL-17 production was significantly downregulated in the group of mice receiving the higher dose of AAV2.hIFN-αwhen compared with PBS treated mice ($p=0.025$), AAV2.GFP treated mice ($p=0.013$) or mice receiving the lower dose of AAV2.hIFN-α ($p=0.018$)

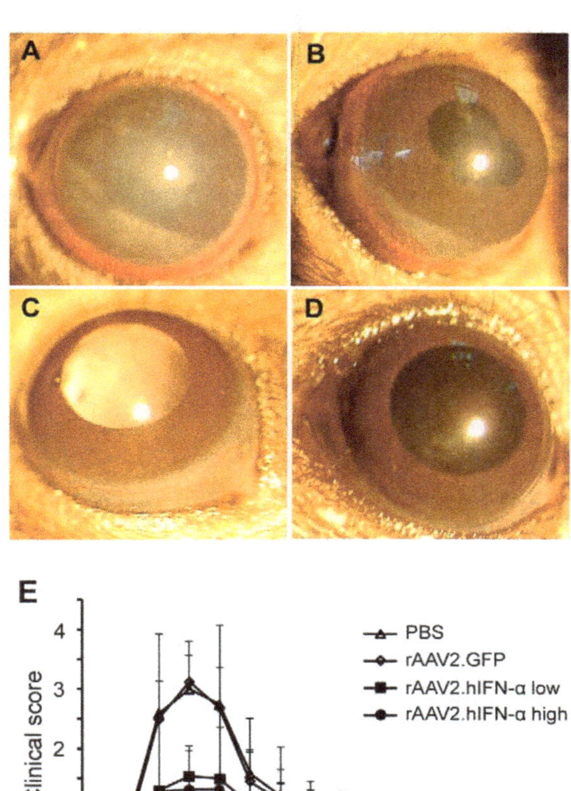

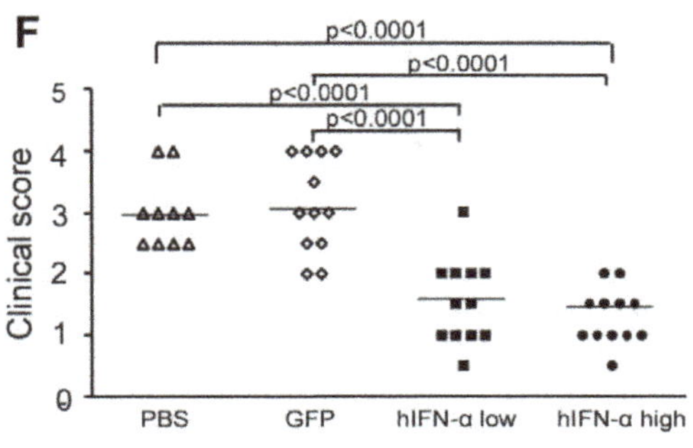

Figure 4. Clinical evaluation of EAU activity. Two doses of AAV2.hIFN-α were subretinally injected into the eye respectively, PBS and AAV2.GFP were used as controls. Three weeks after injection, EAU was induced by immunization with $IRBP_{161-180}$ and ocular inflammation was examined by slit lamp microscopy. Images show significantly severe inflammation in the PBS (A) and AAV2.GFP injected eyes (B) as compared to the AAV2.hIFN-α treated eyes (C, D). Kinetics of EAU (E) reveals that subretinal injection of both doses of AAV2.hIFN-α persistently attenuated ocular inflammation of EAU as compared with PBS and AAV2.GFP. The significant difference was observed consecutively on day 11 to 14 after immunization ($P<0.05$). Data are presented as mean ± standard deviation. Clinical score on day 12 after immunization (F) shows that the PBS injected eyes had a score of 3 (±0.58) and the AAV2.GFP injected eyes reached a mean clinical score of 3.13 (±0.77), the score of AAV2.hIFN-α treated eyes was 1.54 (±0.69, $p<0.0001$, Mann-Whitney U test) in the lower dose treated group and 1.292 (±0.45, $p<0.0001$) in the higher dose group. Each point represents an individual eye. The average scores of each group are denoted by the horizontal bars.

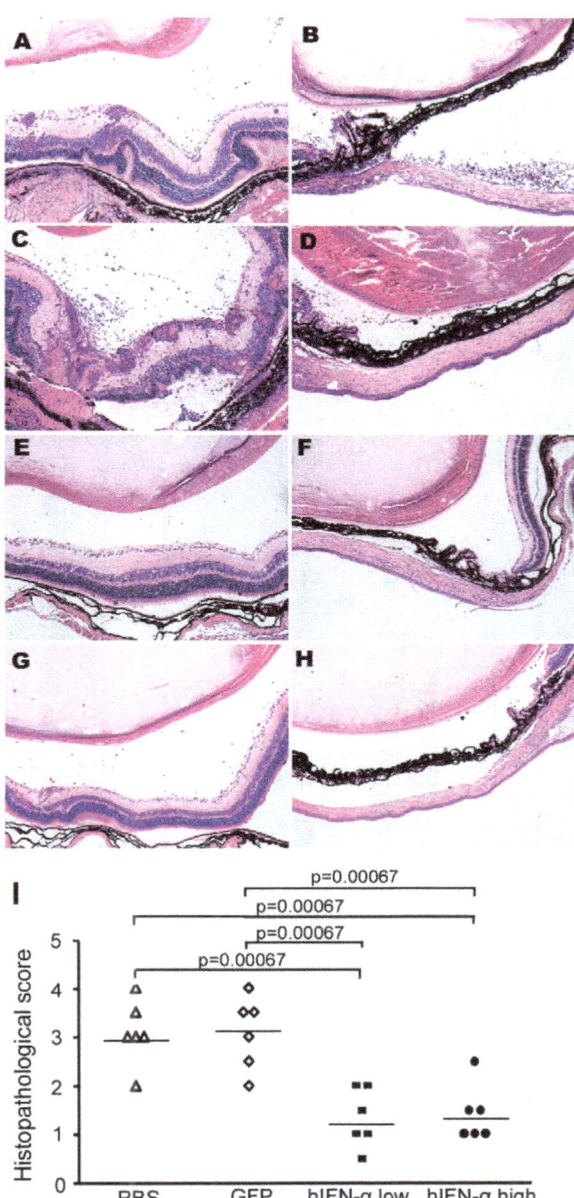

Figure 5. Histological examinations on day 14 of EAU. Images of histological analysis show obvious iris thickening, severe retinal folding, destruction, damage of the photoreceptor layer and massive inflammatory cell infiltration in the iris, vitreous, retina, and subretinal space, as well as intensive vasculitis formation in PBS injected eye (A, B) and AAV2.GFP injected eyes (C, D). However, a minor infiltration of inflammatory cells was observed in the vitreous and retina in both lower (E, F) and higher dose (G, H) of AAV2.hIFN-α treated eyes. (haematoxylin eosin staining, original magnification ×100) Histological grade (I) shows reduced EAU in both doses of AAV2.hIFN-α treated groups as compared with PBS injected and AAV2.GFP injected eyes ($p<0.0001$, Mann-Whitney U test). Each point is the score of an individual eye. The mean scores of each group are denoted by the horizontal bars.

(Figure 6B). Lymphocytes from the tested four groups did not show a detectable proliferation and IL-17 production when cultured with medium alone.

Discussion

In this study, we investigated the effect of an AAV2-based ocular gene therapy designed to make retinal cells secrete a therapeutic molecule, hIFN-α, on the development of EAU in mice. The results showed an effective expression of hIFN-α within the treated eyes following subretinal injection of AAV2.hIFN-α. The distribution of vector DNA was restricted to the injected eye without detectable spreading. Subretinal administration of AAV2.hIFN-α using either a high or low dose of vector (1.5×10^8 vg and 1.5×10^6 vg), both significantly reduced EAU development. The IRBP-specific immune response was not affected following the lower dose vector injection but both IRBP-specific proliferation and IL-17 production were downregulated when the higher vector dose was used.

In an attempt to achieve a successful gene therapy, an effective recombinant viral vector and a feasible gene delivery system in association with a locally effective expression of transgene without

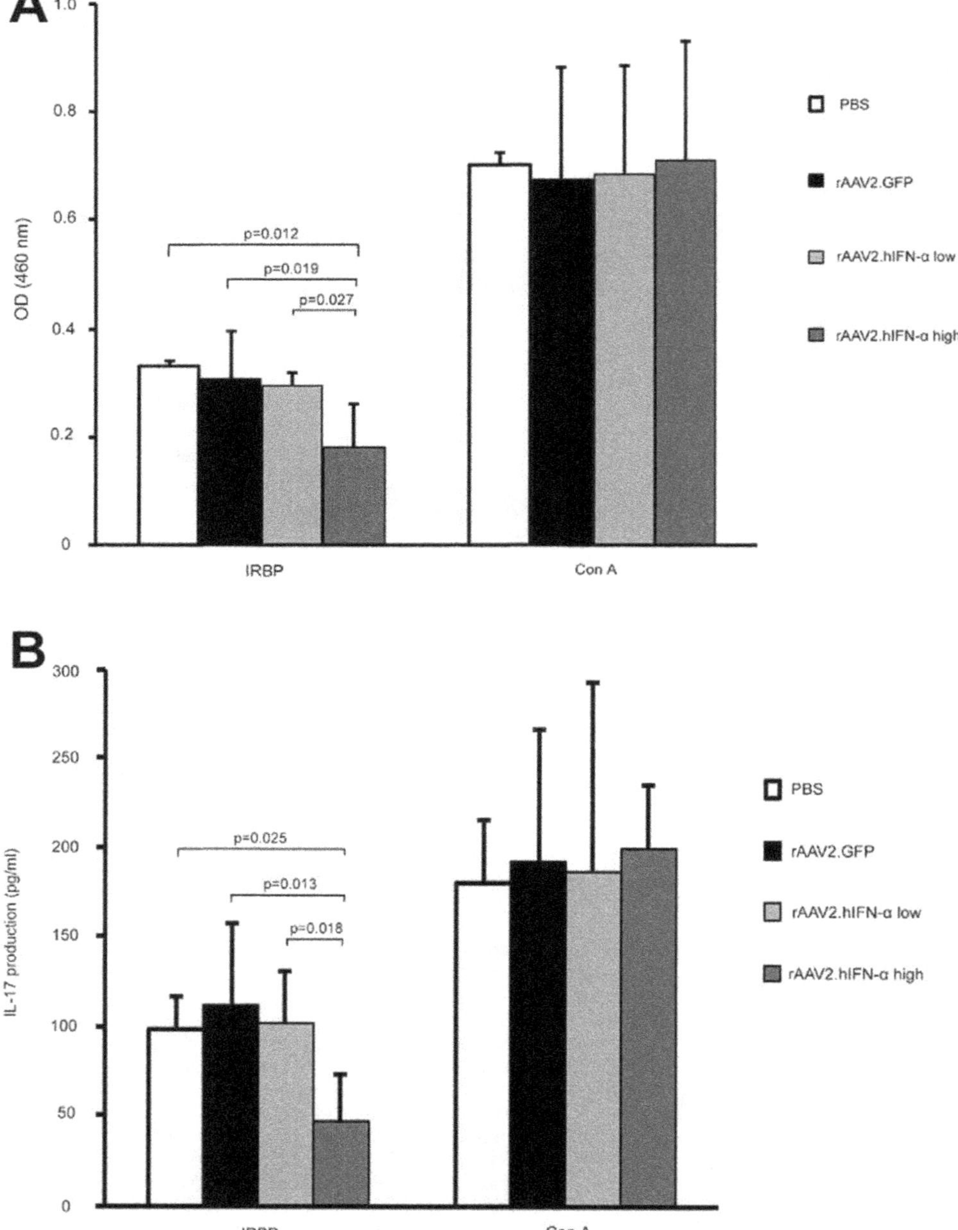

Figure 6. Systemic IRBP-specific immune responses in each group. IRBP-specific lymphocyte proliferation (A) and IL-17 production *in vitro* (B) show no significant difference among lower dose of AAV2.hIFN-α, PBS and AAV2.GFP treated mice ($P>0.05$). A significant decline of lymphocyte proliferation is observed in higher dose of AAV2.hIFN-α treated mice compared with PBS injected ($p=0.012$), AAV2.GFP injected ($p=0.019$) and lower dose of AAV2.hIFN-α treated mice ($p=0.027$). Similarly, the IL-17 production is significantly downregulated in higher dose of AAV2.hIFN-α treated mice as compared with PBS injected ($p=0.025$), AAV2.GFP injected ($p=0.013$) and lower dose of AAV2.hIFN-α treated mice ($p=0.018$). Results are presented as mean ± standard deviation and every experiment was performed three times.

systemic spreading are all necessary. In this study we successfully prepared the recombinant viral vector encoding hIFN-α, an effective immune suppressive cytokine, based on adeno-associated virus, which has been proven to effectively transduce various ocular cell types for a long time. Subretinal injection of AAV2.hIFN-α using two doses resulted in the effective secretion of this cytokine within ocular tissues for at least 70 days. Examination by fluorescence microscopy showed that GFP was expressed by RPE cells and photoreceptors following subretinal injection of AAV2.GFP (data not shown), which are consistent with earlier reports [26,27]. Expression of GFP within the retina suggested that hIFN-α might be secreted predominantly by RPE and cells in the photoreceptor layer. An earlier study by Lai et al [28] revealed that the secreted protein could diffuse into both the posterior and anterior segments of the eye with the natural fluid flow following subretinal injection of AAV2 vectors. It is, therefore, not surprising to note a strikingly diminished inflammatory activity both in the anterior and posterior segments in the AAV2.hIFN-α treated eyes following immunization with $IRBP_{161-180}$ peptide. Another important factor for a successful gene therapy using viral vectors is that the administrated vector should be distributed only in the local tissue [29]. In order to examine whether the injected AAV2 vector entered into other organs, we investigated its dissemination in the contralateral eye and organs distant to the injected site. The result showed that the AAV2 vector DNA was found only in the treated eye but not in the tested organs or in the contralateral eye. This result is consistent with earlier reports in rats [30] and nonhuman primates [31] and this has been attributed to the integrity of the blood-eye barrier. However, early reports showed that AAV2 vector DNA was also detectable in the brain of intravitreally injected dogs [32] and mice [33,34]. This result has been explained by the transport of the AAV2 vector DNA into the brain due to an extremely abundant expression of this DNA in the ganglion cells following intravitreal injection [32]. The experiments with subretinal injection of the recombinant AAV2 vector reported previously by others and the result presented here seem to avoid this unwanted distribution of the injected virus DNA into other organs. It is, therefore, reasonable to presume that subretinal injection of AAV2.hIFN-α may lead to a long-term effect of hIFN-α within the treated eye without, at least, obvious systemic biodistribution of AAV2 vector DNA.

As mentioned above, subretinal injection of AAV2.hIFN-α could lead to a therapeutic concentration of hIFN-α within the eye and was able to significantly inhibit EAU elicited by IRBP administration in the presence of CFA. We subsequently investigated whether a local administration of AAV2.hIFN-α affected the IRBP-specific systemic immune response and whether the inhibitory effect on EAU was associated with a downregulated IRBP-specific systemic immune response. As there was no tracing technique available in this experiment, we adopted a two-dose strategy to identify whether there was a difference in the IRBP-specific systemic immune response as well as an inhibitory effect on EAU following subretinal administration. Our result showed that both doses were able to significantly attenuate the EAU activity although the hIFN-α expression within the eye of the lower dose of AAV2.hIFN-α injected group was thirty-fold lower than that in the higher dose group. A downregulated lymphocyte proliferation and a decreased IL-17 production were only observed in the group of animals receiving the higher dose. However, biodistribution detection showed no dissemination of AAV2 vector DNA in systemic organs and hIFN-α in serum. Additionally, early study showed that subretinal administration of AAV2 vector did not trigger any humoral immune response [27]. Collectively, a likely explanation is that the local immunomodulatory environment in the high dose treated animals is causing local antigen presenting cells to have a less activated phenotype, so that when they migrate to the draining lymph nodes, the T-cells are not as activated and perhaps more anergic or tolerant. In view of these results, it is not likely that the inhibitory effect of hIFN-α on EAU was mediated by a downregulated systemic immune response. However, the downregulated systemic immune response, on one hand, may be useful for uveitis associated systemic diseases. On the other hand, it may lead to unknown and unwanted side effects. More studies are needed to explore and address these issues.

There are some limitations in our study. The production of hIFN-α was only followed for a time period of three months and a prolonged observation is needed to determine the duration of secretion of the transgene product after intraocular administration. Furthermore, the exact mechanisms by which the released hIFN-α exactly inhibits EAU should be explored. In addition, a more effective rAAV2 vector using a promoter modulating the expression of hIFN-α needs to be developed for future studies.

In conclusion, we have now developed an AAV2-mediated long-lasting and effective hIFN-α gene delivery system. The locally secreted hIFN-α following subretinal injection of AAV2.hIFN-α significantly reduced the activity of EAU.

Author Contributions

Conceived and designed the experiments: PY LT BL. Performed the experiments: LT JS QX LW. Analyzed the data: LT CW. Contributed reagents/materials/analysis tools: BL ZP. Wrote the paper: PY LT BL AK.

References

1. Gritz DC, Wong IG (2004) Incidence and prevalence of uveitis in Northern California; the Northern California Epidemiology of Uveitis Study. Ophthalmology 111: 491–500; discussion 500.
2. Goldstein H (1980) The reported demography and causes of blindness throughout the world. Adv Ophthalmol 40: 1–99.
3. Imrie FR, Dick AD (2007) Biologics in the treatment of uveitis. Curr Opin Ophthalmol 18: 481–486.
4. Yeh S, Nussenblatt RB, Levy-Clarke GA (2007) Emerging biologics in the treatment of uveitis. Expert Rev Clin Immunol 3: 781–796.
5. Sobaci G, Erdem U, Durukan AH, Erdurman C, Bayer A, et al. (2010) Safety and effectiveness of interferon alpha-2a in treatment of patients with Behcet's uveitis refractory to conventional treatments. Ophthalmology 117: 1430–1435.
6. Theofilopoulos AN, Baccala R, Beutler B, Kono DH (2005) Type I interferons (alpha/beta) in immunity and autoimmunity. Annu Rev Immunol 23: 307–336.
7. Yang DS, Taylor SR, Lightman SL (2008) Interferon-alpha in the management of patients with Behcet's disease. Br J Hosp Med (Lond) 69: 575–579.
8. Wang W, Edington HD, Rao UN, Jukic DM, Radfar A, et al. (2008) Effects of high-dose IFNalpha2b on regional lymph node metastases of human melanoma: modulation of STAT5, FOXP3, and IL-17. Clin Cancer Res 14: 8314–8320.
9. Mackensen F, Max R, Becker MD (2009) Interferons and their potential in the treatment of ocular inflammation. Clinical ophthalmology (Auckland, N Z) 3: 559–566.
10. Moschen AR, Geiger S, Krehan I, Kaser A, Tilg H (2008) Interferon-alpha controls IL-17 expression in vitro and in vivo. Immunobiology 213: 779–787.
11. Bainbridge JW, Smith AJ, Barker SS, Robbie S, Henderson R, et al. (2008) Effect of gene therapy on visual function in Leber's congenital amaurosis. N Engl J Med 358: 2231–2239.
12. Maguire AM, Simonelli F, Pierce EA, Pugh EN, Jr., Mingozzi F, et al. (2008) Safety and efficacy of gene transfer for Leber's congenital amaurosis. N Engl J Med 358: 2240–2248.
13. Hauswirth WW, Aleman TS, Kaushal S, Cideciyan AV, Schwartz SB, et al. (2008) Treatment of leber congenital amaurosis due to RPE65 mutations by ocular subretinal injection of adeno-associated virus gene vector: short-term results of a phase I trial. Human gene therapy 19: 979–990.
14. Cideciyan AV, Aleman TS, Boye SL, Schwartz SB, Kaushal S, et al. (2008) Human gene therapy for RPE65 isomerase deficiency activates the retinoid cycle of vision but with slow rod kinetics. Proc Natl Acad Sci U S A 105: 15112–15117.

15. Srivastava A, Rajappa M, Kaur J (2010) Uveitis: Mechanisms and recent advances in therapy. Clin Chim Acta 411: 1165–1171.
16. Colella P, Cotugno G, Auricchio A (2009) Ocular gene therapy: current progress and future prospects. Trends Mol Med 15: 23–31.
17. Annear MJ, Bartoe JT, Barker SE, Smith AJ, Curran PG, et al. (2011) Gene therapy in the second eye of RPE65-deficient dogs improves retinal function. Gene Ther 18: 53–61.
18. Barker SE, Broderick CA, Robbie SJ, Duran Y, Natkunarajah M, et al. (2009) Subretinal delivery of adeno-associated virus serotype 2 results in minimal immune responses that allow repeat vector administration in immunocompetent mice. J Gene Med 11: 486–497.
19. Buch PK, Bainbridge JW, Ali RR (2008) AAV-mediated gene therapy for retinal disorders: from mouse to man. Gene Ther 15: 849–857.
20. Broderick CA, Smith AJ, Balaggan KS, Georgiadis A, Buch PK, et al. (2005) Local administration of an adeno-associated viral vector expressing IL-10 reduces monocyte infiltration and subsequent photoreceptor damage during experimental autoimmune uveitis. Mol Ther 12: 369–373.
21. Smith JR, Verwaerde C, Rolling F, Naud MC, Delanoye A, et al. (2005) Tetracycline-inducible viral interleukin-10 intraocular gene transfer, using adeno-associated virus in experimental autoimmune uveoretinitis. Human gene therapy 16: 1037–1046.
22. Lei B, Zhang K, Yue Y, Ghosh A, Duan D (2009) Adeno-associated virus serotype-9 efficiently transduces the retinal outer plexiform layer. Molecular vision 15: 1374–1382.
23. Uchio E, Kijima M, Tanaka S, Ohno S (1994) Suppression of experimental uveitis with monoclonal antibodies to ICAM-1 and LFA-1. Investigative ophthalmology & visual science 35: 2626–2631.
24. Caspi RR (2003) Experimental autoimmune uveoretinitis in the rat and mouse. Current protocols in immunology/edited by John E Coligan [et al] Chapter 15: Unit 15.16.
25. Itano N, Atsumi F, Sawai T, Yamada Y, Miyaishi O, et al. (2002) Abnormal accumulation of hyaluronan matrix diminishes contact inhibition of cell growth and promotes cell migration. Proc Natl Acad Sci U S A 99: 3609–3614.
26. Flannery JG, Zolotukhin S, Vaquero MI, LaVail MM, Muzyczka N, et al. (1997) Efficient photoreceptor-targeted gene expression in vivo by recombinant adeno-associated virus. Proc Natl Acad Sci U S A 94: 6916–6921.
27. Li Q, Miller R, Han PY, Pang J, Dinculescu A, et al. (2008) Intraocular route of AAV2 vector administration defines humoral immune response and therapeutic potential. Molecular vision 14: 1760–1769.
28. Lai YK, Shen WY, Brankov M, Lai CM, Constable IJ, et al. (2002) Potential long-term inhibition of ocular neovascularisation by recombinant adeno-associated virus-mediated secretion gene therapy. Gene Ther 9: 804–813.
29. Rolling F (2004) Recombinant AAV-mediated gene transfer to the retina: gene therapy perspectives. Gene Ther 11 Suppl 1: S26–32.
30. Jacobson SG, Acland GM, Aguirre GD, Aleman TS, Schwartz SB, et al. (2006) Safety of recombinant adeno-associated virus type 2-RPE65 vector delivered by ocular subretinal injection. Mol Ther 13: 1074–1084.
31. Jacobson SG, Boye SL, Aleman TS, Conlon TJ, Zeiss CJ, et al. (2006) Safety in nonhuman primates of ocular AAV2-RPE65, a candidate treatment for blindness in Leber congenital amaurosis. Human gene therapy 17: 845–858.
32. Provost N, Le Meur G, Weber M, Mendes-Madeira A, Podevin G, et al. (2005) Biodistribution of rAAV vectors following intraocular administration: evidence for the presence and persistence of vector DNA in the optic nerve and in the brain. Mol Ther 11: 275–283.
33. Hennig AK, Levy B, Ogilvie JM, Vogler CA, Galvin N, et al. (2003) Intravitreal gene therapy reduces lysosomal storage in specific areas of the CNS in mucopolysaccharidosis VII mice. The Journal of neuroscience : the official journal of the Society for Neuroscience 23: 3302–3307.
34. Hennig AK, Ogilvie JM, Ohlemiller KK, Timmers AM, Hauswirth WW, et al. (2004) AAV-mediated intravitreal gene therapy reduces lysosomal storage in the retinal pigmented epithelium and improves retinal function in adult MPS VII mice. Mol Ther 10: 106–116.

5

In Vivo Safety and Persistence of Endoribonuclease Gene-Transduced CD4+ T Cells in Cynomolgus Macaques for HIV-1 Gene Therapy Model

Hideto Chono[1]*, Naoki Saito[1], Hiroshi Tsuda[1], Hiroaki Shibata[2], Naohide Ageyama[2], Keiji Terao[2], Yasuhiro Yasutomi[2], Junichi Mineno[1], Ikunoshin Kato[1]

1 Center for Cell and Gene Therapy, Takara Bio Inc, Otsu, Shiga, Japan, **2** Tsukuba Primate Research Center, National Institute of Biomedical Innovation, Tsukuba, Ibaraki, Japan

Abstract

Background: MazF is an endoribonuclease encoded by *Escherichia coli* that specifically cleaves the ACA sequence of mRNA. In our previous report, conditional expression of MazF in the HIV-1 LTR rendered CD4+ T lymphocytes resistant to HIV-1 replication. In this study, we examined the *in vivo* safety and persistence of MazF-transduced cynomolgus macaque CD4+ T cells infused into autologous monkeys.

Methodology/Principal Findings: The *in vivo* persistence of the gene-modified CD4+ T cells in the peripheral blood was monitored for more than half a year using quantitative real-time PCR and flow cytometry, followed by experimental autopsy in order to examine the safety and distribution pattern of the infused cells in several organs. Although the levels of the MazF-transduced CD4+ T cells gradually decreased in the peripheral blood, they were clearly detected throughout the experimental period. Moreover, the infused cells were detected in the distal lymphoid tissues, such as several lymph nodes and the spleen. Histopathological analyses of tissues revealed that there were no lesions related to the infused gene modified cells. Antibodies against MazF were not detected. These data suggest the safety and the low immunogenicity of MazF-transduced CD4+ T cells. Finally, gene modified cells harvested from the monkey more than half a year post-infusion suppressed the replication of SHIV 89.6P.

Conclusions/Significance: The long-term persistence, safety and continuous HIV replication resistance of the *mazF* gene-modified CD4+ T cells in the non-human primate model suggests that autologous transplantation of *mazF* gene-modified cells is an attractive strategy for HIV gene therapy.

Editor: John J. Rossi, Beckman Research Institute of the City of Hope, United States of America

Funding: The authors have no support or funding to report.

Competing Interests: Hideto Chono, Naoki Saito, Hiroshi Tsuda, Junichi Mineno and Ikunoshin Kato are employees of Takara Bio Inc. (http://www.takara-bio.co.jp). There are no patents, products in development or marketed products to declare.

* E-mail: chonoh@takara-bio.co.jp

Introduction

Highly active anti-retroviral therapy (HAART) is widely used for human immunodeficiency virus (HIV) therapy and involves the combination of several drugs with different functions that are currently being evaluated in clinical trials; some of these drugs are currently available [1]. HAART treatment reduces plasma viral load to undetectable levels and recovers CD4+ T cells to clinically safe levels. Although HAART therapy has revolutionized the treatment of HIV-1 infection, the need for life-long therapy, difficulties with medication adherence and long-term medication toxicities have led to the search for new treatment strategies that will efficiently reduce the viral load and allow for stable immunological homeostasis. The number of patients who are HAART resistant has significantly decreased in the past 2 years due to newly available drugs, but based on previous experience, drug resistance is likely to increase again. Thus, additional approaches for the management of HIV infection, or approaches performed in combination with HAART therapy, are needed. Gene therapy for HIV-1 infection has been proposed as an alternative to antiretroviral drug regimens [2,3]. A number of different genetic vectors with antiviral payloads have been utilized to combat HIV-1, including antisense RNA against the HIV-1 envelope gene, transdominant protein RevM10, ribozymes, RNA decoys, single chain antibodies, and RNA-interference [4,5]. These protocols use T cells or hematopoietic stem cells as a target for gene modification. Autologous T cell transfer in HIV patients began in the mid 1990's, and since that time, no serious adverse events have been reported to be associated with infusions of autologous T cells, and infusions are well tolerated. The majority of these clinical trials used gene transfer by retrovirus or lentiviral vectors for the delivery of the anti-HIV payloads.

In order to develop a new approach for HIV therapy, we previously constructed an HIV-1 Tat-dependent expression retroviral vector in which the *Escherichia coli* (*E. coli*) endoribonuclease gene *mazF* was fused downstream of the trans-activation response element (TAR) so that the gene expression of *mazF* is induced upon HIV-1 replication [6]. When MazF-transduced cells were infected with HIV-1 IIIB, the replication of HIV-1 was efficiently inhibited without affecting CD4+ T cell growth. MazF-transduced primary CD4+ T cells derived from monkeys also suppressed simian/human immunodeficiency virus (SHIV) replication [6]. Thus, autologous transfer of genetically modified CD4+ T cells conditionally expressing the MazF protein will be a promising strategy for HIV gene therapy. Generally, the shift from the chronic phase to the AIDS phase is due to the balance between viral growth and immune suppression, and the remarkable decrease in CD4+ T cells causes the subsequent deficiency of the immune system, the hallmarks of AIDS. The benefit of the MazF-based gene therapy strategy is that gene-modified CD4+ T cells may be protected from HIV-1-associated cell death and are therefore likely to help the immune system maintain a stable condition.

In this preclinical study, we examined the *in vivo* safety and persistence of MazF-transduced autologous CD4+ T cells (named MazF-Tmac cells) using a non-human primate model. Cynomolgus macaque primary CD4+ T cells were retrovirally transduced with the MazF vector, infused into the autologous monkeys, and the persistence and safety of the MazF-Tmac cells was monitored more than half a year. We found that infused MazF-Tmac cells were detected in the peripheral blood throughout the experimental period. Additionally, experimental autopsy revealed the distribution of the infused lymphocyte in total body.

Results

Manufacturing of MazF-transduced CD4+ T cells using *ex vivo*-expanded cynomolgus macaque CD4+ T cells

In order to infuse more than 1×10^9 MazF-transduced autologous cells, isolated primary CD4+ T lymphocytes were *ex vivo* stimulated, transduced with the MT-MFR-PL2 retroviral vector (Figure 1A), and expanded as described in the Materials and Methods. The resultant MazF-Tmac cells were transplanted into autologous monkeys via intravenous infusion (Figure 1B). We initially used concanavalin A (Con A) for the stimulation of CD4+ T cells (CD4T-1), but Con A only induced a 12-fold cell expansion after 7 days. In order to improve the *ex vivo* expansion, we used anti-CD3/anti-CD28 monoclonal antibody-conjugated beads (anti-CD3/CD28 beads), which are known to yield a more efficient cellular expansion [7,8]. As we expected, the fold expansion of CD4+ T cells (CD4T-2 and CD4T-3) stimulated with anti-CD3/CD28 beads was much higher than with Con A stimulation (Table 1). In order to improve the engraftment efficiency of CD4+ T cells, busulfan was orally administered to the macaques prior to the transplantation, and the gene-modified MazF-Tmac cells were infused into each monkey intravenously at $1.6–2.7 \times 10^9$ cells.

Transduction efficiency and cell surface markers of MazF-Tmac cells

The efficiency of MazF transduction and phenotype of cell surface markers of the MazF-Tmac cells were analyzed using flow cytometry. The MazF vector transduction efficiency of CD4T-2 and CD4T-3 cells was 61.8% and 60.0%, respectively, while only 34.5% for CD4T-1 (Table 1). As shown in Table 2, 99% of the expanded MazF-Tmac cells were CD3 and CD4 double-positive, and in these cells, more than 90% expressed CD95/CD28, which are known central memory phenotype markers [9]. Central memory cells generally have a longer life span compared to effecter memory cells [10]; thus, a higher percentage of central memory cells in MazF-Tmac cells is likely to result in longer persistence after transplantation. Furthermore, to assess the activation status of MazF-Tmac cells, we measured the expression of CD25, which is also known as IL-2 receptor alpha and is an activated T cell marker. CD25 expression of MazF-Tmac cells from CD4T-2 and CD4T-3 was low. In contrast, almost 100% of the CD4+ T cells were found to express CD25 with a higher expression level 2–4 days after stimulation (data not shown). Thus, these data indicate that a large number of MazF-Tmac cells entered into resting or non-activated states during the *ex vivo* culture. CXCR4, a co-receptor for X4 tropic HIV entry, was found to be expressed in expanded CD4T-2 and CD4T-3 MazF-Tmac cells. Furthermore, we observed that there was no significant difference in the measured cell surface markers between Con A- and anti-CD3/CD28 bead-stimulated MazF-Tmac cells (Table 2).

Longitudinal analysis of infused MazF-Tmac cells

To examine the *in vivo* safety and persistence of infused MazF-Tmac cells, peripheral blood from each monkey was collected to monitor the hematological effects and the proviral copy number of the transduced retroviral vector in the genome over six months. There was no significant change in the body weight of the monkeys throughout the experiment (Figure 2A). During the period of 2–4 weeks post-transplantation, severe reduction in the white blood cell (WBC) count, hemoglobin (Hb) concentration, and platelet (PLT) levels were observed in the monkeys CD4T-1 and CD4T-2, while only slight reduction was observed in CD4T-3. These negative effects are considered to be due to the effect of the busulfan treatment, which is known to cause partial bone marrow depletion and functional defects in blood-forming tissues. No other adverse events were observed throughout the experiments. The transient reduction of lymphocytes gradually recovered, and the cell number became stable two months after the transplantation (Figure 2A).

The percentage of persistent MazF-Tmac cells in CD4+ T cells was determined using real-time PCR and flow cytometric analyses. The percentage of MazF-Tmac cells gradually decreased in CD4T-1- and CD4T-2-transplanted monkeys, while in the CD4T-3-transplanted monkey, a drastic reduction of the infused MazF-Tmac cells was observed 3–4 weeks post-transplantation but was not observed at later time points (Figure 2B). Although the levels of MazF-Tmac cells gradually decreased over time, the infused MazF-Tmac cells were detected even after six months post-transplantation. It is reasonable to assume that a population of infused MazF-Tmac cells can persist for a long-term period, likely forming a resting condition.

Detection of anti-MazF antibodies in monkey blood

Although the levels of MazF-transduced CD4+ T cells gradually decreased in the peripheral blood, some were detected throughout the half-year experimental period, suggesting that MazF-Tmac cells showed little or no immunogenicity towards cynomolgus macaques. Because gene therapy for HIV is aimed at reconstituting an HIV-resistant immune system, genetically modified cells must not only inhibit virus replication, but also maintain their expected trafficking behavior and persist *in vivo*. Although the evidence of longitudinal persistence of MazF-Tmac cells supports the low immunogenicity of MazF-Tmac cells, it is important to assess the production of antibodies against MazF. As shown in Figure 3 and Figure S1, we detected no production of anti-MazF antibodies in the CD4T-2 monkey blood after transplantation of the MazF-Tmac cells.

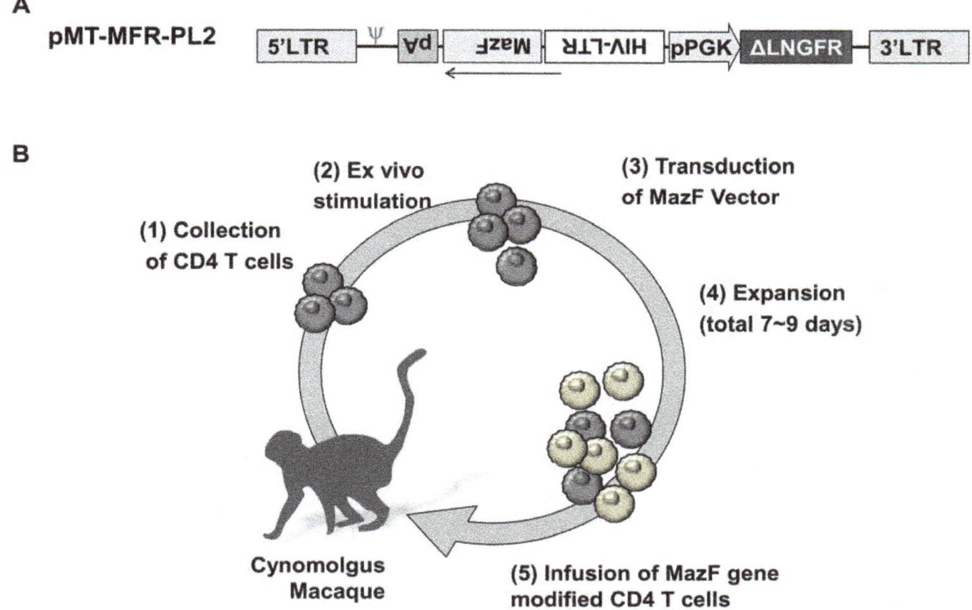

Figure 1. Diagram of autologous CD4+ T cell transplantation using a non-human primate model. (A) Design of gene transfer vector. The MazF gene derived from *E. coli* was inserted directly into the downstream of HIV-LTR sequence. The HIV-LTR-MazF-polyA cassette was introduced in the opposite direction of the MoMLV-LTR. A truncated form of the human ΔLNGFR was also introduced into the retrovirus vector as a surface marker. The ΔLNGFR gene is under the control of the human PGK promoter. (B) Flow diagram of gene-transduced CD4+ T cell manufacture. (1) Peripheral blood was collected by apheresis, (2) CD4+ T cells were selected by positive selection and stimulated *ex vivo* with Con A or anti-CD3/CD28 monoclonal antibody-conjugated beads. (3) The MT-MFR-PL2 vector was transduced twice on days 3 and 4. (4) The transduced cells were expanded for an additional 3–5 days until the total cell number reached more than 10^9. (5) On day 7–9, the expanded cells were collected, washed, and infused to the autologous macaques through venous blood.

In vivo safety of MazF-Tmac cells

It is a great advantage to use primate models for investigating the safety of gene-modified cells, as they can be used for surgical pathological analysis. Therefore, we performed experimental autopsies six months after transplantation. To examine the safety of MazF-Tmac cells, specimens from several organs were fixed in buffered formaldehyde and embedded in plastic. Serial sections were made using a diamond saw. Slides were then stained with hematoxylin-eosin. Histopathological findings of the specimens were contracted with Bozo Research Center (Tokyo, Japan), and no severe adverse events relating to MazF-Tmac cell infusion was observed (Table 3 and Figure S2).

Table 1. Demographic data and summary of expansion fold and transduction efficiency.

	CD4T-1	CD4T-2	CD4T-3
Body Weight (kg)	5.25	5.18	3.7
Method for stimulation	Con A	Anti-CD3/CD28 Beads	Anti-CD3/CD28 Beads
Number of stimulated CD4+ T cells ($\times10^7$ cells)	13.0	1.0	4.6
Days for expansion (days)	7	7	9
Number of infused MazF-Tmac cells ($\times10^9$ cells)	1.6	1.7	2.7
Expansion Fold	12.3	170	58.7
Gene transfer efficiency (%)	34.5	61.8	60.0

Examination of the anti-viral efficacy of MazF-Tmac cells harvested from monkey

In order to examine whether the Tat-dependent expression of MazF and anti-viral efficacy was maintained in the MazF-Tmac cells after infusion, CD4+ T lymphoid cells from a CD4T-1-transplanted monkey (214 days post-infusion of MazF-Tmac cells) were selected and expanded *ex vivo* (Figure 4A). After 7 days of expansion, the genetically modified cells expressing a truncated form of the human low affinity nerve growth factor (ΔLNGFR+) were concentrated with an anti-CD271 monoclonal antibody (Figure 4B). CD271-positive cells and CD271-negative cells were expanded for an additional 4 days. Both groups of expanded cells were infected with SHIV 89.6P [11] at the multiplicity of infection (MOI) of 0.01. Culture supernatants and cell pellets were analyzed at 6 days post-infection. As shown in Figure 4C, the replication of SHIV 89.6P was significantly suppressed in CD271-positive cells

Table 2. Cell surface markers of expanded MazF-Tmac cells.

	CD4T-1	CD4T-2	CD4T-3
CD3(+)/CD4(+) (%)	98.2	98.7	99.9
CD95(−)/CD28(+) (Naïve) (%)	0.7	1.2	0.4
CD95(+)/CD28(+) (CM) (%)	93.0	94.7	91.2
CD95(+)/CD28(−) (EM) (%)	6.2	3.9	8.3
CXCR4 (%)	N/A	92.0	79.4
CD25 (%)	N/A	30.4	24.5

CM: Central Memory, EM: Effector Memory.

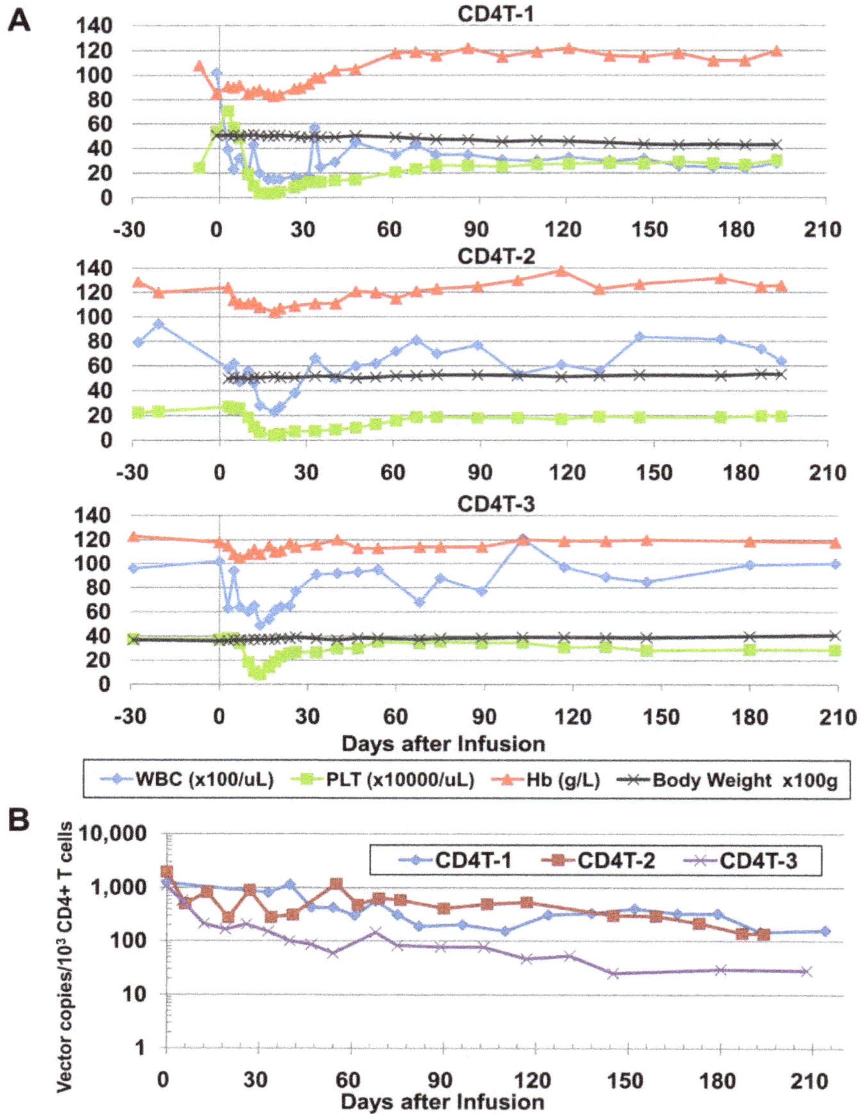

Figure 2. Hematological analysis and engraftment of the MazF-transduced CD4+ T cells. (A) The body weight and several hematological features were measured at the indicated time points, and the number of WBC, Hb, and PLT were represented. Each macaque was monitored throughout the study period. (B) The *in vivo* persistence of retroviral-transduced CD4+ T cells in the peripheral blood. PBMCs were collected at the indicated time points. The percentage of CD4+ T cells was analyzed using flow cytometry, and the proviral MazF vector copy was analyzed using real-time PCR. By compounding these two data, the copy number of the *mazF* gene in CD4+ T cells was calculated.

in comparison with CD271-negative cells. Although western blot analysis managed to detect the expression of MazF, MazF was below the detection limit (data not shown). However, the expression of MazF was clearly induced when the same CD271-positive cells were transduced with the Tat expression retroviral vector M-LTR-Tat-ZG [6] (Figure 4D). These data suggest that the conditional expression system in MazF-Tmac cells is still active at 6 months post-transplantation.

Distribution of MazF-Tmac cells

To examine the distribution and persistence of the infused MazF-Tmac cells in a monkey, lymphocytes isolated from several organs were analyzed using flow cytometry and real-time PCR. As shown in Figure 5A and 5B, ΔLNGFR+ cells were detected in CD4+ T cells isolated from several lymph nodes (LNs), spleen, and peripheral blood. A similar tendency was obtained using real-time PCR (Figure 5C). In contrast, MazF-Tmac cells were not detected in the bone marrow, liver, thymus, and small intestine (data not shown). These data strongly suggest that infused MazF-Tmac cells mainly circulate in the secondary lymphoid organs.

In vivo distribution of MazF-Tmac cells treated with or without retinoic acid

Based on the findings that MazF-Tmac cells were well distributed among secondary lymphoid organs but not in small intestine, we performed additional experiment using one cynomolgus monkey (CD4T-4). In order to investigate the editing effect of the homing receptor to efficiently recruit the gene-modified cells to intestinal tissues in a non-human primate model, the distribution of retinoic acid-treated MazF-Tmac cells was

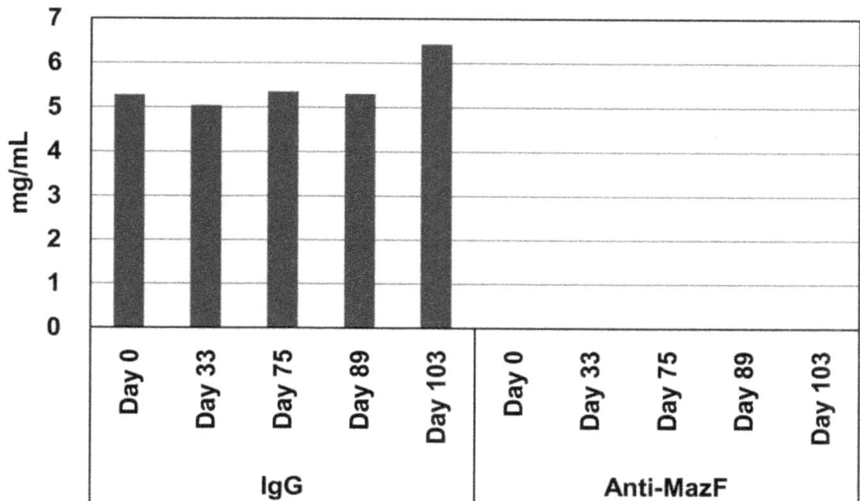

Figure 3. No detection of anti-MazF antibodies in monkey blood after transplantation of MazF-Tmac cells. Plasma samples were isolated from the monkey CD4T-2 at day 0, 33, 75, and 103 after transplantation and were used to detect anti-MazF antibodies on a MazF protein-immobilized microplate. The plasma samples were diluted to 500,000-fold, 50,000-fold, and 10,000-fold and added to each well. After the incubation, antibodies which reacted with immobilized MazF were tried to detect as described in Materials and Methods. No MazF-specific antibodies were detected.

examined in a cynomolgus macaque. The experimental procedure is described in Figure 6A. Non-treated and retinoic acid-treated MazF-Tmac cells were designated as MazF-Tmac-N and MazF-Tmac-R, respectively. Expressions of integrin-α4 and integrin-β7 were remarkably increased in the presence of retinoic acid (Figure 6B). Thereafter, MazF-Tmac-N and MazF-Tmac-R were labeled with carboxyfluorescein diacetate succinimidyl ester (CFSE) and PKH26, respectively. The CFSE-labeled cells were mixed with an equal number of PKH26-labeled cells (Figure 6C), and 6.8×10^8 of the mixed cells were infused into a CD4T-4 monkey. Note that the transduction efficiency of the MazF vector was 65% (data not shown). Three days after the transplantation, experimental autopsy was performed to obtain samples of several organs as described in the Materials and Methods. Both the CFSE- and the PKH26-labeled CD4+ T cells were detected in the peripheral blood and several LNs by FACS analysis (Figure 6D). The percentage of the infused cells in the LNs was low compared to the peripheral blood, indicating that a large number of the infused cells did not migrate to the secondary lymphoid tissues and circulated in the peripheral blood at this time point. In the case of the inguinal and axillary LNs, the percentage of MazF-Tmac-R cells was low compared to MazF-Tmac-N cells. In contrast, a higher percentage of MazF-Tmac-R cells was observed in the mesenteric LN compared to MazF-Tmac-N cells. MazF-Tmac-N cells were evenly distributed in the three LNs analyzed, while the MazF-Tmac-R cells seemed to be preferentially distributed in the mesenteric LNs. Moreover, a large number of MazF-Tmac-R cells were distributed in the small intestine, while MazF-Tmac-N cells were not. To further evaluate the homing effect of the MazF-Tmac cells, the distribution of the labeled-MazF-Tmac cells in cryopreserved organs was analyzed using fluorescence microscopy (Figure 6E). A number of the PKH26-labeled MazF-Tmac-R cells were observed in the mesenteric LNs and in Peyer's patches. Taken together, retinoic acid-treated MazF-Tmac cells seem to be selectively recruited to mesenteric LNs and then transported to Peyer's patches. The distribution of MazF-Tmac-R cells in the intestinal villi remains to be determined.

Table 3. Analysis of *in vivo* safety (Histological finding about autopsy sample).

	CD4T-1	CD4T-2	CD4T-3
Lymph node	±	±	−
Spleen	−	−	±
Bone marrow	++**	−	−
Thymus	N/A	+*	−
Small intestine	−	−	−
Liver	−	−	−
Kidney	−	±	−
Pancreas	−	−	−
Stomach	−	−	±
Lung	−	±	−
Heart	−	−	±

−: No remarkable changes; ±: Minimal; +: Mild; ++: Moderate.
N/A: No equivalent sample available.
*Due to the Aging,
**Side effect due to the busulfan administration.

Discussion

MazF is a toxin encoded by the *E. coli* genome and plays a role in growth regulation under stress conditions in *E. coli* [12]. MazF can act as an endoribonuclease (RNase) that specifically cleaves cellular mRNAs at ACA sequences [13]. Therefore, MazF induction in *E. coli* virtually eliminates almost all cellular mRNAs to completely inhibit protein synthesis. However, MazF-induced cells retain full capacity for protein synthesis, as MazF-induced cells are able to produce a protein at a high level if the prerequisite mRNA is engineered to be devoid of all ACA sequences without altering its amino acid sequence [14]. This indicates that RNA components involved in protein synthesis are protected from

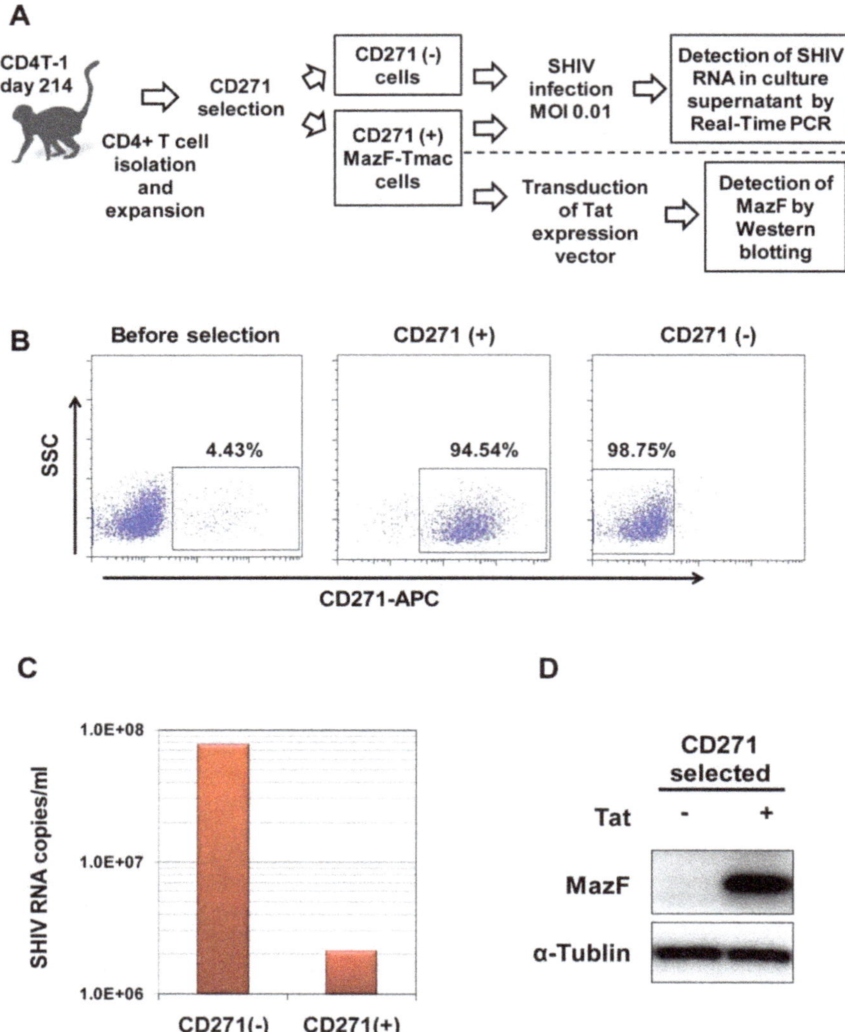

Figure 4. Examination of the anti-viral efficacy of MazF-Tmac cells harvested from the monkey. (A) Flow diagram of the experiment. CD4+ T lymphoid cells from CD4T-1 (214 days post-infusion of the MazF-Tmac cells) were stimulated and expanded *ex vivo*. The genetically modified cells expressing ΔLNGFR+ were concentrated with an anti-CD271 monoclonal antibody and expanded for 4 days. The expanded CD271-enriched cells and CD271-negative cells were infected with SHIV 89.6P. SHIV RNA levels in the culture supernatant were determined using quantitative real-time PCR. Expression of MazF was detected from the cell lysates by western blot analysis. Moreover, CD271-positive cells were transduced with the Tat expression vector. (B) CD271-positive and -negative cells were enriched using an anti-CD271 antibody, and dot plots of the flow cytometry analysis are presented. (C) The suppression of SHIV RNA in the culture supernatant at 6 days after infection was detected by real-time PCR analysis. (D) MazF-Tmac cells transduced with the Tat expression vector were harvested at 20 hours post-transduction and used for western blot analysis. Conditional expression of MazF in a Tat-dependent manner was observed.

MazF cleavage. Indeed, ribosomal RNAs (rRNAs) and transfer RNAs (tRNAs) are protected from MazF cleavage in *E. coli* [15].

RNase-based anti-HIV gene therapy is an attractive strategy to suppress HIV-1 RNA replication. In the case of MazF, there are more than 240 ACA sequences in HIV-1 RNA, suggesting that HIV has almost no chance to gain MazF-related escape mutations. This approach seems to have a substantial advantage over the other known antiviral strategies, including antiviral drug therapy, and RNA-based gene therapies, such as antisense RNA, ribozyme, and siRNA.

MazF overexpressed in mammalian cells preferentially cleaves messenger RNAs (mRNAs), but not ribosomal RNAs [16]. As HIV-1 RNA has more than 240 ACA sequences, we assumed that the viral RNA is highly susceptible to MazF, leading to inhibition of viral replication under a conditional expression system. Indeed, conditional expression of MazF with Tat suppresses replication of both HIV-1 IIIB and SHIV 89.6P without affecting cellular mRNAs, suggesting that this Tat-dependent expression system of MazF is an attractive payload for HIV gene therapy [6]. It is an intriguing phenomenon that viral RNAs are efficiently and preferentially cleaved without affecting cellular mRNAs, and we are now addressing this question. Meanwhile, MazF is a bacterial protein, and its expression is induced by Tat protein; thus, it is important to assess the safety and immunogenicity of *mazF* gene-modified cells *in vivo*. In order to determine the safety of our MazF-retrovirus system *in vivo*, we infused MazF-transduced CD4+ T cells into cynomolgus macaques. In human gene therapy trials, engraftment of 1–2% of genetically modified cells in the peripheral

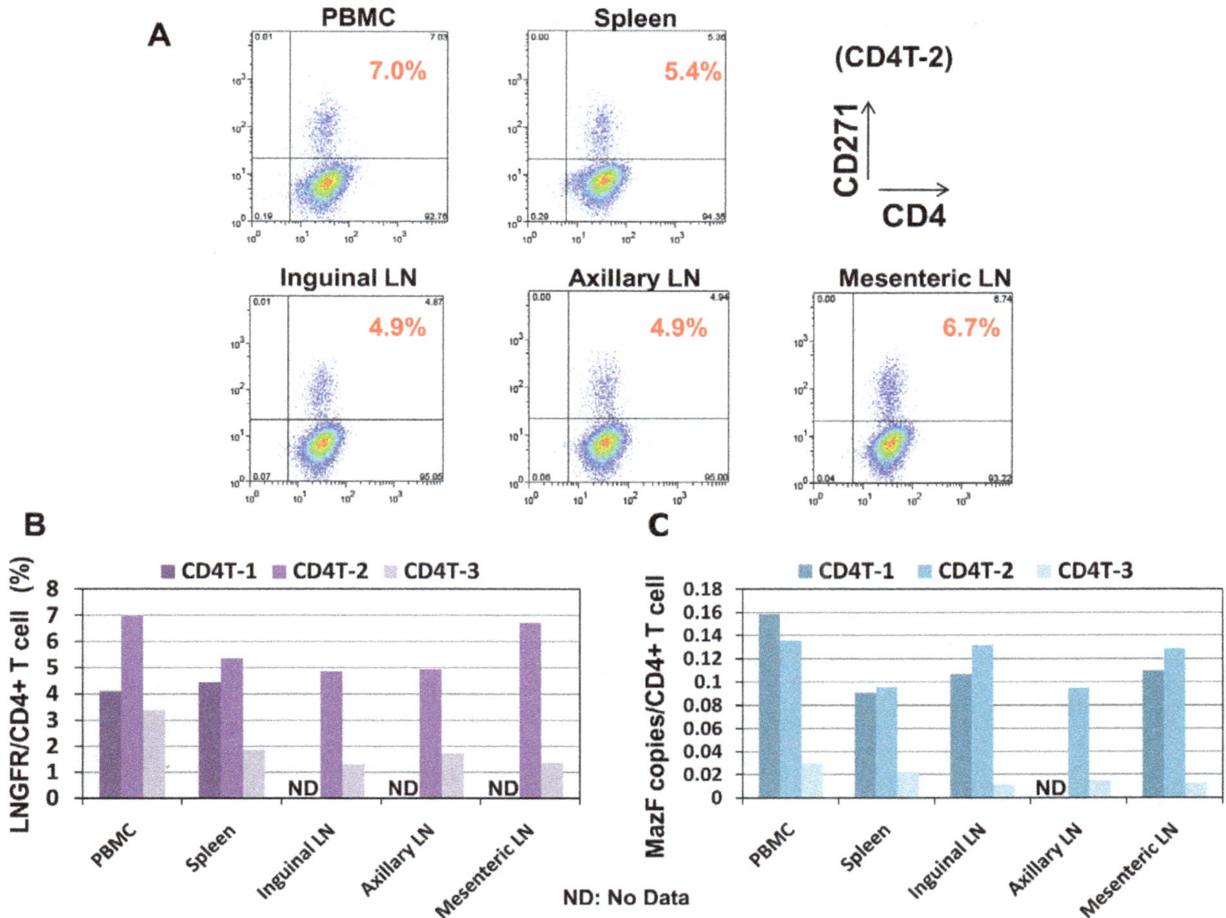

Figure 5. Analysis of the distribution of MazF-Tmac cells in several organs. (A) CD4+ T cells were isolated from lymphocytes separated from several organs, incubated 3–4 days, and stained with anti-CD4 and anti-CD271 antibodies. CD4T-2 is represented by a dot plot. (B) The percentage of CD271+ cells from three macaques is summarized. (C) The Copy number of the MazF gene in CD4+ T cells from each organ was calculated from real-time PCR and flow cytometric data.

circulation has been observed following infusions of about 10 billion cells [17], and higher cell doses results in higher levels of engraftment [18,19]. Infusions of lower than 5×10^9 cells do not reliably result in measurable engraftment levels [19]. Therefore, we decided to infuse more than one billion cells into cynomolgus macaques, reflecting one-tenth of the scale of the human model. Indeed, the *mazF* gene-modified cells were detected over a six month period at a high level, and no histopathological disorders and no MazF-specific antibody production was observed during the experiment, demonstrating that MazF-Tmac cells showed little or no immunogenicity to monkeys. Moreover, MazF-Tmac cells harvested from the CD4T-1-transplanted monkey 6 months post-infusion showed resistance to the replication of SHIV 89.6P, indicating that the long-term persistent MazF-Tmac cells are functional. The expression of MazF in the SHIV-infected MazF-Tmac cells was below the limit of detection due to a low MOI such as 0.01, while in the MazF-Tmac cells transduced with the Tat expression retroviral vector M-LTR-Tat-ZG at 45% efficiency, expression of MazF was clearly induced, indicating that Tat dependent MazF expression system was maintained in the cells even 6 months after the autologous transplantation.

Because gene therapy for HIV is aimed at reconstituting an HIV-resistant immune system, genetically modified cells must inhibit virus replication and maintain persistence *in vivo*. Although *ex vivo* gene therapy targeting CD4+ T cells or CD34+ hematopoietic stem cells has been shown to promote long term persistence of infused cells in peripheral blood in human, it is difficult to obtain information about the distribution pattern of these cells in the whole human body. In order to obtain such information, the monkeys were sacrificed and lymphocytes were isolated from several organs after 6 months of monitoring. Importantly, the infused MazF-Tmac cells were detected in secondary lymphoid tissue, such as several LNs and spleen, and in peripheral blood, although individual differences between CD4T-1, -2, and -3-transplanted monkeys were observed. No histopathological disorders were observed in the organs containing MazF-Tmac cells, indicating that there were no lesions relating to MazF-Tmac cells. The distribution of MazF-Tmac cells in the lymphoid tissues of CD4T-3-transplanted monkey was lower compared to the CD4T-1 and -2-transplanted monkeys. One reason for this phenomenon is likely the lower dosage of busulfan used to treat the CD4T-3-transplated monkey. Busulfan is an alkylating agent with potent effects on hematopoietic stem cells that is commonly used for stem cell transplantation. In rhesus macaques, a low-dose of busulfan has an impact on bone marrow stem/progenitor cells with transient and mild suppression of peripheral blood counts

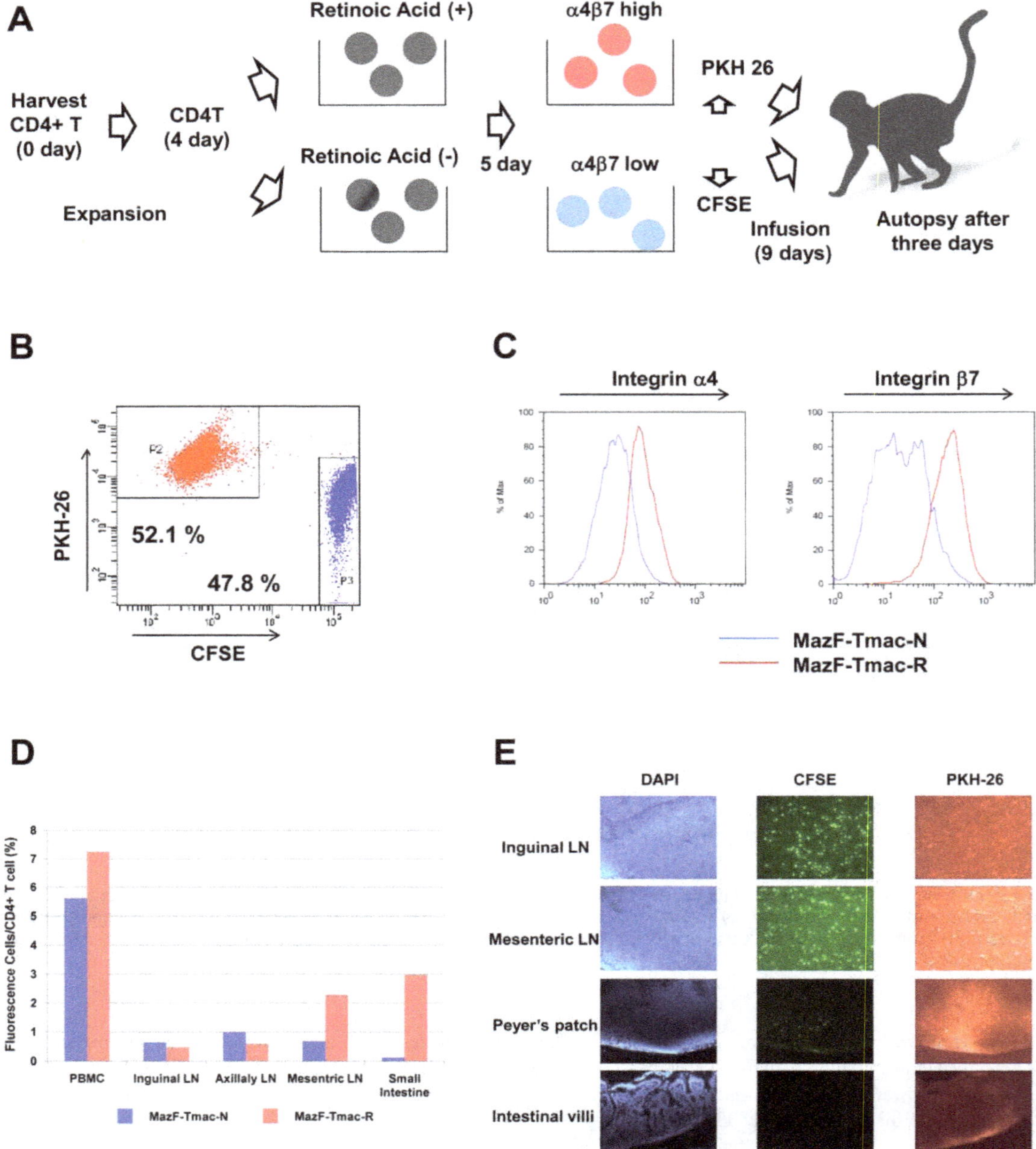

Figure 6. Comparison of the homing effect of MazF-Tmac cells treated with or without retinoic acid. (A) CD4+ T cells from the CD4T-4 monkey were stimulated with anti-CD3/CD28 beads, and MT-MFR-PL2 vector was transduced twice on days 3 and 4. After transduction, total lymphocytes were divided into two culture conditions in which retinoic acid was added to the one. After an additional 5 days of incubation, control and retinoic acid-treated cells were stained with CFSE and PKH26, respectively, mixed at nearly the same numbers, and infused into the autologous CD4T-4. Three days after the transplantation, experimental autopsy was performed. (B) A mixture of the two groups of MazF-Tmac cells stained with CFSE and PKH26 was analyzed using flow cytometry; the ratio of the two groups was almost same. (C) Up-regulation of the homing receptor was confirmed in the MazF-Tmac-R cells. The MazF-Tmac-N and MazF-Tmac-R cells are indicated by the blue line and red line, respectively. (D) Lymphocytes were collected from three lymph nodes (LNs) and small intestines, and a percentage of fluorescently-labeled cells were analyzed by flow cytometry. (E) Fluorescence microscope analysis of distal organ specimens.

[20]. Thus, the lower engraftment efficiency of CD4T-3 (MazF-Tmac) cells might be due to the milder busulfan treatment.

In contrast to the LNs and spleen, a limited number of cells were detected in non-lymphoid tissues such as small intestine and liver. Considering HIV-1 infection, the gastrointestinal (GI) tract, which contains the vast majority of lymphoid tissues in the total body to protect mucosal membranes from foreign antigens, is the dominant site of HIV replication rather than LNs, which were originally thought to be the main infection sites [21]. In GI tract, CD4+ T cells are dramatically decreased during the acute phase of HIV infection [21,22,23]. In rhesus macaques, a similar depletion was also reported during the acute phase of simian immunodeficiency virus (SIV) infection, with CD4+ memory T cells specifically targeted [24,25]. Notably, the rate of mucosal CD4+

T cell depletion in pathogenic SIV-infected monkeys correlates with the disease progression in the rhesus macaque [26]. Indeed, recent studies provide evidence that the depletion of mucosal CD4+ T cells leads to damage of the gut mucosal layer resulting in translocation of microbial products, such as lipopolysaccharide (LPS), ultimately causing chronic and systemic immune activation, which is one of the hallmarks of HIV/SIV infection and one of the predictors of disease progression [27,28]. Although HAART therapy is effective in controlling viral replication and recovering CD4+ T cells in the peripheral blood, restoration of CD4+ T cells is delayed in the GI tract [21,29]. Thus, the repair of depleted CD4+ T cells using gene therapy might attenuate the breakdown of the mucosal layer and prevent mucosal immune system deficiency. To change the tissue distribution of infused CD4+ T cells, the enhancement of homing receptor expression in T lymphocyte is necessary. Integrin $\alpha4\beta7$ is known to facilitate the migration of lymphocytes from gut-inductive sites where immune responses are first induced (Peyer's patches and mesenteric LNs) to the lamina propria [30,31]. Expression of the homing receptor is induced by the addition of retinoic acid [32], which is produced mainly from retinol (vitamin A) by dendritic cells in the mesenteric LNs. As shown in Figure 6D and 6E, although these are preliminary data with only one monkey, editing of the homing receptors integrin-$\alpha4$ and integrin-$\beta7$ by retinoic acid enhanced the recruitment of MazF-Tmac cells to the mesenteric LNs, small intestine, and Peyer's patches. These results may indicate that MazF-Tmac cells treated with retinoic acid selectively accumulate in the mesenteric LNs and then migrate into Peyer's patches. It has been reported that the HIV-1 envelope protein gp120 binds to and signals through the activated form of integrin $\alpha4\beta7$ [33]; however, we expect that retinoic acid-treated MazF-T cells will persist in distal organs without the additional spread of HIV replication because of the HIV-1 resistance observed in the MazF-Tmac cells. Therefore, we speculate that the combination of several culture methods to edit the homing receptor will enhance the recruitment of MazF-Tmac cells to distal lymphoid organs, resulting in a more efficient therapeutic.

In summary, we showed long-term persistence, safety and continuous HIV replication resistance in the *mazF* gene-modified CD4+ T cells in a non-human primate model *in vivo*, suggesting that autologous transplantation of *mazF* gene-modified cells is an attractive strategy for HIV gene therapy.

Materials and Methods

Vector design and viral production

The GALV-enveloped gamma retroviral vector MT-MFR-LP2 was generated as previously described [6]. MT-MFR-PL2 expresses a truncated form of the human low affinity nerve growth factor gene (ΔLNGFR) [34] under the control of a functional PGK promoter and the MazF gene under control of the HIV-LTR promoter (Figure 1A). The ΔLNGFR is a surface marker that allows identification of transduced cells.

Animals

Four cynomolgus macaques (*Macaca fascicularis*, 6–7 years old), CD4T-1, CD4T-2, CD4T-3, and CD4T-4, were used in this experiment and were maintained at the Tsukuba Primate Research Center for Medical Science at the National Institute of Biomedical Innovation (NIBIO, Ibaraki, Japan). The study was conducted according to the Rules for Animal Care and the Guiding Principles for Animal Experiments Using Nonhuman Primates formulated by the Primate Society of Japan [35] and in accordance with the recommendations of the Weatherall report, "The use of non-human primates in research". The protocols for the experimental procedures were approved by the Animal Welfare and Animal Care Committee of the National Institute of Biomedical Innovation (DS18-100). All surgical and invasive clinical procedures were conducted by trained personnel under the supervision of a veterinarian in a surgical facility using aseptic techniques and comprehensive physiologic monitoring. Ketamine hydrochloride (Ketalar, 10 mg/kg; Daiichi-Sankyo, Tokyo, Japan) was used to induce anesthesia for all clinical procedures associated with the study protocol such as blood sampling, gene-modified cell administration, clinical examinations and treatment.

Ex vivo expansion of CD4+ T cells, and transduction of the MazF vector

Peripheral blood from cynomolgus macaques was collected by apheresis as previously described [36]. For the dissolution of red blood lymphocytes, collected blood was treated with ACK lysing buffer (Lonza, Walkersville, MD) and was washed twice with phosphate buffered saline (PBS). Then, CD4+ T cells were isolated using anti-CD4 conjugated magnetic beads (Dynal CD4 Positive Isolation Kit, Invitrogen, Carlsbad, CA) according to the manufacturer's instructions. Isolated CD4+ T cells were cultured at 5×10^5 cells/ml in GT-T503 (Takara Bio, Otsu, Japan) supplemented with 10% FBS (Invitrogen), 200 IU recombinant human interleukin-2 (IL-2; Chiron, Emeryville, CA), 2 mM L-glutamine (Lonza), 2.5 µg/ml Fungizone (Bristol Myers-Squibb, Woerden, The Netherlands) and activated for three days with either 5 µg/ml concanavalin A (Con A, Sigma Chemical, St. Louis, MO) for CD4T-1 or a combination of anti-CD3 clone FN-18 (Biosource, Camarillo, CA, USA) and anti-CD28 clone L293 (BD Biosciences, Franklin Lakes, NJ) monoclonal antibodies conjugated to M-450 epoxy magnetic beads (Invitrogen) at cell-to-bead ratio of 1:1 (CD4T-2 and CD4T-3). On day 3, the activated CD4+ T cells were transduced with the MazF retroviral vector MT-MFR-PL2 in the presence of RetroNectin® (Takara Bio) according to manufacturer's instructions. Transduction was repeated on day 4. CD4+ T cells were further expanded to day 7 to 9 until the total cell number reach more than 10^9. The closed system MazF-Tmac cell manufacturing was performed using gas permeable culture bags; Cultilife 215 (Takara Bio) and Cultilife Eva (Takara Bio) were used for CD4+ T cells expansion and Cultilife spin (Takara Bio) was used for transduction of the MazF retroviral vector.

Transplantation of expanded CD4+ T cells

Prior to the transplantation, each macaque was treated with busulfan (Ohara Pharmaceutical, Shiga, Japan). Busulfan has been used extensively as a preparatory regimen for allogenic hematopoietic stem cell transplantation based on its toxicity to hematopoietic stem cells. Furthermore, it has been reported that in non-human primates, hematopoiesis was significantly decreased after a single, clinically well-tolerated dose of busulfan, with slow, but almost complete, recovery over the next several months [20]. The effects of busulfan on lymphocyte engraftment, however, are not well documented. Although cyclophosphamide is widely used in immune gene therapy trials in humans for lymphocyte transplantation, there is no information available for cyclophosphamides effect on T-cell transplantation in the cynomolgus macaque. It should be noted that we have chosen busulfan for our CD4+ T cell transplantation because busulfan is shown to cause a reduction in the peripheral blood count in human trial [37], we have had success in using busulfan for cynomolgus macaque bone marrow transplantation and according to internal information, busulfan causes a reduction of the peripheral blood count in cynomolgus macaques. Busulfan was orally administered to the macaques twice at 10 mg/kg each (CD4T-1 and CD4T-2) or 6 mg/kg each (CD4T-3) [38]. The expanded cells were harvested, washed three times with PBS, and re-suspended in PBS containing 10% autologous plasma. The collected cells were infused intravenously to monkeys at the speed of 1 ml per minute.

Flow cytometry analysis

The cell surface markers of the expanded cells and peripheral blood mononuclear cells (PBMC) were analyzed using FACSCalibur (BD Bioscience) and FACSCanto (BD Bioscience), and data analysis was performed using CellQuest software (BD Bioscience), FACSDiva software (BD Bioscience) or FlowJo software (Tree Star, Inc., Ashland, OR). The following antibodies were used for staining: anti-CD3 (SP34-2, PerCP), anti-CD4 (L200, FITC), anti-CD25 (2A3, FITC), anti-CD28 (CD28.2, PE), anti-CD95 (DX2, FITC), anti-CXCR4 (12G5, PE) and anti-integrin-β7 (FIB504, PE), which were obtained from BD Bioscience. The anti-CD49d (HP2/1, FITC) antibody was obtained from Beckman Coulter (Fullerton, CA), and the anti-CD271 (LNGFR, PE and APC) antibodies were obtained from Miltenyi Biotec GmbH (Bergisch Gladbach, Germany).

Measurement of hematological data

Two ml of blood was prepared every week. Blood samples were used to measure the white blood cell (WBC) count, red blood cell (RBC) count, hemoglobin (Hb) concentration, hematocrit values, mean corpuscular volume, mean cell hemoglobin concentration and platelet (PLT) count using a Sysmex K-4500 instrument (Toa-iyouddenshi, Kobe, Japan). The concentrations of the biochemical markers in blood samples were also monitored including total proteins, albumin, blood urea nitrogen, glucose, glutamic oxaloacetic transaminase, glutamic pyruvic transaminase, alkaline phosphatase, creatine phosphokinase, lactate dehydrogenase, creatine, sodium, potassium, chlorine and C-reactive protein using an AU400 instrument (Olympus Medical Systems, Tokyo, Japan).

Quantification of gene-modified CD4+ T cells

The existence and persistence of genetically modified CD4+ T cells were monitored by measuring the proviral genome of the transgene using quantitative real-time PCR. DNA samples were extracted from 2×10^6 PBMCs using a Gentra Puregene Blood Kit (QIAGEN, Hilden, Germany). The proviral copy number of the transgene was calculated from 400 ng of genomic DNA with quantitative PCR using a Cycleave RT-PCR Core Kit (Takara Bio) and Provirus Copy Number Detection Primer Set (Takara Bio) according to the manufacturer's instructions. The reaction was performed with the Thermal Cycler Dice Real Time System (Takara Bio), and the data was analyzed using Multiplate RQ software (Takara Bio). For each run, a standard curve was generated from the pMT-MFR-PL2 plasmid, whose copy numbers were already known. Based on the standard curve, the amount of infused cells was quantified.

Detection of anti-MazF antibodies in macaque blood after transplantation of MazF-Tmac cells

To examine whether anti-MazF antibodies can be generated after the transplantation of MazF-Tmac cells, the plasma isolated from the macaques was analyzed. In order to detect anti-MazF antibodies, purified MazF protein or anti-monkey IgG (Nordic Immunological Laboratories, Tilburg, The Netherlands) was pre-coated onto the wells of a 96-well microplate and subsequently blocked with PBS-1% BSA. The plasma samples were isolated from the CD4T-2 at day 0, 33, 75, and 103 after transplantation and were diluted to 500,000-fold, 50,000-fold, and 10,000-fold. Cynomolgus macaque IgG purified from normal macaque plasma with Melon Gel IgG purification Kit (Thermo Fisher Scientific, Rockford, IL, USA) was used as a control for this reaction. The two-fold serial dilutions of the IgG (1 ng/ml to 64 ng/ml) and the diluted plasma samples, as described above, were separately added to each well. After an overnight incubation at 4°C, the wells were washed with PBS-1% BSA. The POD-conjugated anti-monkey IgG (Nordic Immunological Laboratories) was then added to the wells. After 4 hours of incubation at room temperature, the wells were washed three times with PBS-1% BSA followed by the addition of the substrate solution (o-Phenylenediamine, Sigma). The optical density of each well was read at 490/650 nm using a 680XR microplate reader (Bio-Rad Laboratories, Hercules, CA) after stopping the reaction with H_2SO_4 stop solution (Figure S1).

Examination of the anti-viral efficacy of MazF-Tmac cells harvested from a monkey

To examine the function of the *mazF* gene in cells harvested from a MazF-Tmac-transplanted monkey, the frozen lymphoid cells from CD4T-1 at autopsy (214 days post-infusion of MazF-Tmac cells) were recovered, CD4+ T cells were selected using a CD4+ T Cell Isolation Kit (Miltenyi Biotec), stimulated with anti-CD3/CD28 beads at a cell-to-bead ration of 1:1, and expanded in GT-T503 medium supplemented with 10% FBS, 200 IU recombinant human interleukin-2, 2 mM L-glutamine, 2.5 µg/ml Fungizone, 100 units/ml penicillin, and 100 µg/ml streptomycin. After 7 days of expansion, the genetically modified cells expressing ΔLNGFR+ were concentrated with an anti-CD271 monoclonal antibody (CD271 MicroBeads, Miltenyi Biotec) and expanded for 4 days. The cells from the CD271-negative fraction were also harvested and expanded as control non-gene modified CD4+ T cells. The expanded CD271-enriched cells and CD271-negative cells were infected with SHIV 89.6P at the MOI of 0.01 and cultured for 6 more days. Culture supernatants and cell pellets were harvested at 6 days post-infection. RNA in the culture supernatant was recovered with the QIAamp Viral RNA Mini Kit (QIAGEN) and SHIV RNA levels in the culture supernatant were determined by quantitative real-time PCR with a set of specific primers specific for the SHIV *gag* region [39]. In order to detect the Tat-dependent expression of MazF in the CD271-enriched MazF-Tmac cells harvested from the monkey, the cells were transduced with the Tat expression retroviral vector M-LTR-Tat-ZG [6] in the presence of RetroNectin® as per the manufacturer's instruction. Twenty hours after Tat transduction, the cells were harvested, counted by trypan blue exclusion assay, washed twice with PBS, and 5×10^5 cells were suspended in 50 µl of 1× SDS sample buffer. The cell samples were incubated at 95°C for 10 min, and 5 µl of each cell sample was used for western blot analysis. For gel electrophoresis of proteins, the sample solutions described above were loaded into the wells of a 4–20% Tris-Glycine gel (Atto, Tokyo, Japan). After completion of electrophoresis, the gel was transferred to a polyvinylidene fluoride (PVDF) membrane (Millipore, Billerica, MA) with papers containing transfer buffer using the semi-dry method at 60 mA (constant voltage) for 60 min. The membrane was cut in half horizontally around the 20 kDa protein band of the pre-stained protein marker (Bio-Rad Laboratories). The upper part of the membrane was used to detect the α-tubulin (50 kDa) as an internal standard, while the lower part of the membrane was used to detect MazF (12 kDa). After blocking, the membranes were then incubated overnight at 4°C in the blocking buffer (5% skim milk in PBS) containing 1 μg/ml anti-α-tublin antibody (Cell Signaling Technology) and 1 μg/ml anti-MazF polyclonal antibody (rabbit, in-house preparation), respectively. Each membrane was washed three times and subsequently incubated at room temperature for 1 hour in 10 ml of the blocking buffer containing the 10,000-fold diluted goat anti-IgG rabbit antibody (peroxidase conjugated, Thermo Fisher Scientific). The membrane was washed five times by gentle shaking in the washing buffer at room temperature for 5 min. The membrane was soaked at room temperature for 5 min in substrate solution (SuperSignal West Femto Maximum Sensitivity Chemiluminescent Substrate, Thermo Scientific). Protein signals were detected by a CCD camera (LuminoShot 400 Jr, Takara Bio), which captures a digital image of the western blot.

Collection of lymphocyte from several organs

Several organs were collected following euthanasia of the monkeys. After thoracotomy, the right atrium was incised, and 2 L of heparinized PBS was infused into the left ventricle using an 18-gauge needle. After perfusion, several organs were collected, and lymphocytes were separated using the following method: samples of spleen, thymus, liver, bone marrow, and axillary, inguinal and mesenteric LNs were minced and filtered through a 40 μm nylon filter (BD Bioscience); lymphocyte of the small intestine were collected by the Percoll (GE Healthcare, Castle Hill, Australia) density-gradient centrifugation method as described previously [39]; and lymphocytes obtained from each organ were used for the flow cytometric analysis, and extracted DNA was used for quantification PCR.

In vivo homing analysis

CD4T-4 was used for homing analysis. Isolated CD4+ T cells were stimulated with anti-CD3/CD28 beads and cultured in GT-T503 medium supplemented with 10% FBS, 200 IU IL-2, 2 mM L-glutamine, and 2.5 μg/ml Fungizone. After 4 days of expansion, activated CD4+ T cells were divided into two culture bags (ClutiLife Eva), and 10 nM retinoic acid (Sigma) was added to one of the bags. After an additional 5 days of incubation, expanded cells with or without retinoic acid were harvested and labeled with 2 mM PKH26 (Sigma) or 5 μM CFSE (Sigma), respectively, according to the manufacturer's instructions. Thereafter, the cells were washed three times with PBS, mixed in PBS containing 10% autologous plasma and infused into the macaque. Then, CD4T-4 was euthanized at 3 days after transplantation. Lymphocytes from several organs were collected as previously described, and the distributions of labeled lymphocytes were detected by flow cytometric analysis. The specimens from several organs were fixed in buffered formaldehyde and embedded in plastic. Serial sections were made using a diamond saw. The slides were then analyzed under a fluorescence microscope to detect the distribution of the expanded cells in the distal organ specimens.

Acknowledgments

The authors thank the staff of Tsukuba Primate Research Center and Corporation for Production and Research of Laboratory Primates for the kind care and expert handling of the animals. The authors also thank Dr. Keith A. Reimann of Harvard Medical School and Dr. Tomoyuki Miura of Kyoto University for providing the SHIV 89.6P. The authors are also grateful to Dr. Koich Inoue of Takara Bio Inc. for his critical reading of this manuscript and Tomomi Sakuraba of Takara Bio Inc. for conducting the quantitative PCR assay.

Author Contributions

Conceived and designed the experiments: HC NS YY KT JM IK. Performed the experiments: HC NS HT HS NA. Analyzed the data: HC NS HS NA. Contributed reagents/materials/analysis tools: NS HT HS NA. Wrote the paper: HC NS.

References

1. Panel on Antiretroviral Guidelines for Adults and Adolescents. Guidelines for the use of antiretroviral agents in HIV-1-infected adults and adolescents. Department of Health and Human Services. December 1, 2009; 1–161. http://www.aidsinfo.nih.gov/ContentFiles/AdultandAdolescentGL.pdf. Accessed September 16, 2010.
2. Sarver N, Rossi J (1993) Gene therapy: a bold direction for HIV-1 treatment. AIDS Res Hum Retroviruses 9: 483–487.
3. Dropulic B, Jeang KT (1994) Gene therapy for human immunodeficiency virus infection: genetic antiviral strategies and targets for intervention. Hum Gene Ther 5: 927–939.
4. Dropulic B, June CH (2006) Gene-based immunotherapy for human immunodeficiency virus infection and acquired immunodeficiency syndrome. Hum Gene Ther 17: 577–588.
5. Rossi JJ, June CH, Kohn DB (2007) Genetic therapies against HIV. Nat Biotechnol 25: 1444–1454.
6. Chono H, Matsumoto K, Tsuda H, Saito N, Lee K, et al. (2011) Acquisition of HIV-1 Resistance in T Lymphocytes Using an ACA-specific *E. coli* mRNA interferase. Hum Gene Ther 22: 1–9.
7. Onlamoon N, Hudson K, Bryan P, Mayne AE, Bonyhadi M, et al. (2006) Optimization of *in vitro* expansion of macaque CD4 T cells using anti-CD3 and co-stimulation for autotransfusion therapy. J Med Primatol 35: 178–193.
8. Onlamoon N, Plagman N, Rogers KA, Mayne AE, Bostik P, et al. (2007) Anti-CD3/28 mediated expansion of macaque CD4+ T cells is polyclonal and provides extended survival after adoptive transfer. J Med Primatol 36: 206–218.
9. Pitcher CJ, Hagen SI, Walker JM, Lum R, Mitchell BL, et al. (2002) Development and homeostasis of T cell memory in rhesus macaque. J Immunol 168: 29–43.
10. Klebanoff CA, Gattinoni L, Torabi-Parizi P, Kerstann K, Cardones AR, et al. (2005) Central memory self/tumor-reactive CD8+ T cells confer superior antitumor immunity compared with effector memory T cells. Proc Natl Acad Sci U S A 102: 9571–9576.
11. Reimann KA, Li JT, Voss G, Lekutis C, Tenner-Racz K, et al. (1996) An env gene derived from a primary human immunodeficiency virus type 1 isolate confers high in vivo replicative capacity to a chimeric simian/human immunodeficiency virus in rhesus monkeys. J Virol 70: 3198–3206.
12. Engelberg-Kulka H, Hazan R, Amitai S (2005) *mazEF*: a chromosomal toxin-antitoxin module that triggers programmed cell death in bacteria. J Cell Sci 118: 4327–4332.
13. Zhang Y, Zhang J, Hoeflich KP, Ikura M, Qing G, et al. (2003) MazF cleaves cellular mRNAs specifically at ACA to block protein synthesis in *Escherichia coli*. Mol Cell 12: 913–923.
14. Suzuki M, Zhang J, Liu M, Woychik NA, Inouye M (2005) Single protein production in living cells facilitated by an mRNA interferase. Mol Cell 18: 253–261.
15. Baik S, Inoue K, Ouyang M, Inouye M (2009) Significant bias against the ACA triplet in the tmRNA sequence of *Escherichia coli* K-12. J Bacteriol 191: 6157–6166.
16. Shimazu T, Degenhardt K, Nur-E-Kamal A, Zhang J, Yoshida T, et al. (2007) NBK/BIK antagonizes MCL-1 and BCL-XL and activates BAK-mediated apoptosis in response to protein synthesis inhibition. Genes Dev 21: 929–941.
17. Levine BL, Humeau LM, Boyer J, MacGregor RR, Rebello T, et al. (2006) Gene transfer in humans using a conditionally replicating lentiviral vector. Proc Natl Acad Sci U S A 103: 17372–17377.
18. Ranga U, Woffendin C, Verma S, Xu L, June CH, et al. (1998) Enhanced T cell engraftment after retroviral delivery of an antiviral gene in HIV-infected individuals. Proc Natl Acad Sci U S A 95: 1201–1206.

19. van Lunzen J, Glaunsinger T, Stahmer I, von Baehr V, Baum C, et al. (2007) Transfer of autologous gene-modified T cells in HIV-infected patients with advanced immunodeficiency and drug-resistant virus. Mol Ther 15: 1024–1033.
20. Kuramoto K, Follman D, Hematti P, Sellers S, Laukkanen MO, et al. (2004) The impact of low-dose busulfan on clonal dynamics in nonhuman primates. Blood 104: 1273–1280.
21. Brenchley JM, Schacker TW, Ruff LE, Price DA, Taylor JH, et al. (2004) CD4+ T cell depletion during all stages of HIV disease occurs predominantly in the gastrointestinal tract. J Exp Med 200: 749–759.
22. Guadalupe M, Reay E, Sankaran S, Prindiville T, Flamm J, et al. (2003) Severe CD4+ T-cell depletion in gut lymphoid tissue during primary human immunodeficiency virus type 1 infection and substantial delay in restoration following highly active antiretroviral therapy. J Virol 77: 11708–11717.
23. Mehandru S, Poles MA, Tenner-Racz K, Horowitz A, Hurley A, et al. (2004) Primary HIV-1 infection is associated with preferential depletion of CD4+ T lymphocytes from effector sites in the gastrointestinal tract. J Exp Med 200: 761–770.
24. Mattapallil JJ, Douek DC, Hill B, Nishimura Y, Martin M, et al. (2005) Massive infection and loss of memory CD4+ T cells in multiple tissues during acute SIV infection. Nature 434: 1093–1097.
25. Li Q, Duan L, Estes JD, Ma ZM, Rourke T, et al. (2005) Peak SIV replication in resting memory CD4+ T cells depletes gut lamina propria CD4+ T cells. Nature 434: 1148–1152.
26. Picker LJ, Hagen SI, Lum R, Reed-Inderbitzin EF, Daly LM, et al. (2004) Insufficient production and tissue delivery of CD4+ memory T cells in rapidly progressive simian immunodeficiency virus infection. J Exp Med 200: 1299–314.
27. Brenchley JM, Price DA, Schacker TW, Asher TE, Silvestri G, et al. (2006) Microbial translocation is a cause of systemic immune activation in chronic HIV infection. Nat Med 12: 1365–1371.
28. Estes JD, Harris LD, Klatt NR, Tabb B, Pittaluga S, et al. (2010) Damaged intestinal epithelial integrity linked to microbial translocation in pathogenic simian immunodeficiency virus infections. PLoS Pathog 2010 Aug 19;6(8). pii: e1001052. PubMed PMID: 20808901.
29. Guadalupe M, Sankaran S, George MD, Reay E, Verhoeven D, et al. (2006) Viral suppression and immune restoration in the gastrointestinal mucosa of human immunodeficiency virus type 1-infected patients initiating therapy during primary or chronic infection. J Virol 80: 8236–8247.
30. von Andrian UH, Mackay CR (2000) T-cell function and migration. Two sides of the same coin. N Engl J Med 343: 1020–1034.
31. Wagner N, Löhler J, Kunkel EJ, Ley K, Leung E, et al. (1996) Critical role for beta7 integrins in formation of the gut-associated lymphoid tissue. Nature 382: 366–370.
32. Iwata M, Hirakiyama A, Eshima Y, Kagechika H, Kato C, et al. (2004) Retinoic acid imprints gut-homing specificity on T cells. Immunity 21: 527–538.
33. Arthos J, Cicala C, Martinelli E, Macleod K, Van Ryk D, et al. (2008) HIV-1 envelope protein binds to and signals through integrin alpha4beta7, the gut mucosal homing receptor for peripheral T cells. Nat Immunol 9: 301–309.
34. Verzeletti S, Bonini C, Marktel S, Nobili N, Ciceri F, et al. (1998) Herpes simplex virus thymidine kinase gene transfer for controlled graft-versus-host disease and graft-versus-leukemia: clinical follow-up and improved new vectors. Hum Gene Ther 9: 2243–2251.
35. Primate Society of Japan (1986) Guiding principles for animal experiments using nonhuman primates. Primate Res 2: 111–113.
36. Ageyama N, Kimikawa M, Eguchi K, Ono F, Shibata H, et al. (2003) Modification of the leukapheresis procedure for use in rhesus monkeys (*Macaca mulata*). J Clin Apher 18: 26–31.
37. Laurent J, Speiser DE, Appay V, Touvrey C, Vicari M, et al. (2010) Impact of 3 different short-term chemotherapy regimens on lymphocyte-depletion and reconstitution in melanoma patients. J Immunother 33: 723–734.
38. Masuda S, Ageyama N, Shibata H, Obara Y, Ikeda T, et al. (2009) Cotransplantation with MSCs improves engraftment of HSCs after autologous intra-bone marrow transplantation in nonhuman primates. Exp Hematol 37: 1250–1257.
39. Miyake A, Ibuki K, Enose Y, Suzuki H, Horiuchi R, et al. (2006) Rapid dissemination of a pathogenic simian/human immunodeficiency virus to systemic organs and active replication in lymphoid tissues following intrarectal infection. J Gen Virol 87: 1311–1320.

6

Impact of Hydrodynamic Injection and phiC31 Integrase on Tumor Latency in a Mouse Model of MYC-Induced Hepatocellular Carcinoma

Lauren E. Woodard[1], Annahita Keravala[1], W. Edward Jung[1], Orly L. Wapinski[1], Qiwei Yang[2], Dean W. Felsher[2], Michele P. Calos[1]*

1 Department of Genetics, Stanford University School of Medicine, Stanford, California, United States of America, **2** Division of Oncology, Department of Medicine, Stanford University School of Medicine, Stanford, California, United States of America

Abstract

Background: Hydrodynamic injection is an effective method for DNA delivery in mouse liver and is being translated to larger animals for possible clinical use. Similarly, φC31 integrase has proven effective in mediating long-term gene therapy in mice when delivered by hydrodynamic injection and is being considered for clinical gene therapy applications. However, chromosomal aberrations have been associated with φC31 integrase expression in tissue culture, leading to questions about safety.

Methodology/Principal Findings: To study whether hydrodynamic delivery alone, or in conjunction with delivery of φC31 integrase for long-term transgene expression, could facilitate tumor formation, we used a transgenic mouse model in which sustained induction of the human *C-MYC* oncogene in the liver was followed by hydrodynamic injection. Without injection, mice had a median tumor latency of 154 days. With hydrodynamic injection of saline alone, the median tumor latency was significantly reduced, to 105 days. The median tumor latency was similar, 106 days, when a luciferase donor plasmid and backbone plasmid without integrase were administered. In contrast, when active or inactive φC31 integrase and donor plasmid were supplied to the mouse liver, the median tumor latency was 153 days, similar to mice receiving no injection.

Conclusions/Significance: Our data suggest that φC31 integrase does not facilitate tumor formation in this *C-MYC* transgenic mouse model. However, in groups lacking φC31 integrase, hydrodynamic injection appeared to contribute to *C-MYC*-induced hepatocellular carcinoma in adult mice. Although it remains to be seen to what extent these findings may be extrapolated to catheter-mediated hydrodynamic delivery in larger species, they suggest that caution should be used during translation of hydrodynamic injection to clinical applications.

Editor: John E. Tavis, Saint Louis University, United States of America

Funding: PHS Grant Number CA09302, awarded by the National Cancer Institute, DHHS, www.cancer.gov. Amgen Scholars Program through the Stanford Summer Research Program, www.amgenscholars.eu. NIH grant HL068112 to MPC, www.nih.gov. NIH grants CA89305-01A1 and CA034233 to DWF, www.nih.gov. The funders had no role in study design, data collection and analysis, decision to publish, or preparation of the manuscript.

Competing Interests: Michele Calos is an inventor on Stanford-owned patents covering phiC31 integrase and co-founder of Poetic Genetics, a company that has licensed the use of phiC31 integrase for gene therapy purposes.

* E-mail: calos@stanford.edu

Introduction

Hydrodynamic injection of plasmid DNA involves a rapid, high-volume injection of DNA into the tail vein of mice [1,2]. This method can provide delivery of DNA to as many as 40% of hepatocytes and has been widely adopted for delivery of nucleic acids to mouse liver. In addition, catheter-mediated adaptations of the method have been developed for DNA delivery in larger animals, opening the possibility of clinical use for gene therapy [3]. Several groups have reported successful gene delivery to the pig liver [4–7], and a Phase I clinical trial has been conducted in thrombocytopenia patients [6].

Use of φC31 integrase in conjunction with hydrodynamic delivery offers a strategy to make gene delivery in hepatocytes permanent, by bringing about covalent integration of the plasmid DNA into the chromosomes [8,9]. φC31 integrase is a large serine recombinase that is capable of integrating *attB*-containing donor plasmids into pseudo *attP* sites that occur endogenously in mammalian chromosomes [10]. Because its mechanism of integration requires DNA sequence recognition, φC31 integrase has a more restricted integration profile than other integrating vectors such as retroviruses and transposons [11]. The more limited number of potential integration sites may make φC31 integrase less likely to activate an oncogene or disrupt a tumor suppressor gene.

Both hydrodynamic injection and φC31 integrase are relatively new technologies that have not yet been rigorously tested for their potential tumorigenicity. To date, hydrodynamic delivery has not been associated with increased cancer risk. Similarly, φC31 integrase has been used in many pre-clinical gene therapy studies over the years, involving hundreds of animals, without evidence of cancer incidence [10]. In a recent study, φC31-modified human cord-lining epithelial cells failed to form tumors in SCID mice [12]. The same study also analyzed microarray data and found that three tumor suppressor gene transcripts were upregulated in φC31-modified cells [12]. Nevertheless, after prolonged expression of φC31 integrase in cultured cells, chromosomal rearrangements were found by both plasmid rescue and karyotyping [11,13–15]. If such aberrations occurred *in vivo*, they could increase cancer risk by contributing to genomic instability. Therefore, it was of interest to analyze with greater sensitivity whether exposure to hydrodynamic injection or φC31 integrase could stimulate tumorigenesis in an appropriate animal model.

In studies not designed to evaluate cancer risk, cancers have appeared after injection of viral gene therapy vectors *in utero* or in neonatal mice [16,17]. By contrast, in this study we specifically tested whether hydrodynamic injection and/or φC31 integrase were capable of contributing to MYC-induced tumorigenesis in adult mice in a previously validated animal model. This approach is similar to studies that have investigated the potential contribution of various gene therapy vectors to blood cancer formation, which occurred during a clinical trial that employed retroviral vectors to treat children with X-linked severe combined immunodeficiency [18–20]. Small molecule carcinogens, shRNA, and partial hepatectomy have all been demonstrated in separate studies to contribute to MYC-induced hepatocellular carcinoma using the same model and similar methods to those used in this study [21–23].

Mice transgenic for both *TRE-MYC* [24] and *LAP-tTA* [25] have been developed as a mouse model for hepatocellular carcinoma in which the human C-MYC transcription factor is expressed in the liver when doxycycline is absent [26]. In this mouse model, the tumor latency is long enough that subtle oncogenic perturbations would be detectable, yet short enough to be experimentally tractable [23]. *C-MYC* is genomically amplified in up to 50% of human liver tumors, and this amplification can result in C-MYC overexpression [27,28]. The C-MYC transcription factor plays a key role in development by inducing genes that control cell division, growth, and apoptosis [29]. When disregulated in blood cancers, C-MYC has been shown to contribute to the formation of double-strand breaks [30]. Hepatocellular carcinomas initiated in this model were found to regress when C-MYC expression was terminated [26,31]. We asked whether hydrodynamic delivery, either with or without φC31 integrase, might cooperate with C-MYC to accelerate tumor formation in this mouse model.

Materials and Methods

Ethics Statement

The Stanford Administrative Panel on Laboratory Animal Care approved all procedures performed on animals in protocol number 9477, assurance number A3213-01. The Stanford Comparative Medicine program is accredited by the Association for Accreditation and Assessment of Laboratory Animal Care International.

Plasmids

pCS, pCSmI, and pCSI have been described previously [32,33]. Briefly, these plasmids carry ampicillin resistance and contain a CMV promoter and SV40 poly-A tail (pCS), between which either mutant S20F (pCSmI) or wild-type (pCSI) φC31 integrase was cloned. pLiLucB is a liver-specific, luciferase-expressing *attB* donor plasmid that was constructed by digesting pNBL2 [34] with *XhoI* to remove the CMV promoter and digesting pVFB [35] with *EcoRI* to obtain the human alpha-1 antitrypsin promoter with an apolipoprotein enhancer. The ends of both fragments were made blunt by filling in with Klenow polymerase, and the pNBL2 backbone was treated with phosphatase. The construct was ligated using T4 ligase and checked by *XcmI* digestion and sequencing of the promoter region.

Mouse experiments

Genotyped *LAP-tTA* homozygous females were bred to genotyped *TRE-MYC* males (the *TRE-MYC* transgene is on the Y chromosome) to give male mice having one copy of each gene. All mice were on the FVB/N strain background. A solution of doxycycline hyclate (Sigma-Aldrich, St. Louis, MO) was given as drinking water at a concentration of 100 μg/ml from one week before mating cages were set up until after weaning at 7–8 weeks of age. Autoclaved paper tubes were placed in mouse cages to prevent fighting. Mice were randomly assigned to groups in random order. Each experimental group consisted of mice from between 3–8 separate litters. Hydrodynamic injections were carried out as previously described [36] using a heat lamp for tail vein dilation, with the exception that sterile phosphate-buffered saline #20012 (Invitrogen, Carlsbad, CA) was used to dilute the DNA. Live animal imaging was done on the IVIS 200 machine (Caliper Life Sciences, Alameda, CA). Animals in groups given luciferase were imaged on one of eight separate imaging schedules, consisting of between 1–3 experimental groups per imaging schedule. The mice were imaged at Day 1, Week 1, 2, 4, 6, 8, 10, 12, 14, 17, 20, etc. until sacrifice. Mice were monitored weekly for abdominal swelling and/or other signs of distress and sacrificed when it was believed that they would not survive another week. After dissection, portions of the normal liver, liver tumors, and metastatic tumors (if present) were fixed for histology as previously described [36], and snap frozen in a dry ice/isopropanol bath for subsequent genomic DNA and protein analysis.

Luciferase assay

Protein was prepared from tissue samples using the lysis buffer previously described [35] and homogenized with a Kontes pellet pestle motor (VWR, Batavia, IL). Protein prepared from transfected HeLa cells (ATCC, Manassas, VA), producing luciferase from the pNBL2 plasmid after FuGene 6 (Roche, Indianapolis, IN) transfection, was used as the positive control. Protein concentrations were determined by the Bradford method with Protein Assay Reagent (Biorad, Hercules, CA). 15 μg of protein were added per well. The luciferase assay kit procedure was run in quadruplicate on a 96-well plate reader according to the manufacturer's instructions (Promega, Madison, WI).

PCR analysis

Total DNA was prepared from normal-appearing liver and tumor samples using the DNeasy Blood and Tissue Kit according to the manufacturer's directions, including the optional addition of RNase (Qiagen, Valencia, CA). DNA concentrations were measured using the Nanodrop (Thermo Scientific, Wilmington, DE). 200 ng of DNA was added to each PCR reaction, prepared according to manufacturer's directions using illustra puReTaq Ready-To-Go PCR beads (GE Healthcare, Piscataway, NJ). To detect the luciferase-bearing plasmid pLiLucB in the genomic DNA, the forward primer 5′GACCGTGACCTACATCGTC and the reverse primer 5′-CATGTCTGCTCGAAGCGGC were used to amplify the luciferase gene. The template used for the second round in the nested mpsL1 PCR was 1 μl of a 1:10 dilution of the first round PCR reaction. Primers to detect integration at mpsL1 and to detect GAPDH have been previously described [37]. The reactions were carried out at least twice for all samples.

Results

In our previous studies, dozens of wild-type mice have received hydrodynamic injections, with or without integrase [8,35,36,38]. Of these mice, as well as many more mice treated similarly in lab studies that have not been published, no liver tumors have ever been observed. Therefore, for greater sensitivity, a mouse model was used in which all mice would develop tumors. Different groups were tracked to provide survival times that could be compared statistically to determine if the treatments had an effect on the length of time between induction of *C-MYC* expression in the liver and sacrifice due to tumor burden, a time frame defined in this study as "tumor latency." We hypothesized that since φC31 integrase is associated with chromosomal aberrations in tissue culture, its expression might decrease tumor latency in these tumor-prone mice.

LAP-tTA/TRE-MYC double transgenic, male mice were given doxycycline drinking water from conception until 7–8 weeks of age to suppress C-MYC expression in the liver during development, which would have been lethal (**Fig. 1a**) [22]. Complete regulation of C-MYC expression by doxycycline was previously observed to

A

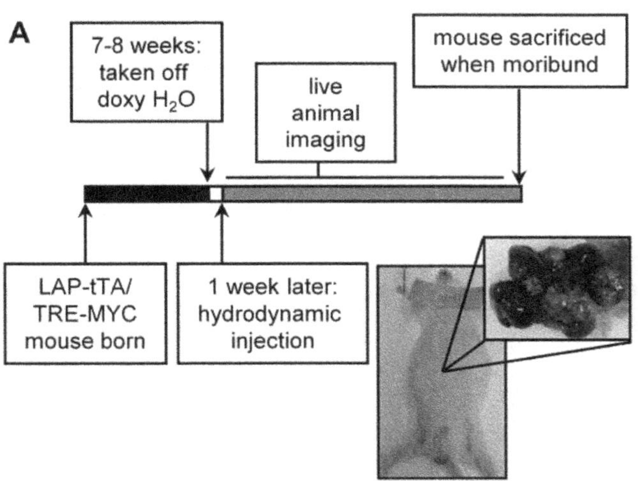

B

Plasmid	Promoter	Transgene
pLiLucB	hAAT/ApoE	luciferase
pCS	CMV	-
pCSmI	CMV	inactive ϕC31
pCSI	CMV	active ϕC31

Figure 1. Experimental design of tumorigenesis assay. (**a**) Transgenic mice were taken off of doxycycline drinking water at 7–8 weeks of age to induce expression of the human *C-MYC* transgene specifically in the liver from the LAP promoter, except for one control group (MYC off). Exactly one week after C-MYC induction, all groups except one control group (MYC on, no injection) were given hydrodynamic injections of phosphate-buffered saline alone or DNA plasmids diluted in phosphate-buffered saline. Mice were monitored weekly, imaged every two or three weeks, and sacrificed when tumors were detectable by gross distention of the abdomen as pictured. Inset shows the dissected liver and tumors from the pictured mouse, which was representative of all mice in all groups. (**b**) The plasmids given by hydrodynamic injection and their features.

have a time scale of four days [22,26]. Therefore, at one week after initiation of sustained C-MYC induction, a hydrodynamic injection [1,2] was administered containing no plasmid (saline only) or 20 μg each of a luciferase-expressing donor plasmid (pLiLucB) and plasmids containing vector backbone alone (pCS), expressing inactive integrase (pCSmI), or active wild-type integrase (pCSI) (**Fig. 1b**). One group was given the active integrase plasmid pCSI alone (20 μg). The DNA dose of 20 μg per plasmid has been used to confer therapeutic levels of hFIX using φC31 integrase in mice [9]. Two groups were not given hydrodynamic injection: one was given doxycycline drinking water for 7–8 weeks, and another was given doxycycline drinking water for one year. Mice that were injected with pLiLucB were imaged the next day to confirm high levels of luciferase expression in the liver, indicating a successful hydrodynamic injection. C-MYC induction preceded integrase expression because the integrase protein can only be detected by Western blot for up to one day after hydrodynamic injection [39].

Mice were monitored weekly for tumor formation. The animals were sacrificed when it was expected that they would not have survived another week, as indicated by swelling in the upper abdomen (**Fig. 1a**) or signs of morbidity. Most of the mice with extensive hepatocellular carcinoma appeared behaviorally normal until the point of sacrifice. At autopsy, mice were dissected, photographed, and examined for the presence of liver tumors. Most tumors were multifocal, presumably arising from different tumor-forming cells (**Fig. 1a**), as has been suggested previously [22,23,26]. No differences in gross type, number, size, mass or distribution of tumors were observed between groups. Imaging was done every 2–3 weeks to monitor whether luciferase expression was observed in locations outside of the liver, indicating a possible luciferase-positive metastasis. Although several cases of metastasis were observed upon dissection (**Table 1**), none were detectable by luciferase imaging.

The seven groups of mice were observed for tumor formation to distinguish the effects of C-MYC induction, hydrodynamic injection, DNA administration, φC31 integrase protein, and φC31 integrase activity (**Fig. 2a**). To make these effects easier to evaluate, we have separated the composite Kaplan-Meier survival curve (**Fig. 2g**) into several plots comparing these effects in a step-wise manner.

Hydrodynamic delivery significantly decreased tumor latency

The survival times of mice in the control groups are compared in Figure 2b. The animals that did not receive C-MYC induction or any injections (yellow) survived until the end of the study, 400

Table 1. Treatment group and number of days from initiation of C-MYC overexpression until sacrifice (survival time) for each case of metastasis.

Group	Number of metastasis	Survival time (days)
no injection	1	209
saline injection	0	
pCS/pLiLucB	0	
pCSmI/pLiLucB	3	111, 139, 329
pCSI/pLiLucB	1	258
pCSI alone	1	164

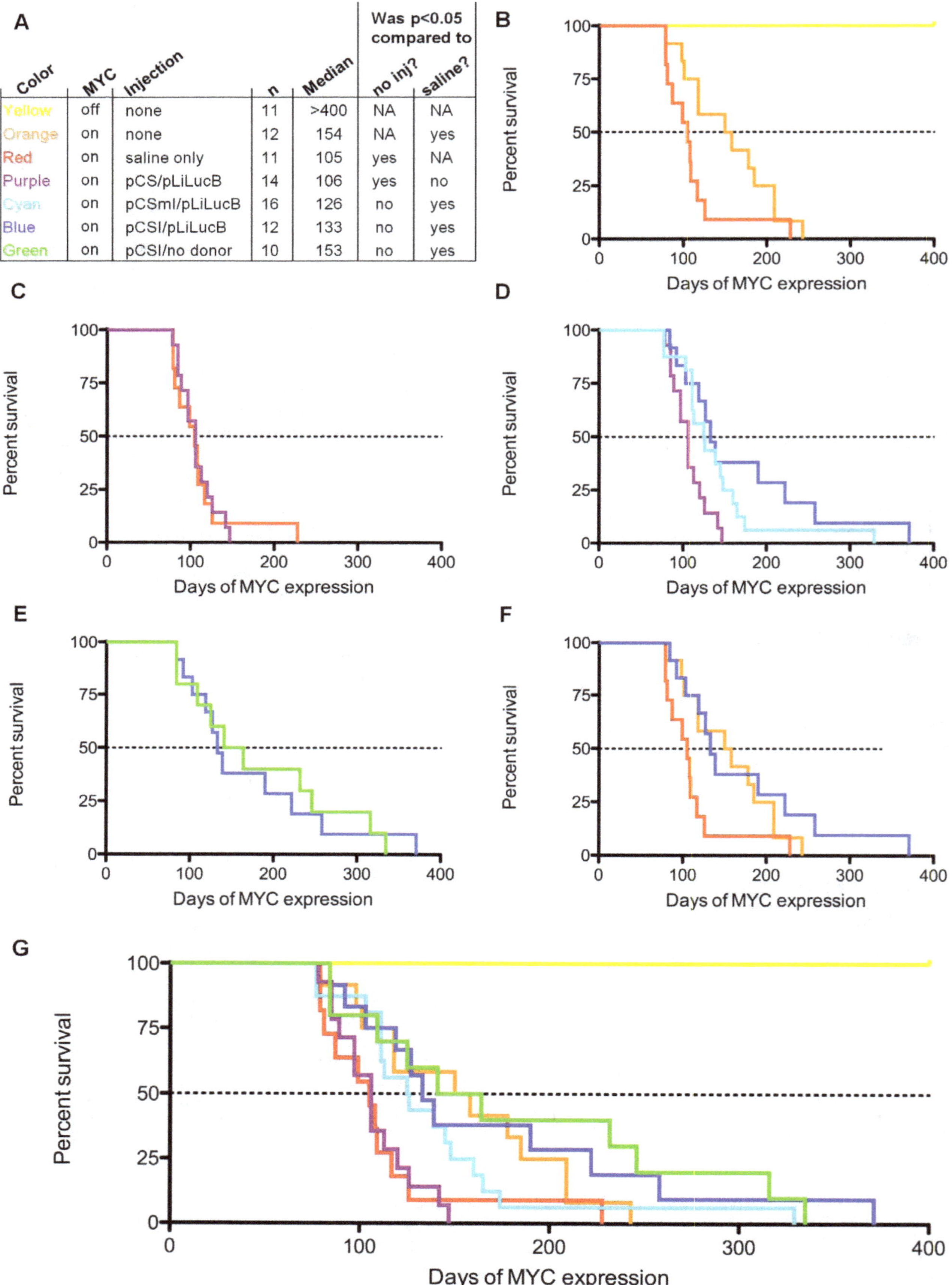

A

Color	MYC	Injection	n	Median	Was p<0.05 compared to no inj?	Was p<0.05 compared to saline?
Yellow	off	none	11	>400	NA	NA
Orange	on	none	12	154	NA	yes
Red	on	saline only	11	105	yes	NA
Purple	on	pCS/pLiLucB	14	106	yes	no
Cyan	on	pCSmI/pLiLucB	16	126	no	yes
Blue	on	pCSI/pLiLucB	12	133	no	yes
Green	on	pCSI/no donor	10	153	no	yes

Figure 2. Survival curves suggest that hydrodynamic injection may contribute to C-MYC-induced tumor formation in the mouse liver. (**a**) Key showing the number of animals (n), median survival time in days (Median), and statistical results for each group. The significance as determined by the Gehan-Breslow-Wilcoxon test comparing each group to the MYC on, no injection (no inj?) or MYC on, saline injection (saline?) control groups is given. (**b**) A comparison of MYC off, no injection (yellow), MYC on, no injection (orange), and MYC on, saline injection (red) survival curves. (**c**) A comparison of MYC on, saline injection and MYC on, pCS/pLiLucB (purple) injection survival curves. (**d**) A comparison of MYC on, pCS/pLiLucB, MYC on, pCSml/pLiLucB (cyan), and MYC on, pCSI/pLiLucB (blue) survival curves. (**e**) The survival curves of groups given pCSI with and without (green) donor plasmid. (**f**) A comparison of pCSI/pLiLucB to the control groups of no injection and saline-only injection. (**g**) The survival curves of all groups shown on the same plot. All plots and statistics were done using GraphPad Prism software.

days after 7–8 weeks of age. In contrast, induction of C-MYC expression in the liver beginning at adulthood (7–8 weeks) resulted in all of the mice being sacrificed prior to the end of the study with a median tumor latency of 154 days. These results confirmed that the *LAP-tTA/TRE-MYC* mouse model allowed for tight oncogene regulation.

Interestingly, in the group of mice that received a hydrodynamic injection of phosphate-buffered saline without any DNA present, the median tumor latency was only 105 days. There was one mouse that survived past 200 days that may have been an exception in some way, for example, by receiving an unsuccessful hydrodynamic injection. Similarly, a single long-surviving mouse was seen in other groups. To keep these outliers from having major effects on statistical significance, we chose the Gehan-Breslow-Wilcoxon statistical test to compare survival times, because this test gives less weight to later events. The group in which *C-MYC* was turned "on" and no treatment was given (orange) was statistically different than the group that had *C-MYC* "on" and received saline-only hydrodynamic injection (red; $p = 0.0359$), indicating that there was a significant decrease in tumor latency associated with the hydrodynamic delivery method.

DNA delivery, luciferase expression, and imaging did not affect tumor latency

To test the effect on tumor latency of DNA without the integrase gene, we gave the transgenic mice hydrodynamic injections containing 20 μg each of pCS and pLiLucB (**Fig. 1b**). Inclusion of this group was intended to control for both the integrase plasmid backbone elements as well as firefly luciferase expression and imaging every 2–3 weeks, which entailed injections of luciferin and anesthesia with isoflurane for a period of approximately 15 minutes. As shown in Figure 2c, the saline-only (red) and pCS/pLiLucB (purple) groups had nearly identical survival curves, except for one late survivor in the saline-only group. The pCS/pLiLucB group was statistically significantly different than the MYC "on", no injection group ($p = 0.014$), again implicating effects of the hydrodynamic injection.

Integrase expression resulted in similar tumor latency to that of untreated mice

To evaluate the effect of φC31 integrase protein expression independent of integration activity, we injected the plasmids pCSmI and pLiLucB (**Fig. 1b**) into a group of C-MYC expressing mice (**Fig. 2d**, cyan). The pCSmI plasmid has a S20F mutation in the catalytic serine, rendering the φC31 integrase made by this plasmid unable to recombine DNA. We observed a statistically significant increase in tumor latency when inactive integrase protein was present, compared to the saline-only group ($p = 0.045$). Again, note that we observed a very late surviving mouse in this group, which lived about twice as long as the second-longest surviving mouse in the group.

When the pCSI construct encoding active integrase (**Fig. 1b**) was administered with the pLiLucB donor plasmid (blue, **Fig. 2d**), the tumor latency also increased compared to the saline only group. According to the Gehan-Breslow-Wilcoxon test of statistical significance, the pCSmI/pLiLucB and pCSI/pLiLucB groups were not significantly different. To test if recombination of plasmid DNA was necessary for the observed survival benefit, we also administered 20 μg of pCSI without any *attB* donor plasmid (green) to a cohort of *TRE-MYC/LAP-tTA* mice. Presence of the *attB*-containing plasmid appeared to have no effect on survival (**Fig. 2e**).

To summarize, the *C-MYC* "on", pCSI/pLiLucB group was not statistically different than the *C-MYC* "on", no injection group (**Fig. 2f**), indicating that the presence of integrase appeared to counteract the tumor acceleration due to hydrodynamic injection. Hydrodynamic injection without integrase expression yielded a survival curve that was significantly different than the uninjected and pCSI/pLiLucB groups. The acceleration of tumor formation in mice that received a hydrodynamic injection appeared to be somehow abrogated by expression of the integrase. All groups are graphed together in **Fig. 2g** on a longer x-axis.

Tumors did not have luciferase activity or φC31 integrase-mediated integration events

In order to investigate further whether φC31 integrase played any role in tumor formation, we analyzed tumors isolated from mice in the pCSI/pLiLucB group. We tested protein extracts from eight tumors and one metastasis from four mice in this group and found that none of them were positive for luciferase activity (**Fig. 3a**). Additionally, we were unable to detect the luciferase gene by PCR in the six tumors from three mice in the pCSI/pLiLucB group that were tested (**Fig. 3b**). This PCR would detect integration at any location in the genome. The tumors that tested negative for luciferase activity included the six tumors that tested negative for the presence of the luciferase gene, suggesting that the luciferase donor plasmid was not integrated and silenced in these tumors. To determine further if φC31 integrase mediated integration of plasmid DNA into the cells that generated tumors, we tested all dissected tumors for integration into the dominant pseudo *attP* site in the mouse liver genome known as mpsL1 [9], using a nested PCR. For each round, one primer was in the mouse genome at mpsL1 while the other primer was the in *attB* sequence in the donor plasmid. PCR analysis was performed on DNA isolated from 19 tumors from 9 mice, including 7 tumors and 1 metastasis that were also tested for luciferase activity and six tumors also tested by PCR for the presence of the luciferase gene. No mpsL1 integration was detected in any tumors. Integration was detected only in DNA isolated from the normal-appearing part of the liver (**Fig. 3c**). A GAPDH control demonstrated that a sufficient amount (200 ng) of genomic DNA was added to each PCR reaction. Thus, no evidence for φC31 integrase activity was found in any of the tumors from mice in the pCSI/pLiLucB group, suggesting that φC31 integrase may not have played a role in tumor formation in the *LAP-tTA/TRE-MYC* transgenic mouse model.

Luciferase imaging data and correlation to tumor latency

Mice were imaged on day 1 and every two weeks thereafter for luciferase expression for the first 14 weeks, followed by every three weeks thereafter. We have shown the luciferase imaging data to

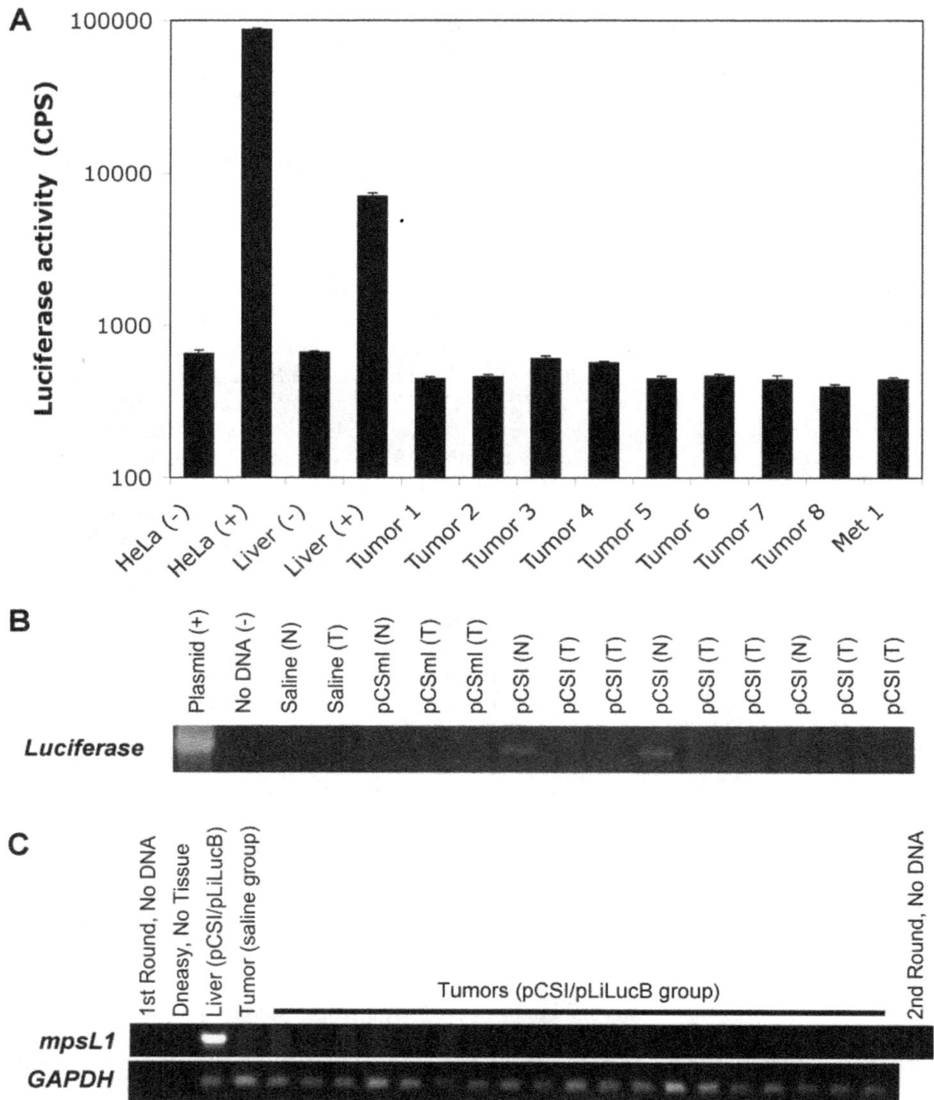

Figure 3. Luciferase activity and PCR analysis of tumors from mice in the pCSI/pLiLucB group provide no evidence of φC31 integrase activity. (**a**) Protein extracts were prepared and the luciferase activity was measured in absolute counts per second (CPS). Controls included HeLa cells given FuGene 6 alone [HeLa (-)] or the CMV-luciferase plasmid pNBL2 via FuGene 6 [HeLa (+)], the normal-appearing part of the tumor-ridden liver taken from either a saline-injected mouse [Liver (-)] and pCSI/pLiLucB-injected mouse [Liver (+)]. Eight tumor samples (Tumor 1 through 8) and one metastasis (Met 1) that were obtained from four animals were also analyzed. The error bars give standard error of the mean for four replicates of each sample. (**b**) PCR analysis to detect the pLiLucB plasmid by amplification of the luciferase transgene. Plasmid DNA (20 ng pLiLucB) and no DNA controls show specific amplification of luciferase only in the reaction containing plasmid. One mouse each from the saline-only and pCSml/pLiLucB groups was analyzed for transgene presence in normal-appearing (N) and tumor (T) tissues (none found). Three mice in the pCSI/pLiLucB group were analyzed for transgene presence in normal-appearing (N) and tumor (T) tissues. Luciferase could be detected in 2/3 normal-appearing liver samples and none of the tumors. (**c**) PCR analysis for integration at the mpsL1 pseudo *attP* site was done on 18 tumors (lanes 5 through 22) and one metastasis (lane 23) taken from nine mice given pCSI/pLiLucB by hydrodynamic injection. Controls included no DNA (1st round, lane 1 and 2nd round, lane 25), and a DNeasy performed on no tissue (lane 2) to show no contamination from the DNA isolation procedure. Normal-appearing liver from a mouse in the pCSI/pLiLucB group (lane 3) served as the positive control. DNA isolated from a tumor in the saline-only group served as the negative control (lane 4). PCR for the *GAPDH* gene showed that sufficient DNA was added to all reactions. Seven tumors and one metastasis were subjected to the analysis in *both* **a** and **c**. Six tumors were analyzed by all assays (**a**, **b** and **c**).

week 10 (**Fig. 4a**), because after week 10 (day 70) animals began to be sacrificed, thus complicating the data with increasing statistical error as the group sizes decreased. Averaged luciferase values were normalized to the day 1 luciferase value to remove variability on account of transfection efficiency. The standard error was calculated using propagation of errors to take this normalization into account. pCSI/pLiLucB gave significantly higher long-term expression than pCSmI/pLiLucB (Student's t-test, $p = 0.014$), demonstrating that φC31 integrase was active in the mouse liver. The pCS/pLiLucB and pCSmI/pLiLucB groups would still retain some luciferase expression due to random integration of the pLiLucB plasmid. The pCS/pLiLucB group maintained luciferase values that were significantly higher than pCSmI/pLiLucB (Student's t-test, $p = 3 \times 10^{-5}$). It is unclear why these groups have

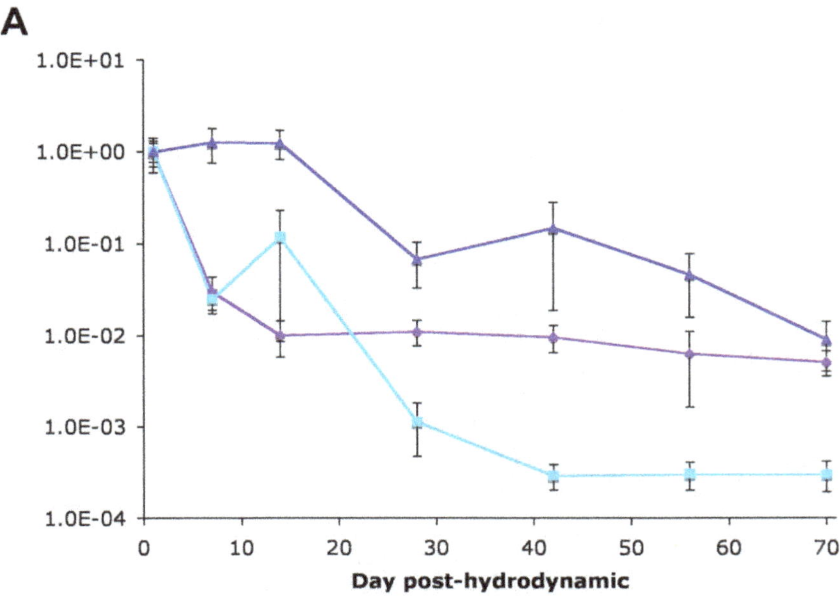

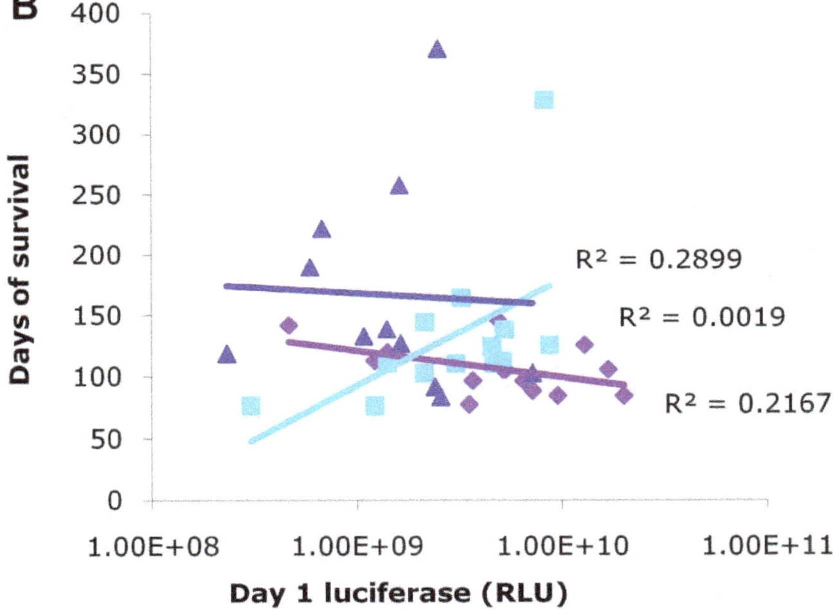

Figure 4. Luciferase expression and the relationship between initial expression values and long-term survival. (**a**) *TRE-MYC/LAP-tTA* transgenic mice given pCS/pLiLucB (purple diamonds), pCSml/pLiLucB (cyan squares), or pCSI/pLiLucB (blue triangles) by hydrodynamic injection were imaged at Day 1, Week 2, 4, 6, 8, and 10. The normalized luciferase levels were obtained by dividing the average luciferase expression in reflective light units (RLU) at each time point by the average level at day 1 for that group. Propagation of errors was used to determine the standard error at each time point given the division calculation (error bars). By student's t-test of the values at day 70, the pCSI/pLiLucB group and pCS/pLiLucB group had a p-value of 0.067, while the pCSI/pLiLucB group and pCS/pLiLucB group were significantly higher than the pCSml/pLiLucB group ($p = 0.014$ and $p = 0.000031$, respectively). (**b**) Each mouse is represented by one point on the scatterplot, using the day 1 luciferase value in reflective light units (RLU) as the x-coordinate and the days of survival as the y-coordinate. The symbols and colors are identical to those used in **a**. The linear line-of-best-fit was calculated by GraphPad Prism and is plotted for each group (R-squared values of pCS/pLiLucB, 0.1065; pCSml/pLiLucB, 0.3839; pCSI/pLiLucB, 0.0033). No R-squared values exceeded 0.95, which would have indicated that there was a trend relating transfection efficiency and survival.

different long-term luciferase levels. One could speculate that since the pCS/pLiLucB group developed tumors faster than the groups given integrase-expressing plasmids, increased numbers of luciferase-positive cells in the liver cause higher long-term luciferase levels. We do not believe that luciferase is an ideal readout for overall levels of transgene expression in the liver, because the levels detected are dependent on the distance from the surface of the animal. In this animal model, tumors formed that may have complicated interpretation of the luciferase levels by displacing the normal liver away from the surface of the animal. It was the possibility of finding metastases that motivated our use of the luciferase transgene in the liver. However, luciferase imaging did not detect any luciferase-positive metastases (**Table 1**).

In order to correlate the efficiency of hydrodynamic injection with tumor latency, the luciferase expression on day 1 was plotted against survival time (**Fig. 4b**). An R-squared value exceeding 0.95 would have indicated a trend correlating transfection efficiency and survival. The R-squared values for all groups were lower than 0.95, regardless of the method used to calculate the trend line, suggesting that variations in transfection efficiency may not have affected tumor latency.

Discussion

This study represents a novel use of a genetic mouse model to provide insights into the safety of new gene therapy methodologies in a solid tissue. Such mouse models are available for most organs that may be targeted by different gene therapy methods. Similar studies using tumor-prone mouse models to investigate the incidence of blood cancers after treatment with various viral vectors have been used to demonstrate that newer vectors containing insulator elements, weaker promoters, and/or lentiviral sequences may be safer than those vectors originally used in clinical trials for X-SCID that became implicated in the formation of leukemias [18,19].

Our data suggested an acceleration in tumor formation due to hydrodynamic injection in combination with C-MYC overexpression. The mechanism whereby hydrodynamic injection stimulated tumor formation is unknown. However, one could speculate that the extensive cellular proliferation that occurred after hydrodynamic injection in wild-type mice [36] may play a role. A comparable level of cellular proliferation induced by partial hepatectomy was reported to cause a similar acceleration in tumor formation in this cancer model [22,23].

We hypothesized that if φC31 integrase were tumorigenic, one would have expected a further decrease in tumor latency when hydrodynamic injection was accompanied by φC31 integrase. Instead, no measurable increase in C-MYC-induced tumor formation was found, suggesting that our hypothesis that φC31 integrase would be tumorigenic in this animal model was incorrect. No tumors taken from mice given active φC31 integrase and the luciferase donor plasmid were found to have integrated at a preferred pseudo *attP* site in the mouse genome, even though one or two out of nineteen might have been expected to be positive by random chance. It is unknown why the presence of either active or inactive φC31 integrase reduced the tumorigenicity of hydrodynamic injection. The recombination activity of φC31 integrase was not likely to be responsible for the significantly longer tumor latency compared to the pCS/pLiLucB and saline groups, because the pCSmI/pLiLucB, pCSI/pLiLucB, and pCSI alone groups were not statistically different from one another. Because the presence of φC31 integrase protein in hepatocytes was correlated with reduced cellular proliferation in a previous study [36], regardless of integrase activity, one possible hypothesis is that the decreased levels of proliferation resulted in reduced tumorigenesis in groups receiving integrase plasmids. We could also speculate that the immune system played a role in the effect, or that interaction of φC31 integrase with cellular proteins [40,41] proved to be anti-tumorigenic. It could be suggested that hydrodynamic injection did not transfect the cells that can go on to become cancer. However, when two oncogenes (*MET* and *ΔN90-CTNNB1*) were administered to the liver of wild-type mice via hydrodynamic injection and integrated with a transposon system, tumors developed in most of the mice within 200 days [42]. Thus, hydrodynamic injection has already been shown to be capable of delivering oncogenes to tumor-forming cells within the liver.

Our mouse model revealed a statistically significant contribution of the hydrodynamic method itself, with or without DNA, to tumor formation. Although significant, it should be noted that the decrease in tumor latency from hydrodynamic delivery alone (**Fig. 2b**) was modest compared to the dramatic one-week median tumor latency when shRNA or small molecule carcinogens such as carbon tetrachloride cooperated with C-MYC in this mouse model [23]. While hydrodynamic injection is perhaps the most robust method of plasmid DNA delivery to mouse liver currently available, adaptations of the method that are less disruptive would be desirable for clinical use. For example, localized, catheter-mediated delivery to the liver has been explored in large animal models [3] and may have a superior safety profile compared to the systemic delivery method used in mice.

Acknowledgments

The authors sincerely thank Shelly Beer, Christopher L. Chavez, Julien Sage, and Jeffrey S. Glenn for their contributions to experimental design and/or interpretation of the results and Sahana Somasegar for assistance with some of the experiments.

Author Contributions

Conceived and designed the experiments: LEW AK DWF MPC. Performed the experiments: LEW AK WEJ OLW QY. Analyzed the data: LEW. Contributed reagents/materials/analysis tools: DWF. Wrote the paper: LEW MPC.

References

1. Liu F, Song Y, Liu D (1999) Hydrodynamics-based transfection in animals by systemic administration of plasmid DNA. Gene Ther 6: 1258–1266. DOI: 10.1038/sj.gt.3300947.
2. Zhang G, Budker V, Wolff JA (1999) High levels of foreign gene expression in hepatocytes after tail vein injections of naked plasmid DNA. Hum Gene Ther 10: 1735–1737. DOI: 10.1089/10430349950017734.
3. Suda T, Kamimura K, Kubota T, Tamura Y, Igarashi M, et al. (2009) Progress toward liver-based gene therapy. Hepatol Res 39: 325–340. DOI: 10.1111/j.1872-034X.2008.00479.x.
4. Fabre JW, Grehan A, Whitehorne M, Sawyer GJ, Dong X, et al. (2008) Hydrodynamic gene delivery to the pig liver via an isolated segment of the inferior vena cava. Gene Ther 15: 452–462. DOI: 10.1038/sj.gt.3303079.
5. Kamimura K, Suda T, Xu W, Zhang G, Liu D (2009) Image-guided, lobe-specific hydrodynamic gene delivery to swine liver. Mol Ther 17: 491–499. DOI: 10.1038/mt.2008.294.
6. Khorsandi SE, Bachellier P, Weber JC, Greget M, Jaeck D, et al. (2008) Minimally invasive and selective hydrodynamic gene therapy of liver segments in the pig and human. Cancer Gene Ther 15: 225–230. DOI: 10.1038/sj.cgt.7701119.
7. Suda T, Suda K, Liu D (2008) Computer-assisted hydrodynamic gene delivery. Mol Ther 16: 1098–1104. DOI: 10.1038/mt.2008.66.
8. Olivares EC, Hollis RP, Chalberg TW, Meuse L, Kay MA, et al. (2002) Site-specific genomic integration produces therapeutic Factor IX levels in mice. Nat Biotechnol 20: 1124–1128. DOI: 10.1038/nbt753.
9. Ehrhardt A, Xu H, Huang Z, Engler JA, Kay MA (2005) A direct comparison of two nonviral gene therapy vectors for somatic integration: in vivo evaluation of the bacteriophage integrase phiC31 and the Sleeping Beauty transposase. Mol Ther 11: 695–706. DOI: 10.1016/j.ymthe.2005.01.010.
10. Calos MP (2006) The phiC31 integrase system for gene therapy. Curr Gene Ther 6: 633–645.
11. Chalberg TW, Portlock JL, Olivares EC, Thyagarajan B, Kirby PJ, et al. (2006) Integration specificity of phage phiC31 integrase in the human genome. J Mol Biol 357: 28–48. DOI: 10.1016/j.jmb.2005.11.098.
12. Sivalingam J, Krishnan S, Ng WH, Lee SS, Phan TT, et al. (2010) Biosafety Assessment of Site-directed Transgene Integration in Human Umbilical Cord-lining Cells. Mol Ther;DOI: 10.1038/mt.2010.61.
13. Liu J, Jeppesen I, Nielsen K, Jensen TG (2006) Phi c31 integrase induces chromosomal aberrations in primary human fibroblasts. Gene Ther 13: 1188–1190. DOI: 10.1038/sj.gt.3302789.
14. Liu J, Skjorringe T, Gjetting T, Jensen TG (2009) PhiC31 integrase induces a DNA damage response and chromosomal rearrangements in human adult fibroblasts. BMC Biotechnol 9: 31. DOI: 10.1186/1472-6750-9-31.

15. Ehrhardt A, Engler JA, Xu H, Cherry AM, Kay MA (2006) Molecular analysis of chromosomal rearrangements in mammalian cells after phiC31-mediated integration. Hum Gene Ther 17: 1077–1094. DOI: 10.1089/hum.2006.17.1077.
16. Themis M, Waddington SN, Schmidt M, von KC, Wang Y, et al. (2005) Oncogenesis following delivery of a nonprimate lentiviral gene therapy vector to fetal and neonatal mice. Mol Ther 12: 763–771. DOI: 10.1016/j.ymthe.2005.07.358.
17. Donsante A, Miller DG, Li Y, Vogler C, Brunt EM, et al. (2007) AAV vector integration sites in mouse hepatocellular carcinoma. Science 317: 477. DOI: 10.1126/science.1142658.
18. Shou Y, Ma Z, Lu T, Sorrentino BP (2006) Unique risk factors for insertional mutagenesis in a mouse model of XSCID gene therapy. Proc Natl Acad Sci U S A 103: 11730–11735. DOI: 10.1073/pnas.0603635103.
19. Montini E, Cesana D, Schmidt M, Sanvito F, Ponzoni M, et al. (2006) Hematopoietic stem cell gene transfer in a tumor-prone mouse model uncovers low genotoxicity of lentiviral vector integration. Nat Biotechnol 24: 687–696. DOI: 10.1038/nbt1216.
20. Ryu BY, Evans-Galea MV, Gray JT, Bodine DM, Persons DA, et al. (2008) An experimental system for the evaluation of retroviral vector design to diminish the risk for proto-oncogene activation. Blood 111: 1866–1875. DOI: 10.1182/blood-2007-04-085506.
21. Beer S, Bellovin DI, Lee JS, Komatsubara K, Wang LS, et al. (2009) Low-level shRNA Cytotoxicity Can Contribute to MYC-induced Hepatocellular Carcinoma in Adult Mice. Mol Ther 20: DOI: 10.1038/mt.2009.222.
22. Beer S, Zetterberg A, Ihrie RA, McTaggart RA, Yang Q, et al. (2004) Developmental context determines latency of MYC-induced tumorigenesis. PLoS Biol 2: e332. DOI: 10.1371/journal.pbio.0020332.
23. Beer S, Komatsubara K, Bellovin DI, Kurobe M, Sylvester K, et al. (2008) Hepatotoxin-induced changes in the adult murine liver promote MYC-induced tumorigenesis. PLoS One 3: e2493. DOI: 10.1371/journal.pone.0002493.
24. Felsher DW, Bishop JM (1999) Reversible tumorigenesis by MYC in hematopoietic lineages. Mol Cell 4: 199–207.
25. Kistner A, Gossen M, Zimmermann F, Jerecic J, Ullmer C, et al. (1996) Doxycycline-mediated quantitative and tissue-specific control of gene expression in transgenic mice. Proc Natl Acad Sci U S A 93: 10933–10938.
26. Shachaf CM, Kopelman AM, Arvanitis C, Karlsson A, Beer S, et al. (2004) MYC inactivation uncovers pluripotent differentiation and tumour dormancy in hepatocellular cancer. Nature 431: 1112–1117. DOI: 10.1038/nature03043.
27. Abou-Elella A, Gramlich T, Fritsch C, Gansler T (1996) c-myc amplification in hepatocellular carcinoma predicts unfavorable prognosis. Mod Pathol 9: 95–98.
28. Kawate S, Fukusato T, Ohwada S, Watanuki A, Morishita Y (1999) Amplification of c-myc in hepatocellular carcinoma: correlation with clinicopathologic features, proliferative activity and p53 overexpression. Oncology 57: 157–163.
29. Donaldson TD, Duronio RJ (2004) Cancer cell biology: Myc wins the competition. Curr Biol 14: R425–R427. DOI: 10.1016/j.cub.2004.05.035.
30. Felsher DW, Bishop JM (1999) Transient excess of MYC activity can elicit genomic instability and tumorigenesis. Proc Natl Acad Sci U S A 96: 3940–3944.
31. Felsher DW (2008) Reversing cancer from inside and out: oncogene addiction, cellular senescence, and the angiogenic switch. Lymphat Res Biol 6: 149–154. DOI: 10.1089/lrb.2008.63403.
32. Portlock JL, Keravala A, Bertoni C, Lee S, Rando TA, et al. (2006) Long-term increase in mVEGF164 in mouse hindlimb muscle mediated by phage phiC31 integrase after nonviral DNA delivery. Hum Gene Ther 17: 871–876. DOI: 10.1089/hum.2006.17.871.
33. Thyagarajan B, Olivares EC, Hollis RP, Ginsburg DS, Calos MP (2001) Site-specific genomic integration in mammalian cells mediated by phage phiC31 integrase. Mol Cell Biol 21: 3926–3934. DOI: 10.1128/MCB.21.12.3926-3934.2001.
34. Thyagarajan B, Calos MP (2005) Site-specific integration for high-level protein production in mammalian cells. Methods Mol Biol 308: 99–106.: 99-106. DOI:10.1385/1-59259-922-2:099.
35. Keravala A, Lee S, Thyagarajan B, Olivares EC, Gabrovsky VE, et al. (2009) Mutational derivatives of PhiC31 integrase with increased efficiency and specificity. Mol Ther 17: 112–120. DOI: 10.1038/mt.2008.241.
36. Woodard LE, Hillman RT, Keravala A, Lee S, Calos MP (2010) Effect of nuclear localization and hydrodynamic delivery-induced cell division on phiC31 integrase activity. Gene Ther 17: 217–226. DOI: 10.1038/gt.2009.136.
37. Bertoni C, Jarrahian S, Wheeler TM, Li Y, Olivares EC, et al. (2006) Enhancement of plasmid-mediated gene therapy for muscular dystrophy by directed plasmid integration. Proc Natl Acad Sci U S A 103: 419–424. DOI: 10.1073/pnas.0504505102.
38. Held PK, Olivares EC, Aguilar CP, Finegold M, Calos MP, et al. (2005) In vivo correction of murine hereditary tyrosinemia type I by phiC31 integrase-mediated gene delivery. Mol Ther 11: 399–408. DOI: 10.1016/j.ymthe.2004.11.001.
39. Chavez CL, Keravala A, Woodard LE, Hillman RT, Stowe TR, et al. (2010) Kinetics and longevity of phiC31 integrase in mouse liver and cultured cells. Hum Gene Ther;DOI: 10.1089/hum.2010.049.
40. Chen JZ, Ji CN, Xu GL, Pang RY, Yao JH, et al. (2006) DAXX interacts with phage PhiC31 integrase and inhibits recombination. Nucleic Acids Res 34: 6298–6304. DOI: 10.1093/nar/gkl890.
41. Wang BY, Xu GL, Zhou CH, Tian L, Xue JL, et al. (2009) PhiC31 integrase interacts with TTRAP and inhibits NFkappaB activation. Mol Biol Rep;DOI: 10.1007/s11033-009-9829-3.
42. Tward AD, Jones KD, Yant S, Cheung ST, Fan ST, et al. (2007) Distinct pathways of genomic progression to benign and malignant tumors of the liver. Proc Natl Acad Sci U S A 104: 14771–14776. DOI: 10.1073/pnas.0706578104.

7

Ovarian Cancer Gene Therapy using HPV-16 Pseudovirion Carrying the HSV-tk Gene

1
Chien-Fu Hung[1,2]*, An Jen Chiang[1,3,4,5], Hsiao-Hsuan Tsai[1], Martin G. Pomper[6], Tae Heung Kang[1], Richard R. Roden[1,2,7], T.-C. Wu[1,2,7,8]

Department of Pathology, Johns Hopkins Medical Institutions, Baltimore, Maryland, United States of America, **2** Department of Oncology, Johns Hopkins Medical Institutions, Baltimore, Maryland, United States of America, **3** Department of Obstetrics and Gynecology, Kaohsiung Veterans General Hospital, Kaohsiung, Taiwan, Division of Obstetrics and Gynecology, National Yang-Ming University School of Medicine, Taipei, Taiwan, **5** Department of Biological Sciences, National Sun Yat-Sen University, Kaohsiung, Taiwan, **6** Department of Radiology, Johns Hopkins School of Medicine, Baltimore, Maryland, United States of America, **7** Department of Obstetrics and Gynecology, Johns Hopkins Medical Institutions, Baltimore, Maryland, United States of America, **8** Department of Molecular Microbiology and Immunology, Johns Hopkins Medical Institutions, Baltimore, Maryland, United States of America

Abstract

Ovarian cancer is the leading cause of death from all gynecological cancers and conventional therapies such as surgery, chemotherapy, and radiotherapy usually fail to control advanced stages of the disease. Thus, there is an urgent need for alternative and innovative therapeutic options. We reason that cancer gene therapy using a vector capable of specifically delivering an enzyme-encoding gene to ovarian cancer cells will allow the cancer cell to metabolize a harmless prodrug into a potent cytotoxin, which will lead to therapeutic effects. In the current study, we explore the use of a human papillomavirus (HPV) pseudovirion to deliver a herpes simplex virus thymidine kinase (HSV-tk) gene to ovarian tumor cells. We found that the HPV-16 pseudovirion was able to preferentially infect murine and human ovarian tumor cells when administered intraperitoneally. Furthermore, intraperitoneal injection of HPV-16 pseudovirions carrying the HSV-tk gene followed by treatment with ganciclovir led to significant therapeutic anti-tumor effects in murine ovarian cancer-bearing mice. Our data suggest that HPV pseudovirion may serve as a potential delivery vehicle for ovarian cancer gene therapy.

Editor: Joseph Najbauer, City of Hope National Medical Center and Beckman Research Institute, United States of America

Funding: This work was supported by the National Cancer Institute Specialized Programs of Research Excellence (http://trp.cancer.gov/) in Cervical Cancer P50 CA098252, CA118790 (Roden), and CA122581 (Roden). The funders had no role in the study design, data collection and analysis, decision to publish, or preparation of the manuscript.

Competing Interests: The authors have declared that no competing interests exist.

* E-mail: chung2@jhmi.edu

Introduction

Ovarian cancer is the leading cause of death from all gynecological cancers and the sixth most common malignancy for women in the United States [1,2]. Although significant advances have occurred in both surgical and chemotherapeutic techniques, the overall 5-year survival rates for all stages of ovarian cancer remain <50% [2,3]. Current therapies (surgery, chemotherapy, and radiotherapy) usually fail to control advanced stages of the disease. Therefore, alternative therapeutic approaches may serve as important methods for controlling these advanced stage ovarian tumors.

One possible approach is the use of suicide gene therapy (SGT). With SGT, the gene for a foreign enzyme (i.e. one from a virus, bacteria, or yeast) is specifically delivered to cancer cells. Gene delivery is followed by systemic administration of a non-toxic prodrug. The infected cancer cells are able to express the foreign enzyme to convert the prodrug into an active cytotoxin, which is able to kill the infected cells. One advantage SGT has over conventional gene therapies is its ability to kill neighboring cells through the bystander effect. The active drug can escape the transduced cells and diffuse into neighboring non-infected cells, ultimately leading to their death as well. The dying cells are also able to induce natural killer (NK) cells and T cells to induce a distant bystander effect. The hope for this approach is to have great specificity for tumor cells, particularly cancer stem cells. This approach should also reduce the toxic side effects associated with conventional cancer therapies due to the increased specificity of both the delivery and activation of the cytotoxin [4].

The most studied suicide gene/prodrug system is the combination of herpes simplex virus thymidine kinase (HSV-tk) with ganciclovir (GCV) [5]. HSV-tk, which has high affinity for ganciclovir, catalyzes the first phosphorylation of GCV that can then be di- and tri-phosphorylated by cellular kinases. Triphosphorylated GCV can be incorporated into replicating DNA, which leads to polymerase inhibition and eventually apoptosis [4–6]. This system has shown some success in the clinic but its utility is limited by its dependence on cell-to-cell contact and gap junctions for the bystander effect [4].

For this study, we use replication-defective human papillomavirus (HPV) pseudovirions to deliver the HSV-tk gene to ovarian tumor cells. Recent studies show DNA plasmids can be packaged into the papillomavirus L1 and L2 capsid proteins to generate the 'pseudovirion' that can efficient deliver the DNA into multiple cell lines [7–9]. The encapsulation also protects the DNA from nucleases and provides a targeted delivery with great stability.

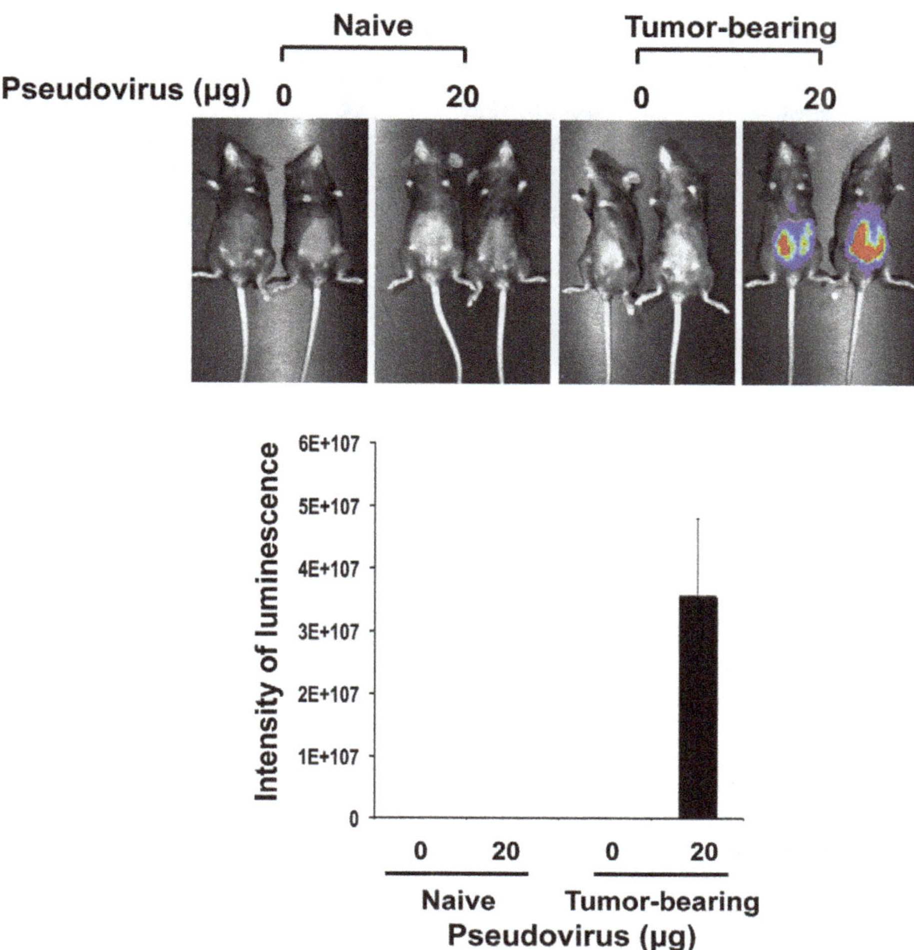

Figure 1. Comparison of HPV pseudovirion infectivity in naïve and murine ovarian tumor-bearing mice. 5–8 weeks old C57BL/6 mice were challenged with MOSEC tumor cells (1×10^6 cells/mouse). One week later, tumor-bearing mice were intraperitoneally injected with or without HPV-16/luc pseudovirions (20 μg HPV-16 L1 protein/mouse, equivalent to 120 ng of DNA/mouse). Naïve mice infected with or without HPV-16/luc pseudovirions served as a control. Mice were imaged by non-invasive luminescence imaging 1 day after infection. Data shown are representative of 2 experiments performed.

Many of the safety concerns associated with the use of live viral vectors are alleviated as the HPV pseudovirions contain a DNA construct different from the natural HPV viral genome. There are also over 100 types of papillomavirus pseudovirions, which allows for repeated boosting using different types since the neutralizing antibodies against one type are usually not cross-reactive with other types.

Here we explore the use of HPV pseudovirions to deliver marker genes and suicidal genes to both murine and human ovarian tumor cells. We found that intraperitoneal injection of HPV-16 pseudovirions led to preferential infection of ectopic and spontaneously occurring murine ovarian cancers in mice. Preferential infection also occurred in human ovarian tumor xenografts of tumor-bearing mice. Intraperitoneal injection of HPV-16 pseudovirions carrying the HSV-tk gene followed by administration of ganciclovir led to significant therapeutic anti-tumor effects in murine-ovarian cancer-bearing mice. Our data shows proof-of-principle that HPV pseudovirions can be useful vectors for delivering therapeutic genes to ovarian cancers.

Materials and Methods

Ethics Statement

This study was carried out in strict accordance with the recommendations of the Guide for the Care and Use of Laboratory Animals of the National Institutes of Health. All procedures were performed with prior approval of the Johns Hopkins Animal Care and Use Committee (protocol MO08M446).

Mice

The C57BL/6 and nude (BALB/c nu/nu) mice were acquired from the National Cancer Institute. *MISIIR-TAG* transgenic mice [10] were kindly provided by Dr. Denise Connolly at the Fox Chase Cancer Center. All animals were maintained under specific pathogen-free conditions, and all procedures were performed according to approved protocols and in accordance with recommendations for the proper use and care of laboratory animals.

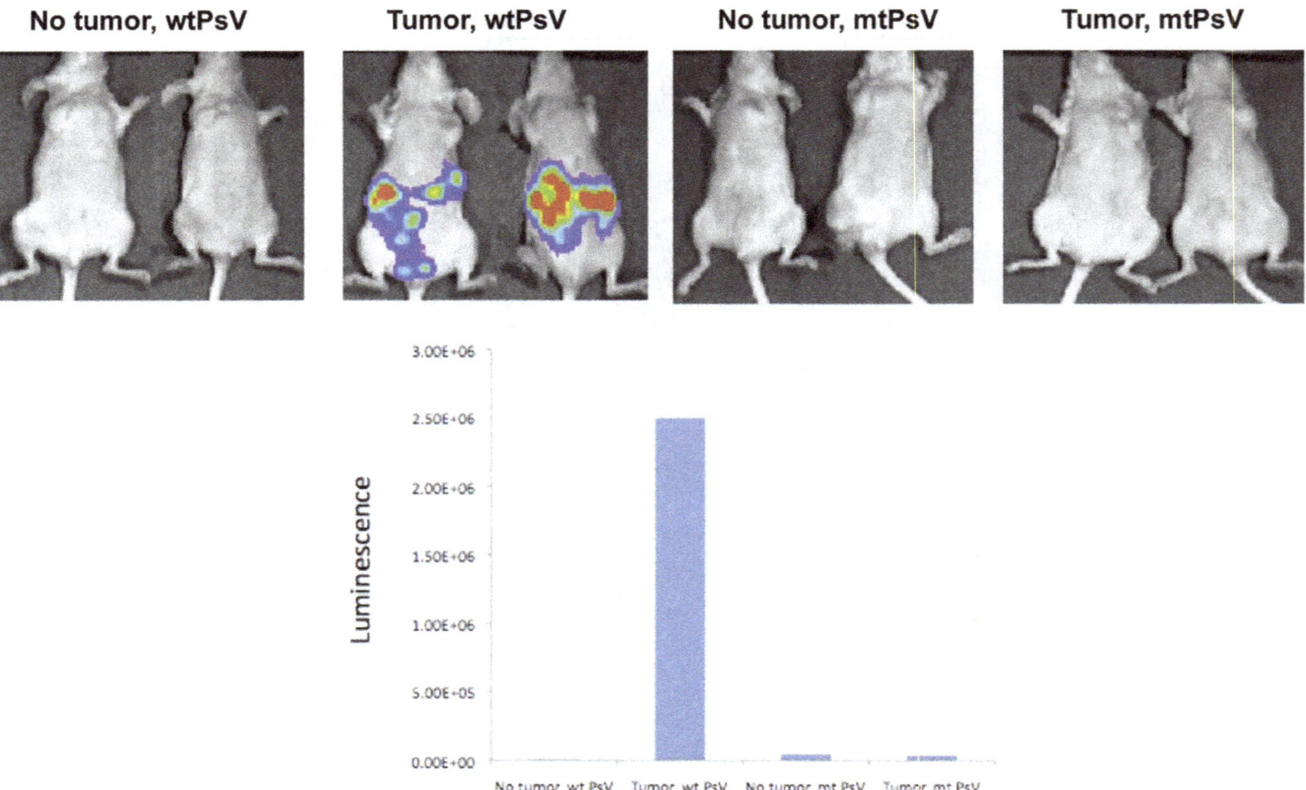

Figure 2. Characterization of the infectivity of HPV pseudovirion in naïve nude mice and human ovarian tumor-bearing nude mice. 5–8 weeks old nude mice were injected intraperitoneally with ES2 human ovarian tumor cells (1×10^6 cells/mouse). One week later, tumor-bearing mice were intraperitoneally injected with wild-type (wt) HPV-16/Luc psV or mutant L2 (mtL2) HPV-16L1mtL2-Luc pseudovirions (20 μg HPV-16 L1 protein/mouse, equivalent to 120 ng of DNA/mouse). Naïve mice infected with wt or mt HPV-16/luc pseudovirions served as controls. Mice were imaged by non-invasive luminescence imaging 1 day after infection. Data shown are representative of 2 experiments performed.

Cell Lines

293TT cells were kindly provided by J Schiller (National Cancer Institute (NCI), National Institutes of Health (NIH)) [11]. The MOSEC cell line (a mouse ovarian cancer cell line) was prepared as described previously [12]. The ES2 cell line (a human ovarian cancer cell line) was purchased from the American Type Culture Collection (ATCC), Manassas, VA. MOSEC/luciferase (MOSEC-luc) cells were generated as described previously [13].

Plasmids

The plasmids encoding HPV16 L1 L2 (pShell16) were kindly provided by Dr. J Schiller (NCI). The point mutation HPV16L1 mtL2 construct is described in our previous study [14]. The generation of the luciferase-expressing plasmid (pcDNA3-luciferase) and the GFP-expressing plasmid (pcDNA3-GFP) has been described previously [15,16]. The pORF-HSVtk plasmid was purchased from InvivoGen.

HPV Pseudovirion Production

HPV16-GFP, HPV16-Luc (luciferase), HPV16-tk (HSVtk Herpes Simplex Virus-Thymidine Kinase) pseudovirions were made using the methods as described previously [11]. Briefly, 293TT cells were cotransfected with HPV expression plasmids pShell16 and the plasmids of choice (such as GFP, luciferase or HSVtk) using Lipofectamine 2000 (Invitrogen). After 48 h, the cells were harvested and washed with Dulbecco's phosphate buffered saline (PBS) (Invitrogen) supplemented with 9.5 mM $MgCl_2$ and antibiotic-antimycotic mixture (DPBS-Mg) (Invitrogen). The cells were suspended in DPBS-Mg supplemented with 0.5% Brij58, 0.2% Benzonase (EMD Chemicals, Gibbstown, NJ, USA), and 0.2% Plasmid Safe (Epicentre Biotechnologies, Madison, WI, USA) at $>100\times10^6$ cells/ml and incubated at 37 C for 24 h for capsid maturation. After maturation, the cell lysate was chilled on ice for 10 min. The salt concentration of the cell lysate was adjusted to 850 mM and incubated on ice for 10 min. The lysate was then clarified by centrifugation, and the supernatant was layered onto an Optiprep gradient. The gradient was spun for 4.5 h at 16 C at 40 000 r.p.m. in a SW40 rotor (Beckman Coulter, Inc., Brea, CA, USA). The purity of HPV pseudovirions was evaluated by running the fractions on 4–15% gradient sodium dodecyl sulfate-polyacrylamide gel electrophoresis. The encapsulated DNA plasmid was quantified by extracting encapsidated DNA from Optiprep factions followed by quantitative real-time PCR comparisons with serial dilutions of naked DNA. The concentrations of plasmids (GFP, luciferase, or HSVtk) in the pseudovirions were determined to be approximately 6.2 ng of DNA per 1 μg of L1 protein.

In vitro Infection of Tumor Cells by HPV16 Pseudovirions

MOSEC or ES2 cells were plated in 96-well plates at a density of 5000 cells/well and grown overnight. The cells were infected with HPV-16/Luc psV (1 μg L1 protein/ml) for 72 hours.

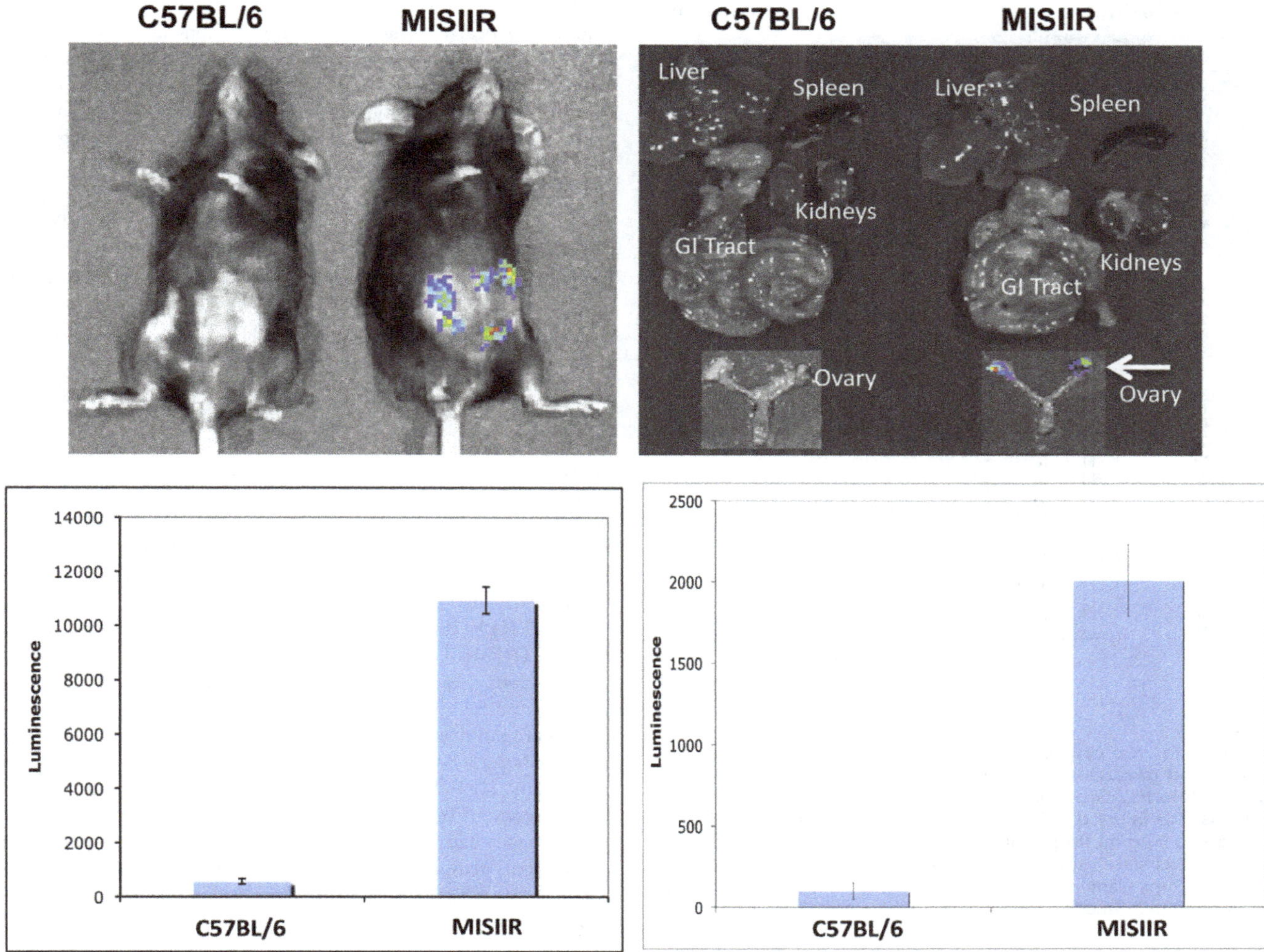

Figure 3. HPV-16/luc psV preferentially infects ovarian tumors in *MISIIR-TAG* transgenic mouse. C57BL/6 mice and *MISIIR-TAG* transgenic mice were injected with 20 μg of HPV-16/luc psV by intraperitoneal injection 10 weeks after birth. Luminescence images were taken 1 day after HPV-16/luv psV injection. *Top,* Representative luminescence images of psV-infected C57BL/6 mice or *MISIIR-TAG* transgenic mice (left) and their harvested organs (right). Note: White arrow indicates only ovarian cancer from MISRII transgenic mice can be infected by HPV-16/luc psV. *Bottom,* Representative bar graphs of luminescence imaging in MISIIR-TAG transgenic mice or C57BL/6 mice. Data representative of 2 experiments performed.

Luciferin (15 μg/ml) was added and incubated for 10 min. An integration time of 10 sec was used for luminescence image acquisition by the IVIS 200 system (Xenogen Corp., Alameda, CA, USA).

Characterization of Tumor Infection by HPV16 Pseudovirions in Mice

C57BL/6 mice (5 per group) were intraperitoneally injected with 1×10^6 MOSEC cells/mouse. One week later, tumor-bearing mice were intraperitoneally injected with HPV-16/Luc psV at a dose of 20 μg HPV-16 L1 protein/mouse (equivalent to 120 ng of DNA/mouse). Luminescence images were recorded the day after the HPV-16/Luc psV injection. An integration time of 2 min was used for luminescence image acquisition.

For the characterization of the infection of human ovarian cancer cells by HPV-16/Luc psV, nude mice were challenged with ES2 human ovarian tumor cells at a dose of 1×10^6 cells/mouse. One week later, tumor-bearing mice were intraperitoneally injected with wild-type (wt) HPV-16/Luc psV or mutant (mt) HPV-16L1mtL2-Luc psV at a dose of 20 μg HPV-16 L1 protein/mouse (equivalent to 120 ng of DNA/mouse). Naïve mice without tumors infected with wt or mt HPV-16/Luc psV served as controls. Luminescence images were taken the day after the HPV-16/Luc psV injection. The mice were injected with 0.2 ml of 15 mg/ml beetle luciferin (potassium salt; Promega). After 10 min, the mice were imaged using the IVIS 200 system (Xenogen Corp., Alameda, CA, USA). An integration time of 30 sec was used for luminescence image acquisition.

In vitro Cytotoxicity Mediated by HPV16-TK Pseudovirions and Ganciclovir

MOSEC-Luc cells were infected HPV16-GFP psV or HPV16-TK psV (1 μg L1 protein/ml) for 48 hours. The infected cells were seeded in 96 well plates. The infected cells were treated with 0 μg/ml, 0.1 μg/ml, 1 μg/ml, or 10 μg/ml of ganciclovir for 72 hours and luciferase expression was examined by IVIS 200 system (Xenogen Corp., Alameda, CA, USA).

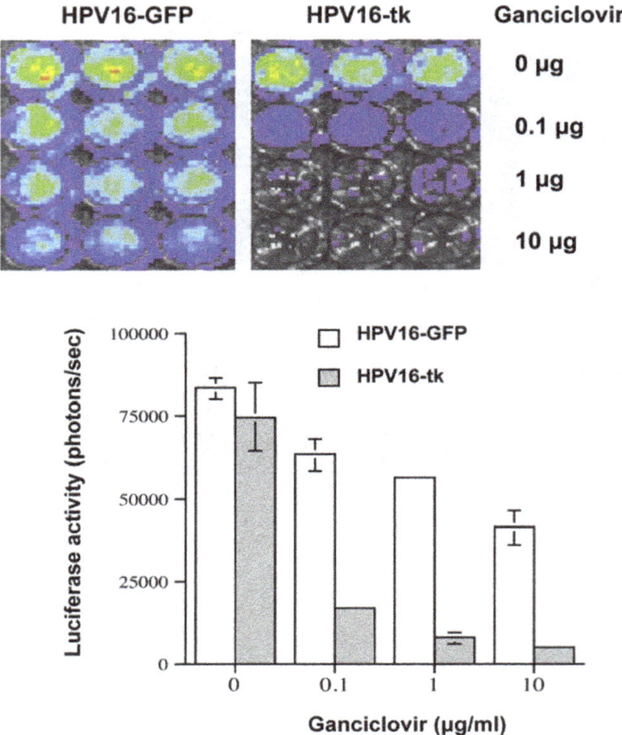

Figure 4. ***In vitro*** **cytotoxicity mediated by HPV16-tk pseudovirions and ganciclovir.** MOSEC-Luc cells were infected HPV16-GFP psV or HPV16/HSV-tk psV at a concentration of 1 µg L1 protein/ml for 48 hours. The infected cells were seeded in 96 well plates and then treated with 0 µg/ml, 0.1 µg/ml, 1 µg/ml, or 10 µg/ml of Ganciclovir for 72 hours. Luciferase expression was examined by the IVIS 200 system (Xenogen Corp., Alameda, CA, USA). Data shown are representative of 2 experiments performed.

In vivo Cytotoxicity Mediated by HPV16-TK Pseudovirions and Ganciclovir

Mice were injected intraperitoneally with 1×10^6 MOSEC-Luc cells/mouse on day 1. Luciferase activity was examined on day 2 as an indication of number of tumors in the mouse. The mice were injected with 0.2 ml of 15 mg/ml beetle luciferin (potassium salt; Promega). After ten minutes, the mice were imaged using the IVIS 200 system (Xenogen Corp., Alameda, CA, USA). An integration time of 2 min was used for luminescence image acquisition. Mice were injected with HPV16-GFP psV (20 µg L1 protein) or HPV16-TK psV (20 µg L1 protein) on day 3. Mice were treated daily with ganciclovir (50 mg/kg) or PBS from day 5 to day 18. Mice were imaged again by non-invasive luminescence imaging on day 20.

Results

Intraperitoneal Injection of HPV-16 Pseudovirions Leads to Preferential Infection of Murine Ovarian Cancer Cells in Tumor-bearing Mice

We initially examined if the HPV-16 pseudovirion carrying the luciferase gene (HPV-16/Luc psV) was capable of infecting the murine ovarian cancer cell line, MOSEC, *in vitro*. As shown in **Figure S1**, HPV-16/Luc psV was able to infect MOSEC tumor cells *in vitro*. To demonstrate if the HPV-16/Luc psV can also infect the murine ovarian cancer cell line in tumor-bearing mice, we first intraperitoneally injected mice with MOSEC tumor cells. The tumor-bearing mice were intraperitoneally injected with HPV-16/Luc psV one week later. As shown in **Figure 1**, while mice without tumors did not show any luciferase activity, tumor-bearing mice intraperitoneally injected with HPV-16/Luc psV demonstrated significant luciferase activity. These data suggest the HPV pseudovirion preferentially infects the tumor cells in tumor-bearing mice.

Intraperitoneal Injection of HPV-16 Pseudovirions Leads to Preferential Infection of Human Ovarian Cancer Cells in Tumor-bearing Nude Mice

We further examined whether the HPV-16/Luc psV was able to infect the human ovarian cancer cell line ES2. As shown in **Figure S2**, ES2 cells infected with HPV-16/Luc psV demonstrated luciferase activity, suggesting that HPV-16/Luc psV was capable of infecting human ovarian cancer cells *in vitro*. We also characterized the *in vivo* infectivity of HPV-16/luc psV in nude mice bearing ES2 human ovarian tumors to determine whether the infectivity of HPV pseudovirions is essential for efficient gene delivery to ovarian tumor cells by HPV pseudovirions. It is now clear that the HPV L2 minor capsid protein is essential for efficient infection of cells by HPV pseudovirions [14,17]. Thus, we have employed HPV-16/Luc psV with a single amino acid mutation in HPV L2 (HPV16L1mtL2-luc psV) that abolishes the infectivity of pseudovirions [14]. As shown in **Figure 2**, only nude mice bearing human ovarian tumors demonstrated significant luminescence compared to the non-tumor-bearing nude mice. Furthermore, only tumor-bearing mice infected by HPV-16/luc psV but not mutant HPV-16/L1mtL2- luc psV demonstrated significant luminescence (**Fig. 2**). Thus, our data show that HPV-16 pseudovirions can also preferentially infect human ovarian tumor cells *in vivo*. Furthermore, our data indicate that intact HPV L2 is essential for efficient delivery of encapsidated genes to ovarian tumor cells by HPV pseudovirions.

HPV-16/luc psV Preferentially Infects Ovarian Tumors in *MISIIR-TAg* Transgenic Mouse

We further examined the preferential infection of ovarian tumor cells by HPV pseudovirions in the *MISIIR-TAg* transgenic mouse, a spontaneously occurring murine ovarian tumor model. This transgenic mouse, which expresses the transforming region of SV40 under the control of the Mullerian inhibitory substance type II receptor gene promoter, has been shown to develop bilateral ovarian tumors. Thus, the spontaneous ovarian cancer model in *MISIIR-TAg* transgenic mice more closely resembles human ovarian cancer than a transplantation model such as MOSEC tumor model. The *MISIIR-TAg* transgenic mouse has been reported to spontaneously develop ovarian carcinoma within 6–13 weeks of birth [10]. In our lab, all of the *MISIIR-TAg* transgenic mice (from a new line acquired from Dr. Connolly) developed ovarian tumors within 4 months of birth. We injected HPV-16/luc psV 10 weeks after birth and we found that HPV-16/Luc psV could also preferentially infect the spontaneously occurring ovarian cancer in the *MISIIR-TAg* transgenic mice (**Fig. 3**). Furthermore, we observed that the vital organs including the lungs, heart, stomach, spleen and kidney were not infected. In addition, no luciferase activity was observed in the normal ovaries of C57BL/6 mice injected with HPV-16/luc psV. Thus, our data indicate that HPV-16 pseudovirions can selectively infect ovarian tumor cells in a spontaneously occurring murine ovarian tumor model.

Infection of HPV-16 Pseudovirions Carrying the HSV-tk Gene followed by Treatment with Ganciclovir Leads to *in vitro* Cytotoxicity of Infected Cells

The preferential infection of HPV-16 pseudovirions in ovarian tumor cells allows for the opportunity to specifically carry therapeutic DNA to ovarian tumor cells for the control of ovarian tumors. Because the initial administration of HPV pseudovirions may not be able to infect all of the ovarian tumor cells, it is important to consider a strategy that allows the ovarian tumor cells not directly infected to also become susceptible. Therefore, we chose the HSV-tk/ganciclovir system, as it is the most widely studied suicide gene therapy system and over two decades of attempts to use the system as an anticancer therapy has shown varying success. To demonstrate if HPV-16/HSV-tk psV can infect ovarian tumor cells and render them susceptible to killing by treatment with ganciclovir, we infected MOSEC-Luc cells with HPV16-GFP psV or HPV16/HSV-tk psV for 48 hours. The infected cells were subsequently treated with different concentrations of ganciclovir and the luciferase expression of the infected cells was measured using the IVIS 200 system. As shown in **Figure 4**, MOSEC-Luc tumor cells infected with HPV-16/HSV-tk psV followed by treatment with ganciclovir led to cell death of the infected cells *in vitro*. This was not observed in cells infected with HPV-16/GFP. We also observed that higher concentrations of ganciclovir led to more cell death. Similar effects were seen when similar assays were conducted with the human ovarian cancer cell line ES2 (see **Figure S3**).

Intraperitoneal Injection of HPV-16 Pseudovirions Carrying the HSV-tk Gene followed by Treatment with Ganciclovir Leads to Significant Antitumor Effects in Murine Ovarian Cancer-bearing Mice

We further determined if MOSEC tumor-bearing mice infected with HPV-16/HSV-tk psV followed by treatment with ganciclovir could exhibit therapeutic antitumor effects. The mice were injected with MOSEC-Luc tumor cells and then treated with HPV-16/HSV-tk psV or HPV-16/GFP psV using regimen as described in **Figure 5**. The mice were subsequently treated with ganciclovir and tumor growth was monitored using a luminescence imaging system. As shown in **Figure 5**, tumor-bearing mice treated with HPV-16/HSV-tk psV followed by treatment with ganciclovir exhibited significantly better therapeutic antitumor effects than mice treated with HPV-16/GFP psV followed by treatment with ganciclovir. These data indicate HPV-16 pseudovirion can be used to effectively deliver the HSV-tk gene to ovarian tumor cells to render ovarian tumor cells more susceptible to treatment with ganciclovir.

Discussion

The successful employment of the HSV-tk gene for ovarian cancer gene therapy using HPV pseudovirions suggests that other suitable candidate genes may also be delivered by HPV pseudovirion to ovarian tumors for ovarian cancer gene therapy. Several candidate genes for enzyme-prodrug combinations for suicide gene therapy have been reported including cytosine deaminase [18,19], nitroreductase [20], carboxylesterase [21], cytochrome p450 [22] and purine nucleoside phosphorylase [23]. Like HSV-tk, the enzymes encoded by these genes can convert the nontoxic prodrugs into drugs capable of blocking DNA synthesis, resulting in eventual cell death as well as bystander effects to kill additional neighboring tumor cells.

For future clinical translation, it will be important to consider safety concerns of both the HSV-tk/GCV system and the delivery vehicle. However, cancer gene therapy using HSV-tk has been extensively used. Many clinical trials using this approach have been conducted in patients with gliomas and no serious adverse events were reported (for review see [24,25]). On the other hand, production of the HPV pseudovirion as DNA delivery vehicles will likely require further developments to improve its safety profile. The current cell line used for generating the pseudovirions contains SV40 large T antigen, which is an oncoprotein, and therefore raises some possible safety concerns. An alternative approach using yeast to produce pseudovirions has been described [26]. The mass production of HPV pseudovirions will also likely require efficient standardized protocols to generate large titers of infectious HPV pseudovirions for clinical translation.

In the current study, we demonstrated preferential infection of murine and human ovarian tumors by HPV-16 pseudovirion. Our findings are consistent with previous studies by Roberts et al. using a nude mouse model for peritoneal dissemination of human ovarian cancer cell line, SHIN3 [27]. They also found that HPV pseudovirion administered intraperitoneally infected ovarian tumor tissues with high specificity while skipping the normal peritoneal tissue surfaces. However, different types of HPV pseudovirion may demonstrate different tumor and/or tissue tropisms. For example, Cerio et al, have shown that an HPV-16, but not HPV-45, pseudovirus could infect SWA-G human ovarian tumor cells *in vitro* [28]. Their data suggest that pseudovirus infection of human tumors may be HPV type- and tumor-specific. Thus, it is important to further identify the right types of HPV pseudovirion for future cancer gene therapy.

The mechanisms for the preferential infection of the ovarian tumor cells by HPV pseudovirions remain unclear. In our study, we showed that an intact L2 is essential for the infectivity of HPV-16 pseudovirion in ovarian tumors (see **Figure 2**). HPV entry to target cells has been shown to be initiated by first binding to heparin sulfonated proteoglycan (HSPG) cell surface attachment factors. The HPV viral particles then undergo a conformational change that exposes the N-terminus of L2 minor capsid protein to furin cleavage [29,30]. The proteolysis of L2 exposes a previously occluded surface of L1 that binds to a currently undetermined cell surface receptor on cells, which is believed to be responsible for particle internalization (for review see [31]). It has also been shown that most ovarian cancer cell lines upregulate furin expression [32]. Thus, it is conceivable that the upregulation of furin expression may contribute to the preferential infection of the ovarian tumor by HPV pseudovirions. We can also exclude the possibility that preferential infection is an artifact of passaging the tumor cells *in vitro* since preferential infection was observed in the spontaneously occurring ovarian tumor model (see **Figure 3**). It will be important to further characterize the mechanisms for the preferential infection of the ovarian tumor cells by HPV pseudovirions. Such information will be useful for improving the specific delivery of gene of interest to ovarian tumor cells using HPV pseudovirions.

In summary, we found that intraperitoneal injection of HPV-16 pseudovirions leads to preferential infection of murine and human ovarian cancer cells in tumor-bearing mice. Furthermore, cancer gene therapy using HPV pseudovirions carrying HSV-tk was capable of specifically targeting the ovarian tumors, resulting potent therapeutic antitumor effects against ovarian tumors. It will be important to further identify the most suitable gene therapy candidates and therapeutic regimens for future studies towards clinical translation.

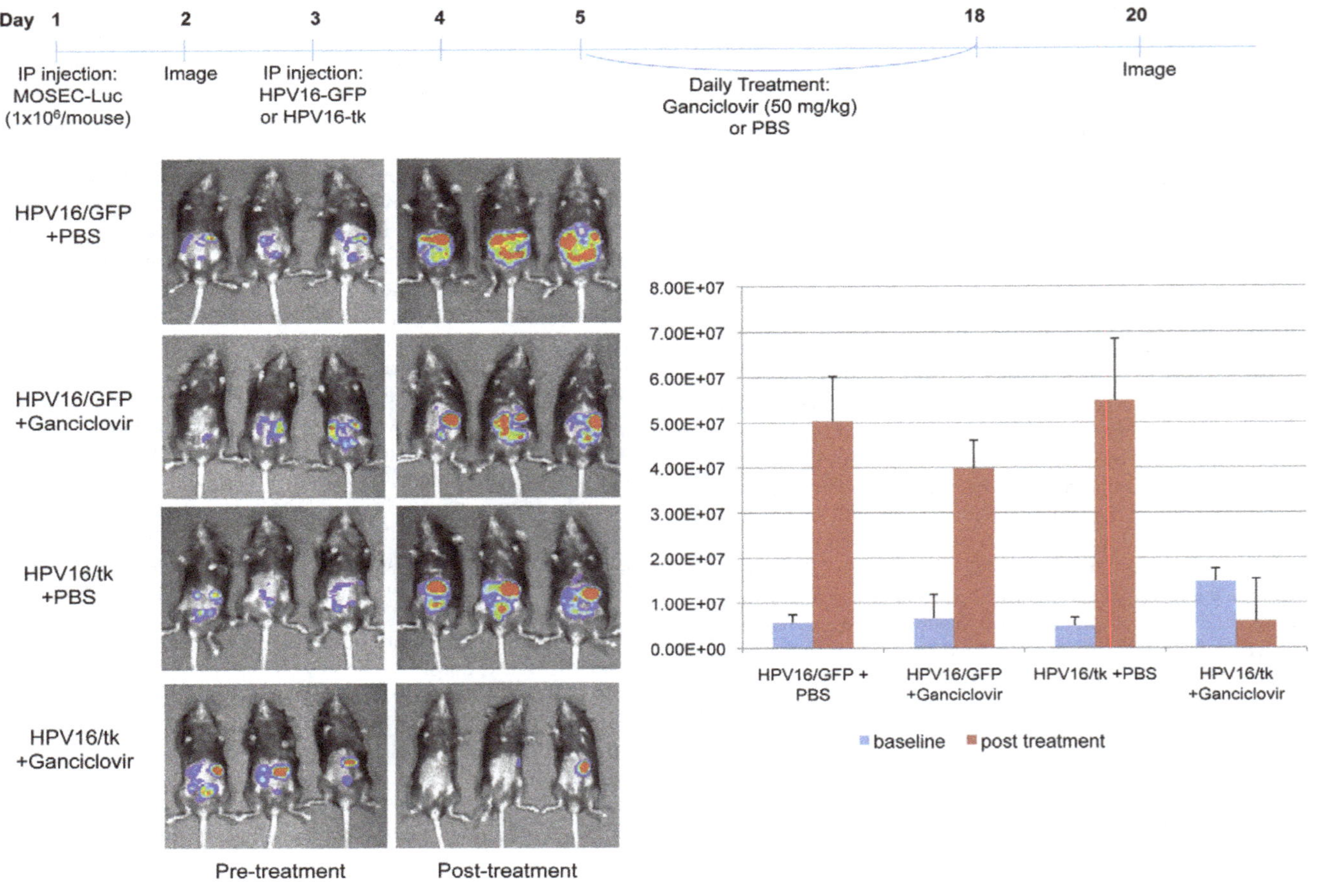

Figure 5. *In vivo* cytotoxicity mediated by HPV16-tk pseudovirions and ganciclovir. C57BL/6 mice (5 per group) were intraperitoneally injected with 1×10^6 MOSEC-Luc cells per mouse on day 1. Luciferase activity was examined on day 2 as indication of number of tumors in the mice. Mice were injected HPV16-GFP psV (L1 protein 20 μg) or HPV16/HSV-tk psV at a dose of L1 protein (20 μg/mouse) on day 3. Mice were treated daily with ganciclovir at a dose of 50 mg/kg or PBS from day 5 to day 18. Mice were imaged by non-invasive luminescence imaging techniques on day 20. Data shown are representative of 2 experiments performed.

Supporting Information

Figure S1 Characterization of the infection of MOSEC tumor cells by HPV-16 pseudovirions *in vitro*. MOSEC cells were seeded into 96-well plates at a density of 5,000 cell/well the night before infection. The seeded MOSEC cells were then infected with HPV-16/Luc psV (1 μg L1 protein/ml) for 72 hours and luciferase expression was examined by the IVIS 200 system (Xenogen Corp., Alameda, CA, USA). Luminescence images of MOSEC ovarian cancer cell line (top). Bar graph depicting the total photon counts for each well (bottom). Note: HPV-16 pseudovirions can efficiently infect MOSEC mouse ovarian cancer *in vitro*. Data shown are representative of 2 experiments performed.

Figure S2 Characterization of the infection of ES2 human ovarian cancer cells by HPV-16 pseudovirions *in vitro*. ES2 human ovarian tumor cells were seeded into 96-well plates at a density of 5,000 cells/well the night before infection. The seeded ES2 cells were then infected with HPV-16/Luc psV (1 μg L1 protein/ml) for 72 hours and luciferase expression was examined by IVIS 200 system (Xenogen Corp., Alameda, CA, USA). Luminescence images of ES2 ovarian cancer cell line (top). Bar graph depicting the total photon counts for each well (bottom). Note: HPV-16 pseudovirions can efficiently infect ES2 human ovarian cancer in vitro. Data shown are representative of 2 experiments performed.

Figure S3 *In vitro* cytotoxicity mediated by HPV16-tk pseudovirions and ganciclovir. ES2-Luc cells were infected HPV16-GFP psV or HPV16/HSV-tk psV at a concentration of 1 μg L1 protein/ml for 48 hours. The infected cells were seeded in 96 well plates and then treated with 0 μg/ml, 0.1 μg/ml, 1 μg/ml, or 10 μg/ml of Ganciclovir for 72 hours. Luciferase expression was examined by the IVIS 200 system (Xenogen Corp., Alameda, CA, USA). Data shown are representative of 2 experiments performed.

Acknowledgments

We would like to thank Katherine Liu (JHMI) for the preparation of the manuscript.

Author Contributions

Conceived and designed the experiments: CFH THK RRR TCW. Performed the experiments: AJC HHT. Analyzed the data: CFH MGP RRR TCW. Wrote the paper: CFH RRR TCW. Edited the manuscript: CFH RRR TCW.

References

1. Greenlee RT, Murray T, Bolden S, Wingo PA (2000) Cancer statistics, 2000. CA: a cancer journal for clinicians 50: 7–33.
2. Jemal A, Siegel R, Ward E, Murray T, Xu J, et al. (2006) Cancer statistics, 2006. CA: a cancer journal for clinicians 56: 106–130.
3. Schwartz PE (2002) Current diagnosis and treatment modalities for ovarian cancer. Cancer treatment and research 107: 99–118.
4. Altaner C (2008) Prodrug cancer gene therapy. Cancer letters 270: 191–201.
5. Morgan RA (2012) Live and Let Die: A New Suicide Gene Therapy Moves to the Clinic. Molecular Therapy 20: 11–13.
6. Moolten FL (1986) Tumor chemosensitivity conferred by inserted herpes thymidine kinase genes: paradigm for a prospective cancer control strategy. Cancer research 46: 5276–5281.
7. Peng S, Monie A, Kang TH, Hung CF, Roden R, et al. (2010) Efficient delivery of DNA vaccines using human papillomavirus pseudovirions. Gene therapy 17: 1453–1464.
8. Gordon SN, Kines RC, Kutsyna G, Ma ZM, Hryniewicz A, et al. (2012) Targeting the vaginal mucosa with human papillomavirus pseudovirion vaccines delivering simian immunodeficiency virus DNA. Journal of immunology 188: 714–723.
9. Peng S, Ma B, Chen SH, Hung CF, Wu T (2011) DNA vaccines delivered by human papillomavirus pseudovirions as a promising approach for generating antigen-specific CD8+ T cell immunity. Cell & bioscience 1: 26.
10. Connolly DC, Bao R, Nikitin AY, Stephens KC, Poole TW, et al. (2003) Female mice chimeric for expression of the simian virus 40 TAg under control of the MISIIR promoter develop epithelial ovarian cancer. Cancer research 63: 1389–1397.
11. Buck CB, Pastrana DV, Lowy DR, Schiller JT (2004) Efficient intracellular assembly of papillomaviral vectors. Journal of virology 78: 751–757.
12. Roby KF, Taylor CC, Sweetwood JP, Cheng Y, Pace JL, et al. (2000) Development of a syngeneic mouse model for events related to ovarian cancer. Carcinogenesis 21: 585–591.
13. Hung CF, Calizo R, Tsai YC, He L, Wu TC (2007) A DNA vaccine encoding a single-chain trimer of HLA-A2 linked to human mesothelin peptide generates anti-tumor effects against human mesothelin-expressing tumors. Vaccine 25: 127–135.
14. Gambhira R, Jagu S, Karanam B, Day PM, Roden R (2009) Role of L2 cysteines in papillomavirus infection and neutralization. Virology journal 6: 176.
15. Hung CF, Cheng WF, Hsu KF, Chai CY, He L, et al. (2001) Cancer immunotherapy using a DNA vaccine encoding the translocation domain of a bacterial toxin linked to a tumor antigen. Cancer research 61: 3698–3703.
16. Lu D, Hoory T, Monie A, Wu A, Wang MC, et al. (2009) Treatment with demethylating agent, 5-aza-2′-deoxycytidine enhances therapeutic HPV DNA vaccine potency. Vaccine 27: 4363–4369.
17. Campos SK, Ozbun MA (2009) Two highly conserved cysteine residues in HPV16 L2 form an intramolecular disulfide bond and are critical for infectivity in human keratinocytes. PLoS ONE 4: e4463.
18. Trinh QT, Austin EA, Murray DM, Knick VC, Huber BE (1995) Enzyme/prodrug gene therapy: comparison of cytosine deaminase/5-fluorocytosine versus thymidine kinase/ganciclovir enzyme/prodrug systems in a human colorectal carcinoma cell line. Cancer research 55: 4808–4812.
19. Hanna NN, Mauceri HJ, Wayne JD, Hallahan DE, Kufe DW, et al. (1997) Virally directed cytosine deaminase/5-fluorocytosine gene therapy enhances radiation response in human cancer xenografts. Cancer research 57: 4205–4209.
20. Bridgewater JA, Springer CJ, Knox RJ, Minton NP, Michael NP, et al. (1995) Expression of the bacterial nitroreductase enzyme in mammalian cells renders them selectively sensitive to killing by the prodrug CB1954. European journal of cancer 31A: 2362–2370.
21. Danks MK, Morton CL, Pawlik CA, Potter PM (1998) Overexpression of a rabbit liver carboxylesterase sensitizes human tumor cells to CPT-11. Cancer research 58: 20–22.
22. Waxman DJ, Chen L, Hecht JE, Jounaidi Y (1999) Cytochrome P450-based cancer gene therapy: recent advances and future prospects. Drug metabolism reviews 31: 503–522.
23. Sorscher EJ, Peng S, Bebok Z, Allan PW, Bennett LL, Jr., et al. (1994) Tumor cell bystander killing in colonic carcinoma utilizing the Escherichia coli DeoD gene to generate toxic purines. Gene therapy 1: 233–238.
24. McCormick F (2001) Cancer gene therapy: fringe or cutting edge? Nature reviews Cancer 1: 130–141.
25. Pulkkanen KJ, Yla-Herttuala S (2005) Gene therapy for malignant glioma: current clinical status. Molecular therapy : the journal of the American Society of Gene Therapy 12: 585–598.
26. Rossi JL, Gissmann L, Jansen K, Muller M (2000) Assembly of human papillomavirus type 16 pseudovirions in Saccharomyces cerevisiae. Human Gene Therapy 11: 1165–1176.
27. Roberts JN, Kines R, Thompson CD, Buck C, Hama Y, et al. (2007) Tropism of HPV pseudoviruses for epithelial surfaces and cancer-derived lines: implications for cytotoxic gene therapy. 24th International Papillomavirus Conference and Clinical Workshop, Beijing, China Abstract 2A-01.
28. Cerio R, Roberts JN, Lowy DR, Schiller JT (2010) HPV pseudoviruses as gene delivery vectors for murine tumors and human ovarian tumor xenografts. 26th International Papillomavirus Conference, Montreal, Canada Abstract P-215.
29. Day PM, Gambhira R, Roden RB, Lowy DR, Schiller JT (2008) Mechanisms of human papillomavirus type 16 neutralization by l2 cross-neutralizing and l1 type-specific antibodies. J Virol 82: 4638–4646.
30. Richards RM, Lowy DR, Schiller JT, Day PM (2006) Cleavage of the papillomavirus minor capsid protein, L2, at a furin consensus site is necessary for infection. Proceedings of the National Academy of Sciences of the United States of America 103: 1522–1527.
31. Schiller JT, Day PM, Kines RC (2010) Current understanding of the mechanism of HPV infection. Gynecologic oncology 118: S12–17.
32. Page RE, Klein-Szanto AJ, Litwin S, Nicolas E, Al-Jumaily R, et al. (2007) Increased expression of the pro-protein convertase furin predicts decreased survival in ovarian cancer. Cellular oncology : the official journal of the International Society for Cellular Oncology 29: 289–299.

8

MicroRNA-Restricted Transgene Expression in the Retina

Marianthi Karali[1]ᵠ, Anna Manfredi[1]ᵠ, Agostina Puppo[1], Elena Marrocco[1], Annagiusi Gargiulo[1], Mariacarmela Allocca[1], Michele Della Corte[5], Settimio Rossi[5], Massimo Giunti[4], Maria Laura Bacci[4], Francesca Simonelli[1,5], Enrico Maria Surace[1], Sandro Banfi[1,3]*, Alberto Auricchio[1,2]*

1 Telethon Institute of Genetics and Medicine (TIGEM), Naples, Italy, **2** Medical Genetics, Department of Pediatrics, University of Naples Federico II, Naples, Italy, **3** Medical Genetics, Department of General Pathology, Second University of Naples, Naples, Italy, **4** Department of Veterinary Medical Science (DSMVET), University of Bologna, Bologna, Italy, **5** Department of Ophthalmology, Second University of Naples, Naples, Italy

Abstract

Background: Gene transfer using adeno-associated viral (AAV) vectors has been successfully applied in the retina for the treatment of inherited retinal dystrophies. Recently, microRNAs have been exploited to fine-tune transgene expression improving therapeutic outcomes. Here we evaluated the ability of retinal-expressed microRNAs to restrict AAV-mediated transgene expression to specific retinal cell types that represent the main targets of common inherited blinding conditions.

Methodology/Principal Findings: To this end, we generated AAV2/5 vectors expressing *EGFP* and containing four tandem copies of miR-124 or miR-204 complementary sequences in the 3′UTR of the transgene expression cassette. These vectors were administered subretinally to adult C57BL/6 mice and Large White pigs. Our results demonstrate that miR-124 and miR-204 target sequences can efficiently restrict AAV2/5-mediated transgene expression to retinal pigment epithelium and photoreceptors, respectively, in mice and pigs. Interestingly, transgene restriction was observed at low vector doses relevant to therapy.

Conclusions: We conclude that microRNA-mediated regulation of transgene expression can be applied in the retina to either restrict to a specific cell type the robust expression obtained using ubiquitous promoters or to provide an additional layer of gene expression regulation when using cell-specific promoters.

Editor: Arto Urtti, University of Helsinki, Finland

Funding: This work was supported by the Fondazione Telethon, the Italian Ministry of Health and the European Commission grants "AAVEYE" (HEALTH-2007-B-223445) and "TREATRUSH" (HEALTH-F2-2010-242013) under the 7th Framework Programme. MK acknowledges financial support by a Marie Curie European Re-integration Grant (grant n. PERG03-GA-2008-231068). The funders had no role in study design, data collection and analysis, decision to publish, or preparation of the manuscript.

Competing Interests: The authors have declared that no competing interests exist.

* E-mail: auricchio@tigem.it (AA); banfi@tigem.it (SB)

ᵠ These authors contributed equally to this work.

Introduction

MicroRNAs (miRNAs) are a class of small 20–25-nucleotide long non-coding RNAs that negatively regulate expression of their target genes by binding to specific sequence elements in the 3′ untranslated region (UTR) of their respective mRNAs [1]. MiRNAs predominantly act to decrease target mRNA levels in animal cells [1] and at least one third of them are expressed in a cell type- or developmental-specific manner [2]. Only recently, endogenous miRNAs have been exploited for the tight post-transcriptional regulation of exogenously delivered (trans)genes in therapeutic and experimental applications [3]. Incorporation of target sites for a specific miRNA (miRTs) at the 3′ end of a transgene cassette has been adapted to provide a means of restricting transgene expression domains to specific cell types, lineages or differentiation states [4,5,6,7,8]. This strategy is particularly useful to further improve transgene specificity, when combined with the transcriptional targeting provided by tissue-specific promoters. A detailed knowledge of the cellular and developmental distribution of miRNAs is a major requisite towards the implementation of this strategy. In one of the first therapeutic applications of this approach, Brown and colleagues [9] combined an hepatocyte-specific promoter with target sequences for a hematopoietic-specific miRNA in a lentiviral-based vector to abolish the immune response generated by the off-target expression of clotting factor IX in the antigen-presenting cells (APCs) of Hemophilia B (ΔF.IX) mice. The dynamic expression of miRNAs has also been exploited to ensure an appropriate restriction of transgene expression across development [10].

Inherited retinal degenerations (IRDs) are a group of conditions that result from mutations in genes encoding proteins with critical functions in retinal pigment epithelium (RPE) or photoreceptor (PR) cells and lead to severe visual deficits and ultimately to blindness [11]. IRDs can greatly benefit from gene therapy using adeno-associated virus (AAV)-derived vectors that transduce non-dividing cells and result in long-term transgene expression [12]. The safety and efficacy of AAV-based gene therapy has been verified in various animal models [13] and in humans [14,15,16,17,18,19,20,21]. Recently, AAV2-mediated gene transfer of *RPE65* in patients affected with Leber's Congenital Amaurosis (LCA, type 2; OMIM 204100) achieved stable improvement of visual and retinal function [14,15,16,17,18, 19,20,21].

Tight spatial and temporal control of transgene expression is desirable in the context of gene therapy. In IRDs, gene transfer should be ideally targeted to either RPE or PRs. This can be in part achieved by selecting the appropriate AAV serotype, as AAVs show variable kinetics of transgene expression and differential tropism for a broad range of ocular cell types [22]. Specificity of transgene expression in the retina can be further enhanced using RPE- or photoreceptor-specific promoter elements [23,24]. However, very often the tissue-specific promoters used in gene therapy vectors do not faithfully recapitulate the patterns of the endogenous promoter. In addition, the levels of transgene expression obtained may either be inadequate for therapeutic purposes or supra-physiological and deleterious for retinal function.

With this study, we aimed to improve controlled transgene expression in the retina by exploiting the post-transcriptional regulation offered by the endogenous miRNA machinery. To this end, we integrated our knowledge on the cellular distribution of miRNAs within the mouse eye [25,26] with the use AAV-mediated strategies for gene transfer to the retina [22]. Here we describe the first paradigm of harnessing retinal-specific miRNAs to delimit transgene expression to the RPE monolayer or the PRs of the adult retina using AAV vectors. We show that efficient restriction of transgene expression can be obtained even at low vector dosages. These findings have implications for the design of gene therapy approaches for hereditary retinopathies as they may improve safety and efficacy of gene transfer.

Results

Use of miR-204 target sites restricts transgene expression to murine PRs *in vivo*

We sought to assess whether post-transcriptional restriction of AAV-mediated transgene expression to PRs could be achieved by exploiting endogenous miRNAs. For this purpose we selected miR-204, a miRNA that is strongly expressed in the RPE from as early as E10.5 to adulthood [25,26] (**Figure 1a**). miR-204 expression was absent from the PRs and was detected by *in situ* hybridization (ISH) at low levels in the inner nuclear layer of the neural retina as well in the ganglion cell layer [26] (**Figure 1a**).

Based on the miR-204 expression pattern in the adult murine retina, we inserted four copies of a sequence that is perfectly complementary to the mature miR-204 (miR204T) immediately downstream of the Woodchuck hepatitis virus Post-transcriptional Regulatory Element (WPRE) in the pAAV2.1-CMV-*EGFP* plasmid (**Figure 1b**; see Materials and Methods). The presence in this plasmid of the ubiquitous CMV promoter drives robust transgene expression in both RPE and PRs [27,28]. The resulting pAAV2.1-CMV-*EGFP*-4xmiR204T plasmid (**Figure 1b**) was used to produce AAV2/5 vectors that efficiently transduce RPE and PRs upon subretinal administration in several species, including mice [29]. Four-week-old C57BL/6 mice (n = 4) were injected with 2.6×10^9 genome copies (GC) (defined as "high dose") of AAV2/5-CMV-*EGFP*-4xmiR204T in one eye, and the same dose of AAV2/5-CMV-*EGFP* as control in the contralateral one. Four weeks after injection, eyes were harvested, retinas were sectioned and retinal sections were analyzed by direct fluorescence microscopy to assess localization of EGFP expression.

The number of EGFP-positive RPE cells in the eyes injected with AAV2/5-CMV-*EGFP*-4xmiR204T (**Figures 2c,d**) was dramatically reduced, compared to contralateral eyes injected with AAV2/5-CMV-*EGFP* (**Figures 2a,b**), indicating efficient suppression of the *EGFP*-miR204T mRNA by endogenous miR-204. Despite the strong reduction of EGFP expression in the RPE, occasional EGFP-positive RPE cells were detected (red arrows in **Figures 2c,d**). We hypothesized that loss of miR-204-mediated regulation in these EGFP-positive RPE cells could result from the saturation of the miRNA activity due to an excess of exogenous miR204Ts. To indirectly test this, we used a 10-fold lower vector dose (2.6×10^8 GC/eye; defined as "low dose"). Analysis of EGFP fluorescence in the low-dose group (n = 4) showed specific restriction of transgene expression to the PRs, while no EGFP expression could be detected within the RPE in any of the sections from the four eyes injected with the miR204T-containing vector (**Figures 2e,f**).

Use of miR-124 target sites restricts transgene expression to murine RPE *in vivo*

To restrict AAV2/5-CMV-mediated transgene expression to the RPE, we exploited miR-124, a miRNA abundantly expressed in differentiated neurons [30]. We and others have shown by ISH that miR-124 stains strongly all retinal cell layers, but is not detected in the RPE [26,31] (**Figure 1a**). Therefore, we cloned four tandem copies of a sequence that is perfectly complementary to the mature miR-124 downstream of the WPRE element in the pAAV2.1-CMV-*EGFP* plasmid (**Figure 1b**). The resulting pAAV2.1-CMV-*EGFP*-4xmiR124T plasmid was used to produce AAV2/5 vectors that were administered to C57BL/6 mice by subretinal injection. Mice (n = 4) received 2.6×10^9 GC (defined as "high dose") of AAV2/5-CMV-*EGFP*-4xmiR124T in one eye, and the same dose of the AAV2/5-CMV-*EGFP* as control in the contralateral one. The animals were sacrificed four weeks after injection. Reporter expression in the transduced retina was evaluated by fluorescence microscopy of retinal sections.

We observed a dramatic reduction in the number of EGFP-positive PRs in eyes injected with the AAV2/5-CMV-*EGFP*-4xmiR124T (**Figures 2g,h**) compared to eyes injected with the control vector (**Figures 2a,b**), suggesting efficient elimination of the miRT-containing transcript by the endogenous miR-124. However, similarly to what observed with the miR204T-containing construct, few scattered EGFP-positive PR cells could be seen in the neural retina (red arrows in **Figures 2g,h**), which implies loss of miRNA-mediated regulation therein. EGFP expression in these cells could result from the saturation of miRNA activity due to an excess of exogenously provided miR124Ts. We then tested a 10-fold decrement in vector dose to assess if off-target expression of the miRT-containing transcript in the transduced PRs would be eliminated. C57BL/6 mice (n = 4) were injected with 2.6×10^8 GC/eye of either virus, and their eyes were analyzed four weeks after injection. We did not observe any EGFP-positive cells in the neural retina of eyes administered with the low dose of AAV2/5-CMV-*EGFP*-4xmiR124T (**Figures 2i,j**), suggesting that at this dose, the presence of the miR124Ts tightly restricts transgene expression to the RPE.

Finally, to exclude that the presence of exogenous miRNA target sequences can interfere with the physiological function of the PRs, we performed electroretinograms (ERG) on mice injected at a high dose (2.6×10^9 GC/eye) with the AAV2/5 vectors harboring the miR-124 or miR-204 target sequences and the control *EGFP* construct. ERG recordings of eyes injected with the miRT-bearing vectors showed no statistically significant differences compared to eyes injected with the *EGFP* control [max a-wave amplitude: EGFP = 336,18 µV (±67,06); miR124T = 350,97 (±132,11) µV; miR204T = 320,70 (±105,09) µV; max b-wave

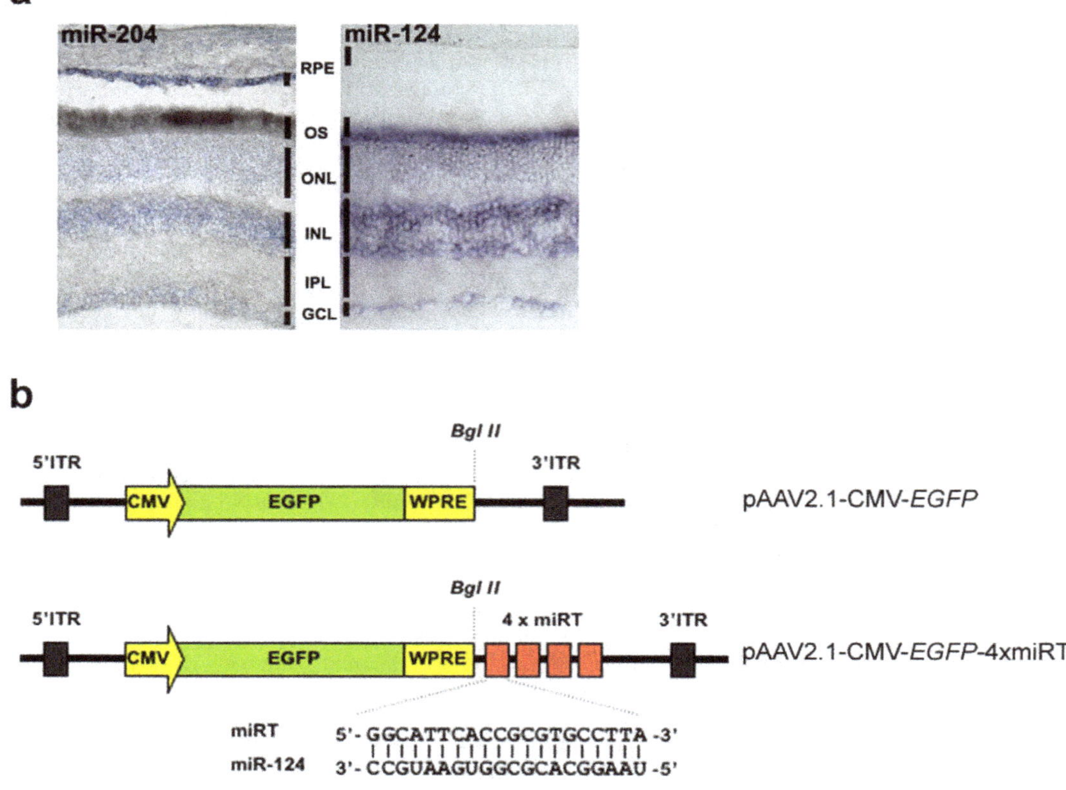

Figure 1. miR-124 and miR-204 expression in retina supports the use of AAV vectors harboring corresponding miRTs. (**a**) Expression profile of miR-204 and miR-124 in retina sections of adult, albino (CD1) mouse as revealed by ISH using LNA-modified probes. miR-124, a neuronal-specific miRNA, is expressed in all layers of the neural retina but is not detected in the RPE. miR-204 is expressed in the GCL and the INL of the neural retina and stains strongly the RPE. RNA ISH for the detection of mature miRNAs was performed using miRCURY LNA™ microRNA Detection Probes (Exiqon, Vedbaek, Denmark) as previously described [26]. (**b**) Schematic representation of the AAV vectors harboring the miRT sites. Four tandem copies (4xmiRT) of a sequence perfectly complementary to the sequence of the mature miR-124 or miR-204 (see alignments) were cloned downstream of the WPRE element in the pAAV2.1-CMV-*EGFP* plasmid. Abbreviations are as follows: CMV, Human Cytomegalovirus promoter; EGFP, Enhanced Green Fluorescence Protein; GCL, Ganglion Cell Layer; INL, Inner Nuclear Layer; IPL, Inner Plexiform Layer; ITR, Inverted Terminal Repeat; miRT, miRNA target site; ONL, Photoreceptor Outer Nuclear Layer; OS, Photoreceptor Outer Segments; RPE, Retinal Pigment Epithelium; WPRE, Woodchuck hepatitis virus Post-transcriptional Regulatory Element.

amplitude: EGFP = 667,83 (±165,47) μV; miR124T = 598,18 (±90,28) μV; miR204T = 690,83 (±143,96) μV].

miRNA-regulation of transgene expression in the porcine retina

We extended our studies to the pig (*Sus scrofa*) as, among non-primate mammals, the porcine retina most closely resembles the human one in terms of size, anatomy, cellular composition and physiology, rendering it a valuable preclinical model system for eye disease and therapy [32]. The mature sequence of miR-124 and miR-204 is identical in pigs and mouse (miRBase, http://www.mirbase.org/; [33]). Given the highly conserved cellular distribution of these two miRNAs across species [26,34,35], we assumed that miR-124 and miR-204 are likely to be expressed in the same porcine retinal layers.

We injected subretinally eleven week-old Large White (LW) female pigs (n = 2 eyes/group) with AAV2/5-CMV-*EGFP*-4xmiR204T and AAV2/5-CMV-*EGFP*-4xmiR124T and compared them with eyes injected with the AAV2/5-CMV-*EGFP* as control. Considering the size proportions of murine and porcine eyes, the dose administered in pigs was equivalent to the low dose injected in mouse (in the mouse eye we administered 1 μl containing 2.6×10^8 GC, in the pig eye 100 μl of a 1:2.6 dilution of the same vector solution, thus containing 1×10^{10} GC). Retinal sections were analyzed, following animal sacrifice six weeks after injection. As shown in Figure 3, the use of target sequences for miR-204 (**Figures 3c,d**) and miR-124 (**Figures 3e,f**) efficiently restricted AAV2/5 mediated *EGFP* expression to the PRs and RPE of the porcine retina, respectively.

Cones are important targets of gene therapy since several blinding conditions, either inherited as monogenic or as complex traits, are due to mutations in genes expressed in cones or are characterized by progressive cone degeneration [36]. Since the porcine retina has a high number of cones compared to the murine one [37], we checked whether both rod and cone PRs were equally transduced following AAV2/5-mediated delivery. Expression of EGFP in cone PRs was confirmed by immunolabelling of porcine retinal sections with the Cone Arrestin antibody

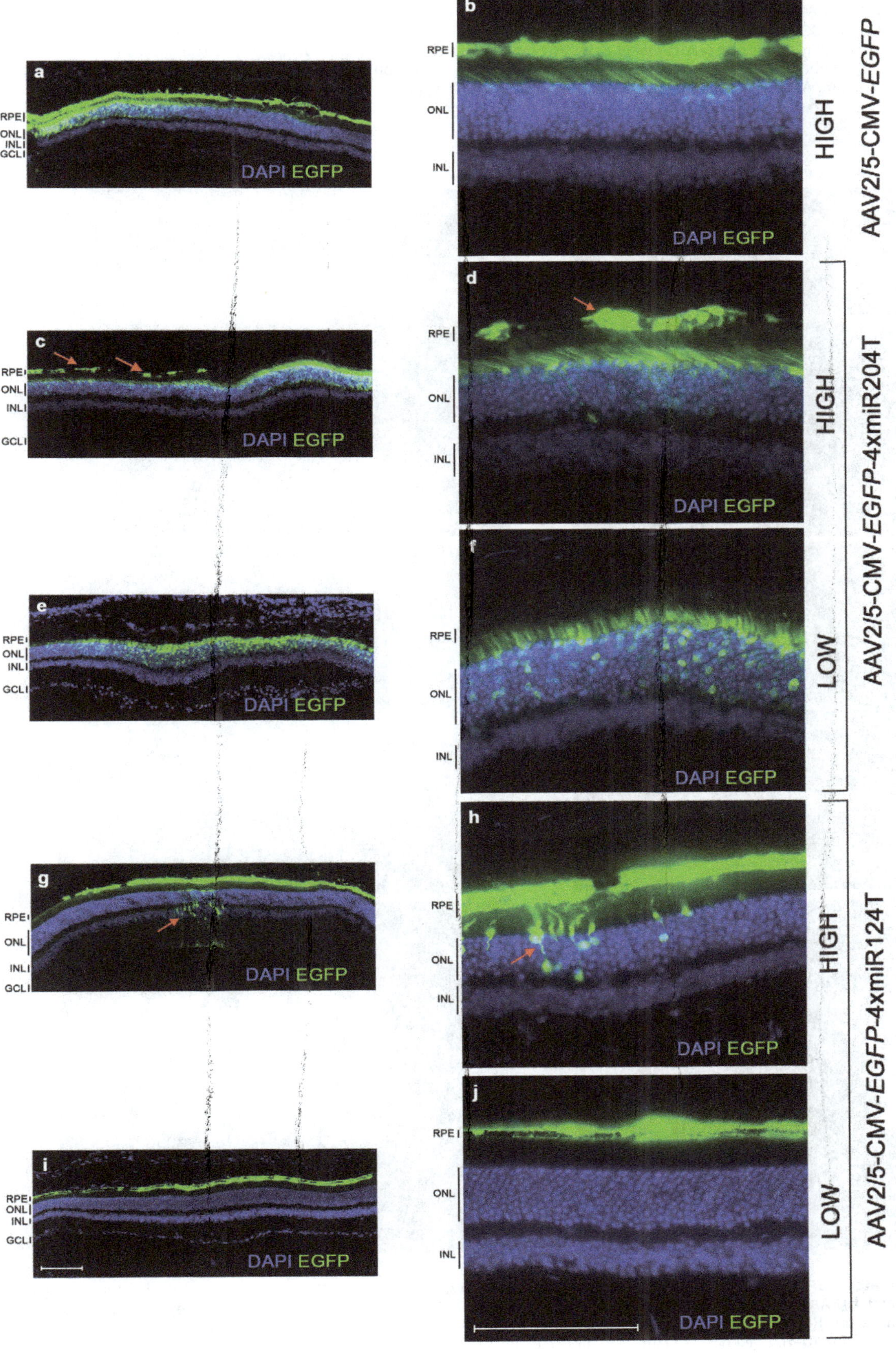
a
RPE
ONL
INL
GCL
DAPI EGFP
b
RPE
ONL
INL
DAPI EGFP
HIGH
AAV2/5-CMV-EGFP
c
RPE
ONL
INL
GCL
DAPI EGFP
d
RPE
ONL
INL
DAPI EGFP
HIGH
e
RPE
ONL
INL
GCL
DAPI EGFP
f
RPE
ONL
INL
DAPI EGFP
LOW
AAV2/5-CMV-EGFP-4xmiR204T
g
RPE
ONL
INL
GCL
DAPI EGFP
h
RPE
ONL
INL
DAPI EGFP
HIGH
i
RPE
ONL
INL
GCL
DAPI EGFP
j
RPE
ONL
INL
DAPI EGFP
LOW
AAV2/5-CMV-EGFP-4xmiR124T

Figure 2. miRNA-regulated *EGFP* expression in the mouse retina. C57BL/6 adult mice (n = 4 eyes/group) were injected subretinally with: 2.6×10^9 GC/eye of AAV2/5-CMV-*EGFP* (**a** and **b**; high dose); 2.6×10^9 GC/eye (**c** and **d**; high dose) or 2.6×10^8 GC/eye (**e** and **f**; low dose) of AAV2/5-CMV-*EGFP*-4xmiR204T; 2.6×10^9 GC/eye (**g** and **h**; high dose) or 2.6×10^8 GC/eye (**i** and **j**; low dose) of AAV2/5-CMV-*EGFP*-4xmiR124T. Mice were sacrificed four weeks after injection, and retinal sections were analyzed by direct fluorescence microscopy. Images at 10X (panels on the left) and 40X magnification (panels on the right) are shown. At high vector doses ectopic EGFP expression (red arrows) was observed in few PR and RPE cells, respectively. Scale bar = 100 μm. Abbreviations: RPE, retinal pigment epithelium; ONL, photoreceptor outer nuclear layer; INL, inner nuclear layer; GCL, ganglion cell layer.

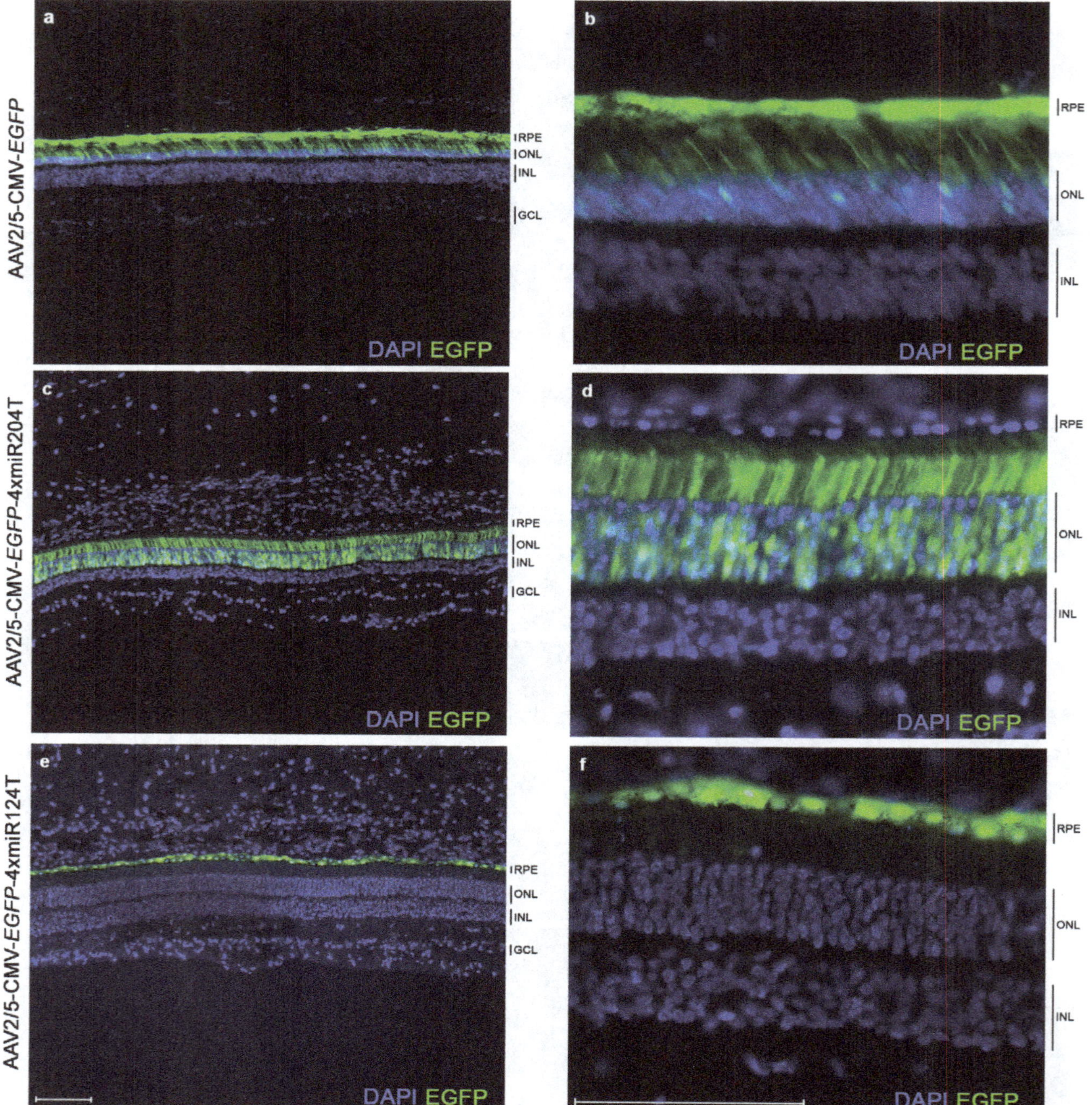

Figure 3. miRNA-regulated *EGFP* expression in the pig retina. Large White (LW) female pigs (n = 2 eyes/group) were injected subretinally with: AAV2/5-CMV-*EGFP* (**a** and **b**); AAV2/5-CMV-*EGFP*-4xmiR204T (**c** and **d**); AAV2/5-CMV-*EGFP*-4xmiR124T (**e** and **f**). All eyes were injected with 1×10^{10} GC/eye of each vector. Retinal cryosections were obtained six weeks after injection and analyzed by direct fluorescence microscopy. Magnification 10X (**a–c**) and 40X (**d–f**). Scale bar = 100 μm. For abbreviations, see Fig. 2 legend.

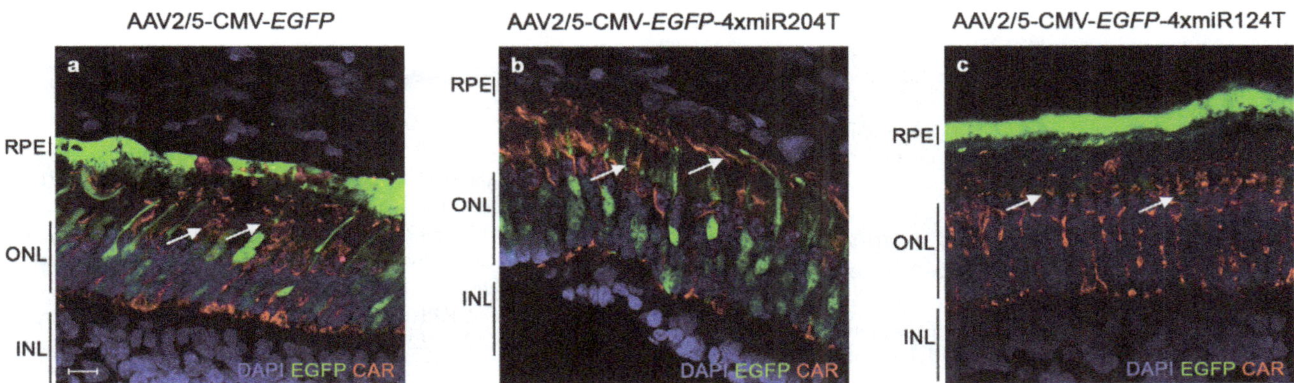

Figure 4. Cone transduction following subretinal administration of AAV vectors bearing miRNA target sites. Retinal cryosections from animals injected subretinally with the various miRNA-regulated vectors as in Fig. 3 were immunolabelled with the cone-specific anti-Cone Arrestin (CAR) antibody (red label). Representative sections of eyes injected with AV2/5-CMV-*EGFP* (**a**), AAV2/5-CMV-*EGFP*-4xmiR204T (**b**) and AAV2/5-CMV-*EGFP*-4xmiR124T (**c**). Colocalization of EGFP and CAR expression is indicated by the arrows. Confocal microscope magnification 63X. Scale bar = 10 μm. For abbreviations, see Fig. 2 legend.

(anti-hCAR) (arrows in **Figure 4**). A weak EGFP fluorescence was detected by confocal microscopy in the PRs of eyes injected with the AAV2/5-CMV-*EGFP*-4xmiR124T (**Figure 4c**).

With the prospect of using this strategy in animal models of inherited retinal degeneration, we included target sequences for miR-204 in an AAV vector encoding the human *AIPL1* gene, mutated in LCA type 4 (OMIM 604393), with the aim to efficiently transfer *AIPL1* to PRs, its main expression site in the retina. We have recently shown that AAV2/8 vectors target murine [27] and porcine PRs [38] more efficiently than AAV2/5. Therefore, we generated an AAV2/8-CMV-*hAIPL1*-4xmiR204T vector. The AAV2/8-CMV-*hAIPL1*-4xmiR204T vector was injected subretinally in two eleven week-old Large White (LW) female pigs along with the control AAV2/8-CMV-*hAIPL1* that lacks the miR-204 target sites in the contralateral eye. The animals were sacrificed six weeks after injection and their eyes were harvested. Retinal cryosections were then analyzed by immunofluorescence with antibodies directed to human, but not porcine, AIPL1 using confocal microscopy. Transgene expression was detected in both PRs and RPE of the porcine retinas injected with the AAV2/8-CMV-*hAIPL1* control vector, while hAIPL1 expression was efficiently restricted to the PRs in retinas injected with the miR204-regulated vector (**Figure 5**).

To assess whether the presence of miRNA target sequences perturbs normal retinal function, ERG recordings were performed on all injected pigs. Both rod and cone isolated and combined

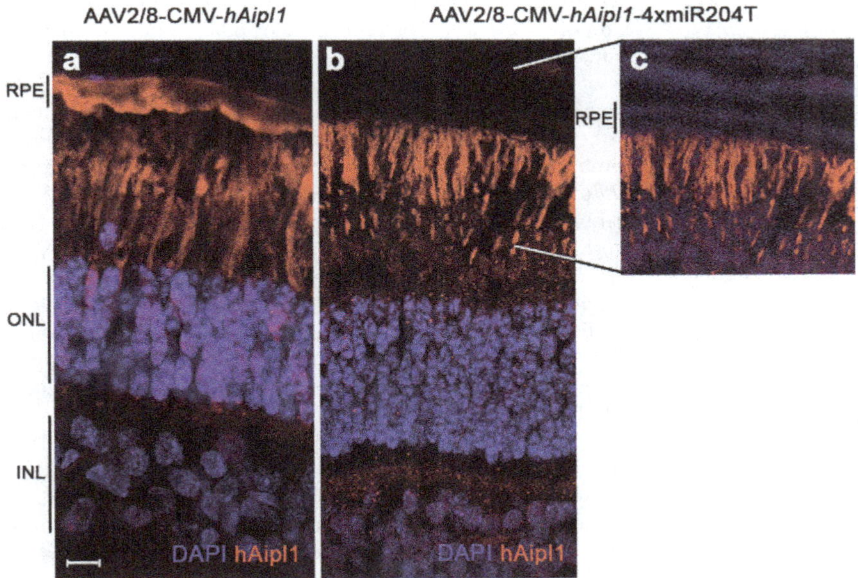

Figure 5. miR204-regulated expression of *hAIPL1* is restricted to the porcine photoreceptors. LW pigs were injected with 1×10^{10} GC/eye with AAV2/8-CMV-*hAIPL1* (**a**) and AAV2/8-CMV-*hAIPL1*-4xmiR204T (**b**) (n = 2 eyes/group). Human AIPL1 immunostaining (red) was performed on pig retinal sections to assess the localization of the transgene expression. The antibody used does not cross-react with the porcine Aipl1. An overexposure of the section in panel (**b**) is shown in (**c**) to highlight that no *hAIPL1* expression was detected in the RPE cells of eyes injected with AAV2/8-CMV-*hAIPL1*-4xmiR204T. Confocal microscope magnification 63X. Scale bar = 10 μm. For abbreviations, see Fig. 2 legend.

responses of treated eyes (n = 2/vector) showed no statistically significant differences compared to baseline measurements [baseline pre-treatment, photopic = 120 (±4,86) μV; scotopic = 44,7 (±0,5) μV and maximal response 196,6 (±9,21) μV; post-treatment, photopic = 130,5 (±5,5) μV; scotopic = 48 (±2,5) μV and maximal 202 (±5) μV] indicating normal retinal function in the injected animals.

Subretinal administrations of AAV vectors harboring miRNA target sites do not significantly perturb endogenous miRNA activity in the eye

As described before, we detected some scattered and discontinuous EGFP-positive areas within the RPE and PR layers (red arrows in **Figures 2c,d,g,h**) of murine retinas injected with high doses (2.6×10^9 GC/eye) of AAV2/5-CMV-*EGFP*-4xmiR204T and AAV2/5-CMV-*EGFP*-4xmiR124T, respectively. We hypothesized that endogenous miRNAs did not completely eliminate the miRT-bearing EGFP transcripts, thus resulting in unexpected EGFP expression. This could be due to miRNA saturation (*i.e.* depletion of levels of the corresponding endogenous miRNA) caused by the presence of an excessive number of exogenously provided miRNA binding sites. Alternatively, the high number of vector-borne miRTs may have elicited a general deregulation of the miRNA/RISC machinery, resulting in a compromised repressive function. When mice were injected with the same vectors at lower doses, we did not detect any ectopic EGFP fluorescence (**Figures 2e,f,i,j**), suggesting that off-target transgene expression was a dosage-dependent phenomenon.

To assess whether expression of exogenous sequences carrying miRTs could interfere with the normal function of the miRNA machinery, we analyzed the endogenous levels of the corresponding miRNAs by qRT-PCR. In particular, we analyzed the expression levels of miR-204 and miR-124, as well as of miR-182. The latter is strongly expressed in the neural retina, predominantly in PRs [25,26], and, to our current knowledge, is unlikely to either be under the direct control of any of the miRNAs tested or have affinity for the miR-204 and miR-124 miRTs. We extracted total RNA either from retinas of AAV2/5-CMV-*EGFP*-4xmiR124T injected mice (n = 4; high dose group) or from the optic cups (including retina, RPE and sclera) of animals injected with AAV2/5-CMV-*EGFP*-4xmiR204T (n = 4; high dose group). As miR-204 is mainly expressed in the RPE and off-target EGFP expression was detected therein, we reasoned that any potential saturation of miR-204 should be assessed in samples that include RPE. We did not observe any significant variation in the endogenous levels of the miRNAs analyzed (**Figure S1a**), implying the absence of a detectable miRNA saturation effect at the level of the whole retinas or optic cups.

To check whether the high number of miRTs could perturb the capacity of miRNAs to regulate their physiological target genes, we analyzed the expression levels of *VAMP3* and *RDH10*, two direct targets of miR-124 [39,40] in retinal samples of animals (n = 4) injected with high doses of either the control AAV2/5-CMV-*EGFP* or the construct bearing the miR-124 binding sites. VAMP3, also known as cellubrevin, is a member of the vesicle-associated membrane protein (VAMP)/synaptobrevin family [41] and is strongly expressed in the retina, according to the BioGPS gene annotation portal (http://biogps.gnf.org/). On the other hand, *RDH10* encodes for retinol dehydrogenase 10 (all-trans) and is primarily expressed in the RPE and the neural retina [42](Mouse Retina SAGE library; [43]). We did not detect any significant variation in the endogenous levels of these target genes (**Figure S1b**), suggesting that the AAV-borne miR124Ts do not interfere with normal miRNA function. Taken together, the above results imply that the exogenously supplied miRTs do not saturate endogenous miRNA levels nor alleviate miRNA repression from its natural targets.

Discussion

Recently, miRNA-mediated regulation of transgene expression has been successfully achieved in the context of somatic gene transfer in specific cell types, lineages or developmental stages [3]. In the present study, we show for the first time that this strategy can be applied to the retina. Subretinal administration of AAV2/5 results in optimal RPE transduction, but also in robust transgene expression in PRs [22]. Here, we demonstrate that subretinal administration of AAV2/5 vectors containing expression cassettes harboring binding sites for miRNAs expressed in specific retinal cell types results in transgene expression tightly restricted to either the RPE or PRs of mice and pigs. In particular, constructs harboring miR-124 binding sites can efficiently de-target reporter expression from the PRs, while the presence of miR-204 sites induces elimination of transgene expression from the RPE. The validation of this approach in the porcine retina confirmed its high clinical potential.

The use of miRNA-regulated vectors can be advantageous in gene therapy for inherited eye diseases: in one instance, when coupled to cell-specific promoters, it adds a layer of regulation to transgene expression. This is desirable as often the promoter elements used in gene therapy vectors do not faithfully recapitulate the expression patterns of the endogenous promoter, probably due to the absence of distant, secondary regulatory elements [9]. For instance, the promoter of *Rhodopsin* - a gene strongly and specifically expressed in rod PRs- induces aberrant reporter expression also in cones [27,44]. In addition, the levels of transgene expression obtained using tissue-specific promoters may not be adequate. For instance, the *Rhodopsin* promoter drives very robust gene expression in PRs. This is not surprising since rhodopsin accounts for more than 70% of PR proteins [45]. While the Rhodopsin promoter element may be desirable if one wants to replace or repress *Rhodopsin* expression, the levels of expression of other transgenes may be supra-physiological or toxic. On the other hand, other retinal-specific promoters, like *RPE65* [23] or *OA1* [46], may provide subtherapeutic levels of transgene expression for some applications in the RPE. Indeed, in one LCA2 clinical trial (ClinicalTrials.gov number, NCT00516477), we have used AAV2/2 vectors expressing *RPE65* from the robust constitutive CBA promoter to obtain therapeutic levels of trangene expression. Assuming that the CBA expression pattern following subretinal administration of AAV2/2 vectors in the human retina is similar to that observed in mice and dogs [47,48], we are presumably misexpressing the *RPE65* in PRs in addition to the RPE. Although this does not appear to be a problem as we did not observe any retinal toxic effect so far [21], ideally we could have tailored *RPE65* expression to RPE if we had included miR-124 target sites in our AAV vector.

A main concern for the application of miRNA-regulated transgene delivery is the potential to saturate their cognate miRNA by exogenously provided miRTs, thus reducing its bioavailability and alleviating control of its natural targets. Interestingly, in all studies that have employed lentiviral platforms for the delivery of miRNA-regulated transgenes, there is no evidence that the excess of exogenously provided miRTs - when engineered according to the principles set for regulated targets [3] - saturates the cognate miRNA [3,4,5,6,9]. Gentner and colleagues showed that only when expression is driven by very strong promoters or when several vector copies are introduced, transgene constructs containing four copies of perfectly complementary miRTs are able to saturate miRNA regulation following lentiviral delivery [49]. In this study, we designed our vectors according to the principles set for regulated targets to prevent miRNA inhibition in the presence of a strong CMV promoter [3]. Indeed, most of the studies applying these parameters report no evidence of miRNA saturation [3]. We observed some scattered, off-target EGFP expression in murine retinas injected with high doses of miRT-bearing vectors, indicative of miRNA inhibition which was not detected when using a ten-fold lower AAV vector dose. However, we did not measure altered levels of neither miRNAs nor their target genes in the retinas treated with high AAV vector doses suggesting that miRNA saturation, if present, occurs at levels below the detection limit of our assay. As an alternative to lowering the dose of viral genome copies administered, the number of miRTs present in the vector construct could be reduced.

The PR- and RPE-restricted pattern of transgene expression at low vector doses was confirmed in the pig retina, which is more similar to the human one in terms of size and anatomy [32]. We can thus expect that a dose similar to the one successfully used in pigs could be applied to humans. Indeed, we have used a similar dose (1.5×10^{10} GC/eye) of AAV2/2 in patients with LCA2 obtaining improvement of visual function [19,20,21]. Our data suggest that administration of low doses of miRT-harboring vectors enables to tailor transgene expression to specific retinal cell types in the absence of off-target effects and deregulation of endogenous miRNA activity.

Ultimately, the efficacy of AAV-mediated miRNA-regulated gene expression in the retina should be proven in animal models of IRDs and, ideally, in non-human primates which possess a cone-enriched macula. Our data suggest that the addition of miRNA target sites to gene therapy vectors enables fine-tuning of transgene expression in the retina possibly rendering gene therapy safer and more efficient.

Materials and Methods

Plasmid construction, AAV vector production and purification

Recombinant AAV vectors containing the EGFP cDNA under the cytomegalovirus (CMV) promoter and four copies of a sequence (referred to as 'miRT') that is perfectly complementary to the miRNAs of interest in the 3′ UTR were constructed by a two-step cloning protocol. Initially, the cassette containing four copies of a sequence which is perfectly complementary to miR-204 (in capital letters) was constructed by annealing the following two sets of oligonucleotides: 5′-ctagatctAGGCATAGGATGACAAAGGGAAcgataggcatAGGATGACAAAGGGAAaagctt-3′, 5′-TTCCCTTTGTCATCCTATGCCTatcgTTCCCTTTGTCATCCTATGCCTAGAT-3′ and 5′-AGGCATAGGATGACAAAGGGAAtcacAGGCATAGGATGACAAAGGGAAagatc-3′, 5′-tcgagatctTCCCTTTGTCATCCTATGCCTgtgaTTCCCTTTGTCATCCTATGCCTaagctt-3′.

Similarly, the cassette containing four copies of a sequence which is perfectly complementary to miR-124 (in capital letters) was constructed by annealing the following two sets of oligonucleotides:

5′-ctagatctGGCATTCACCGCGTGCCTTAcgatGGCATTCACCGCGTGCCTTAaagctt-3′, 5′-TAAGGCACGCGGTGAATGCCatcgTAAGGCACGCGGTGAATGCCagat-3′ and ′-GGCATTCACCGCGTGCCTTAtcacGGCATTCACCGCGTGCCTTAagatc-3′5, 5′-tcgagatctTAAGGCACGCGGTGAATGCCgtgaTAAGGCACGCGGTGAATGCCaagctt-3′. In either case, the resulting double-stranded fragments (each one containing two copies of the respective miRT) were ligated thanks to the presence of phosphorylated 5′ ends. The obtained fragments (containing four copies of the respective miRT) were subcloned in pBluescript II SK(+) previously digested with *Xba* I and *Xho* I. The recombinant clones were digested with *Bgl* II to release the fragment containing the four miRT sites with *Bgl* II protruding ends. The fragment was then cloned into the *Bgl* II site of the pAAV2.1-CMV-*EGFP* plasmid [27] and used for the production of AAV2/5 vectors.

To generate the vectors expressing *hAIPL1*, the coding sequence of the *hAIPL1* gene was amplified from human retina cDNA (BioChain, Hayward, CA) using the primers hAIPL1-NotI-forward (5′-ATATGCGGCCGCCATGGATGCCGCTCTGCTCCT- 3′) and hAIPL1-HindIII-reverse (5′- ACGCGTAAGCTTTTATCAGTGCTGCAGCGAGTGCC- 3′) and cloned into the pAAV2.1-CMV-*EGFP* following digestion with *Not* I and *Hind* III. The final pAAV2.1-CMV-*hAIPL1*-4xmiR204T plasmid was subsequently produced by cloning the fragment containing four miR-204 target sites (released by *Bgl* II digestion of the pAAV2.1-CMV-*EGFP*-4xmiR204T) in the *Bgl* II site of pAAV2.1-CMV-*hAIPL1*.

AAV vectors were produced by triple transfection of 293 cells, purified by two rounds of $CsCl_2$ ultracentrifugation, and titered (in GC/milliliter) using a real-time PCR-based assay TaqMan® (Applied Biosystems, Foster City, CA) and a dot-blot analysis, as previously described [28]. AAV vector production was carried out by the TIGEM AAV vector core.

Animal procedures and vector administration

Ethics Statement. All studies on mice were conducted in strict accordance with the institutional guidelines for animal research and with the Association for Research in Vision and Ophthalmology (ARVO) Statement for the Use of Animal in Ophthalmic and Vision Research. All animal treatments were reviewed and approved in advance by the Ethics Committee of the Centre of Biotechnology, Animal Research Unit, Cardarelli Hospital (Naples, Italy). All procedures on mice were then approved by the Italian Ministry of Health (protocol number: 0000667/11/CB; approval date Sept. 11, 2007).

The experiments involving pigs were conducted according to relevant national and international guidelines. All procedures on pigs were reviewed and approved in advance by the Ethics Committee of the Department of Veterinary Medical Science, University of Bologna (Bologna, Italy) and were then approved by the Italian Ministry of Health (protocol number: 23/2009-B, approval date Feb. 04, 2009). All surgery was performed under anesthesia, and all efforts were made to minimize suffering.

Mice. Four-week old C57BL/6 mice (Harlan, S. Pietro al Natisone, Italy) were anesthetized with an intraperitoneal injection of avertin (1.25% w/v of 2,2,2-tribromoethanol and 2.5% v/v of 2-methyl-2-Butanol; Sigma–Aldrich, St. Louis, MO) at 2 ml/100 g of body weight, and viral vectors were delivered via a trans-scleral transchoroidal approach, as previously described [50]. Mice were injected in the right eye with 2.6×10^9 GC of AAV2/5-CMV-*EGFP*-4xmiRT in the high dose experiments and 2.6×10^8 GC of AAV2/5-CMV-*EGFP*-4xmiRT in the low dose. The same doses of AAV2/5-CMV-*EGFP* were injected in the left eye, as control. Following injection, the extent of transduction was assessed by ophthalmoscopy at days 7 and 28. Eyes were harvested at day 28 after injection.

Pigs. The Large White pigs (LW) used in our study were registered as purebred in the LW Herd Book of the Italian National Pig Breeders' Association. Pigs were starved overnight leaving water *ad libitum*. The anesthetic and surgical procedures for pigs were previously described [38].

Histological analysis

Mice were sacrificed, and their eyeballs were then harvested and fixed overnight by immersion in 4% paraformaldehyde (PFA). Before harvesting the eyeballs, the temporal aspect of the sclerae was marked by cautery in order to orient the eyes with respect to the injection site at the moment of the inclusion. The eyeballs were cut so that the lens and vitreous could be removed leaving the eyecup intact. Mice eyecups were infiltrated with 30% sucrose for cryopreservation, and embedded in tissue freezing medium (O.C.T. matrix, Kaltek, Padua, Italy). For each eye, 150 to 200 serial sections (10 μm-thick) were cut along the horizontal plane and the sections were progressively distributed on 10 slides so that each slide contained 15 to 20 sections, each representative of the whole eye at different levels. The sections were stained with 4′,6′-diamidino-2-phenylindole (Vectashield, Vector Lab Inc., Peterborough, UK) and EGFP was monitored with a Zeiss Axiocam (Carl Zeiss, Oberkochen, Germany) at different magnifications.

Pigs were sacrificed and their eyeballs were harvested and fixed overnight by immersion in 4% PFA. The eyeballs were cut so that the lens and vitreous could be removed, leaving the eyecups in place. The eyecups were cryoprotected by progressive infiltration with 10%, 20% and 30% sucrose. Before embedding, the swine eyecups were analyzed under a fluorescence stereomicroscope (Leica Microsystems GmbH, Wetzlar, Germany) in order to localize the transduced region, whenever an EGFP-encoding vector was administered. Embedding was performed in tissue-freezing medium (O.C.T. matrix, Kaltek, Padua, Italy). For each eye, 200 to 300 serial sections (12 mm-thick) were cut along the horizontal meridian and the sections were progressively distributed on glass slides so that each slide contained 6 to 10 sections. Section staining and image acquisition was performed as described for mice.

Immunofluorescence staining

Frozen retinal sections were washed once with PBS and then fixed for 10 min in 4% PFA. Sections were then permeabilized for 1 hour in PBS containing 0.1% Triton® X-100. Blocking solution containing 10% normal goat serum (Sigma–Aldrich, St. Louis, MO) was applied for 1 hour. Primary antibodies were diluted in PBS and incubated overnight at 4°C. The secondary antibody (Alexa Fluor® 594, anti-rabbit, 1:1000; Molecular Probes, Invitrogen, Carlsbad, CA) was incubated for 45 min. The primary antibodies used were rabbit anti-hAIPL1 (1:700; kindly provided by Michael E. Cheetham, University College London, London, UK) and rabbit anti-hCAR [51] (1:10000; kindly provided by Cheryl M. Craft, University of Southern California, Los Angeles, Ca). Vectashield (Vector Lab Inc., Peterborough, UK) was used to visualize nuclei. Sections were photographed using either a Zeiss Axioplan microscope (Carl Zeiss, Oberkochen, Germany) or a Leica Laser Confocal Microscope System (Leica Microsystems GmbH, Wetzlar, Germany).

Electroretinography

Electrophysiological recordings in mice were performed as detailed in [52] and bilateral ERG evaluations in pigs were carried out as previously described [38].

miRNA and gene expression analysis

MiRNA and gene expression analysis in mice administered with the AAV2/5-CMV-*EGFP*-4xmiR124T and AAV2/5-CMV-*EGFP*-4xmiR204T constructs was performed on samples from whole retinas and optic cups, respectively. Total RNA was extracted using the miRNeasy kit (Qiagen, Inc., Hilden, Germany) according to the manufacturer's instructions and quantified using the NanoDrop 1000 (Thermo Fischer Scientific, Waltham, MA). RNA quality was assessed by gel electrophoresis.

Quantitative (q) Reverse Transcriptase (RT-) PCR-based detection of mature miR-124, miR-182 and miR-204 was performed using the TaqMan® microRNA assays (Applied Biosystems, Foster City, CA). All reactions were performed in triplicate. The qRT-PCR results, recorded as threshold cycle numbers (Ct), were converted to absolute copy number (*i.e.* copies of miRNA per ng of RNA) using a standard curve. To generate the standard curve, serial amounts (ranging from 10^2 to 10^8 copies) of a synthetic RNA oligonucleotide corresponding to miR-124 (5′-UAAGGCACGCGGUGAAUGCC-3′; Sigma–Aldrich, St. Louis, MO) were mixed with 10 ng of total yeast RNA. The samples were analyzed using the TaqMan® microRNA assay and the correlation between threshold cycle numbers (Ct) and copies of miRNA was established.

For the expression analysis of target genes, cDNA synthesis was performed using the Quantitect Reverse Transcription kit (Qiagen, Inc., Hilden, Germany) starting from 1 μg of DNase-treated RNA. In order to unambiguously distinguish spliced cDNA from genomic DNA contamination, exon-specific primers were designed to amplify across introns of the genes tested. All primers were previously tested by reverse transcription (RT)-PCR and no RT control reactions were performed. Primer sequences are the following: MmRdh10_For: 5′-CTAGAGATTAAT-CATGGCCAC-3′; MmRdh10_Rev: 5′-CTCGTGAAAACCCA-CAACTC-3′; MmVamp3_For: 5′-CAGACACAAAATCAAG-TAGATG-3′; MmVamp3_Rev: 5′-CAGTGCATCTGCGCGG-TC-3′. qRT-PCR experiments were performed using the ABI Prism 7900HT Fast Sequence Detection System with ABI Power SYBR Green reagents (Applied Biosystems, Foster City, CA). Real-time PCR results were analyzed using the comparative Ct method normalized against the housekeeping genes *GAPDH* and *ACTB*. The range of expression levels was determined by calculating the standard deviation of the ΔCT.

Supporting Information

Figure S1 AAV vectors harboring miRTs do not detectably perturb miRNA expression and activity in the eye. (**a**) miRNA expression profile analysis in retinas and optic cups of animals injected subretinally with AAV (n = 4 samples/group). Expression levels were determined by qRT-PCR on RNA extracted from retinas injected with AAV2/5-CMV-*EGFP*-4xmR124T and from optic cups of eyes treated with AAV2/5-CMV-*EGFP*-4xmR204T following delivery of a high AAV vector dose (2.6×10^9 GC/eye). Subretinal administration of AAV vectors harboring miRTs does not detectably perturb endogenous miRNA expression in the eye. (**b**) Expression levels of *RDH10* and *VAMP3,* two direct targets of miR-124 in retinas injected with high doses of AAV2/5-CMV-*EGFP*-4xmR124T animals (n = 4). The contralateral eyes injected with the AAV2/5-CMV-*EGFP* control were used as reference. *ACTB* and *HPRT* were used as internal controls. Subretinal administration of AAV vectors harboring miRTs does not detectably perturb endogenous miRNA activity in the eye. Error bars represent the mean plus or minus SEM.

Acknowledgments

We thank Annamaria Carissimo (Bioinformatics Core, TIGEM, Naples, Italy) for help with statistical analyses and the TIGEM AAV Vector Core. We are grateful to Graciana Diez-Roux (TIGEM, Naples, Italy) for critical reading of the manuscript and to Cheryl M. Craft (University of Southern California, Los Angeles, CA) and Michael E. Cheetham (University College London, London, UK) for reagents.

Author Contributions

Conceived and designed the experiments: AA SB MK. Performed the experiments: MK AM AP EM AG MA MDC SR MG. Analyzed the data: MK AM AA SB EMS. Wrote the paper: MK AM MLB FS SB AA.

References

1. Huntzinger E, Izaurralde E (2011) Gene silencing by microRNAs: contributions of translational repression and mRNA decay. Nat Rev Genet 12: 99–110.
2. Landgraf P, Rusu M, Sheridan R, Sewer A, Iovino N, et al. (2007) A mammalian microRNA expression atlas based on small RNA library sequencing. Cell 129: 1401–1414.
3. Brown BD, Naldini L (2009) Exploiting and antagonizing microRNA regulation for therapeutic and experimental applications. Nat Rev Genet 10: 578–585.
4. Brown BD, Gentner B, Cantore A, Colleoni S, Amendola M, et al. (2007) Endogenous microRNA can be broadly exploited to regulate transgene expression according to tissue, lineage and differentiation state. Nat Biotechnol 25: 1457–1467.
5. Colin A, Faideau M, Dufour N, Auregan G, Hassig R, et al. (2009) Engineered lentiviral vector targeting astrocytes in vivo. Glia 57: 667–679.
6. Papapetrou EP, Kovalovsky D, Beloeil L, Sant'angelo D, Sadelain M (2009) Harnessing endogenous miR-181a to segregate transgenic antigen receptor expression in developing versus post-thymic T cells in murine hematopoietic chimeras. J Clin Invest 119: 157–168.
7. Sachdeva R, Jonsson ME, Nelander J, Kirkeby A, Guibentif C, et al. (2010) Tracking differentiating neural progenitors in pluripotent cultures using microRNA-regulated lentiviral vectors. Proc Natl Acad Sci U S A 107: 11602–11607.
8. Xie J, Xie Q, Zhang H, Ameres SL, Hung JH, et al. (2011) MicroRNA-regulated, Systemically Delivered rAAV9: A Step Closer to CNS-restricted Transgene Expression. Mol Ther 19: 526–535.
9. Brown BD, Cantore A, Annoni A, Sergi LS, Lombardo A, et al. (2007) A microRNA-regulated lentiviral vector mediates stable correction of hemophilia B mice. Blood 110: 4144–4152.
10. Gentner B, Visigalli I, Hiramatsu H, Lechman E, Ungari S, et al. (2010) Identification of hematopoietic stem cell-specific miRNAs enables gene therapy of globoid cell leukodystrophy. Sci Transl Med 2: 58ra84.
11. Kaplan J, Rozet J-M, Perrault I, Munnich A Leber Congetital Amaurosis. In: McGraw-Hill, ed. The Online Metabolic & Molecular Bases of Inherited Diseases.
12. Brunetti-Pierri N, Auricchio A (2010) Gene Therapy of Human Inherited Diseases. In: McGraw-Hill, ed. The Online Metabolic & Molecular Bases of Inherited Disease.
13. Colella P, Cotugno G, Auricchio A (2009) Ocular gene therapy: current progress and future prospects. Trends Mol Med 15: 23–31.
14. Bainbridge JW, Smith AJ, Barker SS, Robbie S, Henderson R, et al. (2008) Effect of gene therapy on visual function in Leber's congenital amaurosis. N Engl J Med 358: 2231–2239.
15. Cideciyan AV, Aleman TS, Boye SL, Schwartz SB, Kaushal S, et al. (2008) Human gene therapy for RPE65 isomerase deficiency activates the retinoid cycle of vision but with slow rod kinetics. Proc Natl Acad Sci U S A 105: 15112–15117.
16. Cideciyan AV, Hauswirth WW, Aleman TS, Kaushal S, Schwartz SB, et al. (2009) Human RPE65 gene therapy for Leber congenital amaurosis: persistence of early visual improvements and safety at 1 year. Hum Gene Ther 20: 999–1004.
17. Cideciyan AV, Hauswirth WW, Aleman TS, Kaushal S, Schwartz SB, et al. (2009) Vision 1 year after gene therapy for Leber's congenital amaurosis. N Engl J Med 361: 725–727.
18. Hauswirth WW, Aleman TS, Kaushal S, Cideciyan AV, Schwartz SB, et al. (2008) Treatment of leber congenital amaurosis due to RPE65 mutations by ocular subretinal injection of adeno-associated virus gene vector: short-term results of a phase I trial. Hum Gene Ther 19: 979–990.
19. Maguire AM, High KA, Auricchio A, Wright JF, Pierce EA, et al. (2009) Age-dependent effects of RPE65 gene therapy for Leber's congenital amaurosis: a phase 1 dose-escalation trial. Lancet 374: 1597–1605.
20. Maguire AM, Simonelli F, Pierce EA, Pugh EN, Jr., Mingozzi F, et al. (2008) Safety and efficacy of gene transfer for Leber's congenital amaurosis. N Engl J Med 358: 2240–2248.
21. Simonelli F, Maguire AM, Testa F, Pierce EA, Mingozzi F, et al. (2010) Gene therapy for Leber's congenital amaurosis is safe and effective through 1.5 years after vector administration. Mol Ther 18: 643–650.
22. Surace EM, Auricchio A (2008) Versatility of AAV vectors for retinal gene transfer. Vision Res 48: 353–359.
23. Boulanger A, Liu S, Henningsgaard AA, Yu S, Redmond TM (2000) The upstream region of the Rpe65 gene confers retinal pigment epithelium-specific expression in vivo and in vitro and contains critical octamer and E-box binding sites. J Biol Chem 275: 31274–31282.
24. Flannery JG, Zolotukhin S, Vaquero MI, LaVail MM, Muzyczka N, et al. (1997) Efficient photoreceptor-targeted gene expression in vivo by recombinant adeno-associated virus. Proc Natl Acad Sci U S A 94: 6916–6921.
25. Karali M, Peluso I, Gennarino VA, Bilio M, Verde R, et al. (2010) miRNeye: a microRNA expression atlas of the mouse eye. BMC Genomics 11: 715.
26. Karali M, Peluso I, Marigo V, Banfi S (2007) Identification and characterization of microRNAs expressed in the mouse eye. Invest Ophthalmol Vis Sci 48: 509–515.
27. Allocca M, Mussolino C, Garcia-Hoyos M, Sanges D, Iodice C, et al. (2007) Novel adeno-associated virus serotypes efficiently transduce murine photoreceptors. J Virol 81: 11372–11380.
28. Auricchio A, Kobinger G, Anand V, Hildinger M, O'Connor E, et al. (2001) Exchange of surface proteins impacts on viral vector cellular specificity and transduction characteristics: the retina as a model. Hum Mol Genet 10: 3075–3081.
29. Surace EM, Auricchio A (2003) Adeno-associated viral vectors for retinal gene transfer. Prog Retin Eye Res 22: 705–719.
30. Lagos-Quintana M, Rauhut R, Yalcin A, Meyer J, Lendeckel W, et al. (2002) Identification of tissue-specific microRNAs from mouse. Curr Biol 12: 735–739.
31. Deo M, Yu JY, Chung KH, Tippens M, Turner DL (2006) Detection of mammalian microRNA expression by in situ hybridization with RNA oligonucleotides. Dev Dyn 235: 2538–2548.
32. Guduric-Fuchs J, Ringland LJ, Gu P, Dellett M, Archer DB, et al. (2009) Immunohistochemical study of pig retinal development. Mol Vis 15: 1915–1928.
33. Reddy AM, Zheng Y, Jagadeeswaran G, Macmil SL, Graham WB, et al. (2009) Cloning, characterization and expression analysis of porcine microRNAs. BMC Genomics 10: 65.
34. Wienholds E, Kloosterman WP, Miska E, Alvarez-Saavedra E, Berezikov E, et al. (2005) MicroRNA expression in zebrafish embryonic development. Science 309: 310–311.
35. Conte I, Carrella S, Avellino R, Karali M, Marco-Ferreres R, et al. (2010) miR-204 is required for lens and retinal development via Meis2 targeting. Proc Natl Acad Sci U S A 107: 15491–15496.
36. Mohand-Said S, Hicks D, Leveillard T, Picaud S, Porto F, et al. (2001) Rod-cone interactions: developmental and clinical significance. Prog Retin Eye Res 20: 451–467.
37. Hendrickson A, Hicks D (2002) Distribution and density of medium- and short-wavelength selective cones in the domestic pig retina. Exp Eye Res 74: 435–444.
38. Mussolino C, Della Corte M, Rossi S, Viola F, Di Vicino U, et al. (2011) AAV-mediated photoreceptor transduction of the pig cone-enriched retina. Gene Ther: Mar 17. (Epub ahead of print);doi:10.1038/gt.2011.1033.
39. Karginov FV, Conaco C, Xuan Z, Schmidt BH, Parker JS, et al. (2007) A biochemical approach to identifying microRNA targets. Proc Natl Acad Sci U S A 104: 19291–19296.
40. Arora A, McKay GJ, Simpson DA (2007) Prediction and verification of miRNA expression in human and rat retinas. Invest Ophthalmol Vis Sci 48: 3962–3967.
41. Bernstein AM, Whiteheart SW (1999) Identification of a cellubrevin/vesicle associated membrane protein 3 homologue in human platelets. Blood 93: 571–579.
42. Romand R, Kondo T, Cammas L, Hashino E, Dolle P (2008) Dynamic expression of the retinoic acid-synthesizing enzyme retinol dehydrogenase 10 (rdh10) in the developing mouse brain and sensory organs. J Comp Neurol 508: 879–892.
43. Blackshaw S, Harpavat S, Trimarchi J, Cai L, Huang H, et al. (2004) Genomic analysis of mouse retinal development. PLoS Biol 2: E247.
44. Glushakova LG, Timmers AM, Issa TM, Cortez NG, Pang J, et al. (2006) Does recombinant adeno-associated virus-vectored proximal region of mouse rhodopsin promoter support only rod-type specific expression in vivo? Mol Vis 12: 298–309.
45. Hargrave PA, McDowell JH (1992) Rhodopsin and phototransduction: a model system for G protein-linked receptors. Faseb J 6: 2323–2331.
46. Vetrini F, Auricchio A, Du J, Angeletti B, Fisher DE, et al. (2004) The microphthalmia transcription factor (Mitf) controls expression of the ocular albinism type 1 gene: link between melanin synthesis and melanosome biogenesis. Mol Cell Biol 24: 6550–6559.
47. Acland GM, Aguirre GD, Bennett J, Aleman TS, Cideciyan AV, et al. (2005) Long-term restoration of rod and cone vision by single dose rAAV-mediated gene transfer to the retina in a canine model of childhood blindness. Mol Ther 12: 1072–1082.
48. Bennicelli J, Wright JF, Komaromy A, Jacobs JB, Hauck B, et al. (2008) Reversal of blindness in animal models of leber congenital amaurosis using optimized AAV2-mediated gene transfer. Mol Ther 16: 458–465.
49. Gentner B, Schira G, Giustacchini A, Amendola M, Brown BD, et al. (2009) Stable knockdown of microRNA in vivo by lentiviral vectors. Nat Methods 6: 63–66.

50. Liang F, Anand V, Maguire A, Bennett J (2000) Intraocular delivery of recombinant virus. Meth Mol Med 47: 125–139.
51. Li A, Zhu X, Craft CM (2002) Retinoic acid upregulates cone arrestin expression in retinoblastoma cells through a Cis element in the distal promoter region. Invest Ophthalmol Vis Sci 43: 1375–1383.
52. Allocca M, Manfredi A, Iodice C, Di Vicino U, Auricchio A (2011) AAV-mediated gene replacement either alone or in combination with physical and pharmacological agents results in partial and transient protection from photoreceptor degeneration associated with {beta}PDE deficiency. Invest Ophthalmol Vis Sci: Jan 27. (Epub ahead of print).

9

Pseudotyped AAV Vector-Mediated Gene Transfer in a Human Fetal Trachea Xenograft Model: Implications for *In Utero* Gene Therapy for Cystic Fibrosis

Sundeep G. Keswani[1,2*], Swathi Balaji[1], Louis Le[1], Alice Leung[1], Anna B. Katz[2], Foong-Yen Lim[1,2], Mounira Habli[1], Helen N. Jones[1], James M. Wilson[3], Timothy M. Crombleholme[1,2]

1 Center for Molecular Fetal Therapy, Division of Pediatric, General, Thoracic and Fetal Surgery, Cincinnati Children's Hospital Medical Center and The University of Cincinnati College of Medicine, Cincinnati, Ohio, United States of America, 2 The Children's Institute for Surgical Science, The Children's Hospital of Philadelphia, Philadelphia, Pennsylvania, United States of America, 3 Gene Therapy Program, Department of Pathology and Laboratory Medicine, University of Pennsylvania School of Medicine, Philadelphia, Pennsylvania, United States of America

Abstract

Background: Lung disease including airway infection and inflammation currently causes the majority of morbidities and mortalities associated with cystic fibrosis (CF), making the airway epithelium and the submucosal glands (SMG) novel target cells for gene therapy in CF. These target cells are relatively inaccessible to postnatal gene transfer limiting the success of gene therapy. Our previous work in a human-fetal trachea xenograft model suggests the potential benefit for treating CF *in utero*. In this study, we aim to validate adeno-associated virus serotype 2 (AAV2) gene transfer in a human fetal trachea xenograft model and to compare transduction efficiencies of pseudotyping AAV2 vectors in fetal xenografts and postnatal xenograft controls.

Methodology/Principal Findings: Human fetal trachea or postnatal bronchus controls were xenografted onto immunocompromised SCID mice for a four-week engraftment period. After injection of AAV2/2, 2/1, 2/5, 2/7 or 2/8 with a LacZ reporter into both types of xenografts, we analyzed for transgene expression in the respiratory epithelium and SMGs. At 1 month, transduction by AAV2/2 and AAV2/8 in respiratory epithelium and SMG cells was significantly greater than that of AAV2/1, 2/5, and 2/7 in xenograft tracheas. Efficiency in SMG transduction was significantly greater in AAV2/8 than AAV2/2. At 3 months, AAV2/2 and AAV2/8 transgene expression was >99% of respiratory epithelium and SMG. At 1 month, transduction efficiency of AAV2/2 and AAV2/8 was significantly less in adult postnatal bronchial xenografts than in fetal tracheal xenografts.

Conclusions/Significance: Based on the effectiveness of AAV vectors in SMG transduction, our findings suggest the potential utility of pseudotyped AAV vectors for treatment of cystic fibrosis. The human fetal trachea xenograft model may serve as an effective tool for further development of fetal gene therapy strategies for the *in utero* treatment of cystic fibrosis.

Editor: Nupur Gangopadhyay, University of Pittsburgh, United States of America

Funding: This work is supported in part by grants from the National Institute of Diabetes and Digestive and Kidney Diseases (R01-DK074055, R01-DK072446 and R01-DK59242) (TMC), Wound Healing Foundation 3 M Award, and National Institute of General Medical Sciences (K08 GM098831-01) (SGK). The funders had no role in study design, data collection and analysis, decision to publish, or preparation of the manuscript.

Competing Interests: The authors have read the journal's policy and have the following conflicts: JMW is a consultant to ReGenX Holdings, and is a founder of, holds equity in, and receives a grant from affiliates of ReGenX Holdings. In addition, he is an inventor on patents licensed to various biopharmaceutical companies, including affiliates of ReGenX Holdings. All other authors have declared that no competing interests exist.

* E-mail: sundeep.keswani@cchmc.org

These authors contributed equally to this work.

Introduction

Cystic fibrosis (CF), which is the most common lethal monogenetic disease, results from the absence of a functional cystic fibrosis transmembrane conductance regulator (CFTR) protein [1]. A recently described CFTR−/− porcine model demonstrates a similar phenotype to that of a newborn human with CF. Abdominal lesions dominate the initial presentation, with meconium ileus, pancreatic destruction, early focal biliary cirrhosis, micro gall bladder, and abnormalities in bile ducts [2,3]. These results suggest that CFTR is expressed in several organ systems and site-specific replacement of this single CFTR gene could potentially correct the deficiency, making gene therapy an attractive CF treatment modality.

At birth neither the human patients with CF, nor the new born CFTR−/− piglets, show any evidence of inflammation or morphological abnormalities in the airway or submucosal glands. However, with time the characteristic features of human CF including inflammation, infection, mucus accumulation, tissue remodeling, and airway obstruction manifest. Today, airway infection and inflammation, and associated lung diseases causes much of the morbidities and mortalities associated with CF [4,5]. The airway epithelium and submucosal glands are appealing targets for gene therapy of pulmonary manifestations of CF because they express high levels of CFTR in the tracheobronchial tree (with relatively lower levels of expression found in the respiratory epithelial cells as compared to higher levels in the SMG), and they have been characterized as a potential location of airway stem cells [6–10].

Postnatal gene transfer of a functionally active CFTR gene has been limited by immunologic barriers to viral vectors [11–15]. Also, in the postnatal environment, mucus production and a relatively great distance of the submucosal glands from the trachea lumen have rendered gene therapy ineffective. In clinical trials, CFTR gene transfer was inefficient to either the surface epithelium or submucosal gland cells [16–19]. The discrepancy in gene transfer efficiencies between animal models and human clinical trials may be due to species-specific physiologic differences between humans and lower species [20]. Therefore, an improved model to study gene therapy in cystic fibrosis is necessary to better predict outcomes in clinical trials.

Considering the inefficiencies in postnatal gene transfer, we investigated alternative strategies for cystic fibrosis gene therapy. The fetus presents a potentially favorable environment for CFTR gene transfer including: 1) decreased physical barriers, 2) an immunologically permissive environment, 3) greater access to developing submucosal glands, and 4) the potential to transduce a respiratory-epithelial stem cell population. The development of a human fetal *ex vivo* model would provide the opportunity to screen potential gene transfer modalities in a species specific environment. We have previously reported a postnatal human bronchial xenograft model, where denuded rat tracheas repopulated with human bronchial cells are xenografted into nude mice, developed a fully differentiated pseudo stratified respiratory epithelium with occasional incompletely formed submucosal glands [21]. Applying a similar xenograft strategy to develop a human fetal *ex vivo* model, we implanted whole human fetal tracheas into a subcutaneous pocket in severe combined immuno-deficient (SCID) mice [22–24]. We have recently reported that this model recapitulates normal development of human fetal airway epithelium and tracheal SMG as per the staging system described by Thurlbeck *et al.* [25] after a 4-week engraftment period [24]. Using this xenograft model, we can examine viral-vector-cellular interactions and evaluate transduction efficiencies in a representative human fetal tracheal environment. Our earlier findings of efficient gene transfer in the fetal tracheal environment using adenoviral and pseudo-typed lentiviral-based vectors concurs with the suggestions of others that the fetal trachea may be a conducive environment for gene transfer [26–29].

Due to the limited duration of transgene expression with adenoviruses and the potential risk of insertional mutagenesis with lentiviruses, we chose to examine the effects of adeno-associated viral (AAV) vectors for gene transfer. These AAV vectors have a better safety profile, pose a lower risk for insertional events, and have potential for long term transgene expression [30]. In our previous study, utilizing an *in vitro* human fetal trachea model we reported efficient gene transfer using AAV2/2 to the fetal respiratory epithelium and submucosal glands [21]. Since the capsid is a major determinant of vector tropism, we hypothesized that a pseudotyping strategy, which replaces the capsid of the AAV 2 vector with capsid proteins from other AAV serotypes, could potentially enhance transduction efficiency. AAV serotypes 7 and 8 were isolated from non-human primates. These serotypes are thought to have sufficient homology to retain viral tropism for human target cells, but are divergent enough to avoid detection by pre-existing antibodies generated against commonly found human AAV serotypes [31,32]. The pseudotyping strategy has demonstrated a unique transduction efficiency and tropism profile for each serotype in various tissues, including liver, muscle and skin [31,33–35]. Despite these advantages, postnatal reports indicate that the pseudotyping strategy has not resulted in greatly improved gene transfer to the tracheo-bronchial tree [14,36,37].

In this study, we hypothesize that an AAV pseudotyping strategy in the fetal environment will result in enhanced gene transfer to the target cells of cystic fibrosis gene therapy. To test this hypothesis, using our validated human fetal trachea xenograft model, we compared the transduction efficiency of AAV2 and four AAV pseudotyped vectors (AAV2/1, AAV2/5, AAV2/7, AAV2/8) to the respiratory epithelium and submucosal glands. Further, to assess if it is the fetal environment that is permissive of enhanced gene transfer, we compared fetal transduction efficiencies to postnatal bronchial xenograft controls.

Materials and Methods

Ethics Statement

Human fetal tracheas were obtained from Advanced Bioscience Resources (Alameda, CA). Adult bronchial segments were obtained from The National Disease Research Interchange (Philadelphia, PA). The study protocol, which involves use of anonymous, de-identified, discarded human fetal or adult tissue, was reviewed and granted an exempt status by The Children's Hospital of Philadelphia Institutional Review Board.

All animal procedures were approved by the Institutional Animal Care and Use Committee of The Children's Hospital of Philadelphia. SCID mice were obtained from Charles River Laboratories (Wilmington, MA) ranging in ages 6–8 weeks. Mice were anesthetized with methoxyflurane inhalation for all procedures. After any procedure, mice were allowed to recover in incubators overnight and all efforts were made to minimize suffering.

Pseudotyped Adeno-associated Virus Production

Pseudotyped adeno-associated vectors AAV2/2, 2/1, 2/5, 2/7 and 2/8 were obtained from the Vector Core at the University of Pennsylvania and produced as previously described [31]. The AAV2/2 serotype was constructed by standard transfection protocols and purified by single-step heparin chromatography. A pseudotyping strategy was used to produce AAV2 vectors packaged with the capsid proteins of AAV1, AAV5, AAV7 and AAV8. Briefly, recombinant AAV genomes equipped with AAV2 inverted terminal repeats (ITRs) were packaged by triple transfection of 293 cells with *cis*-plasmid, adenovirus helper plasmid, and a chimeric packaging construct. To create the chimeric packaging constructs, the XhoI site of p5E18 plasmid at 3,169 bp was ablated. The modified plasmid was then restricted with XbaI and XhoI in a complete digestion to remove the AAV2 cap gene and replace it with a 2,267-bp SpeI/XhoI fragment that contains the AAV1, AAV5, AAV7, or AAV8 cap gene. For all AAV vectors, the cDNA bacterial β-galactosidase was inserted as a reporter and driven by a CMV promoter. Pseudotyped recombinant vectors were purified by the standard $CsCl_2$ sedimentation method. Genome copy (GC) titers of AAV vectors were determined by TaqMan (Applied Biosystems, Foster City, CA) analysis, using probes and primers targeting SV40 poly (A) region.

Human Fetal Tracheas

The protocol, which involves use of anonymous, de-identified, discarded human fetal tissue, was reviewed and granted an exempt status by The Children's Hospital of Philadelphia Institutional Review Board. Human fetal tracheas were obtained from Advanced Bioscience Resources (Alameda, CA) from 18 aborted fetuses ranging in age from 18 to 22 weeks based on prenatal ultrasound. The tracheas were placed in Dulbecco's modified Eagle medium (DMEM, Gibco, Carlsbad, CA) containing 10% heat-inactivated fetal bovine serum (Gibco), penicillin 100 IU/mL, and streptomycin 0.1 mg/mL (Gibco). Cultures were incubated at 37°C for 24 hours to exclude infection before transplantation; no tracheas were lost to infection.

SCID-human Fetal Trachea Xenograft Model

All animal procedures were approved by the Institutional Animal Care and Use Committee of The Children's Hospital of Philadelphia. As previously described [24], SCID mice (Charles River Laboratories, Wilmington, MA) ages 6–8 weeks were anesthetized with methoxyflurane inhalation, and all efforts were made to minimize suffering. After a 5-mm incision was made in the right flank, a subcutaneous pouch was created superficial to the panniculus carnosus. Each fetal trachea (mean gestational age 20±0.4 weeks, range 18–22) was implanted into the pouch and secured by a single 8–0 Prolene suture (Ethicon, Somerville, NJ). The skin incision was closed with 5–0 Vicryl sutures (Ethicon) and covered with a transparent dressing (3 M Healthcare, St. Paul, MN).

SCID-human Adult Bronchial Xenografts

The protocol, which involves use of anonymous, de-identified, discarded human tissue, was reviewed and granted an exempt status by The Children's Hospital of Philadelphia Institutional Review Board. Human adult bronchial segments were obtained from the National Disease Research Interchange (Philadelphia, PA). Bronchial segments from a 35-year-old cadaver were sterilely dissected and placed in Dulbecco's modified Eagle medium (Gibco) that contained 10% heat-inactivated fetal bovine serum (Gibco), penicillin 100 IU/mL, and streptomycin 0.1 mg/mL (Gibco). Bronchial segments were then incubated at 37°C for 24 hours to exclude infection before transplantation. After formation of the subcutaneous pockets in 9 SCID mice, the bronchi were placed in the pouch, enveloped by the panniculus carnosus, and secured with an 8–0 prolene (Ethicon). The skin was closed and a sterile transparent dressing was applied (3 M Healthcare). The bronchial segments were engrafted for 1 month.

AAV Vector Delivery to Fetal Trachea and Adult Bronchial Xenografts

All 27 SCID mice tolerated implantation of fetal tracheas and adult bronchi. Four weeks after implantation, the tracheas and bronchi produced mucus, formed an operculum over the openings, and were well vascularized. To deliver vectors, SCID mice were anesthetized with inhalational methoxyflurane. A 1-cm incision was made in the skin at the caudal end of the xenograft. With exposure of the fetal trachea, mucus was extracted by insertion of a disposable microsyringe (Becton Dickinson, Franklin Lakes, NJ) through the operculum of the xenograft. Animals received 1×10^{11}genome copies of AAV-CMV-LacZ, 2/1, 2/2, 2/5, 2/7, 2/8 vectors in 20 μL of phosphate buffered saline (PBS) ($n = 3$/vector) or PBS alone for controls ($n = 3$). The incision was closed and a sterile dressing was applied. One month after vector delivery, trachea xenografts were biopsied or harvested; 2 months later, animals were humanely killed and xenografts were removed for analysis. Similarly in the adult bronchial xenografts at 4 weeks, all specimens produced mucus, which was then extracted by microsyringe (Becton Dickinson) through a superficial incision. 1×10^{11} genome copies of the pseudotyped AAV 2/8 ($n = 3$) or AAV2/2 ($n = 3$) vectors were injected in a total of 20 μL of PBS or PBS alone for 3 controls. One month after vector delivery, adult bronchial xenografts were harvested and transgene expression was quantified in the respiratory epithelium and submucosal gland cells.

Quantification of Transduction

Tracheas or bronchi were cut transversely into 2- to 3-mm pieces, washed in PBS, fixed in 0.5% glutaraldehyde for 15 minutes, and X-gal stained with a solution containing 1 mg/mL of 5-bromo-4-chloro-3-indoyl-β-D-galactopyronidase, 5 mmol/L $K_3Fe(CN)_6$, 5 mmol/L $K_4Fe(CN)_6$, and 1 mmol/L $MgCl_2$ in PBS, pH 7.4. After overnight incubation at 37°C, samples were post-fixed with 10% neutral buffered formalin (Sigma) for 16 hours. Post-fixed X-gal stained tissues were mechanically processed and paraffin embedded. The 5-μm sections obtained were counterstained with 0.5% nuclear fast red. Images were obtained using a Leica microscope and analyzed with computer-assisted image analysis (Scanalytics, Fairfax, VA). A minimum of 9 sections per animal were analyzed for LacZ expression signified by cell specific green staining. Transduction efficiencies were quantified as the percent of positively stained respiratory epithelium and submucosal gland cells.

Immunohistochemistry for AAV2/2 and AAV2/8 Receptors

The 5-μm paraffin sections from 18-week-old fetal tracheas and trachea sections from an adult cadaver (NDRI, Philadelphia, PA) were rehydrated in distilled water, immersed in Tissue Unmasking Fluid, pH 6.2 (Signet Laboratories, Dedham, MA), and microwaved (Ted Pella, Redding, CA) on high for 5 min to facilitate antigen retrieval. Slides were washed with distilled water and transferred to PBS. Samples were blocked using normal 10% goat serum in PBS (30 min at room temperature). Slides were then incubated with a mouse anti-heparan sulfate proteoglycan monoclonal antibody (1:20 dilution, Chemicon, Temecula, CA) with normal 10% rabbit serum (for AAV2/2) or mouse monoclonal antibody for 67-kDa laminin receptor (1:20 dilution, Abcam, Cambridge, MA) with normal 10% rabbit serum (for AAV2/8) for 30 minutes at room temperature and then overnight at 4°C. After slides were washed with PBS containing 0.1% triton, they were incubated for 30 min at room temperature with biotinylated species-specific IgG (1:200, Vector Labs, Burlingame, CA) for AAV2/2 slides and Alexafluor 488 species-specific IgM (1:200, Invitrogen, Carlsbad, CA) for AAV2/8 slides. The AAV2/2 slides were washed with PBS and avidin-biotin complex (Vector Labs) added. The slides were then rinsed in PBS, developed with chromagen 3, 3′-diaminobenzidine (Sigma), lightly stained with hematoxylin, and mounted with xylene-based mounting media. The AAV2/8 slides were washed with PBS and mounted using prolong gold media containing DAPI (Invitrogen).

Statistical Analysis

Paired Student's *t*-test and analysis of variance (ANOVA) were used to compare transduction efficiencies between the five AAV vectors. A p value of <0.05 was considered significant. Data were expressed as mean ± standard error of mean (SEM).

Results

Transduction Efficiency of AAV Pseudotypes in the Xenografted Human Fetal Trachea Model

In evaluating the effect of pseudotyping AAV2 vectors on transduction efficiencies in this model of implanted human fetal tracheas into subcutaneous pockets, all SCID mice tolerated implantation. At four weeks, the tracheas were well vascularized, formed operculum, and produced secretions (Figure 1). 1×10^{11} genome copies of AAV2/2 or pseudotyped vectors AAV2/1, 2/5, 2/7, and 2/8 were individually injected into the lumen of engrafted human fetal tracheas. PBS was injected in control xenografts.

Control xenografts showed no positive LacZ staining at one month after PBS administration. Tracheal biopsies, one month after vector administration demonstrated that AAV2/2 transduced 93±1.5% of the respiratory epithelium and 37±2% of the submucosal gland cells. In xenografts injected with AAV2/1, 2/5 and 2/7, there was minimal LacZ expression in the tracheal biopsies; this finding was confirmed by further analysis on the entire xenograft. At 1 month, both AAV2/1 and AAV2/5 transduced <0.1% of the respiratory epithelium and 0% of the submucosal gland cells, whereas AV2/7 transduced <0.1% of the respiratory epithelium and 2.0±0.1% of the submucosal gland cells. In contrast with the other pseudotyped AAV vectors at 1 month, AAV2/8 transduced 91±1.9% of the respiratory epithelium and 54.4±1.4% of the submucosal gland cells. Specifically, AAV2/8 was significantly more efficient than AAV2/2 in transducing submucosal gland cells (54.4±1.4% vs. 37±2%, respectively) ($p<0.005$). With successful transduction observed only in serotypes AAV2/2 and 2/8, only these xenografts were maintained and harvested for subsequent evaluation. At 3 months, AAV2/2 and 2/8 demonstrated transgene expression >99% in both the respiratory epithelium and submucosal gland cells (Figure 2).

Comparison of Gene Transfer Efficiency in the Adult vs. Fetal Respiratory Epithelium and Submucosal Gland Cells

To confirm that the transduction observed with AAV2/2 and the pseudotyped AAV2/8 was unique to the fetal environment, we developed a postnatal xenograft control by implanting adult bronchial segments into subcutaneous pockets in SCID mice. After a 1 month engraftment period, 1×10^{11} genome copies of AAV2/2 or 2/8 were injected into the bronchial segments. PBS was injected in control xenografts. Transduction efficiency for the respiratory epithelium and submucosal gland cells for AAV2/2 were 16±1.5% and 12±2.1%, respectively. Gene transfer efficiencies for AAV2/8 to the respiratory epithelium and submucosal gland cells were 32±4.1% and 20±1.9%, respectively. PBS controls did not have any LacZ positive staining. Gene transfer with AAV2/8 was significantly greater than with AAV2/2 in both adult respiratory epithelium (32±4.1% vs 16±1.5%; $p<0.01$) and adult submucosal gland cells (20±1.9% vs. 12±2.1%; $p<0.01$) (Figure 3). Transduction by both AAV2/2 and 2/8 were significantly lower in adult bronchial xenografts compared with that observed in the fetal tracheal xenograft in both the respiratory epithelium and submucosal glands. Specifically, in respiratory epithelium, AAV2/2 was 16±1.5% in adult vs. 93±1.5% in fetal ($p<0.0001$), whereas AAV2/8 was 32±4.1% in adult vs. 91±1.9% in fetal ($p<0.0001$). In submucosal gland cells, AAV2/2 was 12±2.1% in adult vs. 37±2% in fetal ($p<0.0001$) and AAV2/8 was 20±1.9% in adult vs. 91±1.9% in fetal ($p<0.0001$) (Figure 3B).

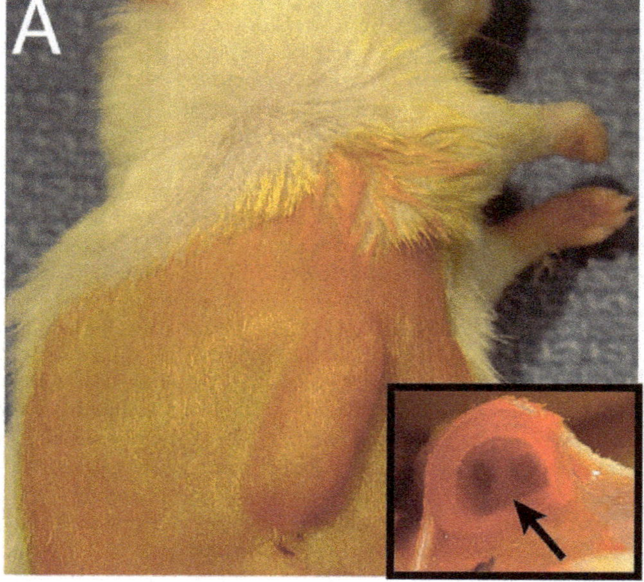

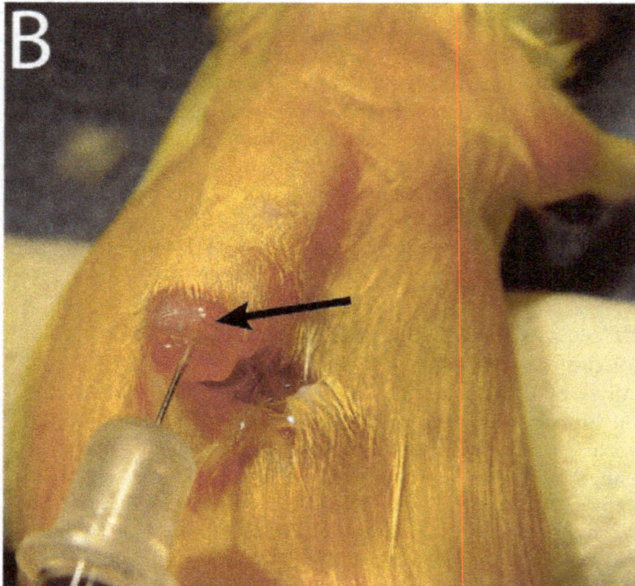

Figure 1. Human fetal trachea xenografts: Human fetal trachea xenografts 4 weeks after subcutaneous implantation in the SCID mice. A) Fetal trachea xenograft model. Inset demonstrates the biopsied cross sectional view of the xenograft with visible carina (arrow) at four weeks after subcutaneous implantation in a SCID mouse. (B) At four weeks after implantation, an operculum is formed over the trachea opening; xenografts produce mucous and are well vascularized (arrow). A microsyringe is inserted through the operculum to extract mucus and inject AAV vectors into the lumen of the xenografts.

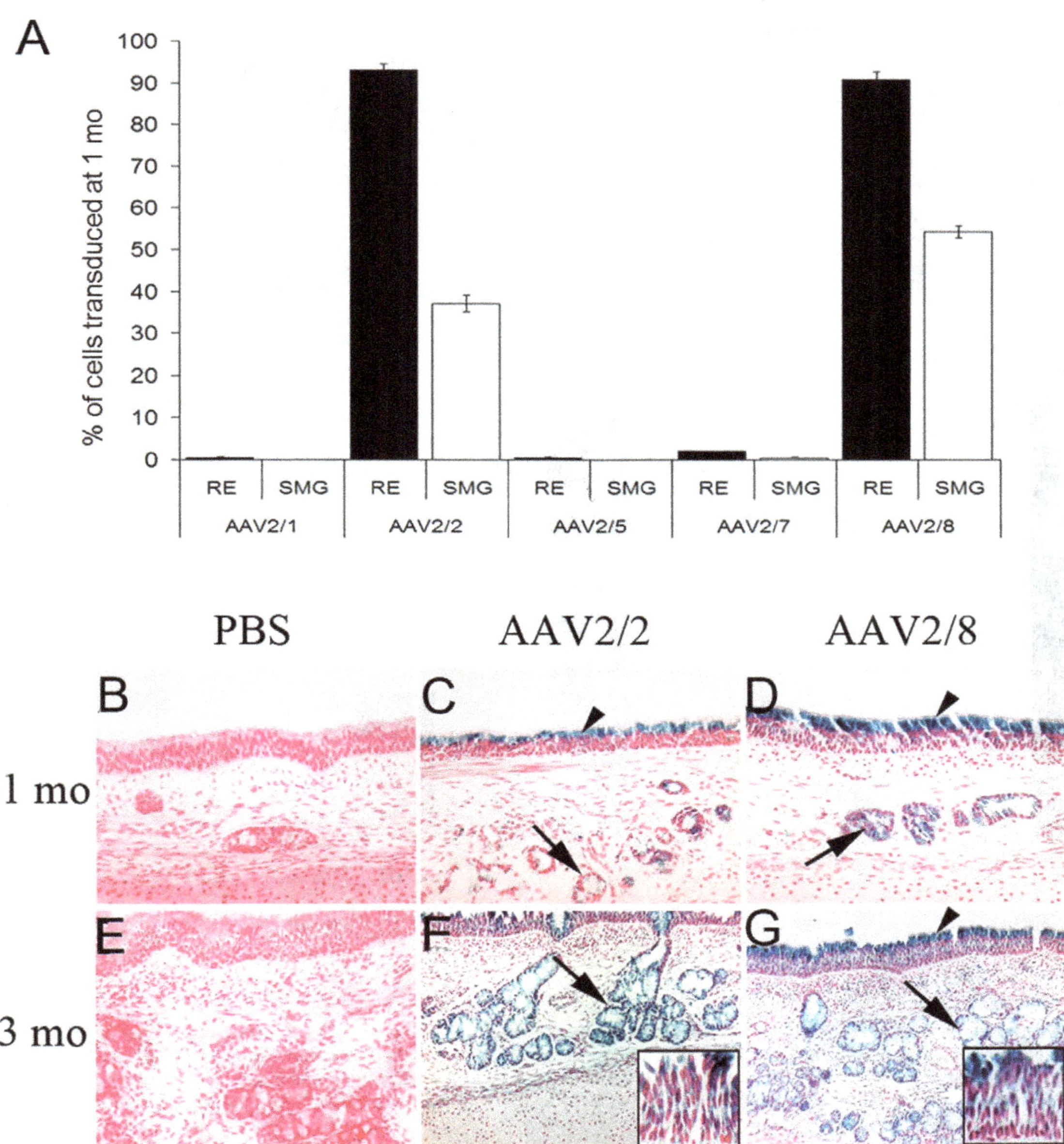

Figure 2. Transduction efficiencies of AAV2 and pseudotyped AAV2 vectors injected in fetal trachea. (A) Graph depicts percent of cell transduction efficiencies at 1 month by AAV2/2 and four pseudotyped AAV2 vectors (AAV2/1, AAV2/5, AAV2/7, AAV2/8) for respiratory epithelium (RE) and submucosal glands (SMGs). Bar plots represent average ± SEM. No LacZ positive cells were found in PBS control xenografts at 1 or 3 months (B, E). Only AAV2/2 (C) and AAV2/8 (D) demonstrate efficient gene transfer to the RE and SMG at 1 month. In comparison, other pseudotyped vectors AAV2/1, AAV2/5 and AAV2/7 minimally transduce the RE and SMG. By 3 months, there is near complete transduction to the RE and SMG by AAV2/2 (F) and AAV 2/8 (G). SMGs (arrow) and RE (arrowheads).

Comparison of AAV2/2 and AAV2/8 Receptors in Adult and Fetal Tracheas

We hypothesized that the significantly enhanced transduction efficiencies observed in the fetal trachea compared to postnatal controls could be due to accessibility of the viral receptors in the fetal trachea. To test this hypothesis, we compared immunostaining patterns between fetal and adult trachea samples for the AAV2 receptor, heparan sulfate proteoglycan (HSPG). Similarly, we performed immuno-histochemistry for a potential AAV2/8 receptor (67 kDa laminin receptor) [38]. Immunostaining in the adult trachea demonstrated expression of HSPG limited to the basolateral surface of the respiratory epithelium. In the fetal trachea, there was a similar basolateral distribution of HSPG expression. Although HSPG distribution was similar in adult and fetal tracheas, fetal submucosal glands are closer to the tracheal lumen and there is a decreased thickness of the fetal respiratory epithelium (Figure 4).

Immunostaining of a proposed AAV2/8 receptor (laminin R) demonstrated enhanced expression in both the respiratory epithelium and submucosal glands in the fetal trachea compared to minimal expression observed in the adult trachea (Figure 5).

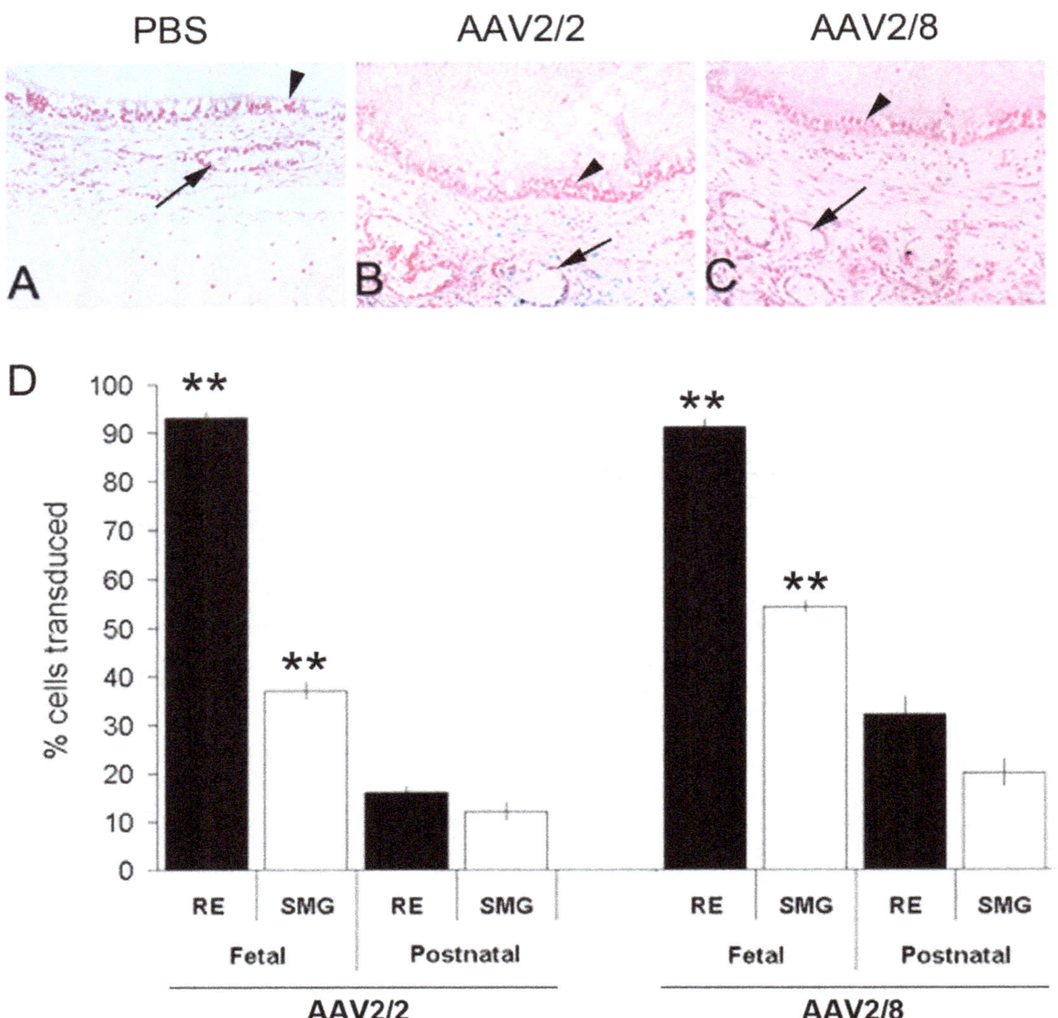

Figure 3. Transduction efficiencies of AAV2/2 and AAV2/8 in adult tracheobronchial xenografts. Transduction efficiencies of AAV2/2 and AAV2/8 were tested in an adult human bronchial xenograft. There was no LacZ positive staining in the PBS control adult xenograft (A). At 1 month, gene transfer to the adult postnatal xenograft with AAV2/2 (B) and AAV 2/8 (C) was minimal to the respiratory epithelium (RE) and submucosal glands (SMG). Arrows indicate SMG and arrowheads point to the RE. (D) Reduced cell transduction efficiency in postnatal xenografts compared to the human fetal trachea xenografts is demonstrated in the bar plot (average±SEM).

Discussion

The purpose of this study is to determine if an AAV pseudotyping strategy in the fetal environment can result in enhanced gene transfer to the target cells of CF gene therapy compared to postnatal controls. Our data demonstrate that AAV serotype 2 and the pseudotyped AAV2/8 vector result in highly efficient gene transfer in the respiratory epithelium and the submucosal gland cells of the fetal trachea compared to postnatal controls in the xenograft model. In light of previous reports of the limited postnatal transduction efficiency and rapid cellular turnover exhibited by the respiratory epithelium, the long term transgene expression with AAV2/2 and AAV2/8 are all the more impressive. At 1 month, transduction of the submucosal gland cells in fetal trachea is more efficient with AAV2/8. However, at 3 months, both AAV2/2 and AAV2/8 achieve highly efficient and stable transduction of the respiratory epithelium and submucosal gland cells. The increased transduction efficiency of AAV2/8 at one month may be related to its previously reported ability to more readily traverse biological barriers. In contrast to AAV2/2 and AAV2/8, the administration of AAV2/1, AAV2/5, and AAV2/7 demonstrate relatively low transduction efficiency in this model compared to AAV2/2 and AAV2/8. In addition, the highly efficient transduction of the submucosal gland cells may have significant implications for the prospective utility of fetal gene therapy to correct cystic fibrosis. The pseudotyped AAV vectors used in this study express a LacZ reporter gene. These are necessary preliminary data to determine the most effective AAV vectors for targeted gene delivery, with the eventual goal of significantly attenuating CF airway manifestations. Goldman *et al.* [21] demonstrated similar levels of transgene expression in human postnatal bronchial xenografts when transduced with either adenoviral CFTR or LacZ vectors. Similarly, we and several other groups have established that genetic reconstitution of CFTR results in functional correction of CF pathology in multiple models of the disease. These studies have also demonstrated a clear relationship between the dose of virus administration, efficacy of gene transfer, and the detected functional improvement, which

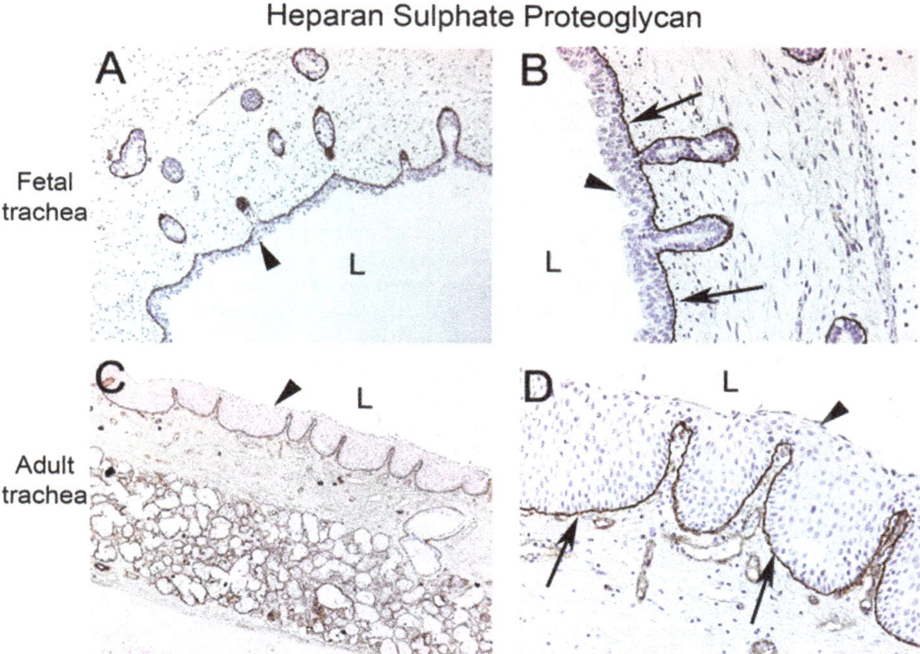

Figure 4. Immunostaining with heparan sulfate proteoglycan (HSPG), the AAV2 receptor on fetal and adult tracheas. Immunostaining at 10× and 40× magnification in fetal (A and B) and adult trachea (C and D) respectively. Expression of HSPG was limited to the basolateral surface of the respiratory epithelium (arrows). There is no staining of the airway epithelium (arrow heads) in either model. Luminal surface of the trachea (L).

partly explains the limited clinical success of postnatal gene therapy. In this context, the goal of this study was not to determine the genetic reconstitution of CFTR using AAV vectors, but to determine if the fetal environment is more permissive of gene transfer, and to further determine if a pseudotyping strategy with AAV vectors may result in enhanced tropism and transduction efficiency profiles. Based on our results, we plan to administer CFTR cDNA with a flag protein sequence or a reporter gene

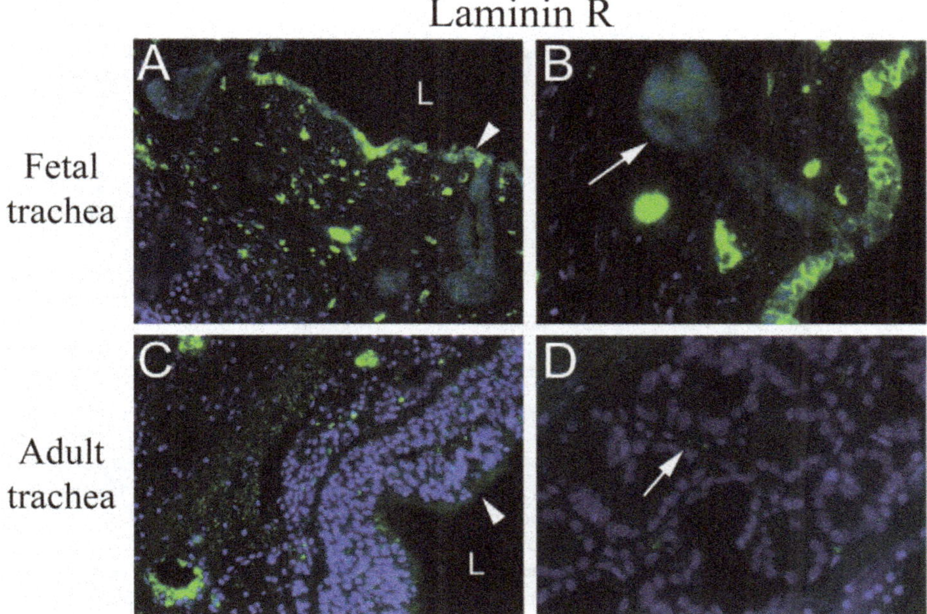

Figure 5. Laminin Receptor (R) staining of fetal and adult tracheas. Immuno fluorescent staining for Laminin R, one of the potential AAV8 receptors on fetal (A and B) and adult tracheas (C and D) at magnification 20× and 40×, repectively, demonstrates expression was most prominent in the surface epithelium (A, arrowheads) and submucosal glands (B, arrows) of the fetal trachea but minimal in the surface epithelium (C) and submucosal glands (D) in the adult trachea. Luminal surface of the trachea (L).

using the AAV serotype 2 and pseudotyped AAV2/8 vectors, and determine the effects on CFTR genetic reconstitution in a human fetal trachea xenograft model.

Efficient gene transfer by AAV2/2 and AAV2/8 was similar to our observations with other viral vectors in the fetal environment, such as adenovirus [28] and lentivirus [26,27]. Despite significant differences in their transduction mechanisms, the excellent gene transfer of the vectors suggests that the fetal trachea may be uniquely permissive to gene transfer strategies. In a similar experiment implanting adult human bronchial segments as a postnatal control, we verified that the efficient transduction observed with AAV2/2 and AAV2/8 was due to unique properties of the fetal trachea and not due to the immuno-compromised SCID xenograft model. We found relatively efficient gene transfer to adult bronchial xenografts compared with previously reported postnatal gene transfer to the tracheobronchial epithelium; this difference was more pronounced in the submucosal gland cells. These results suggest that the xenograft model may favor increased gene transfer efficiency. However, gene transfer with both AAV2/2 and AAV2/8 were significantly lower at 1 month in the postnatal control than in the fetal trachea. Therefore, some differences inherent to the fetal trachea must permit the high efficiency gene transfer with AAV2/2 and AAV2/8. Our findings are consistent with the findings by Tarantal and Lee *et al* [39], who used AAV pesudotyping strategy for fetal gene therapy. Using a fetal monkey model, it was demonstrated that when administered sufficiently early in gestation, fetal gene transfer using AAV pseudotyped vectors results in: 1) site specific long term transgene expression, and 2) offers the possibility of eliminating disease as well as the potential for immune responses to transgene products and/or components of the vector(s). Interestingly, their results also demonstrate that different pesudotyped vectors and different routes of vector administration results in different transduction efficiencies. In a different study, Clemens *et al* [40] studied AAV serotypes 1 and 2, and demonstrated that expression profile of AAV vectors (both levels of transgene being expressed, as well as tissues where transgene expression is detected) after *in utero* gene delivery differs based on the route of administration. Numerous other studies have shown that different AAV serotypes have different tropisms in cell lines based on their surface prevalence of receptors. Zabner *et al* [41] demonstrated that AAV5 was more effective at binding to the apical surface of human airway epithelia and therefore results in better gene transfer as compared to AAV2. Although a few AAV serotypes have shown better transduction compared with the AAV2-based vectors, gene transfer efficiency in human airway epithelium has still not reached therapeutic levels because of pathophysiological barriers in human CF patients [42–44]. A major limitation for this is the lack of efficient vector transduction to airway epithelial cells through the apical surface. Significant progress is being made to achieve high-efficiency transduction of airway epithelium, including using chemicals and a combination of transduction-enhancing compounds after vector transduction [45–47], shortened AAV cassette [48], intramolecular joining of DNA or RNA from independent vectors [49–51], genetic modifications of the AAV capsids [52], and DNA shuffling combined with directed evolution [53]. Taken together with our findings, these studies suggest that AAV vector transduction efficiency and tropism are species specific, and by utilizing strategies such as vector pseudotyping and varying the time and route of vector administration, gene therapy efficiency can be improved. The human xenograft model may provide a very novel and promising tool for clinical/translational/drug efficacy research. In comparison with postnatal gene therapy, *in utero* gene therapy of airway epithelium and SMG for cystic fibrosis offers several potential advantages while posing unique challenges. The delivery of viral vectors directly to the trachea lumen would provide site-specific gene therapy, eliminating the need for systemic vector delivery and thereby decreasing the risks of germ-line transduction. Another advantage is the proximity of potential viral receptors on the respiratory epithelium and the submucosal glands in relation to the trachea lumen. In the pre-immune murine fetal environment, Bouchard *et al* [54] reported that AAV administration has the potential to induce tolerance and allow postnatal re-administration with a partially abrogated immune response. This response suggests that the animal has developed a partial immunologic tolerance to the virus. In previous reports, immunologic tolerance may be developed to the transgene, but not necessarily to the vector. This tolerance may have been due to the limited exposure in the pre-immune fetus to the vector. In contrast, the prolonged exposure to the expressed transgene stimulated a tolerogenic T-cell-mediated response [55,56]. Another report by Boutin *et al* [57] reported that sero-prevalence of antibodies against AAV8 is only moderate in the human population when compared to AAV2, potentially facilitating immune escape of AAV8 vectors *in vivo*. This finding lends additional support to the use of a pseudotyping strategy for CFTR transgene delivery that allows for repeated administration using different capsid serotypes to maximize the efficiency of gene transfer and minimize immunologic reaction. Lastly, *in utero* CFTR replacement has the potential to correct the genetic defect before any manifestations of CF are present.

Despite the unprecedented efficiency of gene transfer observed with multiple vectors in our model, our results must be interpreted cautiously. The SCID mouse cannot mount an immune response, which may prolong transgene expression by the AAV vector. However, we did not observe a significant inflammatory reaction using AAV gene transfer in various models. Furthermore, the formation of membranes at both ends of the trachea provides an enclosed environment and allows prolonged exposure of the virus to the receptors of the fetal trachea. Although impossible to mimic in postnatal airways, this exposure is possible in the fetus because there is no physiologic gas exchange. Potential delivery of vector to the fetal trachea could be performed by endoscopic tracheal occlusion; this is currently being used in human clinical trials in Europe for congenital diaphragmatic hernia [58]. The human fetal trachea xenograft model can be used to screen vectors prior to this type of clinical application and the virus-receptor interaction can be studied in an environment representative of the developing human fetal trachea.

AAV-based vectors were utilized because of their long-term expression and low risk for insertional mutagenesis. However, Li *et al* [59] reported that AAV may randomly integrate at low frequency into mammalian chromosomes, preferentially integrating into transcribed genes in cells that are replicating. The near uniform transgene expression observed with AAV2/2 and AAV2/8 at 3 months after viral gene transfer suggests that integration events may have occurred and that integration into a respiratory stem cell population is likely. If the developing fetal tracheobronchial epithelium is more susceptible to insertional events than postnatal tracheobronchial epithelium, this observation has both positive and negative implications. If integration of AAV vectors occurs more readily in the fetal tracheobronchial stem cells, then correction of the CFTR mutation may be possible with in utero administration of a single site-specific AAV vector with a CFTR transgene. The human fetal trachea SCID xenograft model may be a useful means to study this phenomenon *in vivo* [60]. The downside of AAV integration is the potential of the AAV vector genome to influence chromosomal gene expression, either by inactivation of an adjacent gene, or more worrisome, by activation of an oncogene. Despite this concern, unlike retroviruses, there is recent evidence that demonstrates that AAV vectors are not associated with malignancy [59].

Conclusions

We have shown highly efficient gene transfer by AAV pseudotyping in a validated model representative of human submucosal gland development. The stable expression of transgenes in a rapid cellular turnover environment, such as the trachea, suggests transduction of a stem cell population, possibly with insertional events, that can be easily studied in this model. *In utero* gene therapy for cystic fibrosis has considerable theoretical appeal. AAV vectors and the human fetal trachea SCID xenograft model can be effective tools for studying the mechanisms of efficient AAV transduction of stem cell populations, understanding AAV insertional events, and developing fetal gene therapy strategies for the treatment of cystic fibrosis.

Acknowledgments

We thank Dr. Mary Kemper, University of Cincinnati, for editorial help.

Author Contributions

Conceived and designed the experiments: SGK SB LL AL ABK FYL JMW TMC. Performed the experiments: SGK SB LL AL ABK FYL. Analyzed the data: SGK SB LL AL ABK FYL TMC. Contributed reagents/materials/analysis tools: SGK FYL MH HNJ JMW TMC. Wrote the paper: SGK SB LL AL ABK FYL MH HNJ JMW TMC.

References

1. Ratjen F, Doring G (2003) Cystic fibrosis. Lancet 361: 681–689.
2. Welsh MJ, Rogers CS, Stoltz DA, Meyerholz DK, Prather RS (2009) Development of a porcine model of cystic fibrosis. Trans Am Clin Climatol Assoc 120: 149–162.
3. Ostedgaard LS, Meyerholz DK, Chen JH, Pezzulo AA, Karp PH, et al. (2011) The DeltaF508 mutation causes CFTR misprocessing and cystic fibrosis-like disease in pigs. Sci Transl Med 3: 74ra24.
4. Flume PA (2011) Pneumothorax in cystic fibrosis. Curr Opin Pulm Med 17: 220–225.
5. Stenbit AE, Flume PA (2011) Pulmonary exacerbations in cystic fibrosis. Curr Opin Pulm Med 17: 442–447.
6. Engelhardt JF, Yankaskas JR, Ernst SA, Yang Y, Marino CR, et al. (1992) Submucosal glands are the predominant site of CFTR expression in the human bronchus. Nature genetics 2: 240–248.
7. Borthwick DW, Shahbazian M, Krantz QT, Dorin JR, Randell SH (2001) Evidence for stem-cell niches in the tracheal epithelium. American journal of respiratory cell and molecular biology 24: 662–670.
8. Duan D, Sehgal A, Yao J, Engelhardt JF (1998) Lef1 transcription factor expression defines airway progenitor cell targets for in utero gene therapy of submucosal gland in cystic fibrosis. American journal of respiratory cell and molecular biology 18: 750–758.
9. Driskell RA, Engelhardt JF (2003) Current status of gene therapy for inherited lung diseases. Annual review of physiology 65: 585–612.
10. Xie W, Fisher JT, Lynch TJ, Luo M, Evans TI, et al. (2011) CGRP induction in cystic fibrosis airways alters the submucosal gland progenitor cell niche in mice. The Journal of clinical investigation.
11. Beck SE, Jones LA, Chesnut K, Walsh SM, Reynolds TC, et al. (1999) Repeated delivery of adeno-associated virus vectors to the rabbit airway. Journal of virology 73: 9446–9455.
12. Davies JC, Geddes DM, Alton EW (2001) Gene therapy for cystic fibrosis. The journal of gene medicine 3: 409–417.
13. Grubb BR, Pickles RJ, Ye H, Yankaskas JR, Vick RN, et al. (1994) Inefficient gene transfer by adenovirus vector to cystic fibrosis airway epithelia of mice and humans. Nature 371: 802–806.
14. Halbert CL, Rutledge EA, Allen JM, Russell DW, Miller AD (2000) Repeat transduction in the mouse lung by using adeno-associated virus vectors with different serotypes. Journal of virology 74: 1524–1532.
15. Weiss DJ (2004) Delivery of DNA to lung airway epithelium. Methods in molecular biology 246: 53–68.
16. Harvey BG, Leopold PL, Hackett NR, Grasso TM, Williams PM, et al. (1999) Airway epithelial CFTR mRNA expression in cystic fibrosis patients after repetitive administration of a recombinant adenovirus. The Journal of clinical investigation 104: 1245–1255.
17. Zuckerman JB, Robinson CB, McCoy KS, Shell R, Sferra TJ, et al. (1999) A phase I study of adenovirus-mediated transfer of the human cystic fibrosis transmembrane conductance regulator gene to a lung segment of individuals with cystic fibrosis. Human gene therapy 10: 2973–2985.
18. Hida K, Lai SK, Suk JS, Won SY, Boyle MP, et al. (2011) Common gene therapy viral vectors do not efficiently penetrate sputum from cystic fibrosis patients. PloS one 6: e19919.
19. Griesenbach U, Alton EW (2009) Cystic fibrosis gene therapy: successes, failures and hopes for the future. Expert review of respiratory medicine 3: 363–371.
20. Flotte TR, Fischer AC, Goetzmann J, Mueller C, Cebotaru L, et al. (2010) Dual reporter comparative indexing of rAAV pseudotyped vectors in chimpanzee airway. Molecular therapy : the journal of the American Society of Gene Therapy 18: 594–600.
21. Goldman MJ, Yang Y, Wilson JM (1995) Gene therapy in a xenograft model of cystic fibrosis lung corrects chloride transport more effectively than the sodium defect. Nature genetics 9: 126–131.
22. Peault B, Tirouvanziam R, Sombardier MN, Chen S, Perricaudet M, et al. (1994) Gene transfer to human fetal pulmonary tissue developed in immunodeficient SCID mice. Human gene therapy 5: 1131–1137.
23. Wang X, Zhang Y, Amberson A, Engelhardt JF (2001) New models of the tracheal airway define the glandular contribution to airway surface fluid and electrolyte composition. American journal of respiratory cell and molecular biology 24: 195–202.
24. Keswani SG, Le LD, Morris LM, Lim FY, Katz AB, et al. (2011) Submucosal gland development in the human fetal trachea xenograft model: implications for fetal gene therapy. Journal of pediatric surgery 46: 33–38.
25. Thurlbeck WM, Benjamin B, Reid L (1961) Development and distribution of mucous glands in the foetal human trachea. Br J Dis Chest 55: 54–64.
26. Lim FY, Kobinger GP, Weiner DJ, Radu A, Wilson JM, et al. (2003) Human fetal trachea-SCID mouse xenografts: efficacy of vesicular stomatitis virus-G pseudotyped lentiviral-mediated gene transfer. Journal of pediatric surgery 38: 834–839.
27. Lim FY, Martin BG, Sena-Esteves M, Radu A, Crombleholme TM (2002) Adeno-associated virus (AAV)-mediated gene transfer in respiratory epithelium and submucosal gland cells in human fetal tracheal organ culture. Journal of pediatric surgery 37: 1051–1057; discussion 1051–1057.
28. Knight AK, Martin BG, Crombleholme TM (1999) Screening of adenoviral and HSV gene therapy vectors for in utero treatment of cystic fibrosis using fetal tracheal organ culture. Surg Forum: 509–511.
29. Keswani SG, Crombleholme TM (2004) Gene transfer to the tracheobronchial tree: implications for fetal gene therapy for cystic fibrosis. Seminars in pediatric surgery 13: 44–52.
30. Lu Y (2004) Recombinant adeno-associated virus as delivery vector for gene therapy–a review. Stem cells and development 13: 133–145.
31. Gao GP, Alvira MR, Wang L, Calcedo R, Johnston J, et al. (2002) Novel adeno-associated viruses from rhesus monkeys as vectors for human gene therapy. Proceedings of the National Academy of Sciences of the United States of America 99: 11854–11859.
32. Arbetman AE, Lochrie M, Zhou S, Wellman J, Scallan C, et al. (2005) Novel caprine adeno-associated virus (AAV) capsid (AAV-Go.1) is closely related to the primate AAV-5 and has unique tropism and neutralization properties. Journal of virology 79: 15238–15245.
33. Hildinger M, Auricchio A, Gao G, Wang L, Chirmule N, et al. (2001) Hybrid vectors based on adeno-associated virus serotypes 2 and 5 for muscle-directed gene transfer. Journal of virology 75: 6199–6203.
34. Keswani SG, Balaji S, Le L, Leung A, Lim FY, et al. (2012) Pseudotyped adeno-associated viral vector tropism and transduction efficiencies in murine wound healing. Wound Repair Regen 20: 592–600.
35. Michelfelder S, Varadi K, Raupp C, Hunger A, Korbelin J, et al. (2011) Peptide Ligands Incorporated into the Threefold Spike Capsid Domain to Re-Direct Gene Transduction of AAV8 and AAV9 In Vivo. PloS one 6: e23101.
36. Halbert CL, Allen JM, Miller AD (2001) Adeno-associated virus type 6 (AAV6) vectors mediate efficient transduction of airway epithelial cells in mouse lungs compared to that of AAV2 vectors. Journal of virology 75: 6615–6624.
37. Halbert CL, Standaert TA, Aitken ML, Alexander IE, Russell DW, et al. (1997) Transduction by adeno-associated virus vectors in the rabbit airway: efficiency, persistence, and readministration. Journal of virology 71: 5932–5941.
38. Akache B, Grimm D, Pandey K, Yant SR, Xu H, et al. (2006) The 37/67-kilodalton laminin receptor is a receptor for adeno-associated virus serotypes 8, 2, 3, and 9. Journal of virology 80: 9831–9836.
39. Tarantal AF, Lee CC (2010) Long-term luciferase expression monitored by bioluminescence imaging after adeno-associated virus-mediated fetal gene delivery in rhesus monkeys (Macaca mulatta). Human gene therapy 21: 143–148.
40. Bilbao R, Reay DP, Li J, Xiao X, Clemens PR (2005) Patterns of gene expression from in utero delivery of adenoviral-associated vector serotype 1. Human gene therapy 16: 678–684.

41. Zabner J, Seiler M, Walters R, Kotin RM, Fulgeras W, et al. (2000) Adeno-associated virus type 5 (AAV5) but not AAV2 binds to the apical surfaces of airway epithelia and facilitates gene transfer. Journal of virology 74: 3852–3858.
42. Carter BJ (2005) Adeno-associated virus vectors in clinical trials. Human gene therapy 16: 541–550.
43. Aitken ML, Moss RB, Waltz DA, Dovey ME, Tonelli MR, et al. (2001) A phase I study of aerosolized administration of tgAAVCF to cystic fibrosis subjects with mild lung disease. Human gene therapy 12: 1907–1916.
44. Wagner JA, Moran ML, Messner AH, Daifuku R, Conrad CK, et al. (1998) A phase I/II study of tgAAV-CF for the treatment of chronic sinusitis in patients with cystic fibrosis. Human gene therapy 9: 889–909.
45. Duan D, Yue Y, Yan Z, Yang J, Engelhardt JF (2000) Endosomal processing limits gene transfer to polarized airway epithelia by adeno-associated virus. The Journal of clinical investigation 105: 1573–1587.
46. Ding W, Yan Z, Zak R, Saavedra M, Rodman DM, et al. (2003) Second-strand genome conversion of adeno-associated virus type 2 (AAV-2) and AAV-5 is not rate limiting following apical infection of polarized human airway epithelia. Journal of virology 77: 7361–7366.
47. Yan Z, Zak R, Zhang Y, Ding W, Godwin S, et al. (2004) Distinct classes of proteasome-modulating agents cooperatively augment recombinant adeno-associated virus type 2 and type 5-mediated transduction from the apical surfaces of human airway epithelia. Journal of virology 78: 2863–2874.
48. Ostedgaard LS, Rokhlina T, Karp PH, Lashmit P, Afione S, et al. (2005) A shortened adeno-associated virus expression cassette for CFTR gene transfer to cystic fibrosis airway epithelia. Proceedings of the National Academy of Sciences of the United States of America 102: 2952–2957.
49. Nakai H, Storm TA, Kay MA (2000) Increasing the size of rAAV-mediated expression cassettes in vivo by intermolecular joining of two complementary vectors. Nat Biotechnol 18: 527–532.
50. Halbert CL, Allen JM, Miller AD (2002) Efficient mouse airway transduction following recombination between AAV vectors carrying parts of a larger gene. Nat Biotechnol 20: 697–701.
51. Pergolizzi RG, Ropper AE, Dragos R, Reid AC, Nakayama K, et al. (2003) In vivo trans-splicing of 5′ and 3′ segments of pre-mRNA directed by corresponding DNA sequences delivered by gene transfer. Molecular therapy : the journal of the American Society of Gene Therapy 8: 999–1008.
52. White AF, Mazur M, Sorscher EJ, Zinn KR, Ponnazhagan S (2008) Genetic modification of adeno-associated viral vector type 2 capsid enhances gene transfer efficiency in polarized human airway epithelial cells. Human gene therapy 19: 1407–1414.
53. Gray SJ, Blake BL, Criswell HE, Nicolson SC, Samulski RJ, et al. (2010) Directed evolution of a novel adeno-associated virus (AAV) vector that crosses the seizure-compromised blood-brain barrier (BBB). Molecular therapy : the journal of the American Society of Gene Therapy 18: 570–578.
54. Bouchard S, MacKenzie TC, Radu AP, Hayashi S, Peranteau WH, et al. (2003) Long-term transgene expression in cardiac and skeletal muscle following fetal administration of adenoviral or adeno-associated viral vectors in mice. The journal of gene medicine 5: 941–950.
55. Jerebtsova M, Batshaw ML, Ye X (2002) Humoral immune response to recombinant adenovirus and adeno-associated virus after in utero administration of viral vectors in mice. Pediatric research 52: 95–104.
56. Colletti E, Lindstedt S, Park PJ, Almeida-Porada G, Porada CD (2008) Early fetal gene delivery utilizes both central and peripheral mechanisms of tolerance induction. Experimental hematology 36: 816–822.
57. Boutin S, Monteilhet V, Veron P, Leborgne C, Benveniste O, et al. (2010) Prevalence of serum IgG and neutralizing factors against adeno-associated virus (AAV) types 1, 2, 5, 6, 8, and 9 in the healthy population: implications for gene therapy using AAV vectors. Human gene therapy 21: 704–712.
58. Jani JC, Nicolaides KH, Gratacos E, Valencia CM, Done E, et al. (2009) Severe diaphragmatic hernia treated by fetal endoscopic tracheal occlusion. Ultrasound in obstetrics & gynecology : the official journal of the International Society of Ultrasound in Obstetrics and Gynecology 34: 304–310.
59. Li H, Malani N, Hamilton SR, Schlachterman A, Bussadori G, et al. (2011) Assessing the potential for AAV vector genotoxicity in a murine model. Blood 117: 3311–3319.
60. Conese M, Ascenzioni F, Boyd AC, Coutelle C, De Fino I, et al. (2011) Gene and cell therapy for cystic fibrosis: from bench to bedside. Journal of cystic fibrosis : official journal of the European Cystic Fibrosis Society 10 Suppl 2: S114–128.

Enhanced Collateral Growth by Double Transplantation of Gene-Nucleofected Fibroblasts in Ischemic Hindlimb of Rats

Ziyang Zhang[1,2*], Alex Slobodianski[2], Wulf D. Ito[3], Astrid Arnold[2], Jessica Nehlsen[2], Shaoxiang Weng[4,5], Natalie Lund[5], Jihong Liu[6], José-Tomás Egaña[1,7], Jörn A. Lohmeyer[1], Daniel F. Müller[1], Hans-Günther Machens[1]

1 Department of Plastic Surgery and Hand Surgery, Faculty of Medicine, University Hospital Rechts der Isar, Technische Universität München, Munich, Germany, **2** Department of Plastic Surgery and Hand Surgery, University of Lübeck, Lübeck, Germany, **3** Cardiovascular Center Oberallgaeu, Academic Teaching Hospital, University of Ulm, Immenstadt, Germany, **4** Department of Cardiovascular Diseases, School of Medicine, Sir Run Run Shaw Hospital, Zhejiang University, Hangzhou, China, **5** Experimental Angiology, Medical Department II, University Hospital Lübeck, Lübeck, Germany, **6** Department of Urology, Tongji Hospital, Huazhong University of Science and Technology, Wuhan, China, **7** Facultad de Ciencias, Center for Genome Regulation, Universidad de Chile, Santiago, Chile

Abstract

Background: Induction of neovascularization by releasing therapeutic growth factors is a promising application of cell-based gene therapy to treat ischemia-related problems. In the present study, we have developed a new strategy based on nucleofection with alternative solution and cuvette to promote collateral growth and re-establishment of circulation in ischemic limbs using double transplantation of gene nucleofected primary cultures of fibroblasts, which were isolated from rat receiving such therapy.

Methods and Results: Rat dermal fibroblasts were nucleofected *ex vivo* to release bFGF or VEGF165 in a hindlimb ischemia model *in vivo*. After femoral artery ligation, gene-modified cells were injected intramuscularly. One week post injection, local confined plasmid expression and transient distributions of the plasmids in other organs were detected by quantitative PCR. Quantitative micro-CT analyses showed improvements of vascularization in the ischemic zone (No. of collateral vessels via micro CT: 6.8 ± 2.3 vs. 10.1 ± 2.6; $p<0.05$). Moreover, improved collateral proliferation (BrdU incorporation: 0.48 ± 0.05 vs. 0.57 ± 0.05; $p<0.05$) and increase in blood perfusion (microspheres ratio: gastrocnemius: 0.41 ± 0.10 vs. 0.50 ± 0.11; $p<0.05$; soleus ratio: soleus: 0.42 ± 0.08 vs. 0.60 ± 0.08; $p<0.01$) in the lower hindlimb were also observed.

Conclusions: These results demonstrate the feasibility and effectiveness of double transplantation of gene nucleofected primary fibroblasts in producing growth factors and promoting the formation of collateral circulation in ischemic hindlimb, suggesting that isolation and preparation of gene nucleofected cells from individual accepting gene therapy may be an alternative strategy for treating limb ischemia related diseases.

Editor: Carlo Gaetano, Istituto Dermopatico dell'Immacolata, Italy

Funding: This work was supported by grants from Innovations fund Schleswig-Holstein and University Hospital rechts der Isar, Technische Universität München to HGM; a clinic research grant from Technische Universität München to ZZ (KKF. No. 8744556); German Research Council (DFG) IT-13/1, IT- 13/2, IT-13/3 to WDI and FONDAP (Nr. 15090007) to JTE. ZZ was supported by a scholarship from the China Scholarship Council. The funders had no role in study design, data collection and analysis, decision to publish, or preparation of the manuscript.

Competing Interests: The authors have declared that no competing interests exist.

* E-mail: zhangziyang776@googlemail.com

These authors contributed equally to this work.

Introduction

Lower extremity ischemia causes many clinic disorders. Patients suffer from a slight muscle pain or walking problems to lower leg ulceration and gangrene or even amputation. Although surgical procedures can help some patients with arterial occlusions, new treatment approaches are still needed for the patients who are not suitable for surgery [1]. Therapeutic neovascularization based on proangiogenic growth factors has been suggested as a possible clinical approach [2,3,4,5]. In this regard, the use of recombinant proangiogenic growth factors has been tested in both pre-clinic and clinical trials in previous studies. For example, Baffour R et al. proved that recombinant bFGF could enhance angiogenesis and growth of collaterals by *in vivo* administration in a rabbit hindlimb ischemic model [6]. In addition, VEGF was found to improve neovascularization in a hindlimb ischemia model [7]. However, although some of the results were encouraging from the past researches and randomized placebo-controlled double-blind clinical trials with recombinant proteins, there are still some sub-optimal results which are needed to be addressed. In particular, Lederman et al. reported that an improvement occurred in peak walking time 90 days after treatment in TRAFFIC trial with bFGF. However, this therapeutic effect was not observed at other time points [8]. In a randomized VEGF clinical trial (RAVE trial) with AdVEGF-121, there was no clinical therapeutic effects observed [9]. One of the possible explanations for failure of growth factor delivery in those studies could be owing to the direct administration of single growth factor, which could not induce enough therapeutic effects.

The combined administration of both bFGF and VEGF has been tested recently and found to have synergistic effects. In 1995, Asahara et al. proved for the first time that such synergistic effects of bFGF and VEGF enhanced collateral growth in a rabbit hindlimb ischemia model when they were administrated with a ratio of around 1:50 (bFGF:VEGF) [10]. However, the usual limitations of protein therapies are the low half life of the recombinant proteins (VEGF: 3 to 6 minutes *in vivo* and bFGF 1.5 minutes to 3 minutes *in vivo* [11,12,13]) and the possible side effects associated with high doses of exogenous proteins (apart from the possible tumorigenic effects because of inducement of angiogenesis, high dose VEGF could cause edema due to an increased microvascular permeability[14,15], high dose bFGF could cause hypotension related to a dose-dependent vasodilating effect [16]).

Currently, gene therapy has emerged as a rational approach to constantly produce and release proangiogenic molecules in the ischemic area [17,18,19]. In this regard, Lee et al. demonstrated that injection of both bFGF and VEGF plasmids together intramuscularly improved the therapeutic effects in ischemic damage. However, the short biological half life of the both factors owing to the immune clean effects was found to lead to failure of long-term therapeutic efficacy. To improve the efficiency of gene transfection, many previous studies used viral vector to enhance transfection efficiency by direct delivery of gene construct or via injection of cells transfect with viral vectors. Kondoh et al. reported that virus-based *ex vivo* gene transfer method [20] increased transfection efficiency; in addition, high efficiency of adenovirus-based *ex vivo* fibroblast gene transfer was also established for bFGF and VEGF genes. However, owing to the biohazard associated with the use of viral vectors, viral gene therapy is not yet widely accepted for clinical use.

In the present study, we developed a new strategy using *ex vivo* gene transfer of autologous cells via non-viral nucleofection technique to maximize the bFGF and VEGF expression in *in vitro* and *in vivo* experiments. This strategy was proven to have the highest transfection efficiency when compared to other classic non-viral methods, including the original nucleofection method. In the animal model of hindlimb ischemia, the delivered primary fibroblasts remarkably increased the formation of collateral vessels and improved blood supply to ischemic tissue area, as measured by micro-CT 3D reconstructions of microvascular networks and quantification of arteriogenesis and angiogenesis.

Materials and Methods

Cell isolation and characterization

Fibroblasts were isolated from skin obtained from the back of inbred rats. Briefly, the samples were cut into 4 cm×1 mm strips and then incubated with Dispase-2 (Roche, Penzberg, Germany). Subsequently, the epidermal layer was carefully removed and the dermis was minced and then incubated for 3 hours under magnetic rotation with 0.1% collagenase (Roche, Penzberg, Germany). After that, the mixture was filtered through a 100-µm Cell Strainer (BD biosciences, Hamburg, Germany) to obtain the primary cells. For characterization, cytospinned cells and normal cells seeded for 48 hours were fixed in ice-cooled ethanol for 30 minutes. Subsequently, the cells were stained with anti fibroblast antibody (Prolyl 4-hydroxylase subunit beta: P4H beta, Acris, Heidelberg, Germany) and tetramethyl rhodamine isothiocyanate conjugated phalloidin (Sigma-Aldrich, MO, USA) according to the manufacturer's instructions. Then, the cells were mounted in Prolong-containing DAPI (Invitrogen, Oregon, USA). Afterwards, cell morphology was analyzed by phase-contrast/ fluorescence microscopy (Nikon, eclipse te2000-s).

High-efficient *ex vivo* nucleofection

Nucleofection was performed under different conditions, and 1×10^6 primary rat skin fibroblasts (passage 2, 80–90% confluent) were trypsinized and harvested by centrifugation at 100×g for 10 min. The original nucleofection protocol was conducted following the suggested instructions (Basic Primary Mammalian Fibroblast Nucleofector® Kit, Lonza, Cologne, Germany). The supernatant was removed and the cell pellets were resuspended in 100 µl of nucleofection solution or 100 µl of Dulbecco's Modified Eagle Medium(DMEM) supplemented with 10% Fetal Calf Serum (FCS) for the purpose of comparing different nucleofection solutions. Afterwards, 4 µg of pmaxGFP® plasmids (Lonza) were mixed with the cells and subsequently transferred into nucleofection cuvettes. We also tested different transfection cuvettes and found that Eppendorf electroporation cuvettes (4-mm gap, Eppendorf, Hamburg, Germany) were as efficient as Amaxa cuvettes (2-mm gap, Amaxa, Cologne, Germany). Subsequently, the cells were nucleofected by using the U30 program from the nucleofection device and 500 µl of pre-warmed culture medium was immediately added to the cells. The cells were trypsinized and analyzed with a CASY® system (Innovatis AG, Reutlingen, Germany) for cell number and cell viability 48 hours after transfection. Transfection efficiency and apoptosis were quantified by fluorescent activated cell sorting (FACS; Cytomation MoFlo® Flow Cytometer, Dako, Denmark). DMEM+10% FCS, Eppendorf cuvettes (4-mm gap, Eppendorf, Hamburg, Germany) and U30 program were chosen for the *in vitro* and *in vivo* study. Plasmids encoding for VEGF165 and bFGF were constructed based on pmaxGFP® backbone (Lonza). The modified VEGF165 nucleofection protocol was as following: 1) Fibroblasts (3×10^6, passage 2) were mixed with 12 µg of VEGF165 plasmid and 100 µl of nucleofection solution (DMEM+10% FCS); 2) the mixture was then transferred into Eppendorf electroporation cuvettes (4-mm gap) and nucleofected with single electropulse program U30. After that, cells were transferred into a T25 culture flask and 4 ml DMEM+10% FCS were added; 3) the above two steps were repeated for 5 times with a total of 15×10^6 cells. 4) After 24 hours, VEGF165 nucleofected cells were collected and counted, only 5×10^6 cells were obtained for *in vivo* administration. The bFGF nucleofection protocol was conducted at the same time as VEGF165 nucleofection with another 15×10^6 cells to obtain 5×10^6 bFGF nucleofected cells. Cells (5×10^6 with bFGF and 5×10^6 with VEGF165) were then mixed before *in vivo* cell administration.

Growth-factor production

Transfected cells (1.4×10^5) were seeded in 12-well plates and cultured in 1.5 ml of DMEM + 10% FCS. Subsequently, medium was changed and collected daily. Concentrations of VEGF165 and bFGF were quantified by Bio-Plex Suspension Array System, following manufacturer's instructions (Bio-Rad, Hamburg, Germany).

Hindlimb ischemia model

Experiments were performed on male Lewis inbred rats (weight 200 grams, Charles River Laboratories, Sulzfeld, Germany).

Femoral artery ligation was performed as described previously [21]. All *in vivo* procedures were approved by animal committee of Luebeck University (No.1/1m/09).

Cell administration

Animals were randomly divided into 2 groups of treated and control animals. Directly after ligation of the right femoral artery, the cells (1×10^7) transfected with VEGF165 or bFGF (5×10^6 each) were intramuscularly injected into the gracilis muscle and adductor muscles in the middle part of the thigh because it has been demonstrated that this is the site of major collateral growth in the rat model employed but also in other animal models [21,22]. This is also the site of major collateral growth in humans when the superficial femoral artery is occluded and was consequently chosen as main injection site in the TAMARIS and WALK trials [23]. The same number of cells without transfection was injected into the same site in control group.

Quantitative micro-CT system

High-resolution desktop X-ray micro-CT system (SkyScan1072, SkyScan, Belgium) was used to visualize and quantify the vascular networks. Seven days after femoral artery ligation, micro-CT angiographies were performed as described before with modifications [21], After perfusion with the contrast medium, the ischemic zone of limbs was reconstructed from Z-axis cross section slices. After visualization and reconstruction of the vascular networks in the ischemic zone, collateral vessels were quantified and compared between the control and treated animals as described earlier [21]. Typical corkscrew-like collateral vessels were counted in 3D view. Compared to X-ray view, collaterals were easier to identify. After 3D reconstructions, the bone structures were subtracted and the vessel volume was quantified. Voxel number information from reconstruction slices of the ischemia zone (600 cross-sections below the proximal end of the ligation point) was collected for quantification of blood volume (see Materials and Methods S1 for detailed protocol).

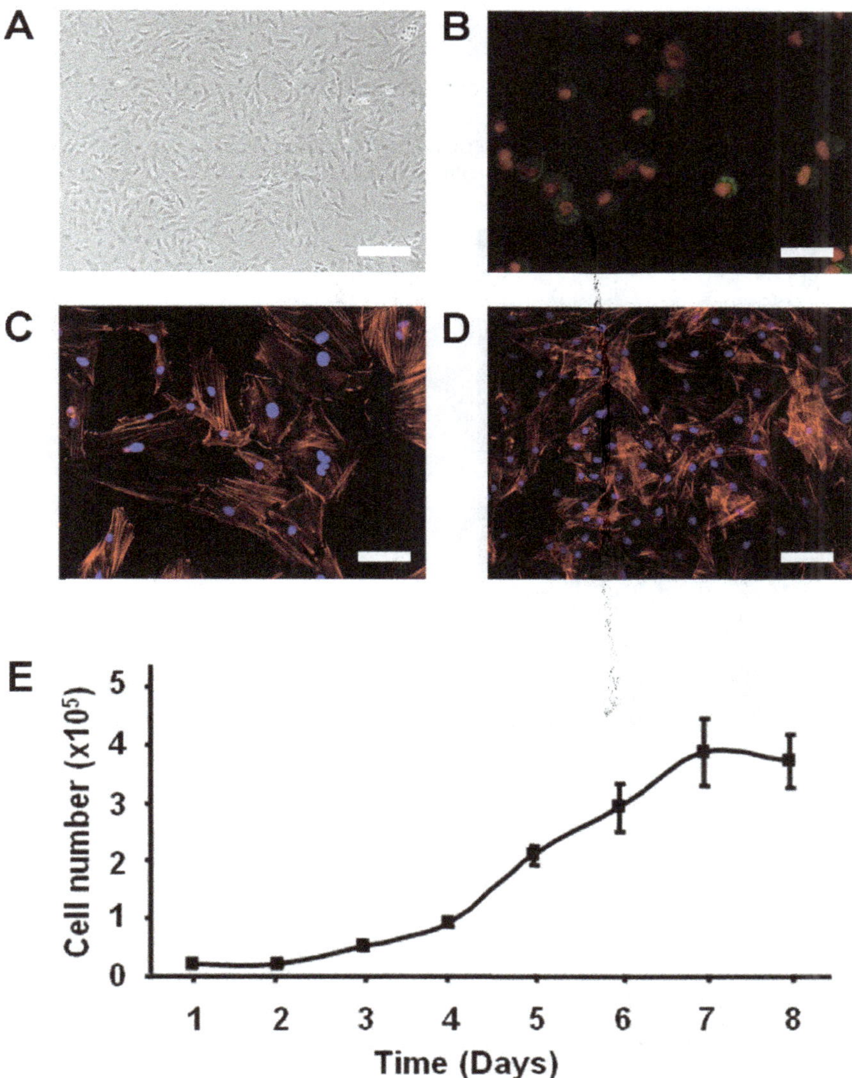

Figure 1. Preparation and characterization of rat primary fibroblasts. (A) Morphology of rat dermal primary fibroblasts (passage 2) was shown under phase contract microscope. (B) Characterization of isolated fibroblast with anit-fibroblast antibody (Prolyl 4-hydroxylase subunit beta: P4H beta), green: P4Hbeta; red: PI nucleus staining. (C) Morphology of fibroblasts under subconfluent and (D) confluent conditions was analyzed by phalloidin (red) and DAPI (blue) staining. (E) Primary rat dermal fibroblasts (passage 2) growth curve. Scale bar represents 200 µm in A, 100 µm in B and D, 50 µm in C.

Plasmid pharmacokinetics

The distribution of the plasmid was assessed by real-time PCR detecting the pmaxGFP® plasmid backbone sequences. At day 3, 7, 14, and 28 after injections, animals were sacrificed and organs were carefully collected and frozen for plasmid detection. Afterwards, the DNA was isolated with NucleoSpin® Tissue kit (MACHEREY-NAGEL, Dueren, Germany) and detected with specific primer for the plasmid backbone (see Materials and Methods S1 for detailed protocol).

Local gene expression

Seven days post injection, animals were sacrificed and samples were obtained from the muscles of the treated and control animals. Total RNA was then isolated with NucleoSpin® RNA II kit (MACHEREY-NAGEL, Dueren, Germany) according to the manufacturer's instructions. VEGF165 and bFGF mRNA expression was detected with specific primer for both the genes (see Materials and Methods S1 for detailed protocol).

Collateral proliferation and blood perfusion ratio

Animals were sacrificed, the middle zone of the collaterals on day 7 including the surrounding tissues were taken, and proliferation assays were performed as described previously [21,24]. Proliferation of the collateral artery was detected by 5-Bromo-2′-Deoxyuridine (BrdU) labeling and detection Kit 2 (Roche Diagnostics, Penzberg, Germany). The proliferative index was calculated as the number of BrdU-positive nuclei to the total number of nuclei inside the vessel wall. Blood flow in the lower hindlimb was detected on day 7 after ligation by FluoSpheres polystyrene microspheres (15 μm, red-fluorescent, Invitrogen, USA). The microspheres were injected via catheters through the carotid artery of rats running on a treadmill. After injection, rats were sacrificed and gastrocnemius and soleus from both hindlimbs were taken. Blood flow was expressed as ratios of occluded and non-occluded hindlimb perfusion (microspheres numbers) of the soleus and gastrocnemius (see Materials and Methods S1 for detailed protocol).

Statistical analysis

All data were evaluated by at least 3 independent experiments. The data were shown as Mean ± SEM. Statistical comparisons between 2 groups were performed with two-tail Student's *t*-test. One-way ANOVA followed by post-hoc analyses was used for comparison of differences within multiple groups. The differences between the groups were considered significant when $p<0.05$.

Results

Isolation and characterization of primary dermal fibroblasts

Isolated rat dermal fibroblasts were spindle-shaped and adhered rapidly to the culture flasks (Figure 1A). The characteristics of

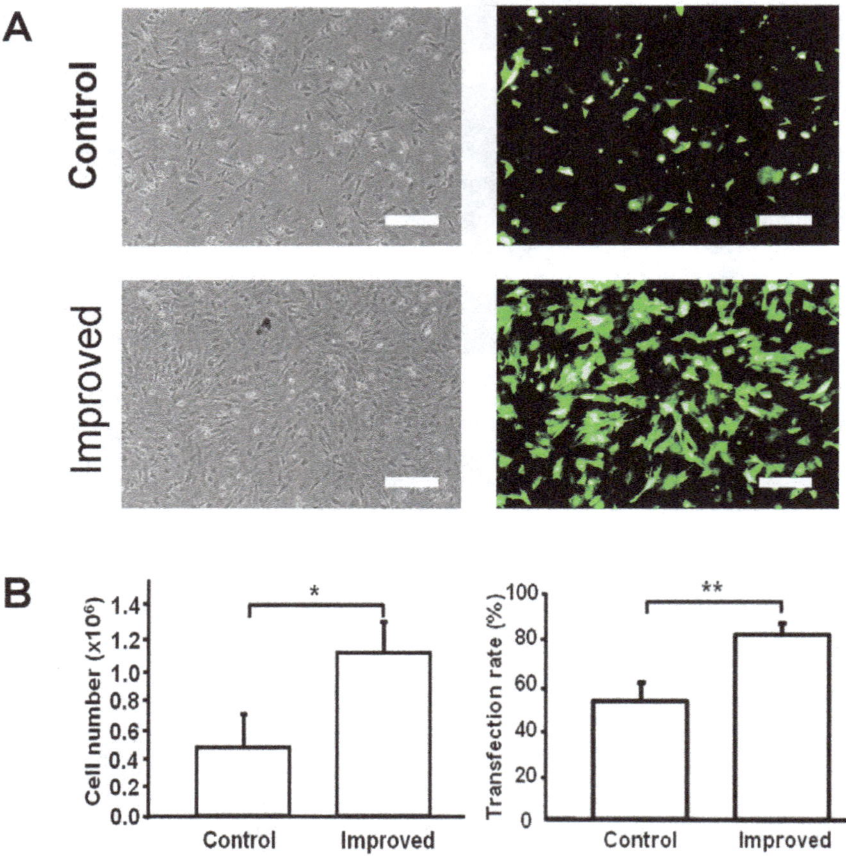

Figure 2. Optimization of nucleofection in primary cultures of fibroblasts. (**A**) Improved method (improved) and original method (control) were compared under fluorescence microscope to show optimization of nucleofection. Representative pictures of each method are shown in this panel. Scale bar represents 100 μm. (**B**) Cell number and transfection rate were significantly enhanced by the improved method (experiment was repeated for more than 5 times; * $p<0.05$; ** $p<0.01$).

these primary fibroblasts were detected by cytospin for the expression of prolyl 4-hydroxylase subunit beta (P4H beta). A fluorescent microscopic imaging for the expression of P4H beta is presented (Figure 1B). In addition, the actin cytoskeleton morphology of the fixed and permeabilized cells was also examined by FITC-label phalloidin under sub-confluent and confluent conditions (Figure 1 C and D), which indicated the nature of smooth muscle cells. The cell growth curve was obtained with normal culture medium (DMEM+10%FCS), showing an active cell replication with a doubling time of 24–48 hours. Cell growth was linear during the first 7 days and then reached a plateau phase on day 8 (Figure 1E).

Optimization of nucleofection with improved reagents

We first examined transfection efficiency with six nucleofector programs (including A24, T16, U12, U23, U30, and V13). The cells were transfected with commercial protocol provided by the manufacturer. The highest transfection efficiency (around 60%) and cell viability (>95%) were obtained with program U30. Therefore, program U30 was chosen for further *in vitro* and *in vivo* experiments.

To achieve the maximal therapeutic effects, nucleofection reagents were modified to improve gene transfection efficiency in primary cell cultures of fibroblasts (details described in Materials and Methods). Two days after nucleofection, the total number of cells significantly decreased in the control group, in which commercial kit reagents were used (Figure 2A, upper panels). When transfected reagents were modified, transfection efficiency, as shown by more GFP-positive cells, was enhanced (Figure 2A, lower panels). With such improved reagents, 2 days after nucleofection, more transfected cells were obtained in contrast to the control standard protocol (Figure 2B, left panel: 0.42±0.35 (Improved) vs. 1.07±0.29 (Control); *$p<0.05$). By FACS, we found that the use of modified solution did not affect cell growth, but induced higher transfection rate (Figure 2B, right panel: 80. 5±5.0 (Improved) vs. 51.5±7.9 (Control); **$p<0.01$).

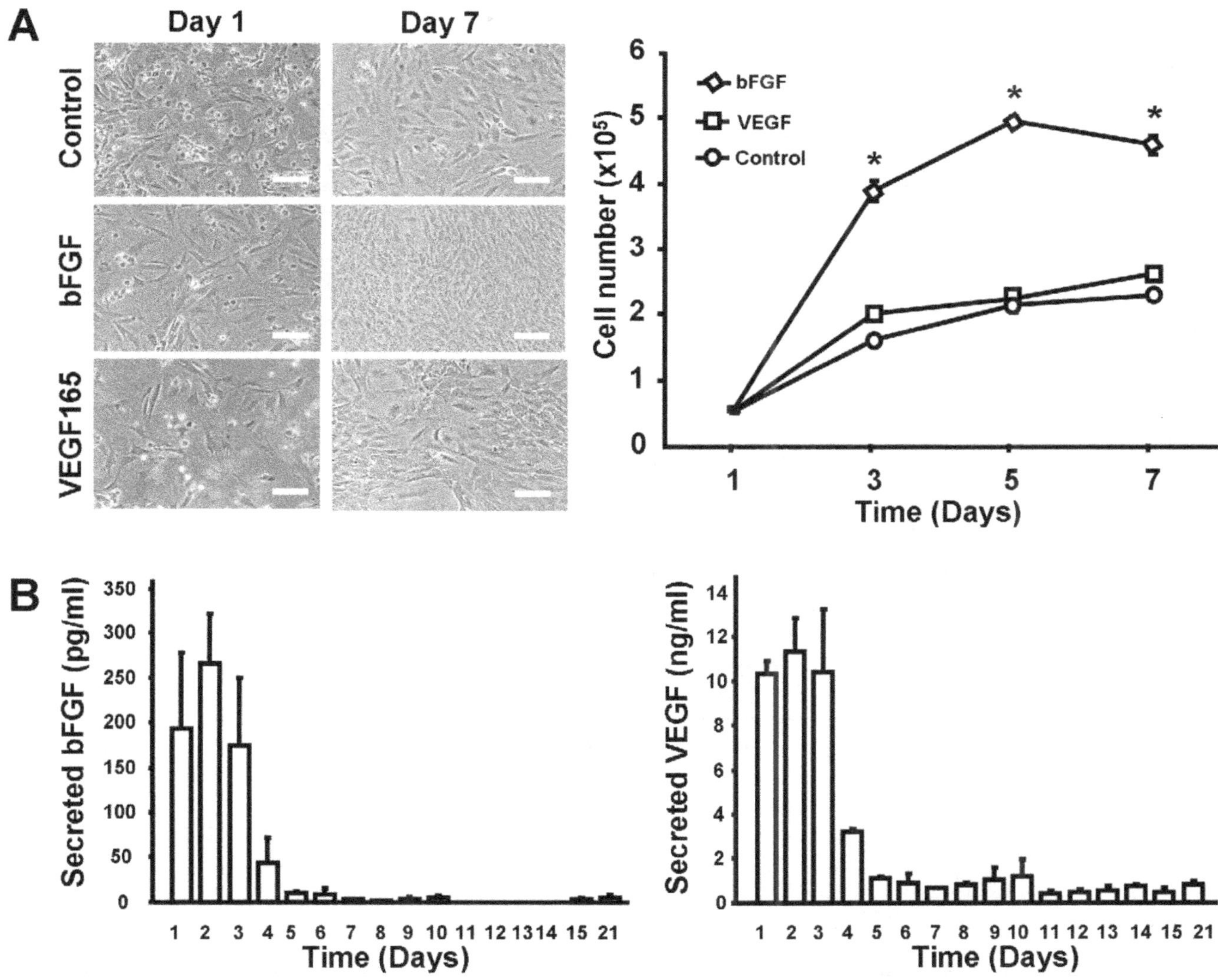

Figure 3. Cell growth and gene expression in primary cultures of fibroblasts transfected with bFGF and VEGF plasmids. After Nucleofection, 1.4×10^5 cells were seeded in a 12 wells plate, 1.5 ml of the culture medium was changed every day. (**A**) 7 days after Nucleofection, more cells were observed in transfected groups. Quantification showed that significant differences were found between bFGF nucleofected group and control group (* $P<0.05$). (**B**) Recombinant growth factors were detected for up to 21 days in the culture media. Scale bar represents 100 μm.

Dermal fibroblast nucleofection with VEGF and bFGF plasmid

After optimization with pmaxGFP vector, VEGF165 and bFGF sequences were inserted into the pmaxGFP® backbone as coding sequences. Seven days later, significantly more cells were observed in the group transfected with plasmids expressing bFGF when compared with the control (Figure 3A). Next, the growth-factor release was evaluated daily for 21 days (Figure 3B). Long-term expressions of both VEGF165 and bFGF proteins were found after nucleofection, and the dynamics of their release were similar. Both growth factors reached the expression or release peak at the first week. However, the amount of secreted growth factors was different between both the groups, with about 50-fold higher release of VEGF165 than bFGF.

In vivo gene-delivery efficiency by nucleofected primary dermal fibroblasts

After administration of genetically modified fibroblasts, distribution of the plasmids in the peripheral tissues or organs was detected by real-time PCR. No plasmid could be detected in any organs of the control rats injected with nonmodified cells. The plasmid was detected for more than 28 days at the site of injection (Figure 4A). The peak of expression at the injection site was on day 3, and then remained at a fairly high level. From day 3 to day 7, the plasmid concentration dropped rapidly. After day 7, the local concentration was maintained at the level of 10^5 copies/100 ng DNA, and then deceased to the order of 10^3 copies/100 ng DNA on day 28. Expression of bFGF and VEGF165 was also detected by PCR at the site of injection. On day 7 post injection, the expression of both angiogenic growth factors in the muscles was more than 100-folds higher than that in the control group (Figure 4B). In all peripheral tissues and organs from the experimental rats, no plasmid was detected after day 14 (Figure 4C).

Administration of nucleofected fibroblasts enhanced angiogenesis and arteriogenesis in the ischemic zone

After cell administration, the ischemic zone was reconstructed (Figure 5A) and the collateral was counted in 3D reconstruction views (Figure 5B). A significant increase in the number of vessels was triggered by the injection of nucleofected cells (Figure 6A and B; $*p<0.05$). Quantification was conducted after reconstruction of the ischemic zone (Figure 7A). Both angiogenesis (Figure 7B, right upper panel; 3.61 ± 0.56 *vs.* 5.13 ± 1.08 $*p<0.05$) and arteriogenesis (Figure 7B, right lower panel; 1.33 ± 0.09 *vs.* 1.63 ± 0.06, $*p<0.05$) increased, indicating an improvement in the medium-size vessel and related small and thin vascular networks.

Increased collateral growth and blood flow in ischemic hindlimbs treated with nucleofected fibroblasts

To further examine the effects of nucleofected cells on collateral growth, collateral proliferation index was analyzed after local administration of nucleofected cells. The results showed an enhanced collateral proliferation in the same model (Figure 8A, BrdU incorporation: 0.48 ± 0.05 vs. 0.57 ± 0.05; $*p<0.05$). Re-establishment of a collateral circulation in ischemic lower hindlimbs was detected by fluorescent microspheres. These microspheres were trapped inside the lumen of the small arteries and the number of the microspheres inside each muscle is related to the blood flow (Figure 8B, left panel). Microspheres from both soleus and gastrocnemius (ligated and nonligated hindlimbs) were

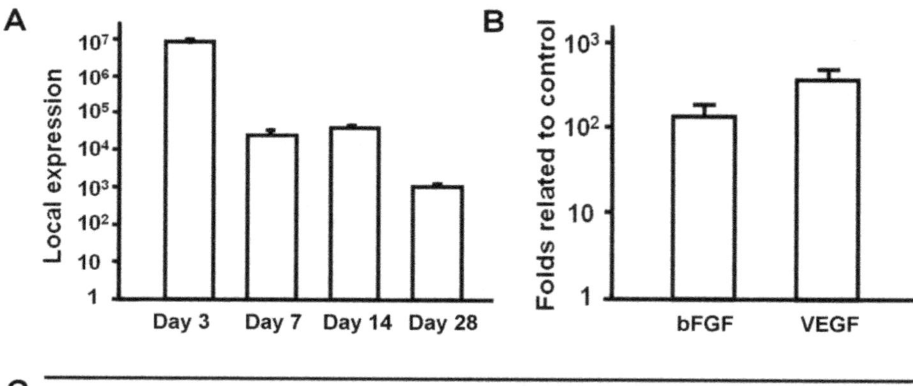

C

Tissue	Day 3	Day 7	Day 14	Day 28
Testis	5.8 ± 0.2	9.6 ± 0.1	N	N
Kidney	6.6 ± 3.4	9.6 ± 5.3	N	N
Heart	86.9 ±34.5	N	N	N
Spleen	10.3 ± 7.8	117.5 ± 56.2	N	N
Liver	1.9 ±3.2	N	N	N

Figure 4. Gene delivery efficiency and expression *in vivo* by modified primary dermal fibroblasts. (**A**) High levels of plasmids were detected in the injected area for more than 28 days. (**B**) 7 days after cell injection, gene expressions of bFGF and VEGF165 from injected area were measured. Results showed that the expressions of both bFGF and VEGF165 were 100 times increased related to the control group. (**C**) After cell administration, organs or tissues were collected at 4 different time points (experimental group: n = 3; control group: n = 3) and the sequence of the plasmid backbone was used for detection of its distribution. Results are shown as the average value obtained from 100 ng DNA of each organ or tissue. N represents that no plasmids were detected.

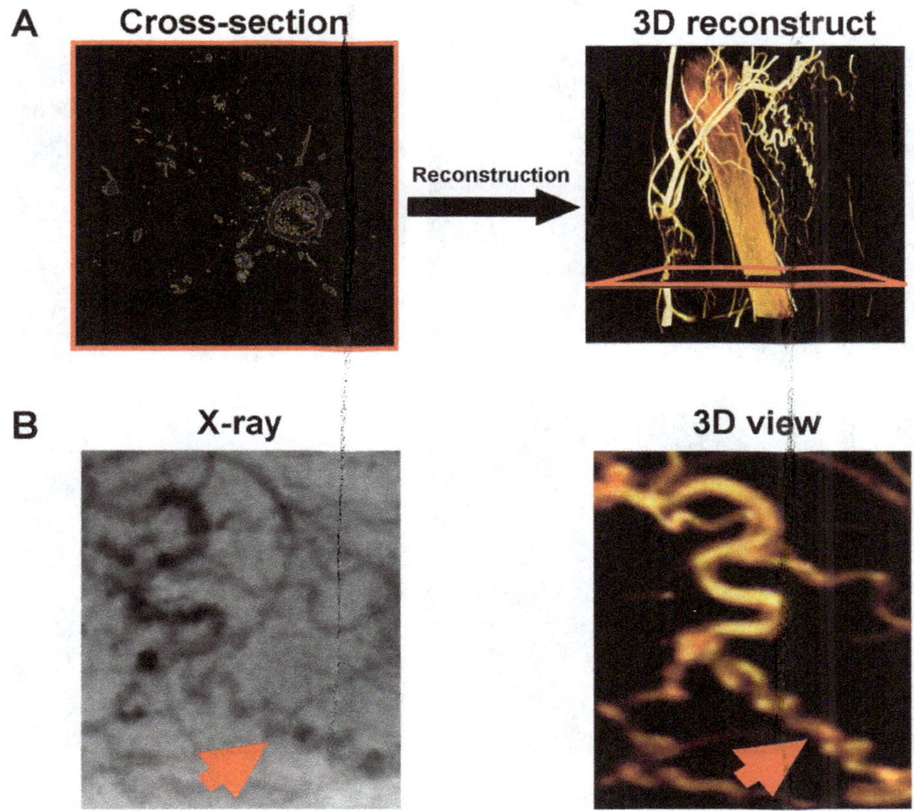

Figure 5. Comparison of micro-CT 3 dimensional collateral detection with planar method. (**A**) Ischemic hindlimb was reconstructed through 1024 Z-axis slices (left panel). (**B**) Vessels in 3 dimensional (3D) reconstruction views were analyzed. Red arrows show the same corkscrew collateral vessel in both X-ray review and 3D reconstruction view.

counted under fluorescent microscope to obtain the perfusion ratio from each animal. Blood flow from soleus and gastrocnemius significantly increased after administration of nucleofected cells (Figure 8B, right; microspheres ratio: gastrocnemius: 0.41±0.10 vs. 0.50±0.11; $*p<0.05$; soleus ratio: soleus: 0.42±0.08 vs. 0.60±0.08; $**p<0.01$).

Discussion

Although several technologies of gene therapy have been extensively applied in animal models of ischemia, their use in clinical settings is still limited [25]. Among the main reasons behind the poor clinical translation of animal studies into humans

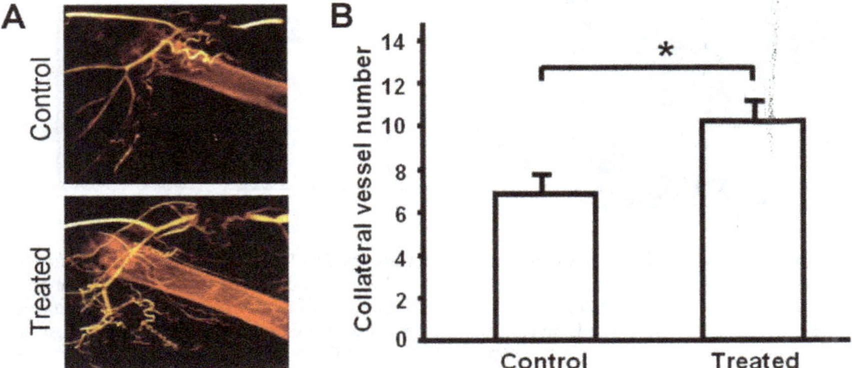

Figure 6. Increased 3D collateral vessels in ischemic hindlimbs treated with nucleofected fibroblasts. (**A**) One week after cell administration, micro-CT angiography was performed and the ischemic zone from both treated and control samples were reconstructed. (**B**) Summarized data showed that injection of transfected cells increased the number of visible collateral vessels (treated group: n = 7; control group: n = 6 $*p<0.05$).

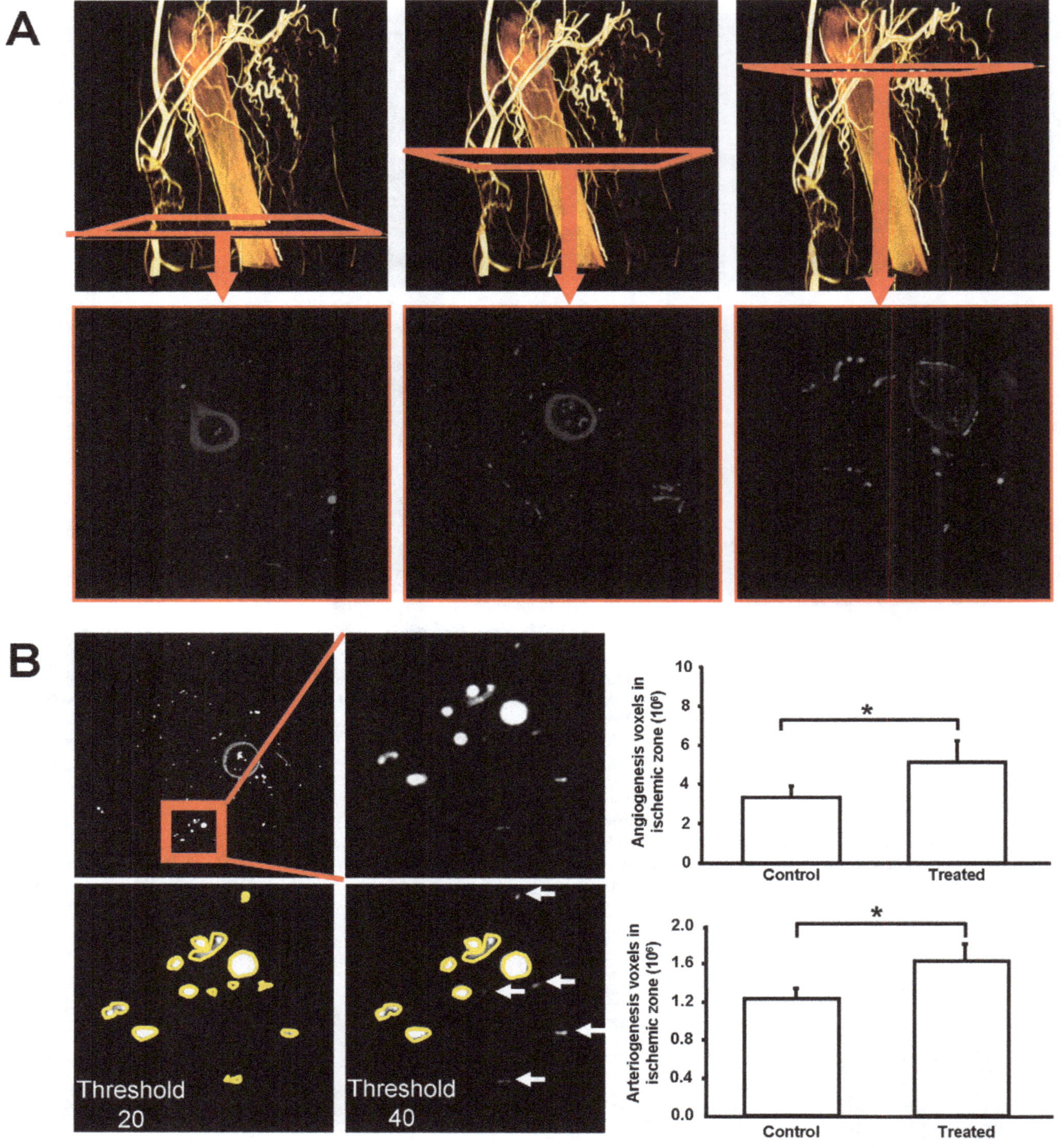

Figure 7. Increased vascular volume in ischemic hindlimbs treated with nucleofected fibroblasts. (**A**) The ischemic zone was defined as 600 slices below the proximal ligation point (slices from the left panel to right panel), including the distal ligation point in the middle panel. (**B**) Quantification was done with 2 different thresholds: T20 and T40. With threshold 20, all vessels (angiogenesis and arteriogenesis related) were counted. Threshold 40 was used to quantify only vessels with higher caliber (arteriogenesis related). (**C and D**) Vessels related to angiogenesis and arteriogenesis were significantly enhanced after nucleofected fibroblasts injection (treated group: n = 7; control group: n = 6; Angiogenesis: * $p<0.05$, Arteriogenesis: *$p<0.05$).

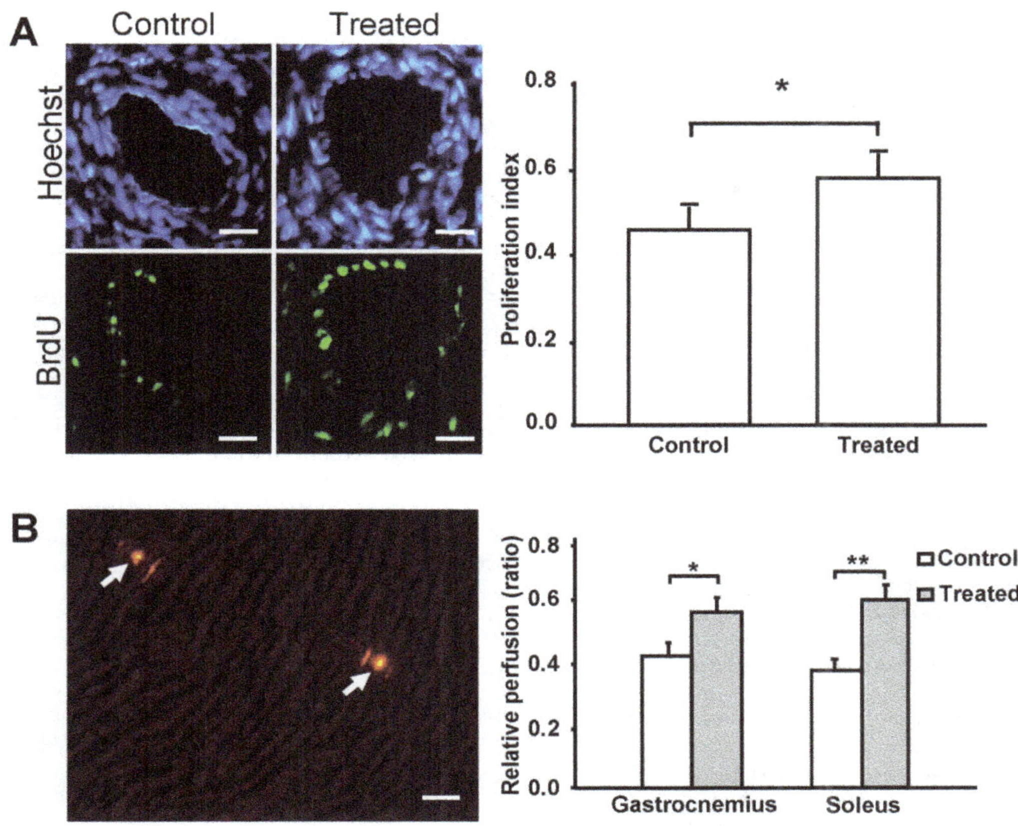

Figure 8. Increased collateral growth and blood flow in ischemic hindlimbs treated with nucleofected fibroblasts. (**A**) One week after cell administration, collateral growth was detected and quantified by BrdU and Hoechst staining. The proliferation index is expressed as BrdU (green) positive nuclei *vs.* total (Hoechst/blue). Quantification showed that proliferation index was significantly enhanced by the injection of transfected cells (Experimental group: n = 8; control group: n = 7,* $p<0.05$). Scale bar represents 50 μm. (**B**) Blood flow was analyzed by FluoSpheres® blood flow detection method. Cryosections were analyzed by fluorescent microscopy and the numbers of the microspheres per muscle sample were counted (left panel). The white arrows show the fluorescent microspheres trapped in the small capillaries. Blood flow ratio was calculated as numbers of microspheres trapped in the ligated muscle *vs.* the number trapped in the same part of the non-ligated leg in the same animal. Results are shown as gastrocnemius perfusion ratio between control and experimental group; soleus perfusion ratio between control group and experimental group (right panel). In both muscles, the blood flow was significantly improved (Experimental group: n = 8; control group: n = 7 soleus: **$p<0.01$ gastrocnemius *$p<0.05$). Scale bar represents 50 μm.

is the lack of both a highly efficient gene delivery system and relatively easy procedures for the clinical translation. Here, we described a modified nucleofection technology based on alternative reagents which owns a high transfection efficiency (>80%) and also a relatively easy operation procedures.

Nucleofection technology is a newly developed nonviral transfection method based on electroporation technology. It could be useful for applications in gene therapy with autologous cells [26,27,28]. Different approaches have been used for nucleofection based gene transfer into primary culture cells [29,30]. Several previous studies have demonstrated the possibility of using this technology to promote neovascularization in ischemic tissues. Aluigi et al. have reported that nucleofection of human mesenchymal stem cells *in vitro* could produce gene expression for more than 20 days [26]. Although stem/progenitor cells were considered to be better candidates for *ex vivo* transfection, uncontrolled differentiation that could lead to a serious side effect was always a concern. Thus, in our study, the physiological stable autologous fibroblasts were used to deliver targeted genes into the ischemic tissue to demonstrate the efficiency of gene therapy. Compared with a recent study by Mueller et al., who demonstrated that a high-efficiency *ex vivo* rat dermal fibroblast transfection with VEGF nucleofection technology could induce local neovascularization effects in a rat skin flap model [31], our findings at least overcame two major drawbacks, namely the relative high cost (Our method cost only 10 folder less than the original method) and the low transfection efficiency (550 pg/ml peak expression of VEGF in the previous study[31] and 10 ng/ml peak expression of VEGF in our present study). Thus, improved reagents for nucleofection in the present study will largely reduce the cost for high efficiency of nucleofection. This modified nucleofection may direct toward the development of similar protocols for human autologous cell gene therapy. However, it should be noted that much work may be needed to translate the findings from the present study to a clinical setting. Most importantly, there is a need to establish efficient protocols for preparation of primary cell cultures from human tissues and to establish the nucleofection efficiency of related genes into such cell cultures. In addition, the applicability for different ischemic diseases in human needs more careful evaluation because the ischemic changes or stages observed in the animal model we used in the present study may be not necessarily seen under human conditions. Certainly there are a number of promising candidates and promising ways of therapeutic application [32,33,34,35]. In the light of previously published studies, the complex mechanism of collateral growth and last not least the results of the present study we think a gene therapy with combination of different growth factors may be likely to have a sustained effect in the treatment of lower extremity ischemia. However, as pointed out above, it is still a very long way to clinical application.

The delivery of our cells directly into the middle part of the thigh is also another important aspect which may favor the therapeutic effects while lower the possible systematic side effects. Our results also confirmed a possible localized expression pattern. It was found that the plasmid can be detected for more than 28 days in the injected area, but it was undetectable in other organs after 14 days. The peak of expression of the plasmid *in vivo* was determined to occur on day 3 (Figure 4A), which is consistent with the *in vitro* data (Figure 3B). Although most of the previous studies showed that less than 10% of the plasmid can reach the general circulation after direct plasmid intramuscular injection [36,37], it was reported that plasmid can be detected by PCR up to 1 year in mice [38]. Here, we showed that the use of *ex vivo* transfection has substantially decreased this time. When compared with the local plasmid concentration, the plasmids in the other organs were fairly low. On day 7, plasmid accumulation in the spleen could be explained by "cleaning effects" of the circulating plasmid by the immune system. All these findings indicate that autologous cell gene delivery can make sustained gene expression in the injected area locally.

After injections of gene-modified fibroblasts into an ischemia model, we also analyzed the neovascularization effects using a 3D micro-CT system. This technology was used here because it presents several advantages when compared to the planar area measurement methods. In our previous studies, angiographies had to be taken from different angles to obtain sufficient information about the collateral vessels [21,24]. Even under the best circumstances, reliable collateral vessel counting is difficult to perform. In the present study, we were able to easily reconstruct the 3D structures of the ligated hindlimbs and quantify the collateral vessels in 3D views (Figure 5A and B). With the use of this method, we were also able to quantify the blood volume by voxel rendering in the reconstruction sections. Vessels related to arteriogenesis and angiogenesis were analyzed separately (Figure 7), and both were found to be improved after cell administration. This result was confirmed by measuring the blood flow in lower hindlimb (Figure 8). Using this technique, we analyzed the efficiency of this autologous cell therapy with gene delivery in the hindlimb ischemia model. Our results strongly suggest that autologous cell therapy with mixture of VEGF165 and bFGF nucleofected cells is very efficient to promote the formation and growth of collateral vessels and re-establish circulation in ischemic area of hindlimb.

In summary, we established a gene delivery method based on highly efficient modified nucleofection approach using double transplantation of nucleofected primary fibroblasts. This technology owns 2 major advantages over other local application: 1) No exogenous vectors are needed; 2) High transfection efficiency with a relatively low cost. This technology might have the potential to be used in the future clinically.

Acknowledgments

The authors gratefully acknowledge the support of the TUM's Thematic Graduate Center/Faculty Graduate Center of Medical Life Science and Technology at Technische Universität München. The authors would like to thank Dr. Zou for his helpful advices and critical revision of the manuscript.

Author Contributions

Conceived and designed the experiments: ZZ AS WDI HGM. Performed the experiments: ZZ AA JN SW NL. Analyzed the data: ZZ AA JN. Contributed reagents/materials/analysis tools: ZZ JAL DFM JL. Wrote the paper: ZZ JTE JAL DFM JL HGM.

References

1. Beard JD (2000) Chronic lower limb ischemia. West J Med 173: 60–63.
2. Holzbach T, Vlaskou D, Neshkova I, Konerding MA, Wortler K, et al. (2010) Non-viral VEGF(165) gene therapy–magnetofection of acoustically active magnetic lipospheres ('magnetobubbles') increases tissue survival in an oversized skin flap model. J Cell Mol Med 14: 587–599.
3. Spanholtz T, Maichle A, Niedworok C, Stoeckelhuber BM, Kruger S, et al. (2009) Timing and targeting of cell-based VEGF165 gene expression in ischemic tissue. J Surg Res 151: 153–162.
4. Harder Y, Amon M, Laschke MW, Schramm R, Rucker M, et al. (2008) An old dream revitalised: preconditioning strategies to protect surgical flaps from critical ischaemia and ischaemia-reperfusion injury. J Plast Reconstr Aesthet Surg 61: 503–511.
5. Spanholtz TA, Theodorou P, Holzbach T, Wutzler S, Giunta RE, et al. (2010) Vascular Endothelial Growth Factor (VEGF(165)) Plus Basic Fibroblast Growth Factor (bFGF) Producing Cells induce a Mature and Stable Vascular Network-a Future Therapy for Ischemically Challenged Tissue. J Surg Res.
6. Baffour R, Berman J, Garb JL, Rhee SW, Kaufman J, et al. (1992) Enhanced angiogenesis and growth of collaterals by in vivo administration of recombinant basic fibroblast growth factor in a rabbit model of acute lower limb ischemia: dose-response effect of basic fibroblast growth factor. J Vasc Surg 16: 181–191.
7. Takeshita S, Isshiki T, Ochiai M, Eto K, Mori H, et al. (1998) Endothelium-dependent relaxation of collateral microvessels after intramuscular gene transfer of vascular endothelial growth factor in a rat model of hindlimb ischemia. Circulation 98: 1261–1263.
8. Lederman RJ, Mendelsohn FO, Anderson RD, Saucedo JF, Tenaglia AN, et al. (2002) Therapeutic angiogenesis with recombinant fibroblast growth factor-2 for intermittent claudication (the TRAFFIC study): a randomised trial. Lancet 359: 2053–2058.
9. Rajagopalan S, Mohler ER, 3rd, Lederman RJ, Mendelsohn FO, Saucedo JF, et al. (2003) Regional angiogenesis with vascular endothelial growth factor in peripheral arterial disease: a phase II randomized, double-blind, controlled study of adenoviral delivery of vascular endothelial growth factor 121 in patients with disabling intermittent claudication. Circulation 108: 1933–1938.
10. Asahara T, Bauters C, Zheng LP, Takeshita S, Bunting S, et al. (1995) Synergistic effect of vascular endothelial growth factor and basic fibroblast growth factor on angiogenesis in vivo. Circulation 92: II365–371.
11. George ML, Eccles SA, Tutton MG, Abulafi AM, Swift RI (2000) Correlation of plasma and serum vascular endothelial growth factor levels with platelet count in colorectal cancer: clinical evidence of platelet scavenging? Clin Cancer Res 6: 3147–3152.
12. Lazarous DF, Shou M, Stiber JA, Dadhania DM, Thirumurti V, et al. (1997) Pharmacodynamics of basic fibroblast growth factor: route of administration determines myocardial and systemic distribution. Cardiovasc Res 36: 78–85.
13. Mullane EM, Dong Z, Sedgley CM, Hu JC, Botero TM, et al. (2008) Effects of VEGF and FGF2 on the revascularization of severed human dental pulps. J Dent Res 87: 1144–1148.
14. Yasuhara T, Shingo T, Muraoka K, wen Ji Y, Kameda M, et al. (2005) The differences between high and low-dose administration of VEGF to dopaminergic neurons of in vitro and in vivo Parkinson's disease model. Brain Res 1038: 1–10.
15. Harrigan MR, Ennis SR, Masada T, Keep RF (2002) Intraventricular infusion of vascular endothelial growth factor promotes cerebral angiogenesis with minimal brain edema. Neurosurgery 50: 589–598.
16. Cuevas P, Carceller F, Ortega S, Zazo M, Nieto I, et al. (1991) Hypotensive activity of fibroblast growth factor. Science 254: 1208–1210.
17. Ferraro B, Cruz YL, Coppola D, Heller R (2009) Intradermal delivery of plasmid VEGF(165) by electroporation promotes wound healing. Mol Ther 17: 651–657.

18. Nikol S (2007) Viral or non-viral angiogenesis gene transfer-New answers to old questions. Cardiovasc Res 73: 443–445.
19. Bonadio J, Smiley E, Patil P, Goldstein S (1999) Localized, direct plasmid gene delivery in vivo: prolonged therapy results in reproducible tissue regeneration. Nat Med 5: 753–759.
20. Kondoh K, Koyama H, Miyata T, Takato T, Hamada H, et al. (2004) Conduction performance of collateral vessels induced by vascular endothelial growth factor or basic fibroblast growth factor. Cardiovasc Res 61: 132–142.
21. Herzog S, Sager H, Khmelevski E, Deylig A, Ito WD (2002) Collateral arteries grow from preexisting anastomoses in the rat hindlimb. Am J Physiol Heart Circ Physiol 283: H2012–2020.
22. Ito WD, Arras M, Scholz D, Winkler B, Htun P, et al. (1997) Angiogenesis but not collateral growth is associated with ischemia after femoral artery occlusion. Am J Physiol 273: H1255–1265.
23. Nikol S (2008) Gene therapy of cardiovascular disease. Curr Opin Mol Ther 10: 479–492.
24. Khmelewski E, Becker A, Meinertz T, Ito WD (2004) Tissue resident cells play a dominant role in arteriogenesis and concomitant macrophage accumulation. Circ Res 95: E56–64.
25. Choo PW, Rand CS, Inui TS, Lee ML, Ma CC, et al. (2000) A pharmacodynamic assessment of the impact of antihypertensive non-adherence on blood pressure control. Pharmacoepidemiol Drug Saf 9: 557–563.
26. Aluigi M, Fogli M, Curti A, Isidori A, Gruppioni E, et al. (2006) Nucleofection is an efficient nonviral transfection technique for human bone marrow-derived mesenchymal stem cells. Stem Cells 24: 454–461.
27. Cesnulevicius K, Timmer M, Wesemann M, Thomas T, Barkhausen T, et al. (2006) Nucleofection is the most efficient nonviral transfection method for neuronal stem cells derived from ventral mesencephali with no changes in cell composition or dopaminergic fate. Stem Cells 24: 2776–2791.
28. Jacobsen F, Mertens-Rill J, Beller J, Hirsch T, Daigeler A, et al. (2006) Nucleofection: a new method for cutaneous gene transfer? J Biomed Biotechnol 2006: 26060.
29. Zeitelhofer M, Vessey JP, Thomas S, Kiebler M, Dahm R (2009) Transfection of cultured primary neurons via nucleofection. Curr Protoc Neurosci Chapter 4: Unit4 32.
30. Kang J, Ramu S, Lee S, Aguilar B, Ganesan SK, et al. (2009) Phosphate-buffered saline-based nucleofection of primary endothelial cells. Anal Biochem 386: 251–255.
31. Mueller CK, Thorwarth MW, Schultze-Mosgau S (2010) Angiogenic gene-modified fibroblasts for induction of localized angiogenesis. J Surg Res 160: 340–348.
32. Doi K, Ikeda T, Marui A, Kushibiki T, Arai Y, et al. (2007) Enhanced angiogenesis by gelatin hydrogels incorporating basic fibroblast growth factor in rabbit model of hind limb ischemia. Heart Vessels 22: 104–108.
33. Fujita M, Ishihara M, Shimizu M, Obara K, Nakamura S, et al. (2007) Therapeutic angiogenesis induced by controlled release of fibroblast growth factor-2 from injectable chitosan/non-anticoagulant heparin hydrogel in a rat hindlimb ischemia model. Wound Repair Regen 15: 58–65.
34. Marui A, Tabata Y, Kojima S, Yamamoto M, Tambara K, et al. (2007) A novel approach to therapeutic angiogenesis for patients with critical limb ischemia by sustained release of basic fibroblast growth factor using biodegradable gelatin hydrogel: an initial report of the phase I-IIa study. Circ J 71: 1181–1186.
35. Olea FD, Vera Janavel G, Cuniberti L, Yannarelli G, Cabeza Meckert P, et al. (2009) Repeated, but not single, VEGF gene transfer affords protection against ischemic muscle lesions in rabbits with hindlimb ischemia. Gene Ther 16: 716–723.
36. Gravier R, Dory D, Laurentie M, Bougeard S, Cariolet R, et al. (2007) In vivo tissue distribution and kinetics of a pseudorabies virus plasmid DNA vaccine after intramuscular injection in swine. Vaccine 25: 6930–6938.
37. Parker SE, Monteith D, Horton H, Hof R, Hernandez P, et al. (2001) Safety of a GM-CSF adjuvant-plasmid DNA malaria vaccine. Gene Ther 8: 1011–1023.
38. Bembenek A, Lotterer E, Machens A, Cario H, Krause U, et al. (1998) Neuroendocrine tumor of the common hepatic duct: a rare cause of extrahepatic jaundice in adolescence. Surgery 123: 712–715.

11

Separating Lentiviral Vector Injection and Induction of Gene Expression in Time, does not Prevent an Immune Response to rtTA in Rats

David M. Markusic, Dirk R. de Waart, Jurgen Seppen*

Academic Medical Center, Tytgat Institute for Liver and Intestinal Research, Amsterdam, The Netherlands

Abstract

Background: Lentiviral gene transfer can provide long-term expression of therapeutic genes such as erythropoietin. Because overexpression of erythropoietin can be toxic, regulated expression is needed. Doxycycline inducible vectors can regulate expression of therapeutic transgenes efficiently. However, because they express an immunogenic transactivator (rtTA), their utility for gene therapy is limited. In addition to immunogenic proteins that are expressed from inducible vectors, injection of the vector itself is likely to elicit an immune response because viral capsid proteins will induce "danger signals" that trigger an innate response and recruit inflammatory cells.

Methodology and Principal Findings: We have developed an autoregulatory lentiviral vector in which basal expression of rtTA is very low. This enabled us to temporally separate the injection of virus and the expression of the therapeutic gene and rtTA. Wistar rats were injected with an autoregulatory rat erythropoietin expression vector. Two or six weeks after injection, erythropoietin expression was induced by doxycycline. This resulted in an increase of the hematocrit, irrespective of the timing of the induction. However, most rats only responded once to doxycycline administration. Antibodies against rtTA were detected in the early and late induction groups.

Conclusions: Our results suggest that, even when viral vector capsid proteins have disappeared, expression of foreign proteins in muscle will lead to an immune response.

Editor: Jacques Zimmer, Centre de Recherche Public de la Santé (CRP-Santé), Luxembourg

Funding: This research was partially funded by NWO (http://www.zonmw.nl/), 016.026.012, to JS. The funders had no role in study design, data collection and analysis, decision to publish, or preparation of the manuscript.

Competing Interests: The authors have declared that no competing interests exist.

* E-mail: j.seppen@amc.uva.nl

Introduction

Many forms of gene therapy will require the ability to modulate the expression of therapeutic genes to maintain expression levels within a therapeutic window or adjust expression levels based on disease progression within the patient [1]. Lentiviral vectors derived from HIV-1 are a well-suited vehicle for the treatment of a variety of inherited and acquired diseases. They can deliver a relatively large therapeutic cassette into both dividing and non-dividing cells and integrate into the host cell genome providing life long expression of the therapeutic gene [2–4].

Because the tetracycline (Tet-On) inducible system [5] has been extensively used to regulate gene expression *in vitro* and *in vivo* [6–8], it is an attractive candidate to develop regulated gene therapy. The Tet-On system is composed of a chimeric reverse tetracycline transactivator (rtTA) composed of the herpesvirus VP16 transcription activating domain and a mutant tetracycline repressor protein from *Escherichia coli.* Furthermore, the system contains a minimal CMV promoter fused to several copies of the tetracycline operator sequence (tetO). In the presence of tetracycline or doxycycline, rtTA binds to the tetO and thus initiates transcription.

Early versions of the Tet-On system required high concentration of doxycycline for activation (100 ng/ml to 1000 ng/ml), which are easily obtained in cell culture but not *in vivo.* Novel rtTA variants derived from viral evolution were recently described that are responsive to as little as 10 ng/ml doxycycline [9], making them potentially better suited for *in vivo* use.

Although there have been significant improvements made in the basal activity and sensitivity of rtTA, this chimeric bacterial and viral protein can be a potent immunogen. Indeed, in studies performed in mice [10] and non-human primates [11,12], the development of rtTA antibodies and cytotoxic T cell mediated clearance of rtTA expressing cells was observed.

Immune responses to therapeutic proteins and clearance of corrected cells is a major obstacle to the clinical implementation of gene therapy. The Danger Model proposed by Matzinger suggests that the immune system does not function solely based on detection of self and non-self, but additionally requires a danger signal to activate antigen presenting cells (APC) leading to an immune response [13,14]. The Danger Model predicts that presentation of the antigen in the absence of danger signals would lead to either elimination or anergization of T cells and induce a temporary state of tolerance. In regards to gene therapy, the injection of a viral vector introduces large amounts of foreign proteins and is a potent trigger for the activation of danger signals [15].

We have previously described a single Tet-on inducible lentiviral vector with autoregulatory expression of rtTA [16]. This vector is characterised by very low basal expression levels of rtTA in the absence of doxycycline stimulation. Only when doxycycline is administrated, expression of rtTA and the therapeutic or marker gene is induced[16].

Mathematical modelling predicts that this type of synthetic gene circuit exhibits bimodal expression; the regulated gene can only be in a "on" or "off" state, without intermediary expression levels, and this was indeed verified experimentally[17]. However, the absolute magnitude of expression levels will vary between individual integrated vector genomes[17].

We showed in cell culture that our autoregulatory vector has lower background and higher induction than vectors in which there is constitutive expression of rtTA[16]. This vector also performed better *in vivo* in immunocompromised mice. Human hematopoietic stem cells were transduced with an autoregulatory or constitutive rtTA vector and transplanted into immune deficient mice[18]. Only cells transduced with the autoregulatory vector differentiated into multiple lineages and several cycles of GFP expression could be induced by doxycycline administration[18].

These data indicate that autoregulatory lentiviral vectors perform better than vectors in which there is constitutive expression of rtTA. Likely because constitutive expression of rtTA is toxic and also leads to higher background expression of the regulated gene.

We have previously shown that lentiviral vectors can be used for the stable long term expression of erythropoietin (Epo) in rats [19]. Erythropoietin gene therapy would be an alternative to treatment with recombinant Epo in patients with kidney failure. However, because over expression of Epo and the resulting high hematocrits will lead to a variety of clinical problems, Epo gene therapy must be carefully regulated.

To test our autoregulatory lentiviral vector system with a therapeutic gene in immunocompetent animals, we constructed an inducible rat Epo vector. This allowed us to determine if induction of rtTA expression in absence of the danger signals associated with the injection of viral particles, would avoid an immune response to rtTA and allow for repeated rounds of doxycycline stimulation.

Results

Construction and in vitro evaluation of TREAutoR4rEPO

Our previously described single doxycycline inducible lentiviral vector TREAutoR3 [16] was modified by replacing the d2eGFP gene with the cDNA coding for rat erythropoietin and introduction of a novel rtTA variant, V16 (V9I F67S R171K) [9] with a 10 fold increased sentivity to doxycycline to make TREAutoR4rEPO. We selected a rat muscle cell line, H9C2, to evaluate the function of the system *in vitro*. H9C2 cells were transduced with concentrated TREAutoR4rEPO virus and allowed to expand. Following expansion, cells were stimulated with 10 ng/ml doxycycline and 72 hours later media was collected and cell lysates were prepared to determine basal and induced EPO and rtTA expression levels respectively. Western blot of H9C2 cell lysates showed undetectable levels of rtTA expression in the absence of doxycycline (Figure 1 lane 3), rtTA expression was only detected following treatment with 10 ng/ml doxycycline (Figure 1 lane 4). Control cells showed no detectable rtTA expression in the absence or presence of doxycycline (Figure 1

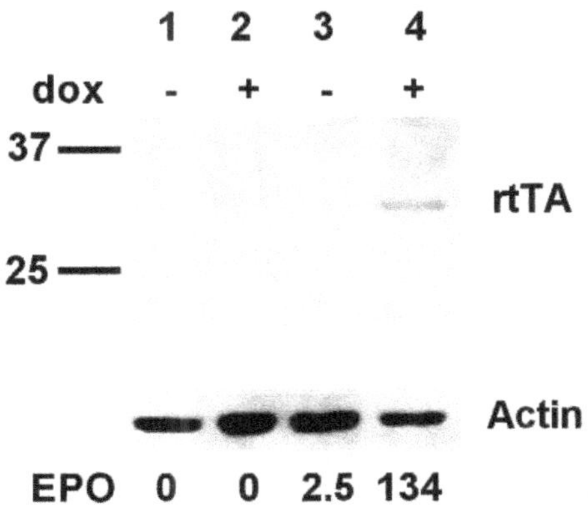

Figure 1. *In vitro* regulation of Epo expression in H9c2 rat myoblasts. A Western blot on control and transduced H9c2 cells was performed to detect rtTA expression. Expression of actin was used as a loading control. Simultaneously, the corresponding levels of Epo secreted into the cell culture media were measured by ELISA and are reported as mIU/mL below the Western blot. Lanes 1 and 2 control H9c2 lysates, 3 and 4 H9c2 cells transduced with TREAutoR4rEPO. Lanes 2 and 4 contain lysates of cells that were induced by the addition of doxycycline.

lanes 1). Epo was not detected in the media of mock transduced cells. (Figure 1 lower panel lanes 1 and 2). A low basal level of Epo was detected in the media of unstimulated cells transduced with the TREAutoR4rEPO vector (Figure 1 lower panel lane 3). Following stimulation with 10 ng/ml doxycycline we detected an strong increase in Epo levels (Figure 1 lower panel lanes 4) of 53 fold.

Constitutive expression of rat Epo

We previously demonstrated long term expression of Epo delivered by an intramuscular injection of a lentiviral vector in Fisher 344 rats [19]. To confirm similar long-term expression in Wistar rats, a lentiviral vector with a constitutive CMV promoter driving expression of Epo was injected into the hind leg of Wistar rats and blood samples were collected every two weeks. An increase in hematocrit was observed two weeks following virus injection to 60%, reaching a plateau level of approximately 75% by week ten (Figure 2), confirming long term Epo expression. These data indicate that lentiviral vectors with constitutive expression of rat Epo are not silenced or cleared by the immune system in rat muscle.

Inducible expression or rat Epo

In total 16 rats received an IM injection of 0.4ug p24 of TREAutoR4rEPO virus in 100 µl PBS into the right hind leg. The animals were divided into two groups: early induction, receiving doxycycline in the drinking water two weeks following virus injection, and late induction getting doxycycline in the drinking water six weeks following virus injection. One rat from the early induction group and two from the late induction group did not have any response to doxycycline stimulation and were classified as non-responders. Blood was collected every two weeks for hematocrit determination. Two weeks following doxycycline administration the average hematocrit of the early induction group increased from 51% to 67% (Figure 3). Unexpectedly, after four weeks of doxycycline treatment the average hematocrit dropped down to 59%. Since the mean life span of erythrocytes in the Wistar rat is approximately 60 days [20], this rapid decrease in

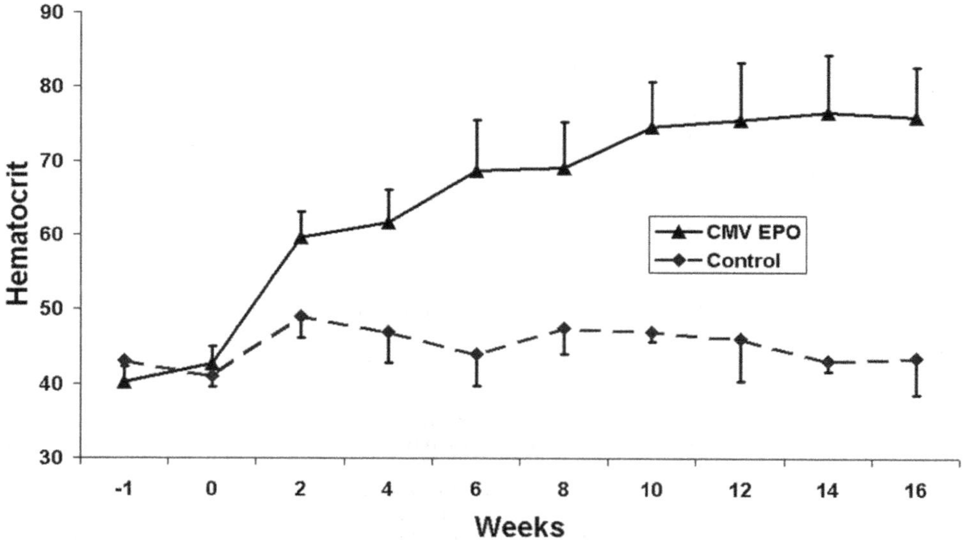

Figure 2. Constitutive lentiviral expression of Epo. Wistar rats were injected with CMV Epo (n = 11) or vehicle (n = 2) at t = 0. A sustained elevated hematocrit was observed in all CMV Epo injected animals.

hematocrit suggests that there was a loss of Epo expression shortly after initiation of doxycycline administration. At the four and six week time points there was a significant difference ($p<0.005$) in hematocrit between untreated and doxycycline treated rats. A second round of stimulation with doxycycline was performed ten weeks following virus injection and no change in hematocrit was detected in all rats in the early induction group.

At six weeks following virus injection the early induction group was placed on normal water while the late induction group received its first doxycycline in the drinking water for a period of four weeks. Two weeks following doxycycline stimulation we observed an increase in hematocrit in the late induction group to approximately 62% ($p<0.005$) compared to virus injected rats on normal water. Because the magnitude in increase in hematocrit of the early and late induction groups were comparable, this demonstrated that transduced, non-induced cells persist for six weeks without being eliminated or silenced. As with the early induction group, we observed a rapid decrease in hematocrit after four weeks treatment

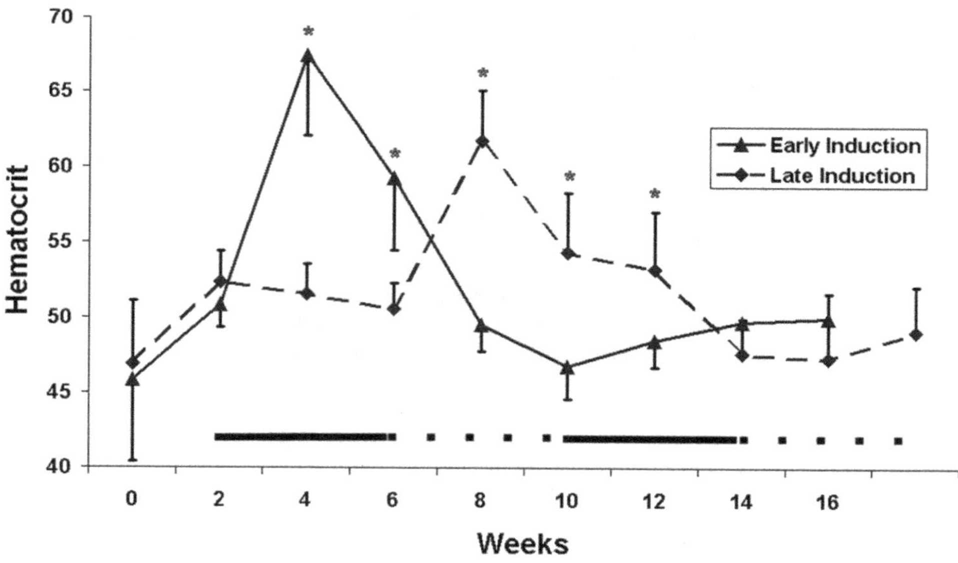

Figure 3. Inducible lentiviral expression of Epo. Wistar rats were injected with TREAutoR4rEpo at t = 0. Early induction rats (n = 7) were given doxycycline in the drinking water for two periods of four weeks starting at weeks 2 and 10 (solid line). Late induction rats (n = 5) were given doxycycline in the drinking water for two periods of four weeks starting at weeks 6 and 14 (dashed line). The solid and dashed lines below indicate the starting points for doxycycline administration for the early and late induction groups respectively. * Indicates a statistical significant difference $p<0.05$ between the early and late induction groups.

with doxycycline, again suggesting a rapid elimination of transduced cells upon induction of Epo expression. A second round of doxycycline stimulation at week 14 failed to raise hematocrit levels as observed with the early induction group (Figure 3).

Interestingly, one rat, R15, within the late induction group was capable of undergoing multiple rounds of induction with doxycycline (Figure 4) and was not included in the data analysis for the late induction group. The kinetics of hematocrit changes of this rat were also markedly different. High hematocrits were maintained longer after doxycycline administration was halted. These observations provide more evidence that the rapid decrease in hematocrits in most animals induced by doxycycline was due to elimination of transduced cells.

Detection of rtTA antibodies in plasma is independent of early or late induction

Plasma from rats at two, six, and ten weeks after viral injection was analyzed for the presence of rtTA antibodies in the early induction, late induction, and non-responder groups. No antibodies were detected in the plasma of animals from each group at the two weeks time point. At the ten week time point no difference was seen in the total number of animals positive for rtTA antibodies between the early and late induction groups (Table 1). This suggests that there is no benefit in delaying induction for preventing a humoral immune response.

Influx of immune cells detected within the area of viral injection

Rats were injected with a lentiviral GFP vector to better understand the local immunological response to an intramuscular injection. Animals were sacrificed at one and two weeks following injection and muscle was collected for immunostaining with an antibody directed against rat CD45 to detect the presence of infiltrating immune cells. One week following lentiviral vector injection we observed massive infiltration of CD45 positive cells in areas with remnants of GFP expression. (Figure 5A,B) and not in areas negative for GFP expression (Figure 5C) or in the PBS injected muscle (Figure 5D). Only punctuate GFP expression was detected, these are likely remnants of GFP expressing muscle cells. The muscle tissue with immune cell infiltration appeared damaged, also suggesting the clearance of transduced cells. No GFP positive muscle cells were detected two weeks following viral injection (data not shown). These data indicate that rats do mount a vigorous immune response to immunogenic antigens delivered by lentiviral vectors.

Discussion

The ability to regulate the expression level of a therapeutic gene is vital for the advancement of gene therapy into the clinic. In addition to concerns over safety, expression levels of the therapeutic gene may require modulation in response to the disease progression of the patient[1]. Lentiviral vector mediated gene therapy is well suited for the long-term expression of a therapeutic gene. We have previously described an autoregulatory lentiviral vector that uses the tetracycline inducible system and is characterised by low basal expression of rtTA and regulated genes in the absence of doxycycline stimulation [16]. To test our system with a therapeutically relevant gene *in vivo* we constructed a vector in which Erythropoietin (Epo) expression could be regulated. This vector also included a new rtTA variant [9] which is 100 times more sensitive to doxycycline than the originally described rtTA.

We confirmed that by using this vector rtTA protein expression was undetectable on western blot of transduced muscle cells in the absence of doxycycline (Figure 1). We also showed that this vector mediates a robust induction of the therapeutic gene Epo *in vitro*.

Wistar rats were injected with the inducible Epo vector and doxycycline was administrated two weeks (early induction) or six weeks (late induction) after vector injection.

In both early and late and induction groups we observed a similar pattern, an initial increase in hematocrit at two weeks following doxycycline treatment followed by a reduction in hematocrit levels at four weeks on doxycycline (Figure 3). Given that the estimated life span of Wistar rat erythrocytes is 59 days

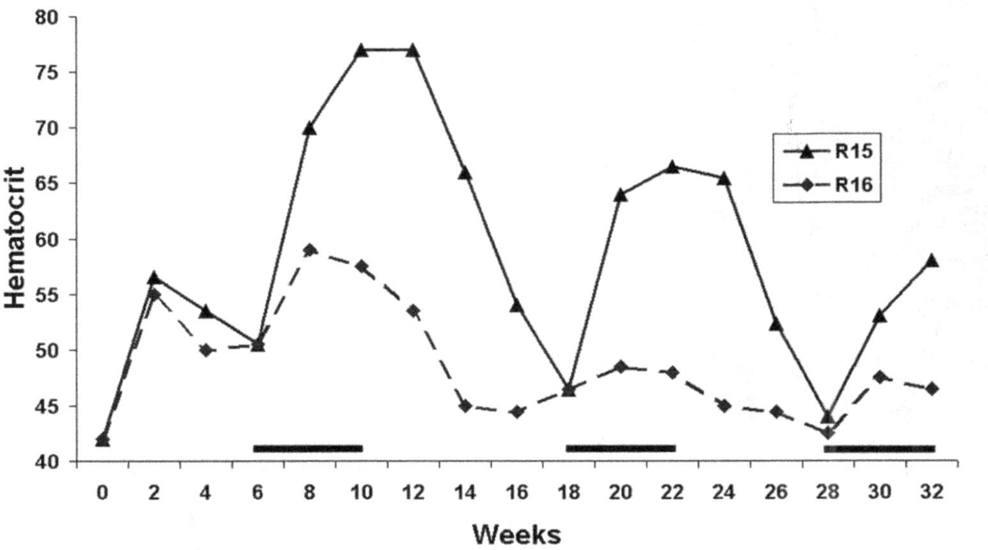

Figure 4. Multiple cycles of Epo expression. Wistar rats were injected with TREAutoR4rEpo at t = 0. Rats were given doxycycline in the drinking water for three periods of four weeks starting at weeks 6, 18 and 28 (solid line). In one rat (R15), hematocrits could be increased with each of three successive rounds of doxycycline administration. The cage and litter mate (R16) only responded once to doxycycline.

Table 1. Antibodies directed against rtTA.

	Weeks following virus administration		
Group	**2**	**6**	**10**
Early Induction (n = 3)	0/3	2/3	3/3
Late Induction (n = 3)	0/3	1/3	3/3
Non responders (n = 2)	0/2	2/2	2/2

Eight animals were analyzed for the presence of circulating antibodies to rtTA by ELISA.
At 2 weeks following virus administration no animals had received doxycycline.
At 6 weeks the Early induction group had been given doxycycline in the drinking water for 4 weeks and were subsequently placed on normal water. At 10 weeks the Late induction group had been given doxycycline in the drinking water for 4 weeks. The Non responders consist of one animal each from the Early and Late induction groups.
All animals developed antibodies to rtTA.

[20], this suggests that immediately following doxycycline administration there is a rapid loss in exogenously expressed Epo. Silencing of vector is unlikely since rats injected with a constitutive Epo vector show long term expression without reduction in therapeutic effect (Figure 2) and because rats can be induced as efficiently two or six weeks after vector injection. Furthermore, in human hematopoietic cells grafted in immune deficient mice, multiple rounds of induction with a comparable autoregulatory GFP vector are also possible[18].

The most likely explanation of the loss of Epo expressing cells is therefore an cytotoxic immune response against the transduced muscle cells. This hypothesis is strengthened by the appearance of antibodies to rtTA in the injected animals. However, only direct detection of rtTA specific cytotoxic T cells will conclusively prove that the loss of Epo expression is immune mediated.

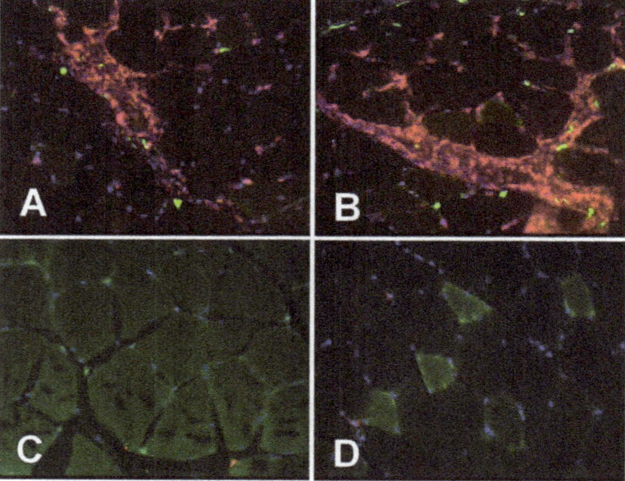

Figure 5. Histochemistry of rat muscle injected with GFP lentiviral vector. Wistar rats were injected with a lentiviral GFP expression vector (A-C) or saline control (D). (A,B) Areas with remnants of GFP expressing cells (green) show co-localization with CD45 stained (red) infiltrating immune cells. (C) Areas without GFP expression within the same piece of tissue are devoid of infiltrating immune cells. (D) Control injected muscle is negative for both GFP expression and infiltrating immune cells.

Interestingly, one animal in the late induction group was capable of undergoing multiple inductions (Figure 4), while the other animals were not responsive to a second round of doxycycline stimulation (Figure 3). Whether this was a consequence of the late induction is unclear and will require further investigations. No difference was observed in the development of antibodies against rtTA between non-responders, early induction, and late induction groups at ten weeks following virus injection (Table 1). This suggests that delaying induction has no benefit for the prevention of a humoral immune response.

A strong immune response was observed following intramuscular injected lentiviral vector expressing GFP. Muscle harvested one week following vector injection showed sporadic expression of GFP that was accompanied by massive infiltration of immune cells (Figure 5A and 5B). No GFP positive cells or areas of infiltrating immune cells were detected in an animal sacrificed two weeks following vector injection (data not shown), further suggesting a rapid clearance of GFP expressing muscle cells. These data show that rats have a vigorous immune response to lentiviral vectors expressing GFP from a ubiquitous promoter and might be a better animal model for pre clinical gene therapy studies than the commonly used murine models.

Several factors, including contaminants from the concentration of viral preparation [21] and efficient transduction of professional antigen presenting cells (APC) [22,23], may play a role in the short term expression observed following intramuscular injection of lentiviral vectors. Introduction of muscle specific promoters have been shown to improve long term adenoviral [24] and AAV [25] mediated expression. A muscle specific promoter driving rtTA expression was required to obtain long term regulation using an adenoviral vector [26]. Together, this suggests that gene transfer to antigen presenting cells within the muscle and subsequent expression and presentation of the transgene may be a critical factor in the initiation of an immune response.

In summary, we have shown that the low basal level of rtTA expressed in our autoregulatory vector is not sufficient to avoid an immune response to rtTA.

Our results therefore suggest that danger signals associated with the injection of a viral vector are not essential for the development of an immune response. However, since our autoregulatory vector has, by definition, a low level of basal expression, we therefore cannot completely exclude the possibility that the immune system is primed at the moment of injection.

Further modifications are required to translate this system into clinical applications.

Materials and Methods

Plasmid construction

The constitutive rat Epo lentiviral vector was constructed by cloning rat Epo as an EcoR1 fragment in prrlcpptCMVPRE[27].

An expression plasmid containing the rtTA variant V16 (V9I F67S R171K), rtTA4, was digested with XbaI and XmaI and subcloned into a XbaI and XmaI digest of pRRLcpptMCSIRESrtTA3LTRTetO to make pRRLcpptMCSIRESrtTA4LTRTetO and was verified by sequencing. An expression plasmid for d2eGFP and pRRLcpptMCSIRESrtTA4LTRTetO were digested with BamHI and EcoRI and the resulting d2eGFP fragment was cloned into pRRLcpptMCSIRESrtTA4LTRTetO to make pRRLcpptd2eGFPIRESrtTA4LTRTetO. A BamHI and EcoRV digest was performed to liberate a fragment containing d2eGFPIRESrtTA4 and was subcloned into a BamHI and

EcoRV digest of pBSK to make pBSK d2eGFPIRESrtTA4. An AgeI and XhoI digest was performed on pBSK d2eGFPIRESrtTA4 and TREAutoR3 and the new fragment d2eGFPIRESrtTA4 was cloned into the TREAutoR3 backbone to make TREAutoR4. The gene coding for rat erythropoietin was recovered by an EcoRI digest of the pRRLcpptCMVEpo plasmid cloned into the backbone of an EcoRI digest of TREAutoR4 to make TREAutoR4rEPO.

Cell lines and culturing

Human embryonic kidney (HEK) 293T, HeLa, and H9c2 rat DB1X heart myoblasts were originally obtained from ATCC (http://www.atcc.org/), cultured in standard DMEM supplemented with 10% fetal bovine serum, 100 U/ml penicillin, 100 μg/ml streptomycin, 2 mM glutamine at 37°C in 10% CO_2.

Lentiviral vector preparation

Lentiviral vectors were produced as previously reported [27]. Briefly, HEK 293T cells were transiently transfected by calcium phosphate precipitation using a third generation lentiviral vector system [28,29]. Twenty-four hours following transfection, fresh media supplemented with 25 mM HEPES buffer pH 7.4 was added. Virus containing supernatent was harvested 48 and 72 hours following transfected, filtered through 0.45 μm Millipore filters and concentrated by ultra centrifugation using a Beckman SW-28 rotor 20,000 RPM for 2 hours at 4°C. Viral pellets were resuspended in PBS and frozen at −80°C.

Viral transduction

The p24 antigen content of concentrated TREAutoR4rEpo lentivirus was determined using a commercial ELISA kit from Perkin Elmer (NEK050A). H9C2 cells were seeded out at 1×10^5 per well and were transduced for four hours in the presence of 10 μg/ml DEAE Dextran. Gene expression was induced by the addition of 10 ng/ml doxycycline (Sigma). Epo secretion into media was determined using a commercial ELISA kit from R&D Systems (DEP00). Viral titers of LVpgkGFP were determined by serial dilution on HeLa cells. GFP expression in transduced HeLa cells was determined by flow cytometry 72 hours following transduction.

Ethics statement

All animal experiments were performed approved by the Animal Ethical Committee at the Academic Medical Center of Amsterdam.

Intramuscular injection of CMV rEPO, TREAutoR4rEPO and LVpgkGFP

Male Wistar rats weighing approximately 300 g were anesthetized by isoflurane gas inhalation. The right hind leg was injected with a total of 100 μl of CMVrEpo, TREAutoR4rEPO virus (0.4 μg p24) or 100 μl of LVpgkGFP (0.4 μg p24, corresponding to 1×10^7 HeLa transducing units) in three separate injections.

Doxycycline administration, blood collection, and analysis

Drinking water was prepared containing 200 ug/ml doxycycline, 1% sucrose pH 6.0. Blood was collected every two weeks via the tail vein under isoflurane gas anaesthesia. Hematocrit levels were determined using a glass capillary following standard protocols. Plasma was frozen at −20°C for determining rtTA antibody titers.

ELISA for rat antibodies to rtTA

RtTA was expressed in 293T cells by calcium phosphate coprecipitation. Expression of rtTA was confirmed by western blotting. ELISA plates (Nunc) were coated overnight with 5 ug cellular lysate (rtTA or control) per well in 50 mM carbonate buffer pH 9.6. The wells were blocked with 1% gelatine in PBS, washed and incubated with serial dilutions of rat plasma collected at 2, 6, and 10 weeks following virus injection. After washing, rat immunoglobins were detected with anti-rat IgG peroxidase (Nordic) and o-phenylenediamine tablets (Sigma).

ELISA's were always performed in duplicate with the same samples applied to rtTA and control (293T cell lysate). To correct for a specific binding, the absorbance of the control plate was subtracted from rtTA coated plate. Rat plasma was considered to be positive for rtTA antibodies when the absorption of samples diluted 800 times was above the background.

Immunostaining

In vivo formaldehyde fixed and sucrose embedded muscle tissue was snap frozen in liquid nitrogen. Sections of 7 μm were prepared and kept at −20°C prior to use. Sections were allowed to equilibrate at room temperature and washed three times in PBS for 5 minutes each. Subsequently sections were incubated for hour with a 1:100 dilution of mouse anti rat CD45 (MCA43R AbD Serotec) in PBS/0.05% Tween-20/5% Normal goat serum/5% Rat plasma. Then sections were washed three times, five minutes each in PBS/0.05% Tween-20. A 1:500 dilution of goat anti mouse IgG Alexa 594 in PBS/0.05% Tween-20/5% Normal goat serum/5% Rat plasma was performed for one hour followed by three wash steps in PBS five minutes each. Sections were mounted with Vectashield with DAPI (Vector laboratories H-1200). Images were captured at (200×) magnification using a fluorescent microscope (Leica DMRA2).

SDS-PAGE and Western blotting

H9c2 cell lysates (50 μg) were separated on 10% SDS-PAGE and blotted onto nitrocellulose using the Bio-Rad Miniprotean III system. An antibody directed against the rtTA (TET02 MoBiTec) was used at a 1:1000 dilution. An antibody directed against actin was purchased from NeoMarkers (Ab-5) and used at a dilution of 1:1000. A 1:1000 dilution of goat anti mouse HRP (Bio-Rad 170–6516) was used as the secondary antibody. Detection of reactive bands on western blot was performed using the Lumi-Light Western Blot Substrate (Roche 12 015 200 001) and blots were analyzed using a Lumi Imager F1 and Lumi Analyst 3.1 software (Roche).

Statistical analysis

Statistical analysis was performed using SPSS 11.0 software using the Mann-Whitney U test. Values were determined to be significantly different with $p<0.05$.

Acknowledgments

We thank B. Berkhout and A. Das, Department of Experimental Virology, Academic Medical Center, Amsterdam, for providing us with rtTA variant V16.

We thank C. Kunne, J. Hiralall and R. van der Rijt, AMC Liver Center, Amsterdam, for technical assistence.

Author Contributions

Conceived and designed the experiments: DMM DdW JS. Performed the experiments: DMM DdW JS. Analyzed the data: DMM DdW JS. Wrote the paper: DMM JS.

References

1. Clackson T (2000) Regulated gene expression systems. Gene Ther 7: 120–125.
2. Ailles LE, Naldini L (2002) HIV-1-derived lentiviral vectors. Curr Top Microbiol Immunol 261: 31–52.
3. Trono D (2000) Lentiviral vectors: turning a deadly foe into a therapeutic agent. Gene Ther 7: 20–23.
4. Galimi F, Verma IM (2002) Opportunities for the use of lentiviral vectors in human gene therapy. Curr Top Microbiol Immunol 261: 245–254.
5. Gossen M, Bujard H (1992) Tight control of gene expression in mammalian cells by tetracycline-responsive promoters. Proc Natl Acad Sci U S A 89: 5547–5551.
6. Agha-Mohammadi S, Lotze MT (2000) Regulatable systems: applications in gene therapy and replicating viruses. J Clin Invest 105: 1177–1183.
7. Corbel SY, Rossi FM (2002) Latest developments and in vivo use of the Tet system: ex vivo and in vivo delivery of tetracycline-regulated genes. Curr Opin Biotechnol 13: 448–452.
8. Goverdhana S, Puntel M, Xiong W, Zirger JM, Barcia C, et al. (2005) Regulatable gene expression systems for gene therapy applications: progress and future challenges. Mol Ther 12: 189–211.
9. Zhou X, Vink M, Klaver B, Berkhout B, Das AT (2006) Optimization of the Tet-On system for regulated gene expression through viral evolution. Gene Ther 13: 1382–1390.
10. Ginhoux F, Turbant S, Gross DA, Poupiot J, Marais T, et al. (2004) HLA-A*0201-restricted cytolytic responses to the rtTA transactivator dominant and cryptic epitopes compromise transgene expression induced by the tetracycline on system. Mol Ther 10: 279–289.
11. Favre D, Blouin V, Provost N, Spisek R, Porrot F, et al. (2002) Lack of an immune response against the tetracycline-dependent transactivator correlates with long-term doxycycline-regulated transgene expression in nonhuman primates after intramuscular injection of recombinant adeno-associated virus. J Virol 76: 11605–11.
12. Latta-Mahieu M, Rolland M, Caillet C, Wang M, Kennel P, et al. (2002) Gene transfer of a chimeric trans-activator is immunogenic and results in short-lived transgene expression. Hum Gene Ther 13: 1611–20.
13. Matzinger P (2002) The danger model: a renewed sense of self. Science 296: 301–305.
14. Matzinger P (1994) Tolerance, danger, and the extended family. Annu Rev Immunol 12: 991–1045.
15. Brown BD, Lillicrap D (2002) Dangerous liaisons: the role of "danger" signals in the immune response to gene therapy. Blood 100: 1133–1140.
16. Markusic D, Oude-Elferink R, Das AT, Berkhout B, Seppen J (2005) Comparison of single regulated lentiviral vectors with rtTA expression driven by an autoregulatory loop or a constitutive promoter. Nucleic Acids Res 33: e63.
17. May T, Eccleston L, Herrmann S, Hauser H, Goncalves J, et al. (2008) Bimodal and hysteretic expression in mammalian cells from a synthetic gene circuit. PLoS One 3: e2372.
18. Centlivre M, Zhou X, Pouw SM, Weijer K, Kleibeuker W, et al. (2010) Autoregulatory lentiviral vectors allow multiple cycles of doxycycline-inducible gene expression in human hematopoietic cells in vivo. Gene Ther 17: 14–25.
19. Seppen J, Barry SC, Harder B, Osborne WR (2001) Lentivirus administration to rat muscle provides efficient sustained expression of erythropoietin. Blood 98: 594–596.
20. Derelanko MJ (1987) Determination of erythrocyte life span in F-344, Wistar, and Sprague-Dawley rats using a modification of the [3H]diisopropylfluorophosphate ([3H]DFP) method. Fundam Appl Toxicol 9: 271–276.
21. Scherr M, Battmer K, Eder M, Schule S, Hohenberg H, et al. (2002) Efficient gene transfer into the CNS by lentiviral vectors purified by anion exchange chromatography. Gene Ther 9: 1708–14.
22. VandenDriessche T, Thorrez L, Naldini L, Follenzi A, Moons L, et al. (2002) Lentiviral vectors containing the human immunodeficiency virus type-1 central polypurine tract can efficiently transduce nondividing hepatocytes and antigen-presenting cells in vivo. Blood 100: 813–22.
23. Esslinger C, Chapatte L, Finke D, Miconnet I, Guillaume P, et al. (2003) In vivo administration of a lentiviral vaccine targets DCs and induces efficient CD8(+) T cell responses. J Clin Invest 111: 1673–1681.
24. Hartigan-O'Connor D, Kirk CJ, Crawford R, Mule JJ, Chamberlain JS (2001) Immune evasion by muscle-specific gene expression in dystrophic muscle. Mol Ther 4: 525–533.
25. Cordier L, Gao GP, Hack AA, McNally EM, Wilson JM, et al. (2001) Muscle-specific promoters may be necessary for adeno-associated virus-mediated gene transfer in the treatment of muscular dystrophies. Hum Gene Ther 12: 205–215.
26. Lena AM, Giannetti P, Sporeno E, Ciliberto G, Savino R (2005) Immune responses against tetracycline-dependent transactivators affect long-term expression of mouse erythropoietin delivered by a helper-dependent adenoviral vector. J Gene Med 7: 1086–1096.
27. Seppen J, Rijnberg M, Cooreman MP, Oude Elferink RP (2002) Lentiviral vectors for efficient transduction of isolated primary quiescent hepatocytes. J Hepatol 36: 459–65.
28. Dull T, Zufferey R, Kelly M, Mandel RJ, Nguyen M, et al. (1998) A third-generation lentivirus vector with a conditional packaging system. J Virol 72: 8463–71.
29. Zufferey R, Dull T, Mandel RJ, Bukovsky A, Quiroz D, et al. (1998) Self-inactivating lentivirus vector for safe and efficient in vivo gene delivery. J Virol 72: 9873–9880.

12

Insights into Phosphate Cooperativity and Influence of Substrate Modifications on Binding and Catalysis of Hexameric Purine Nucleoside Phosphorylases

Priscila O. de Giuseppe[1], Nadia H. Martins[1], Andreia N. Meza[1], Camila R. dos Santos[1], Humberto D'Muniz Pereira[2], Mario T. Murakami[1]*

1 Laboratório Nacional de Biociências (LNBio), Centro Nacional de Pesquisa em Energia e Materiais, Campinas, São Paulo, Brazil, 2 Instituto de Física de São Carlos, Grupo de Cristalografia, Universidade de São Paulo, São Carlos, São Paulo, Brazil

Abstract

The hexameric purine nucleoside phosphorylase from *Bacillus subtilis* (BsPNP233) displays great potential to produce nucleoside analogues in industry and can be exploited in the development of new anti-tumor gene therapies. In order to provide structural basis for enzyme and substrates rational optimization, aiming at those applications, the present work shows a thorough and detailed structural description of the binding mode of substrates and nucleoside analogues to the active site of the hexameric BsPNP233. Here we report the crystal structure of BsPNP233 in the apo form and in complex with 11 ligands, including clinically relevant compounds. The crystal structure of six ligands (adenine, 2′deoxyguanosine, aciclovir, ganciclovir, 8-bromoguanosine, 6-chloroguanosine) in complex with a hexameric PNP are presented for the first time. Our data showed that free bases adopt alternative conformations in the BsPNP233 active site and indicated that binding of the co-substrate (2′deoxy)ribose 1-phosphate might contribute for stabilizing the bases in a favorable orientation for catalysis. The BsPNP233-adenosine complex revealed that a hydrogen bond between the 5′ hydroxyl group of adenosine and Arg^{43*} side chain contributes for the ribosyl radical to adopt an unusual C3′-*endo* conformation. The structures with 6-chloroguanosine and 8-bromoguanosine pointed out that the Cl^6 and Br^8 substrate modifications seem to be detrimental for catalysis and can be explored in the design of inhibitors for hexameric PNPs from pathogens. Our data also corroborated the competitive inhibition mechanism of hexameric PNPs by tubercidin and suggested that the acyclic nucleoside ganciclovir is a better inhibitor for hexameric PNPs than aciclovir. Furthermore, comparative structural analyses indicated that the replacement of Ser^{90} by a threonine in the *B. cereus* hexameric adenosine phosphorylase (Thr^{91}) is responsible for the lack of negative cooperativity of phosphate binding in this enzyme.

Editor: Andreas Hofmann, Griffith University, Australia

Funding: This work was supported by the following research funding agencies: FAPESP [www.fapesp.br/] (grants numbers 2007/00194-9, 2010/51890-8) and CNPq [www.cnpq.br/]. The funders had no role in study design, data collection and analysis, decision to publish, or preparation of the manuscript.

Competing Interests: The authors have declared that no competing interests exist.

* E-mail: mario.murakami@lnbio.org.br

Introduction

Purine nucleoside phosphorylases (PNPs; EC 2.4.2.1) are versatile enzymes that catalyze the reversible phosphorolysis of purine (2′deoxy)ribonucleosides producing bases and (2′deoxy)ribose 1-phosphate [1]. Their key role in the purine salvage pathway made PNPs attractive targets for drug design against several pathogens, such as *Mycobacterium tuberculosis* [2,3], *Plasmodium falciparum* [4–7], *Trichomonas vaginalis* [8–10] *and Schistosoma mansoni* [11,12], which lacks the *de novo* pathway for purine nucleotides synthesis. Due to their catalytic function, PNPs have also been investigated for the synthesis of nucleoside analogues (NAs) [13] and the activation of prodrugs in anti-cancer gene therapies [14].

NAs can be used in the treatment of a range of human viral infections, such as those caused by HIV, herpesvirus and hepatitis B/C virus [15–19]. They are among the first cytotoxic molecules to be used in the treatment of cancer [20] and have been studied as potential drugs against tuberculosis [21,22], malaria [7,23], trichomoniasis [24] and schistosomiasis [25]. The chemical synthesis of these compounds is generally a costly multistep process that includes several protection and deprotection stages [13,26]. This has encouraged the development of new methods for the synthesis of NAs using PNPs and other enzymes as biocatalysts [13,27,28]. The main advantages of this approach are the higher stereospecificity, regioselectivity and efficiency of enzymes, whose employment usually dispenses group protection and purification steps, optimizing the process [13].

The differences in substrate specificity regarding trimeric and hexameric PNPs have allowed the development of suicide gene therapies strategies against solid tumors [14,29]. Trimeric PNPs are mainly found in mammalian species and are specific for guanine and hypoxanthine (2′-deoxy)ribonucleosides whereas hexameric PNPs are prevalent in bacteria and accept adenine as well as guanine and hypoxanthine (2′-deoxy)ribonucleosides as substrates [1]. Thus, nontoxic adenosine analogues, which are poor substrates for human PNP, can be cleaved to cytotoxic bases specifically in tumor cells transfected with the bacterial hexameric

PNP gene [14]. Main advances in this field have been achieved with the *E. coli* PNP [30–33].

In this context, the aim of the present work was to shed light on how a diverse set of substrate modifications affects its binding and catalysis by hexameric PNPs using a structural approach. For this purpose, we choose the hexameric PNP (BsPNP233) from the model specie *Bacillus subtilis*, which displays great biotechnological potential to produce NAs, including the antiviral drug ribavirin [34]. We have solved the crystal structure of BsPNP233 in the apo form and in complex with 11 ligands comprising sulfate, bases, natural nucleosides and NAs, including clinically relevant compounds. The crystal structure of six ligands (adenine, 2′deoxyguanosine, aciclovir, ganciclovir, 8-bromoguanosine, 6-chloroguanosine) in complex with a hexameric PNP are presented for the first time.

Besides providing a broad structural basis for studies aiming at the rational design of BsPNP233 and its homologues for biotechnological applications, this work also bring new insights into the distinct kinetic models for phosphate binding in hexameric PNPs. Furthermore, the structural information showed here may also be instrumental for the development of new inhibitors against hexameric PNPs from pathogens such as *Plasmodium falciparum* and *Trichomonas vaginalis* [5,6,8,9] and for the combined design of both hexameric PNPs and prodrugs to improve specificity and efficiency of anti-cancer PNP gene therapies [14].

Materials and Methods

Chemicals

Adenine (Ade), adenosine (Ado), 2-fluoradenosine (F-Ado), tubercidin (TBN), 2′-deoxyguanosine (dGuo), hypoxanthine (Hyp), ganciclovir (GCV), aciclovir (ACV), 8-bromoguanosine (Br-Guo) and 6-chloroguanosine (Cl-Guo) were all purchased from Sigma-Aldrich.

Expression and Purification of Recombinant BsPNP233

BsPNP233 was expressed in *E. coli* cells and purified by immobilized metal affinity and size-exclusion chromatographies as described in [35]. The protein concentration was determined by absorption spectroscopy at 280 nm using the theoretical molar extinction coefficient of 16 515 $M^{-1}cm^{-1}$ calculated by the program ProtParam [36].

Crystallization

BsPNP233 at 11 mg/ml in 20 mM Tris–HCl pH 7.0, 50 mM NaCl and 1 mM DTT was crystallized by sitting-drop vapor-diffusion technique according to conditions previously described [35]. The crystals belong to the space groups $P32_1$, $P6_322$, $P2_12_12_1$ and $H32$ with one, two or six monomers per asymmetric unit depending on symmetry and cell dimensions.

Preparation of BsPNP233-ligand Complexes

The protein-ligand complexes were prepared by adding 0.1 µl of 50 mM ligand, dissolved in DMSO, to 1 µl crystallization drops at least 12 h prior to data collection. The ligands used were nucleosides, purine bases and NAs (Table S1). This procedure was performed in drops containing BsPNP233 crystals grown in 0.1 M sodium acetate pH 4.6, 3.2 M sodium chloride, 5% *(v/v)* glycerol at 291 K.

X-ray Data Collection and Processing

X-ray diffraction experiments were performed on the W01B-MX2 beamline at the Brazilian Synchrotron Light Laboratory (Campinas, Brazil). The data collection was carried out using crystals soaked in a cryoprotectant solution composed by the mother liquor and 20% *(v/v)* glycerol and flash-cooled in a nitrogen-gas stream at 100 K. The radiation wavelength was set to 1.458 Å and a MAR Mosaic 225 mm CCD detector was used to record the X-ray diffraction data. Data were indexed, integrated and scaled using the HKL-2000 suite [37] or the programs MOSFLM [38] and SCALA [39] from the CCP4 package [40]. Data processing statistics are summarized in Table S1.

Structure Determination and Refinement

The structures were solved by molecular replacement using the programs MOLREP [41] or PHASER [42], both from the CCP4 suite [40]. The first BsPNP233 structure was determined using the atomic coordinates of *B. anthracis* PNP (PDB code 1XE3) [43] as a search model. The subsequent BsPNP233 structures were solved using the atomic coordinates of BsPNP233 solved at 1.7 Å resolution (BsPNP233-GCV dataset, Table S1) as template. Refinement was carried out using the programs REFMAC5 [44] and COOT [45]. After 20 cycles of rigid body refinement in REFMAC5 [44], the models were refined alternating cycles of restrained isotropic refinement in REFMAC5 [44] and manual rebuilding and real space refinement in COOT [45]. Water molecules were added after refinement of the protein model at chemically reasonable places using COOT [45]. Subsequently, the ligands were added to the model and refined as described above using library descriptions generated by the program SKETCHER from the CCP4 suite [40]. The intensity based twin refinement of REFMAC5 was applied to refine the structures of BsPNP233 in complex with adenosine, 2-fluoradenosine and adenine. The majority of models for the BsPNP233 protein included all but the first and last residues (1 and 233). In the electron density map of the crystal structure solved in the space group $P2_12_12_1$ the residue 1 and additional eight residues from the N-terminal his-tag were clearly defined and added to the model. Ramachandran analysis carried out by Molprobity [46] showed that all residues from all models are found in allowed regions (except Gly^{121} of the BsPNP233-Ade structure, chain B). Refinement statistics are detailed in Table S1. Weighted 2Fo-Fc maps (2mFo-DFcalc) of ligands as well as a table of interactions between ligands and protein residues are presented in the supplementary material (Figure S1, Table S2). The atomic coordinates and structure factors of form I (4D8V), form II (4D8X), form III (4D8Y), form IV (4D98) and the complexes of BsPNP233 with Hyp (4DAB), Ade (4DAO), Ado (4D9H), dGuo (4DA0), F-Ado (4DAN), Cl-Guo(4DAE), Br-Guo (4DA8), TBN (4DAR), GCV (4DA6) and ACV (4DA7) have been deposited in the Protein Data Bank, Research Collaboratory for Structural Bioinformatics, Rutgers University, New Brunswick, NJ (http://www.rcsb.org/).

Figure Preparation

The figures of structures were prepared using PyMOL [47].

Structural Alignment

All structural comparisons were performed using the SSM algorithm [48] available at the program COOT [45] or at the PDBeFold server [49].

Results and Discussion

BsPNP233 Conserves the Quaternary Structure and Topology of Hexameric PNPs

The crystal structure of BsPNP233 confirmed that it is a homohexamer with D_3 symmetry as observed for other hexameric PNPs (Figure 1A) [50,51]. It was solved by X-ray crystallography in four distinct space groups ($P321$, $P2_12_12_1$, $P6_322$ and $H32$). The crystal contacts are similar in the crystal structures solved in $P321$, $P2_12_12_1$ and $P6_322$ but differ in the $H32$ space group. In the later, we observed additional crystallographic interfaces, resulting from a more compact crystal packing with a lower solvent content (41%) than crystals belonging to other space groups (~56%) (Figure S2) [35].

The BsPNP233 subunits surround a central axis and alternate in an up/down fashion forming a disc-shaped structure with six active sites: three located at the top face and other three at the bottom face. Analogously to other hexameric PNPs, BsPNP233 is a trimer of dimers where each subunit interacts with the adjacent subunits forming two interfaces: the catalytic, which contains the active site, and the inter-dimeric, involved in hexamer stabilization (Figure 1A). The inter-dimeric interface is larger than the catalytic interface and both are mainly maintained by hydrophobic interactions. In the ligand-free crystal structure (form II), the inter-dimeric and the catalytic interface areas are 1711 and 1554 Å^2, respectively.

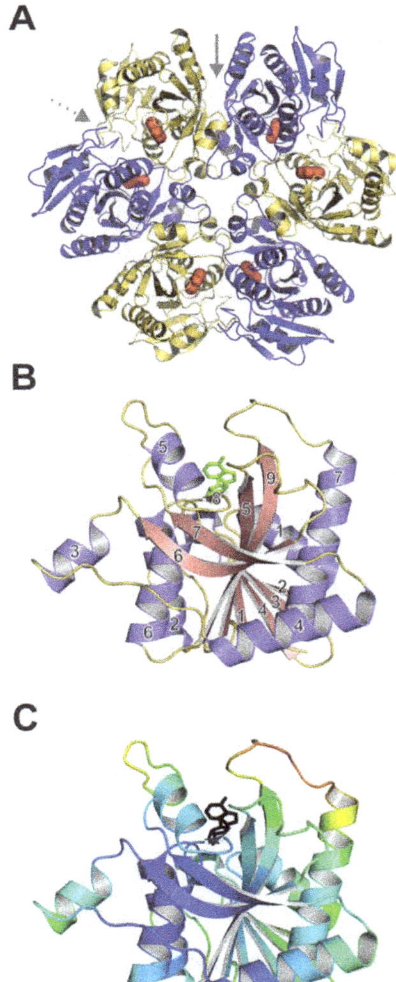

Figure 1. Overall structure of BsPNP233. A. Cartoon representation of the hexamer BsPNP233 with adenine (red spheres) bound in the active site. Solid and dashed grey arrows indicate the inter-dimeric and catalytic interfaces, respectively. B. Cartoon representation of BsPNP233 protomer in complex with adenosine (*green* stick). Loops, α-helices and β-strands are shown in *yellow*, *blue* and *pink*. The α-helices and β-strands were numbered according to the Mao and colleagues notation [50]. C. BsPNP233 protomer colored by B-factors from *dark blue* (lowest) to *red* (highest). Adenosine is represented by a *black* stick.

The BsPNP233 subunit conserves the *E. coli* hexameric PNP (EcPNP) subunit topology with few exceptions. Its central mixed β-sheet lacks the short β10 strand observed in EcPNP [50] and is surrounded by eight (instead of seven) α-helices (Figure 1B). The extra 5-residues α-helix connects the strands β2 and β3 and is not labeled to preserves the Mao and colleagues notation [50]. BsPNP233 and EcPNP subunits share sequence identity of 58% (PDB code 1ECP, [50]) and superpose with a r.m.s.d of 0.93 Å for 231 Cα atoms aligned (Figure S3). Structural alignment of BsPNP233 subunit with hexameric PNPs subunits from other *Bacillus* species resulted in a r.m.s.d of 0.80 Å - 0.94 Å for 231 Cα atoms aligned and an average sequence identity of 71% (Figure S3).

Analysis of the B-factor distribution in the apo BsPNP233 crystal structure shows that the loop connecting β9 and α7 as well as the N-terminal portion of α7 present the highest B-factor values, highlighting its intrinsic flexibility. As this region surround the active site, its flexibility may be important for catalysis (Figure 1C).

Free Purine Bases Adopt Alternative Conformations in the Active Site

The crystal structures of BsPNP233 in complex with hypoxanthine (Hyp) and adenine (Ade) showed that the purine-binding site consists of residues Cys^{91}, Gly^{92}, Phe^{159}, Val^{177} and Met^{179}. Hydrophobic interactions are predominant in the stabilization of both ligands (Figure 2A).

The BsPNP233-Ade binary complex was solved with (BsPNP233-Ade-SO_4) or without (BsPNP233-Ade) sulfate ion and represent the first of their kind to be reported for hexameric PNPs. Two subunits were observed in the asymmetric unit of both crystal structures and all of them exhibited clear density for the ligand in the active site (Figure S1).

Superposition of BsPNP233-Ade and BsPNP233-Ade-SO_4 complexes showed a preferential orientation of Ade in the base-binding site, except in one case where it is rotated by 49° around an axis perpendicular to the base plane (Figure 2B). This alternative orientation is not followed by significant conformational changes in the active-site residues (Figure 2B); however, it alters the solvation of the active-site pocket. In the alternative orientation, a crystallographic water molecule in the ribose-binding site is absent. This solvent molecule mediates a hydrogen bond between the AdeN^9 atom and the carbonyl group of Ser^{90} in the presence of sulfate ion (Figure 2B).

Interestingly, the Hyp adopts an orientation similar to the alternative conformation of Ade (Figure 2C). In this case, a glycerol molecule is located in the ribose-binding site and seems to induce the displacement of Hyp, avoiding a steric clash with the HypN^9 atom. This observation, along with those described above, suggests that binding of the co-substrate ribose-1-phoshate might contribute for stabilizing the base in the favorable orientation for catalysis.

The Hydrogen Bond between the 5′ Hydroxyl Group of Ado and Arg^{43*} Side Chain Contributes for a Ribosyl C3′-endo Conformation

The base moiety of adenosine (Ado) binds to the BsPNP233 active site in a very similar fashion to that seen in homologous PNPs (Figure 3). However, the ribosyl group adopts a C3′-*endo* form instead of the C4′-*endo* or O4′-*exo* conformations usually observed in Ado complexes with hexameric PNPs (PDB codes

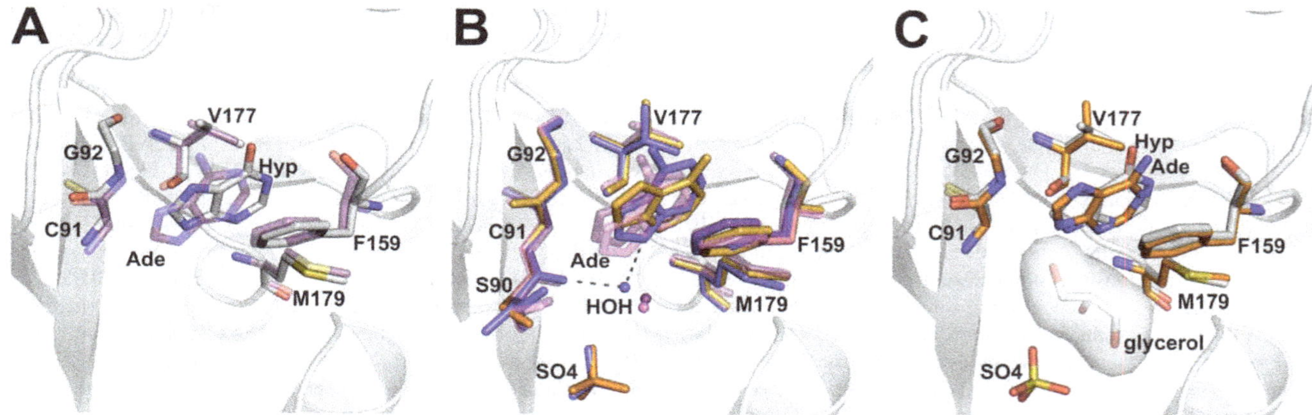

Figure 2. Comparison of free bases bound to the BsPNP233 active site. A. Structural comparison of a representative BsPNP233-Ade complex (*purple* carbon atoms) with the BsPNP233-Hyp complex (*grey* carbon atoms). B. The structure of the four BsPNP233-Ade complexes solved independently are superimposed. The sulfate-free Ade-complexes are colored in *purple* (chain A) and *pink* (chain B) whereas the two independent complexes solved with sulfate bound (dataset I) are colored in *orange* (chain A) and *blue* (chain B). C. The structure of the Ade-complex where Ade presents an alternative conformation (carbon atoms in *orange*) is superimposed in the structure of Hyp-complex (carbon atoms in *grey*). The surface of the glycerol molecule present at the Hyp-complex is shown to evidence the influence of this molecule in the position and orientation of Hyp in the active site. The hydrogen bonds are shown as *dashed lines.*

3UAW, [52]; 1ODI, [53]; 1PK7, [54]; 3U40, [55]; 1Z37, [51]; 1VHW, [56]) (Figure 3). This unusual conformation may be explained by a hydrogen bond between the 5′ hydroxyl group of Ado and Arg^{43*} side chain (residues from the adjacent subunit are designated by an asterisk) not observed in other Ado complexes (Figure 3). Typically, the 5′-OH group of Ado is found interacting with one or two water molecules not observed in BsPNP233-Ado complex, suggesting that the hydration of the active site may influence the ribosyl conformation.

In sulfate/phosphate free complexes of hexameric PNPs with Ado, an O4′*–exo* conformation is usually found. However, in all complexes where the phosphate-binding site is occupied by a sulfate or phosphate, the ribosyl group shows a C4′*–endo* conformation, except for the *Thermus thermophilus* (TtPNP)-Ado complex (PDB code 1ODI, [53]). Since the side chain of Arg^{43*} participates in phosphate binding, the presence of this co-substrate and the hydration of the active site probably prevent the interaction between Ado 5′-OH group and Arg^{43*} side chain observed in BsPNP233-Ado complex favoring the ribose to adopt a C4′*–endo* conformation.

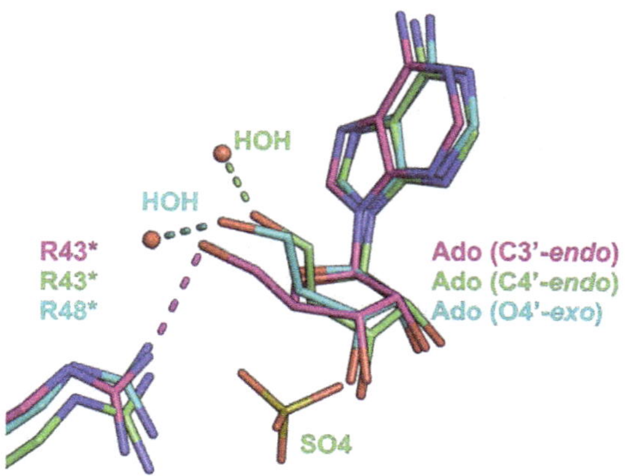

Figure 3. The different conformations of Ado ribosyl radical. Structural superposition of BsPNP233-Ado (*magenta* carbon atoms), *B. cereus* adenosine phosphorylase (BcAdoP)-Ado-SO_4 (*green* carbon atoms, PDB code 3UAW [52]) and *Entamoeba histolytica* PNP-Ado (*cyan* carbon atoms, PDB code 3U40 [55]) complexes. The different puckers adopted by the ribose moiety of adenosine are labeled and the hydrogen bonds involving the 5′-OH group of Ado in each complex are represented by *dashed lines*. The sugar puckers were assigned by the pucker.py script of PyMOL [47].

2′-deoxyguanosine Binding Mode Resembles to that Observed for Adenosine

In the BsPNP233-(2′-deoxyguanosine) complex structure, the base of 2′-deoxyguanosine (dGuo) binds to the active site in a similar manner to that observed for Ado (Figure 4). Neither the extra amino group at position 2 nor the carbonyl group at position 6 was observed making hydrogen bonds with the protein residues. A hydrogen bond between $dGuoN^7$ and $Ser^{202}O^{\gamma}$ atoms slightly rotates the base and brings the residue Ser^{202} closer to the substrate (Figure 4B). The lack of the 2′-OH group in dGuo is counterbalanced by extra hydrophobic interactions between $dGuoC^{2'}$ and Glu^{178} carbon atoms (Figure 4A). Comparisons between BsPNP233-dGuo and *T.* vaginalis PNP (TvPNP)-(2′-deoxyinosine) complexes showed that the deoxyribosyl group of both ligands conserves the binding mode, whereas the base assumes a little different orientation induced by the $dGuoN^7$-$Ser^{202}O^{\gamma}$ hydrogen bond exclusively observed in BsPNP233-dGuo complex (Figure 4C).

BsPNP233 can be Explored as an Alternative in Gene Therapy Approaches using 2-Fluoradenosine as Prodrug

The compound 2-fluoradenosine (F-Ado) is an adenosine analogue which liberates the toxic metabolite 2-fluoradenine when cleaved. Its deoxy form has been studied as a prodrug in an anti-tumor gene therapy approach based on a modified human PNP [57]. The crystal structure of BsPNP233-(F-Ado) complex had two BsPNP233 subunits per asymmetric unit and both presented clear electronic density for the ligand (Figure S1). In the two independent active sites, F-Ado was found in the same orientation, similar to that of Ado (Figure 4E). The extra fluorine atom at position 2 is allocated in a hydrophobic micro-

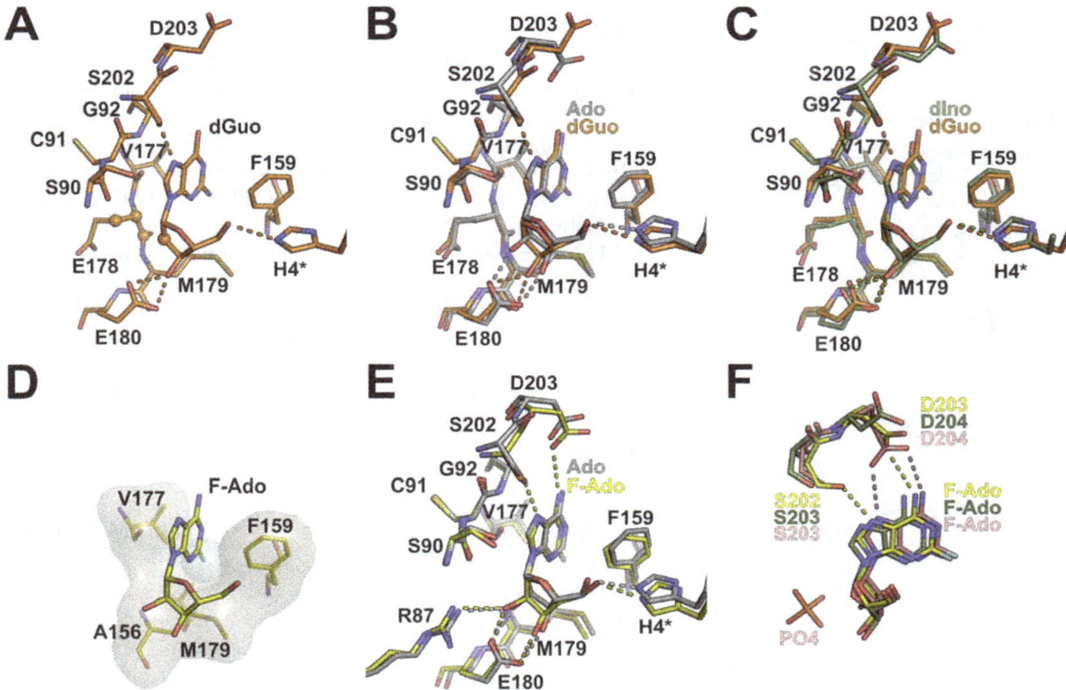

Figure 4. The binding mode of 2′ deoxyguanosine and 2-fluoradenosine. A. Representation of the BsPNP233 residues that interact with dGuo showing as spheres the atoms involved in hydrophobic interactions with dGuo $C^{2'}$ atom. B. Structural alignment between the dGuo-complex (carbon atoms in *orange*) and the Ado-complex (carbon atoms in *grey*). C The structure of dGuo-complex and TvPNP-(2′-deoxyinosine) complex (carbon atoms in *green*, PDB code 1Z39, [51]) are superimposed. D. Representation of F-Ado complex showing the residues involved in van der Waals interactions with F^2 atom (*light blue* sphere). E. Structural comparison of F-Ado complex (carbon atoms in *yellow*) with the Ado-complex (carbon atoms in *grey*). F. The structures of F-Ado complex, EcPNP-F-Ado-PO_4 complex (carbon atoms in *pink*, PDB code 1PK9 [54]) and TvPNP-F-Ado complex (carbon atoms in *green*, PDB code 1Z35, [51]) are superimposed. In all panels hydrogen bonds are represented by *dashed lines* and color coded according to their respective structures.

environment consisting of Ala^{156}, Phe^{159}, Val^{177} and Met^{179} (Figure 4D). This motif is fully conserved in EcPNP, which has been tested in anti-tumor gene therapy by activating produgs like F-ado [30].

Two hydrogen bonds (N^6-$Asp^{203}O^{\delta}$ and N^7-$Ser^{202}O^{\gamma}$) observed in BsPNP233-F-Ado complex, but not in BsPNP233-Ado complex, contribute for subtle changes in nucleoside position and base orientation (Figure 4E). The F-Ado ribosyl moiety adopts the catalytically favorable C4′-*endo* conformation supported by tight hydrogen bonds of nucleoside sugar hydroxyl groups with His^{4*}, Arg^{87} and Glu^{180} side chains (Figure 4E). Structural comparisons among BsPNP233-F-Ado, TvPNP-F-Ado (PDB code 1Z35) and EcPNP-F-Ado (PDB code 1PK9) complexes showed a similar binding mode. However, the presence of phosphate in the EcPNP-(F-Ado) complex displaces by about 0.5 Å the ribosyl moiety, disrupts the N^7-$Ser^{202}O^{\gamma}$ hydrogen bond and leads the N^7 atom closer to the Asp^{203} side chain, favoring the catalysis (Figure 4F).

Since F-Ado binds to the BsPNP233 active site in a manner similar to that of the natural substrate Ado, placing the F^2 atom in a hydrophobic pocket conserved in EcPNP, our structural data indicate that, as well as EcPNP [54], BsPNP233 is able to convert 2-fluoradenosine in the cytotoxic 2-fluoradenine. Thus, we concluded that BsPNP233 can be explored as an alternative in the development of anti-tumors gene therapy approaches using this prodrug or the less toxic 2-fluoro-2′-deoxyadenosine [57].

The Cl^6 Substituent of 6-chloroguanosine Induces a Ribose C3′-exo Conformation and May Prevent Catalysis

The NA 6-chloroguanosine (Cl-Guo) can be used for the synthesis of 2-amino-6-chloro-9-(2,3-dideoxy-3-fluoro-beta-D-erythro-pentofuranosyl)purine, a compound with anti-HBV effects [58]. In addition, the free base 6-chloroguanine is an inhibitor of the trimeric PNP from *Schistosoma mansoni* [59]. Here we report the first crystal structure of a PNP in complex with Cl-Guo.

The molecule Cl-Guo displays a similar binding mode to that observed for dGuo (Figure 5A). However, as the chlorine van der Waals radius is larger than that of oxygen, the Cl^6 substituent pushes the base in the direction of the ribosyl moiety to avoid steric clashes with $Gly^{92}C^{\alpha}$, $Val^{205}C^{\gamma 2}$, and $Asp^{203}O^{\delta 1}$ atoms. This base displacement induces the ribosyl group to adopt an unusual C3′-*exo* conformation.

The C3′-*exo* pucker was already observed in the nucleoside 9-β-D-xylofuranosyladenine bound to EcPNP (PDB code 1PR6, [54]) and it is considered incompatible with the sugar conformation required for PNP catalysis [54]. Moreover, structural comparisons with the EcPNP-Ado-PO_4 complex (PDB code 1PK7, [54]) showed that the chlorine atom may prevent the Asp^{203} side chain to approach to the N^7 atom to donate a proton during catalysis (Figure 5B). Thus, these findings suggest that Cl-Guo as well as other NAs with 6-substituents heavier than chlorine cannot be cleaved by BsPNP233 and other hexameric PNPs.

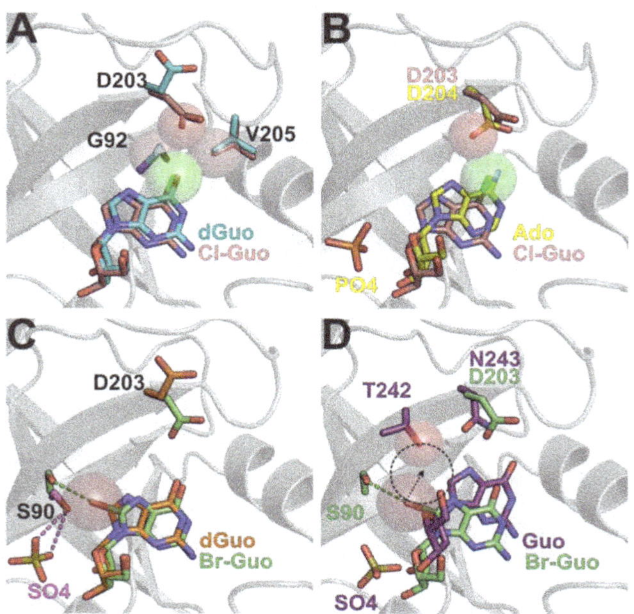

Figure 5. The influence of Cl^6 and Br^8 modifications in catalysis and nucleoside binding. A. Structural alignment of Cl-Guo complex (*pink* carbon atoms) and dGuo complex (*cyan* carbon atoms). Spheres represent the van der Waals radius of Cl^6, $Gly^{92}C^{\alpha}$, $Asp^{203}O^{\delta 1}$ and $Val^{205}C^{\gamma 2}$ atoms. B. Superposition of Cl-Guo complex and EcPNP-Ado-PO_4 complex (*yellow* carbon atoms, PDB code 1PK7 [54]). Spheres represent the van der Waals radius of Cl^6 and EcPNP $Asp^{204}O^{\delta 1}$ atoms to highlight the steric conflict imposed by the Cl^6 atom. C. The Br-Guo complex (carbon atoms in *green*), dGuo complex (carbon atoms in *orange*) and sulfate complex (carbon atoms in *magenta*, form IV, chain B) structures are superimposed. The sphere represents the van der Waals radius of Br^8 and the dashed lines represent hydrogen bonds colored according to the respective structures. D. Structural comparison of Br-Guo complex and the trimeric HsPNP-Guo-SO_4 complex (*purple* carbon atoms, PDB code 1RFG, [63]). The spheres represent the van der Waals radius of Br^8 and HsPNP $Thr^{242}O^{\gamma 1}$ atoms. The dashed circle has the same radius of Br^8 and indicates the steric clash that would occur if BrGuo was placed at the Guo position in the HsPNP active site.

The Br^8 Substituent Displaces Ser^{90} Away from the Phosphate Binding Site and Might be Detrimental for Catalysis

The 8-bromoguanosine (Br-Guo) is a "poor substrate" of the trimeric PNP from calf spleen [60]. Its first crystallographic portrayal in complex with a protein is described here. The addition of a bromine radical at the C^8 atom of guanosine results in the formation of a halogen bond between Br^8 and $Ser^{90}O^{\gamma}$ atoms, which implicates in both positional and rotational displacement of the base by 0.3 Å and 7°, respectively (Figure 5C). The ribosyl moiety of Br-Guo presents a typical C4′*–endo* conformation and binds to the active site in a very similar fashion to that seen for 2′deoxyguanosine (Figure 5C).

In BsPNP233-(Br-Guo) complex, the side chain of the catalytic residue Asp^{203} is facing the O^6 and N^7 atoms of Br-Guo and the Ser^{90} side chain is pushed away from the active site in order to accommodate the bromine atom (Figure 5C). In hexameric PNPs, the hydroxyl group of Ser^{90} participates in the coordination of phosphate [61]. The position that it assumes in BsPNP233-sulfate and EcPNP-Ado-PO_4 complexes (PDB code 1PK7 [54]) is incompatible with the presence of Br^8 atom because of steric hindrance (Figure 5C). Thus, the bromine radical probably prevents the phosphate-Ser^{90} interaction being detrimental for binding and correct orientation of phosphate.

Site-directed mutations of human PNP phosphate binding site leads to a decrease in catalytic efficiency ranging from 25- to 185-fold [62]. Likewise, impairment of any phosphate interaction in the hexameric PNP active site may reduce the catalytic activity. As Br-Guo probably prevents the phosphate-Ser^{90} interaction it might be a "poor substrate" or even an inhibitor of BsPNP233 and other hexameric PNPs as well.

This interpretation cannot be applied for trimeric PNPs because Ser^{90} is not structurally conserved in trimeric PNPs. However, structural comparisons between BsPNP233-(Br-Guo) and human PNP in complex with guanosine and sulfate (PDB code 1RFG, [63]) indicate that Br-Guo is probably a "poor substrate" for trimeric PNPs because of steric hindrance involving the bromine and the side chain of Thr^{242}, which would hinder the displacement of the N^7 atom towards Asn^{243} side chain for stabilization of the transition state [64] (Figure 5D).

Corroboration of the Competitive Inhibition Mechanism of Hexameric PNP by Tubercidin

Tubercidin (7-deazaadenosine) is an adenosine analogue which presents antiviral, antischistosomal and antifungal properties as well as antitumor activity [65–68]. Furthermore, tubercidin and other 7-deazapurine nucleosides are inhibitors of EcPNP [69,70].

TBN presented an interaction mode very similar to that seen for the natural substrate adenosine (Figure 6). Slightly differences were observed in its ribosyl moiety that assumed an O4′*–exo* pucker instead of the C3′*-exo* conformation of Ado in complex with BsPNP233 (Figure 6). The C^7 substituent in TBN makes hydrophobic and van der Waals interactions with residues Cys^{91} and Ser^{202}. The ribosyl moiety is stabilized by a conserved network of hydrogen bonds involving His^{4*}, Glu^{180} and Arg^{87} side chains and by hydrophobic interactions with Glu^{178} (C^{α} and C^{β} atoms) and $Met^{179}C^{\gamma}$ atom (Figure 6). Our structural data corroborate the competitive inhibition mechanism of hexameric PNP by TBN defined by *in vitro* studies [69]. The substitution of N^7 by a carbon prevents the protonation step of the N^7 atom required for catalysis [70], making TBN a non-cleavable adenosine analogue by EcPNP and probably by other PNPs.

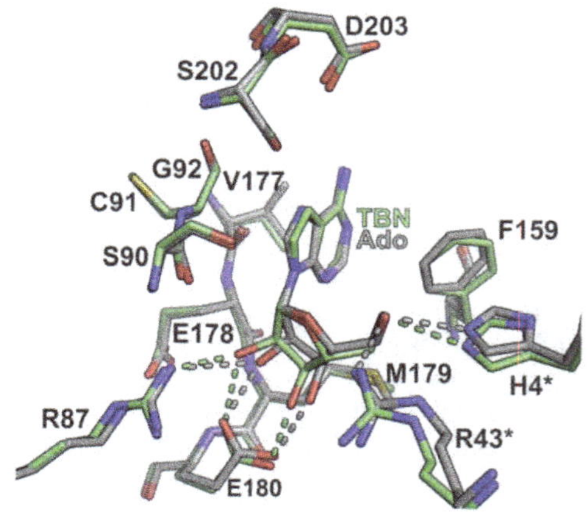

Figure 6. The binding mode of tubercidin. Structural comparison between the BsPNP233-TBN (carbon atoms in *green*) and BsPNP233-Ado (carbon atoms in *grey*) complexes. Dashed lines indicate hydrogen bonds and are colored according to their respective complexes.

Ganciclovir Inhibits Both Trimeric and Hexameric PNPs

Ganciclovir (GCV) is an acyclic NA used to treat cytomegalovirus infections [17]. It is also used together with herpes simplex virus thymidine kinase in a suicide gene therapy system that has been studied for the treatment of hepatocellular carcinoma [71]. GCV is an inhibitor of the human PNP (trimeric) [72] and probably has inhibitory effects on hexameric PNPs as well. Our structural data support this hypothesis revealing that GCV binds to the nucleoside binding site of BsPNP233 (Figure 7).

The guanine moiety of GCV conserves the position observed for the 2′-deoxyguanosine base but it is rotated by about 10° to accommodate the acyclic chain in the ribose-binding site (Figure 7A–B). A water molecule mediates hydrogen bonds between the ligand O^6 atom and the side chains of Ser^{202} and Asp^{203}. The N^7 atom interacts with $Ser^{202}O^{\gamma}$ and $Gly^{92}N$ atoms, and the base is stabilized by hydrophobic contacts with Ser^{90}, Cys^{91}, Ser^{202} and Phe^{159} (Figure 7A).

Interestingly, the three oxygens of the acyclic radical occupy similar positions to those observed for the three oxygens of dGuo ribosyl group, mimetizing its binding mode (Figure 7B). From the three hydrogen bonds observed for dGuo ribosyl moiety, the GCV acyclic radical conserves two, involving the His^{4*} and Glu^{180} side chains. Moreover, the $C^{4'}$ atom of the GCV acyclic moiety preserves the hydrophobic interactions with $Met^{179}C^{\beta}$ and $Met^{179}C^{\gamma}$ atoms performed by the dGuo $C^{3'}$ atom (Figure 7B). Therefore our data indicate that GCV is also a competitive inhibitor for hexameric PNPs.

Aciclovir Acyclic Chain Adopts Two Conformations in the BsPNP233 Ribosyl Binding Site

Aciclovir (ACV) is an antiviral drug used to treat herpes virus infections [73] and has modest inhibitory effects on human PNP [74]. Here, we present for the first time the crystal structure of a hexameric PNP with ACV. This structure revealed differences in the aciclovir binding mode, which can be explored for drug design targeting hexameric PNPs from pathogens such as *P. falciparum* [6] and *T. vaginalis* [8].

Aciclovir binds to the BsPNP233 nucleoside binding site and is stabilized by hydrophobic interactions and a hydrogen-bonding network mediated by solvent molecules (Figure 7C–D). Interestingly, the acyclic tail assumes two alternative conformations that, seen simultaneously, resemble the conformation observed for the ganciclovir acyclic radical (Figure 7C–E). In one of these conformations, the 3′ hydroxyl group of ACV is attached to the carboxyl group of Glu^{180} side chain while the carbon atoms make hydrophobic contacts with the main chain of Glu^{178} and with the $Met^{179}C^{\beta}$ and $Met^{179}C^{\gamma}$ atoms (Figure 7C). A phosphate ion, modeled with half occupancy based on difference maps, also makes a hydrogen bond with the ligand 3′ hydroxyl group (Figure 7C). The other conformation is stabilized by a hydrogen bond between the 3′-OH group of ACV and the His^{4*} side chain (Figure 7D).

The ACV guanine moiety assumes a different position and orientation from that observed for GCV (Figure 7E), getting closer to the Phe^{159} side chain. The main chain of Cys^{91} and the side chain of Val^{177} also contribute with hydrophobic interactions to the base (Figure 7C–D). The O^6 atom makes water mediated hydrogen bonds with the Asp^{203} side chain and with the Phe^{159} carbonyl oxygen (Figure 7C and D). The same is observed for N^1 and N^2 atoms, which interact through a water molecule with the Gln^{158} carbonyl oxygen; for N^7 atom, which makes water mediated hydrogen bonds with Asp^{203} side chain, and; for N^9 atom, whose interaction with both Ser^{90} and Ser^{202} hydroxyl groups is also mediated by a solvent molecule (Figure 7C–D).

Structural comparison between BsPNP233-ACV and human PNP (HsPNP)-ACV (PDB code 1PWY, [74]) complexes showed differences in the binding mode. In the HsPNP-ACV complex, the base N^1, N^2, N^7 and O^6 atoms interact directly with active-site residues through hydrogen bonds. In addition, the acyclic chain adopts a different conformation, which is stabilized by hydrophobic interactions with Phe^{200} side chain and Ala^{116}/Ala^{117} main chains (Figure 7F). To investigate if differences in the interaction mode of aciclovir with BsPNP233 and HsPNP may result in different binding affinities, we estimated the strength of protein–ligand interactions using the rerank score function of MOLEGRO [75]. According to this analysis, ACV presented similar predicted binding affinities in both complexes, which was slightly higher (lower rerank score value) for the BsPNP233 complex (Table S3). The same analysis was performed for GCV whose predicted binding affinity was considerable higher than that observed for ACV (Table S3). This result indicates that GCV is a better inhibitor for hexameric PNPs than ACV.

Structural Basis of Distinct Kinetic Models for Phosphate Binding in Hexameric PNPs

The asymmetric unit of the BsPNP233 crystal structure belonging to the *H*32 space group presented a catalytic dimer whose protomers adopt an open and a closed conformation, respectively (Figure 8A). The electron density map clearly showed a tetrahedral molecule in the active site of both subunits (Figure S1). As the crystallization condition was phosphate free and contained high concentrations of ammonium sulfate, we modeled sulfate ions in both sites.

The open and closed conformations of BsPNP233-sulfate complex were already observed in EcPNP-sulfate/phosphate structures and have been associated with two dissociation constants that characterize phosphate binding to EcPNP [61,76]. The closed conformation is defined by a disruption of helix α7 and subsequent displacement of its N-terminal portion and the precedent loop towards the active site (Figure 8A). This conformation seems to be triggered by the interaction of Arg^{24} side chain with phosphate and results in an approximation of Arg^{216} to the catalytic residue Asp^{203} (Figure 8A) [61]. As BsPNP233 protomers are able to adopt open and closed conformations like EcPNP subunits, this suggests that the negative cooperativity of phosphate binding demonstrated for EcPNP [61] is also applied for BsPNP233.

Comparison between BsPNP233-sulfate and *Bacillus cereus* adenosine phosphorylase (BcAdoP)-sulfate complexes (PDB codes 3UAV, 3UAW, 3UAX, 3UAY, 3UAZ, [52]) showed that BcAdoP assumes an intermediate conformation where only the first turn of helix α7 is disrupted (Figure 8A). In the BcAdoP-sulfate complex structure (PDB code 3UAW, [52]), Arg^{217} (corresponding to BsPNP233-Arg^{216}) points to the active site but it is not able to approach Asp^{204} (BsPNP233-Asp^{203}) such as BsPNP233-Arg^{216} (Figure 8A).

The apparent inability of BcAdoP to adopt the closed conformation seems to be caused by a steric hindrance imposed by Thr^{91} to the conformational change that Phe^{221} (BsPNP233-Phe^{220}) undergoes for the closed conformation being achieved (Figure 8B). In BsPNP233 and EcPNP this threonine residue is replaced by a serine, which allows Phe^{220} side chain to adopt the rotamer observed in the closed conformation (Figure 8C). These analyses suggest that the negative cooperativity model of phosphate binding displayed by EcPNP cannot be applied for BcAdoP, as BcAdoP apparently presents only one conformational state. This hypothesis is supported by functional studies, which showed that BcAdoP obeys Michaelis–Menten kinetics [77].

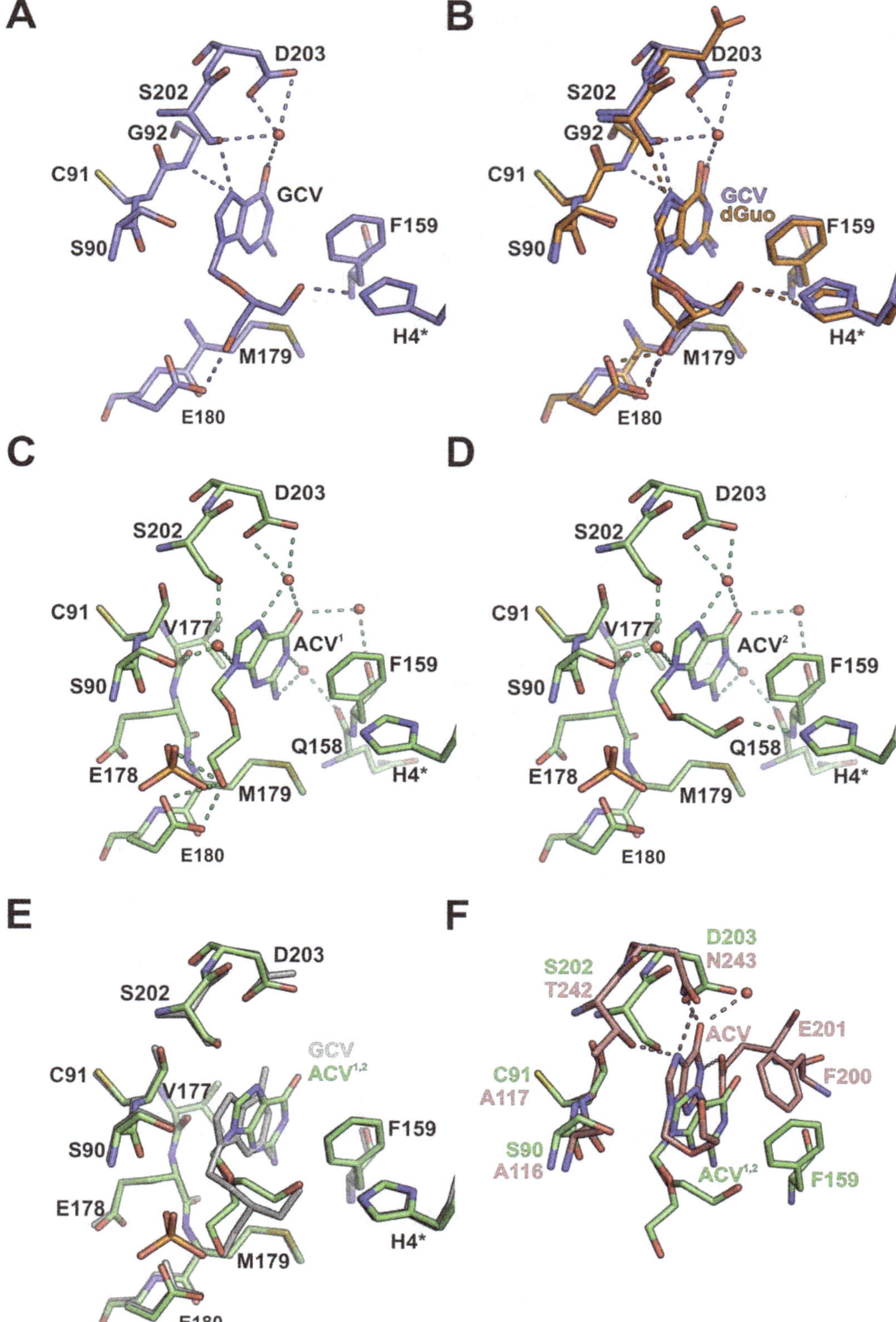

Figure 7. The binding mode of acyclic nucleosides. A. Stick representation of GCV bound in the BsPNP233 active site. B. Structural comparison of GCV-complex (*blue* carbon atoms) with dGuo-complex (*orange* carbon atoms). C and D show the stick representation of the two conformations of ACV (ACV[1] and ACV[2]) bound to the BsPNP233 active site. E. The structures of GCV-complex (*grey*) and ACV[1,2]-complex (*green* carbon atoms) are superimposed. F. Structural alignment of ACV[1,2]-complex with HsPNP-ACV complex (*pink* carbon atoms, PDB code 1PWY [74]). In all panels dashed lines indicate hydrogen bonds and are color coded according to their respective complexes.

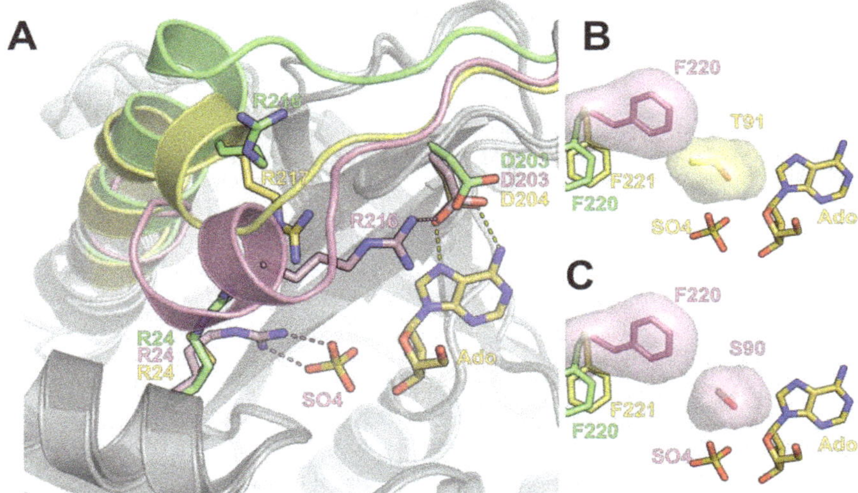

Figure 8. Structural basis of distinct kinetic models for phosphate binding in hexameric PNPs. A. Structural superposition of BsPNP233-sulfate open (*green*) and closed (*pink*) conformations with the BcAdoP-Ado complex (*yellow*, PDB code 3UAW, [52]). The cartoon representation highlights the conformational differences observed in the main chain of the β9-α7 loop and the N-terminal portion of helix α7 in the three structures. Dashed lines represent hydrogen bonds and follow the color code of their respective structures. B. The surface representation of BsPNP233 Phe^{220} in the closed conformation (*pink*) and of the BcAdoP Thr^{91} evidence the steric hindrance imposed by the $Thr^{91}C^{\gamma 2}$ atom to that Phe^{220} rotamer. C. The surface representation of BsPNP233 Phe^{220} and Ser^{90} in the closed conformation shows that the Ser^{90} side chain allows the Phe^{220} side chain to perform the conformational change needed for the closed conformation takes place.

A previous work reported that BsPNP233 is specific for 6-aminopurine nucleosides [78]. However, Xie and coworkers [34] recently showed that BsPNP233 (named PNP_{702}) exhibits a broad substrate specificity and present comparable activity towards both guanosine (6-oxopurine nucleoside) and adenosine (6-aminopurine nucleoside). Our structural data is in agreement with Xie and coworkers data indicating that BsPNP233 conserves the same catalytic mechanism proposed for EcPNP [76], where catalysis occurs in the closed conformation (Figure 8A).

Conclusion

This report provided a broad description of how the hexameric PNP from *B. subtilis* interacts with natural substrates and the impact of modifications in such substrates on binding and catalysis. The structural analysis reported here can be instrumental for studies aiming to optimize BsPNP233 or other hexameric PNPs for biotechnological applications such as industrial synthesis of nucleoside analogues or gene therapy against solid tumors. An initiative of this sort has been taken for *E. coli* PNP to optimize the cleavage of the prodrug Me(*talo*)-MeP-R with great success [29].

The crystal structure of six ligands (adenine, 2′deoxyguanosine, aciclovir, ganciclovir, 8-bromoguanosine and 6-chloroguanosine) in complex with a hexameric PNP are presented for the first time. The information extracted from these structures can be extended to homologous hexameric PNPs to help the development of new inhibitors against pathogens such as *T. vaginalis* [8] and *P. falciparum* [6] as well as new prodrugs for gene therapies against tumors [30,79].

In addition, our results and comparative analyses shed light on distinct kinetic models for phosphate binding in hexameric PNPs. According to our model the substitution of the conserved residue Ser^{90} by a threonine disrupts the open/close mechanism of hexameric PNPs subunits, which results in the loss of the negative cooperativity of phosphate binding.

Supporting Information

Figure S1 Weighted 2Fo-Fc map (2mFo-DFcalc) of the ligands (*ball and stick*) bound to the BsPNP233 active site. A. Ade-complex (chain A). B. Ade-SO_4 complex, evidencing only Ade (form I, chain A). C. Hyp-complex. D. Ado-complex (chain A). E. F-Ado complex (chain A). F. dGuo complex. G. Cl-Guo complex. H. Br-Guo complex. I. TBN complex. J. GCV complex. K. ACV complex. L. SO_4 complex (form IV, chain A).

Figure S2 Crystallographic interfaces (*dark grey*) observed at the crystal structures solved at space groups $P32_1$, $P2_12_12_1$, $P6_322$ (A) and at $H32$ space group (B).

Figure S3 Structural alignment of BsPNP233 subunit with homologous hexameric PNPs protomers. The regions with the highest r.m.s.d. values are colored: BsPNP233 (*green*), BaPNP (*blue* - PDB 1XE3/F), BcPNP (*yellow* - PDB 2AC7/B), EcPNP (*red* - PDB 1ECP/A).

Table S1 Data collection and refinement statistics.

Table S2 Distances (Å) between the ligand atoms and interacting BsPNP233 atoms. Potential hydrogen bonds are highlighted by grey boxes. In the case of crystal structures containing more than one complex per asymmetric unit, only one of them is shown in the table. For the ligand adenine a representative structure of the preferential§ (BsPNP233-Ade complex, chain A) and alternative¥ (form I, chain A) conformations are presented.

Table S3 *In silico* prediction of ligand binding affinity using the rerank score function of MOLEGRO [75]. ¥ The two values of BsPNP233-ACV complex correspond to the ACV[1] and ACV^2 alternative conformations, respectively. § HsPNP-ACV (PDB CODE: 1PWY).

Acknowledgments

We gratefully acknowledge the Brazilian Biosciences National Laboratory (CNPEM, Campinas, Brazil) and Brazilian Synchrotron Light Laboratory (CNPEM, Campinas, Brazil) for the use of the crystallization (RoboLab) and X-ray diffraction (MX2 beamline) facilities.

Author Contributions

Conceived and designed the experiments: ANM CRS HDP MTM NHM POG. Performed the experiments: ANM CRS NHM POG. Analyzed the data: CRS MTM NHM POG. Contributed reagents/materials/analysis tools: HDP MTM. Wrote the paper: MTM POG.

References

1. Pugmire MJ, Ealick SE (2002) Structural analyses reveal two distinct families of nucleoside phosphorylases. Biochem J 361: 1–25.
2. Basso LA, Santos DS, Shi W, Furneaux RH, Tyler PC, et al. (2001) Purine nucleoside phosphorylase from Mycobacterium tuberculosis. Analysis of inhibition by a transition-state analogue and dissection by parts. Biochemistry 40: 8196–8203.
3. Caceres RA, Timmers LFSM, Ducati RG, da Silva DON, Basso LA, et al. (2012) Crystal structure and molecular dynamics studies of purine nucleoside phosphorylase from Mycobacterium tuberculosis associated with acyclovir. Biochimie 94: 155–165. doi:10.1016/j.biochi.2011.10.003.
4. Lewandowicz A, Schramm VL (2004) Transition State Analysis for Human and Plasmodium falciparum Purine Nucleoside Phosphorylases†. Biochemistry 43: 1458–1468. doi:10.1021/bi0359123.
5. Shi W, Ting L-M, Kicska GA, Lewandowicz A, Tyler PC, et al. (2004) Plasmodium falciparum purine nucleoside phosphorylase: crystal structures, immucillin inhibitors, and dual catalytic function. J Biol Chem 279: 18103–18106. doi:10.1074/jbc.C400068200.
6. Madrid DC, Ting L-M, Waller KL, Schramm VL, Kim K (2008) Plasmodium falciparum purine nucleoside phosphorylase is critical for viability of malaria parasites. J Biol Chem 283: 35899–35907. doi:10.1074/jbc.M807218200.
7. Cassera MB, Hazleton KZ, Merino EF, Obaldia N 3rd, Ho M-C, et al. (2011) Plasmodium falciparum parasites are killed by a transition state analogue of purine nucleoside phosphorylase in a primate animal model. PLoS ONE 6: e26916. doi:10.1371/journal.pone.0026916.
8. Munagala N, Wang CC (2002) The purine nucleoside phosphorylase from Trichomonas vaginalis is a homologue of the bacterial enzyme. Biochemistry 41: 10382–10389.
9. Munagala NR, Wang CC (2003) Adenosine is the primary precursor of all purine nucleotides in Trichomonas vaginalis. Mol Biochem Parasitol 127: 143–149.
10. Rinaldo-Matthis A, Wing C, Ghanem M, Deng H, Wu P, et al. (2007) Inhibition and structure of Trichomonas vaginalis purine nucleoside phosphorylase with picomolar transition state analogues. Biochemistry 46: 659–668. doi:10.1021/bi061515r.
11. Pereira HD, Franco GR, Cleasby A, Garratt RC (2005) Structures for the potential drug target purine nucleoside phosphorylase from Schistosoma mansoni causal agent of schistosomiasis. J Mol Biol 353: 584–599. doi:10.1016/j.jmb.2005.08.045.
12. Castilho MS, Postigo MP, Pereira HM, Oliva G, Andricopulo AD (2010) Structural basis for selective inhibition of purine nucleoside phosphorylase from Schistosoma mansoni: kinetic and structural studies. Bioorg Med Chem 18: 1421–1427. doi:10.1016/j.bmc.2010.01.022.
13. Patel RN (2006) Biocatalysis in the pharmaceutical and biotechnology industries. CRC Press. 924 p.
14. Zhang Y, Parker WB, Sorscher EJ, Ealick SE (2005) PNP anticancer gene therapy. Curr Top Med Chem 5: 1259–1274.
15. De Clercq E (2007) Acyclic nucleoside phosphonates: past, present and future. Bridging chemistry to HIV, HBV, HCV, HPV, adeno-, herpes-, and poxvirus infections: the phosphonate bridge. Biochem Pharmacol 73: 911–922. doi:10.1016/j.bcp.2006.09.014.
16. De Clercq E (2009) Anti-HIV drugs: 25 compounds approved within 25 years after the discovery of HIV. International Journal of Antimicrobial Agents 33: 307–320. doi:10.1016/j.ijantimicag.2008.10.010.
17. Faulds D, Heel RC (1990) Ganciclovir. A review of its antiviral activity, pharmacokinetic properties and therapeutic efficacy in cytomegalovirus infections. Drugs 39: 597–638.
18. Morfin F, Thouvenot D (2003) Herpes simplex virus resistance to antiviral drugs. J Clin Virol 26: 29–37.
19. Paeshuyse J, Dallmeier K, Neyts J (2011) Ribavirin for the treatment of chronic hepatitis C virus infection: a review of the proposed mechanisms of action. Curr Opin Virol 1: 590–598. doi:10.1016/j.coviro.2011.10.030.
20. Galmarini CM, Mackey JR, Dumontet C (2002) Nucleoside analogues and nucleobases in cancer treatment. The Lancet Oncology 3: 415–424. doi:10.1016/S1470–2045(02)00788-X.
21. Long MC, Allan PW, Luo M-Z, Liu M-C, Sartorelli AC, et al. (2007) Evaluation of 3-deaza-adenosine analogues as ligands for adenosine kinase and inhibitors of Mycobacterium tuberculosis growth. J Antimicrob Chemother 59: 118–121. doi:10.1093/jac/dkl448.
22. Van Calenbergh S, Pochet S, Munier-Lehmann H (2012) Drug design and identification of potent leads against mycobacterium tuberculosis thymidine monophosphate kinase. Curr Top Med Chem 12: 694–705.
23. Evans GB, Furneaux RH, Kelly PM, Schramm VL, Tyler PC (2007) Transition state analogue inhibitors of N-ribosyltransferases: new drugs by targeting nucleoside processing enzymes. Nucleic Acids Symp Ser (Oxf): 63–64. doi:10.1093/nass/nrm032.
24. Wright JM, Dunn LA, Kazimierczuk Z, Burgess AG, Krauer KG, et al. (2010) Susceptibility in vitro of clinically metronidazole-resistant Trichomonas vaginalis to nitazoxanide, toyocamycin, and 2-fluoro-2′-deoxyadenosine. Parasitol Res 107: 847–853. doi:10.1007/s00436-010-1938-3.
25. el Kouni MH, Messier NJ, Cha S (1987) Treatment of schistosomiasis by purine nucleoside analogues in combination with nucleoside transport inhibitors. Biochemical Pharmacology 36: 3815–3821. doi:10.1016/0006–2952(87)90443-6.
26. Pinheiro E, Vasan A, Kim JY, Lee E, Guimier JM, et al. (2006) Examining the production costs of antiretroviral drugs. AIDS 20: 1745–1752. doi:10.1097/01.aids.0000242821.67001.65.
27. Ubiali D, Rocchietti S, Scaramozzino F, Terreni M, Albertini AM, et al. (2004) Synthesis of 2′-Deoxynucleosides by Transglycosylation with New Immobilized and Stabilized Uridine Phosphorylase and Purine Nucleoside Phosphorylase. Advanced Synthesis & Catalysis 346: 1361–1366. doi:10.1002/adsc.200404019.
28. Rocchietti S, Ubiali D, Terreni M, Albertini AM, Fernández-Lafuente R, et al. (2004) Immobilization and stabilization of recombinant multimeric uridine and purine nucleoside phosphorylases from Bacillus subtilis. Biomacromolecules 5: 2195–2200. doi:10.1021/bm049765f.
29. Bennett EM, Anand R, Allan PW, Hassan AEA, Hong JS, et al. (2003) Designer gene therapy using an Escherichia coli purine nucleoside phosphorylase/prodrug system. Chem Biol 10: 1173–1181.
30. Parker WB, Allan PW, Hassan AEA, Secrist JA 3rd, Sorscher EJ, et al. (2003) Antitumor activity of 2-fluoro-2′-deoxyadenosine against tumors that express Escherichia coli purine nucleoside phosphorylase. Cancer Gene Ther 10: 23–29. doi:10.1038/sj.cgt.7700520.
31. Martiniello-Wilks R, Dane A, Voeks DJ, Jeyakumar G, Mortensen E, et al. (2004) Gene-directed enzyme prodrug therapy for prostate cancer in a mouse model that imitates the development of human disease. J Gene Med 6: 43–54. doi:10.1002/jgm.474.
32. Parker WB, Allan PW, Ealick SE, Sorscher EJ, Hassan AEA, et al. (2005) DESIGN AND EVALUATION OF 5′-MODIFIED NUCLEOSIDE ANALOGS AS PRODRUGS FOR AN E. COLI PURINE NUCLEOSIDE PHOSPHORYLASE MUTANT. Nucleosides, Nucleotides and Nucleic Acids 24: 387–392. doi:10.1081/NCN-200059807.
33. Tai C-K, Wang W, Lai Y-H, Logg CR, Parker WB, et al. (2010) Enhanced efficiency of prodrug activation therapy by tumor-selective replicating retrovirus vectors armed with the Escherichia coli purine nucleoside phosphorylase gene. Cancer Gene Therapy 17: 614–623. doi:10.1038/cgt.2010.17.
34. Xie X, Xia J, He K, Lu L, Xu Q, et al. (2011) Low-molecular-mass purine nucleoside phosphorylase: characterization and application in enzymatic synthesis of nucleoside antiviral drugs. Biotechnol Lett: 1107–1112. doi:10.1007/s10529-011-0535-6.
35. Martins NH, Meza AN, Santos CR, de Giuseppe PO, Murakami MT (2011) Molecular cloning, overexpression, purification, crystallization and preliminary X-ray diffraction analysis of a purine nucleoside phosphorylase from Bacillus subtilis strain 168. Acta Crystallogr Sect F Struct Biol Cryst Commun 67: 618–622. doi:10.1107/S1744309111010414.
36. Gasteiger E, Hoogland C, Gattiker A, Duvaud S, Wilkins MR, et al. (2005) Protein Identification and Analysis Tools on the ExPASy Server. The Proteomics Protocols Handbook. Humana Press. 571–607.
37. Otwinowski Z, Minor W (1997) [20] Processing of X-ray diffraction data collected in oscillation mode. Macromolecular Crystallography Part A. Academic Press, Vol. Volume 276. 307–326.
38. Leslie AGW (2006) The integration of macromolecular diffraction data. Acta Crystallogr D Biol Crystallogr 62: 48–57. doi:10.1107/S0907444905039107.
39. Kabsch W (1988) Evaluation of single-crystal X-ray diffraction data from a position-sensitive detector. Journal of Applied Crystallography 21: 916–924. doi:10.1107/S0021889888007903.
40. Collaborative Computational Project, Number 4 (1994) The CCP4 suite: programs for protein crystallography. Acta Crystallographica Section D Biological Crystallography 50: 760–763. doi:10.1107/S0907444994003112.

41. Vagin A, Teplyakov A (1997) MOLREP: an Automated Program for Molecular Replacement. Journal of Applied Crystallography 30: 1022–1025. doi:10.1107/S0021889897006766.
42. McCoy AJ, Grosse-Kunstleve RW, Adams PD, Winn MD, Storoni LC, et al. (2007) Phaser crystallographic software. J Appl Crystallogr 40: 658–674. doi:10.1107/S0021889807021206.
43. Grenha R, Levdikov VM, Fogg MJ, Blagova EV, Brannigan JA, et al. (2005) Structure of purine nucleoside phosphorylase (DeoD) from Bacillus anthracis. Acta Crystallogr Sect F Struct Biol Cryst Commun 61: 459–462. doi:10.1107/S174430910501095X.
44. Murshudov GN, Vagin AA, Dodson EJ (1997) Refinement of macromolecular structures by the maximum-likelihood method. Acta Crystallogr D Biol Crystallogr 53: 240–255. doi:10.1107/S0907444996012255.
45. Emsley P, Cowtan K (2004) Coot: model-building tools for molecular graphics. Acta Crystallogr D Biol Crystallogr 60: 2126–2132. doi:10.1107/S0907444904019158.
46. Chen VB, Arendall WB, Headd JJ, Keedy DA, Immormino RM, et al. (2010) MolProbity: all-atom structure validation for macromolecular crystallography. Acta Crystallogr D Biol Crystallogr 66: 12–21. doi:10.1107/S0907444909042073.
47. DeLano WL (2002) The PyMOL Molecular Graphics System. Available:http://www.pymol.org.
48. Krissinel E, Henrick K (2007) Inference of macromolecular assemblies from crystalline state. J Mol Biol 372: 774–797. doi:10.1016/j.jmb.2007.05.022.
49. Krissinel E, Henrick K (2004) Secondary-structure matching (SSM), a new tool for fast protein structure alignment in three dimensions. Acta Crystallogr D Biol Crystallogr 60: 2256–2268.
50. Mao C, Cook WJ, Zhou M, Koszalka GW, Krenitsky TA, et al. (1997) The crystal structure of Escherichia coli purine nucleoside phosphorylase: a comparison with the human enzyme reveals a conserved topology. Structure 5: 1373–1383.
51. Zang Y, Wang W-H, Wu S-W, Ealick SE, Wang CC (2005) Identification of a subversive substrate of Trichomonas vaginalis purine nucleoside phosphorylase and the crystal structure of the enzyme-substrate complex. J Biol Chem 280: 22318–22325. doi:10.1074/jbc.M501843200.
52. Dessanti P, Zhang Y, Allegrini S, Tozzi MG, Sgarrella F, et al. (2012) Structural basis of the substrate specificity of Bacillus cereus adenosine phosphorylase. Acta Crystallogr D Biol Crystallogr 68: 239–248. doi:10.1107/S090744491200073X.
53. Tahirov TH, Inagaki E, Ohshima N, Kitao T, Kuroishi C, et al. (2004) Crystal structure of purine nucleoside phosphorylase from Thermus thermophilus. J Mol Biol 337: 1149–1160. doi:10.1016/j.jmb.2004.02.016.
54. Bennett EM, Li C, Allan PW, Parker WB, Ealick SE (2003) Structural basis for substrate specificity of Escherichia coli purine nucleoside phosphorylase. J Biol Chem 278: 47110–47118. doi:10.1074/jbc.M304622200.
55. Hewitt SN, Choi R, Kelley A, Crowther GJ, Napuli AJ, et al. (2011) Expression of proteins in Escherichia coli as fusions with maltose-binding protein to rescue non-expressed targets in a high-throughput protein-expression and purification pipeline. Acta Crystallogr Sect F Struct Biol Cryst Commun 67: 1006–1009. doi:10.1107/S1744309111022159.
56. Badger J, Sauder JM, Adams JM, Antonysamy S, Bain K, et al. (2005) Structural analysis of a set of proteins resulting from a bacterial genomics project. Proteins 60: 787–796. doi:10.1002/prot.20541.
57. Afshar S, Sawaya MR, Morrison SL (2009) Structure of a mutant human purine nucleoside phosphorylase with the prodrug, 2-fluoro-2′-deoxyadenosine and the cytotoxic drug, 2-fluoroadenine. Protein Sci 18: 1107–1114. doi:10.1002/pro.91.
58. Torii T, Onishi T, Izawa K, Maruyama T, Demizu Y, et al. (2006) Synthesis of 6-arylthio analogs of 2′,3′-dideoxy-3′-fluoroguanosine and their effect against hepatitis B virus replication. Nucleosides Nucleotides Nucleic Acids 25: 655–665. doi:10.1080/15257770600686394.
59. Postigo MP, Guido RVC, Oliva G, Castilho MS, da R Pitta I, et al. (2010) Discovery of New Inhibitors of Schistosoma mansoni PNP by Pharmacophore-Based Virtual Screening. J Chem Inf Model 50: 1693–1705. doi:10.1021/ci100128k.
60. Bzowska A, Kulikowska E, Darzynkiewicz E, Shugar D (1988) Purine nucleoside phosphorylase. Structure-activity relationships for substrate and inhibitor properties of N-1-, N-7-, and C-8-substituted analogues; differentiation of mammalian and bacterial enzymes with N-1-methylinosine and guanosine. J Biol Chem 263: 9212–9217.
61. Mikleušević G, Štefanić Z, Narczyk M, Wielgus-Kutrowska B, Bzowska A, et al. (2011) Validation of the catalytic mechanism of Escherichia coli purine nucleoside phosphorylase by structural and kinetic studies. Biochimie 93: 1610–1622. doi:10.1016/j.biochi.2011.05.030.
62. Erion MD, Takabayashi K, Smith HB, Kessi J, Wagner S, et al. (1997) Purine nucleoside phosphorylase. 1. Structure-function studies. Biochemistry 36: 11725–11734. doi:10.1021/bi961969w.
63. Canduri F, Silva RG, dos Santos DM, Palma MS, Basso LA, et al. (2005) Structure of human PNP complexed with ligands. Acta Crystallogr D Biol Crystallogr 61: 856–862. doi:10.1107/S0907444905005421.
64. Ho M-C, Shi W, Rinaldo-Matthis A, Tyler PC, Evans GB, et al. (2010) Four generations of transition-state analogues for human purine nucleoside phosphorylase. Proc Natl Acad Sci USA 107: 4805–4812. doi:10.1073/pnas.0913439107.
65. Acs G, Reich E, Mori M (1964) BIOLOGICAL AND BIOCHEMICAL PROPERTIES OF THE ANALOGUE ANTIBIOTIC TUBERCIDIN. Proc Natl Acad Sci U S A 52: 493–501.
66. el Kouni MH, Diop D, Cha S (1983) Combination therapy of schistosomiasis by tubercidin and nitrobenzylthioinosine 5′-monophosphate. Proc Natl Acad Sci U S A 80: 6667–6670.
67. Hwang BK, Ahn SJ, Moon SS (1994) Production, Purification, and Antifungal Activity of the Antibiotic Nucleoside, Tubercidin, Produced by Streptomyces-Violaceoniger. Canadian Journal of BotanyRevue Canadienne De Botanique 72: 480–485.
68. OWEN SP, SMITH CG (1964) CYTOTOXICITY AND ANTITUMOR PROPERTIES OF THE ABNORMAL NUCLEOSIDE TUBERCIDIN (NSC-56408). Cancer Chemother Rep 36: 19–22.
69. Perlman ME, Davis DG, Koszalka GW, Tuttle JV, London RE (1994) Studies of inhibitor binding to Escherichia coli purine nucleoside phosphorylase using the transferred nuclear Overhauser effect and rotating-frame nuclear Overhauser enhancement. Biochemistry 33: 7547–7559.
70. A Bzowska ZK (1998) 7-Deazapurine 2′-deoxyribofuranosides are noncleavable competitive inhibitors of Escherichia coli purine nucleoside phosphorylase (PNP). Acta biochimica Polonica 45: 755–768.
71. Krohne TU, Shankara S, Geissler M, Roberts BL, Wands JR, et al. (2001) Mechanisms of cell death induced by suicide genes encoding purine nucleoside phosphorylase and thymidine kinase in human hepatocellular carcinoma cells in vitro. Hepatology 34: 511–518. doi:10.1053/jhep.2001.26749.
72. Ray AS, Olson L, Fridland A (2004) Role of Purine Nucleoside Phosphorylase in Interactions between 2′,3′-Dideoxyinosine and Allopurinol, Ganciclovir, or Tenofovir. Antimicrob Agents Chemother 48: 1089–1095. doi:10.1128/AAC.48.4.1089–1095.2004.
73. Thiers BH (1990) Acyclovir in the treatment of herpesvirus infections. Dermatol Clin 8: 583–587.
74. dos Santos DM, Canduri F, Pereira JH, Vinicius Bertacine Dias M, Silva RG, et al. (2003) Crystal structure of human purine nucleoside phosphorylase complexed with acyclovir. Biochem Biophys Res Commun 308: 553–559.
75. Thomsen R, Christensen MH (2006) MolDock: a new technique for high-accuracy molecular docking. J Med Chem 49: 3315–3321. doi:10.1021/jm051197e.
76. Koellner G, Bzowska A, Wielgus-Kutrowska B, Luić M, Steiner T, et al. (2002) Open and closed conformation of the E. coli purine nucleoside phosphorylase active center and implications for the catalytic mechanism. J Mol Biol 315: 351–371. doi:10.1006/jmbi.2001.5211.
77. Sgarrella F, Frassetto L, Allegrini S, Camici M, Carta MC, et al. (2007) Characterization of the adenine nucleoside specific phosphorylase of Bacillus cereus. Biochim Biophys Acta 1770: 1498–1505. doi:10.1016/j.bbagen.2007.07.004.
78. Jensen KF (1978) Two purine nucleoside phosphorylases in Bacillus subtilis. Purification and some properties of the adenosine-specific phosphorylase. Biochim Biophys Acta 525: 346–356.
79. Sorscher EJ, Peng S, Bebok Z, Allan PW, Bennett LL Jr, et al. (1994) Tumor cell bystander killing in colonic carcinoma utilizing the Escherichia coli DeoD gene to generate toxic purines. Gene Ther 1: 233–238.

13

Minicircle-oriP-IFNγ: A Novel Targeted Gene Therapeutic System for EBV Positive Human Nasopharyngeal Carcinoma

Yufang Zuo[1], Jiangxue Wu[1], Zumin Xu[1,3], Shiping Yang[1¤], Haijiao Yan[1], Li Tan[1], Xiangqi Meng[1], Xiaofang Ying[1], Ranyi Liu[1], Tiebang Kang[1], Wenlin Huang[1,2*]

1 State Key Laboratory of Oncology in South China, Cancer Center, Sun Yat-Sen University, Guangzhou, People's Republic of China, **2** Institute of Microbiology, Chinese Academy of Science, Beijing, People's Republic of China, **3** Department of Radiation Oncology, Cancer Center, Sun Yat-Sen University, Guangzhou, People's Republic of China

Abstract

Background: Nonviral vectors are attractively used for gene therapy owing to their distinctive advantages. Our previous study has demonstrated that transfer of human *IFNγ* gene into nasopharyngeal carcinoma (NPC) by using a novel nonviral vector, minicircle (mc), under the control of cytomegalovirus (CMV) promoter was effective to inhibit tumor growth. However, therapies based on CMV promoter cannot express the targeted genes in cancer tissues. Previous studies indicated that the development of human NPC was closely associated with Epstein-Barr virus (EBV) and demonstrated the transcriptional enhancer function of oriP when bound by EBV protein. Therefore, the present study is to explore the targeted gene expression and the anti-tumor effect of a novel tumor-specific gene therapeutic system (mc-oriP-*IFNγ*) in which the transgene expression was under the transcriptional regulation of oriP promoter.

Methodology/Principal Findings: Dual-luciferase reporter assay and ELISA were used to assess the expression of luciferase and IFNγ. WST assay was used to assess the cell proliferation. RT-PCR was used to detect the mRNA level of EBNA1. RNAi was used to knockdown the expression of EBNA1. NPC xenograft models in nude mice were used to investigate the targeted antitumor efficacy of mc-oriP-*IFNγ*. Immunohistochemistry was used to detect the expression and the activity of the IFNγ in tumor sections. Our results demonstrated that mc-oriP vectors mediated comparable gene expression and anti-proliferative effect in the EBV-positive NPC cell line C666-1 compared to mc-CMV vectors. Furthermore, mc-oriP vectors exhibited much lower killing effects on EBV-negative cell lines compared to mc-CMV vectors. The targeted expression of mc-oriP vectors was inhibited by EBNA1-siRNA in C666-1. This selective expression was corroborated in EBV-positive and -negative tumor models.

Conclusions/Significance: This study demonstrates the feasibility of mc-oriP-*IFNγ* as a safe and highly effective targeted gene therapeutic system for the treatment of EBV positive NPC.

Editor: Maria G. Masucci, Karolinska Institutet, Sweden

Funding: Funding was provided by the National Basic Research Program of China (973 Program, Nos. 2010CB529904 and 2010CB912201), the National Natural Science Foundation of China (Nos. 30801360 and 30973448), the Key Project of Chinese Ministry of Education (No. 109124), the Science Fund for Young Scholar of Cancer Center of Sun Yat-Sen University, the Science Fund for Young Teacher of Sun Yat-Sen University (2009267), a grant from Chinese Academy of Sciences KSCX1-YW-10, and by support from the Guangdong Recruitment Program of Creative Research Groups. The funders had no role in study design, data collection and analysis, decision to publish, or preparation of the manuscript.

Competing Interests: The authors have declared that no competing interests exist.

* E-mail: hwenl@mail.sysu.edu.cn

These authors contributed equally to this work.

¤ Current address: Department of Radiation Oncology, Hainan Provincial People's Hospital, Haikou, Hainan, People's Republic of China

Introduction

The goal of cancer treatment is to selectively eliminate malignant cells while leaving normal tissues intact [1]. Therefore, targeted strategies are needed to be implemented for future therapies to ensure efficient activity at the site of patients' primary tumors or metastases without causing intolerable side effects. To this end, cellular mechanisms of gene regulation have been successfully exploited to direct therapeutic gene expression into cancer cells [2,3,4]. Transcriptional targeting is feasible because the tissue- or cancer-specific promoter can be activated in the targeted cancer cells in the presence of proper subset of activators while remaining silent in the non-targeted cells [5].

Nasopharyngeal carcinoma (NPC) is prevalent in South China, North Africa, and among Alaskan Eskimos. A unique feature of NPC is that nearly 100% of anaplastic or poorly differentiated nasopharyngeal carcinomas contain Epstein-Barr virus genomes and express EBV proteins [6], which are expressed exclusively in the malignant tissues but not in the surrounding normal tissues. This difference provides an exploitable opportunity for tumor-specific targeting. Initial genetic dissections of EBV identified one viral protein, Epstein-Barr Nuclear Antigen 1 (EBNA1), and one region of the viral genome, termed latent origin of plasmid replication (oriP), as being necessary and sufficient for replication of the viral plasmid. Previous studies have determined that EBNA1 is essential for regulating the transcription of the transforming genes of EBV [7,8,9]. Additionally, EBNA-1, the only viral protein required for the replication of EBV in latently-infected cells, is found in all EBV-associated malignancies [10]. The oriP is composed of two separable *cis* elements, the Family of Repeats (FR) and Dyad Symmetry element (DS) [11]. The FR element consists of 20 tandem 30-bp repeats and acts as a transcriptional enhancer for heterologous promoters when it is bound by EBNA1. Based on these features, the oriP-CMV promoter has been exploited for targeted gene therapy in EBV-positive NPC [12].

Our laboratory has investigated the potential effect of minicircle-mediated *IFNγ* gene therapy in human nasopharyngeal carcinoma. Our data indicated that *IFNγ* gene transfer produced an antiproliferative effect on NPC cells *in vitro* and a profound antitumor effect *in vivo* [13,14]. We also demonstrated that minicircle-CMV-*IFNγ* was more efficient than corresponding conventional plasmids due to its capability of mediating long-lasting, high level of *IFNγ* gene expression [13]. The CMV promoter, however, is ubiquitously expressed without tumor-targeting activity; thus the application of this promoter is limited due to the potential side effects caused by unwanted expression of a therapeutic gene in normal tissues [15]. Furthermore, the persistence of transgene expression from the minicircle can be achieved in cells with low turnover rates, such as hepatocytes and skeletal muscle cells [16]. These issues are especially critical when the therapeutic gene is delivered systemically, such as by intravenous injection.

To solve these problems, we have developed a novel minicircle (mc) vector in which transgene expression is under the transcriptional regulation of the oriP-CMV promoter (hereinafter to be referred as oriP promoter). The binding of EBNA1 to the FR domain in oriP region activates the transcription of downstream genes. Selective expression of the therapeutic gene is successfully achieved both *in vitro* and *in vivo*, indicating the feasibility of mc-oriP-*IFNγ* as a safe and highly effective gene therapy system for the treatment of NPC. To our knowledge, this is the first report on a non-viral minicircle vector used in targeted gene therapy and is the first time that the oriP promoter has been combined with the minicircle system for NPC-targeted therapy. This strategy lays the foundation for targeted gene therapy of metastatic NPC by intravenous delivery of therapeutic genes.

Results

Selective expression of luciferase in EBV-positive C666-1 cells mediated by oriP-vectors

To determine the transgene expression provided by the novel EBNA1-regulated minicircle vectors in EBV-negative cells (293, NP69, CNE-1 and CNE-2 cells) and the only available EBV-positive NPC cell line (C666-1), the minicircle-luci was compared with its parent plasmid p2ΦC31-luci and the intermediate plasmid from which p2ΦC31-luci was derived (pSP72). All these plasmids contained a luciferase expression cassette driven by an oriP promoter or cytomegalovirus promoter (Figure 1A). Luciferase activity was assessed 48 h (72 h for C666-1 since its low growth rate) after transfection using the dual-luciferase reporter assay system. Luciferase activities were 10–60 fold lower when driven by oriP promoter than by CMV promoter in EBV-negative cells ($p<0.001$; Figure 2A). In contrast, luciferase activity was 2–5 fold higher when driven by oriP promoter than by CMV promoter in the EBV-positive C666-1 cells ($p<0.01$; Figure 2A). Occasionally, low levels of luciferase activity were detected in some EBV-negative cells when driven by the oriP promoter, which suggested the basal expression induced by the minimal CMV IE promoter included in oriP promoter. This observation is consistent with a previous study [12]. The expression levels of the minicircle groups were significantly higher than those of the corresponding parent groups, demonstrating that the minicircle is more efficient in mediating transgene expression *in vitro*. ($p<0.05$; Figure 2A). There was no consistent difference when minicircle groups were compared with pSP72 groups in different cell lines in the short term (48 hrs or 72hrs), which may be due to the size of the pSP72 vector is close to the minicircle vector.

Selective expression of IFNγ in EBV-positive C666-1 cells mediated by oriP-vectors

To investigate whether mc-oriP-*IFNγ* can mediate efficient expression of the *IFNγ* gene in EBV-positive NPC cells, the minicircle-*IFNγ* was compared with its parent plasmid p2ΦC31-*IFNγ* and the intermediate plasmid from which p2ΦC31-*IFNγ* was derived (pSP72). All of these plasmids contained an IFNγ expression cassette driven by an oriP promoter or CMV promoter (Figure 1A). 293 cells, NP69 cells, and three NPC cell lines were transfected according to the regimen shown in Table 1. The culture supernatant of each treatment was collected to investigate the cumulative production of IFNγ over the indicated time course using ELISA. No IFNγ was found in the culture medium from p2ΦC31-transfected cells (data not shown). The expression level of IFNγ was obviously lower when driven by oriP promoter than by CMV promoter in EBV-negative cells ($p<0.05$; Figure 2B). However, there was no significant difference in IFNγ expression level when driven by the oriP or CMV promoter in EBV-positive C666-1 cells ($p>0.05$; Figure 2B). The expression levels of the minicircle groups were significantly higher than those of the corresponding parent plasmid groups ($p<0.05$; Figure 2B). There was no consistent difference when the minicircle groups were compared with the pSP72 groups in different cell lines.

Mc-oriP-IFNγ selectively inhibits the growth of EBV-positive C666-1 cells

The killing effects of mc-oriP-*IFNγ* on NPC cells compared with mc-CMV-*IFNγ* were assessed using the WST assay. The WST assay was performed with Cell Counting Kit-8 (CCK-8) by using Dojindo's highly water-soluble tetrazolium salt WST-8. WST-8 is reduced by dehydrogenases in cells to give a yellow colored product (formazan), which is soluble in the tissue culture medium. The amount of the formazan dye generated by the activity of dehydrogenases in cells is directly proportional to the number of living cells. The detection sensitivity of CCK-8 is higher than other tetrazolium salts such as MTT, XTT, MTS or WST-1 (Cell Counting Kit-8 Technical Manual). Transfection of NPC cells with the mc-CMV-*IFNγ* resulted in significantly reduced cell viability in both EBV-negative cells (CNE-1, CNE-2) and EBV-positive C666-1 cells ($p<0.05$; Figure 3). However, mc-oriP-*IFNγ* caused a significant reduction of C666-1 cell viability but no impact on EBV-negative cells. Treatment of C666-1 cells with mc-oriP-*IFNγ* or mc-CMV-*IFNγ* achieved a similar extent of toxicity (relative growth rate of 48.89±1.7% and 46.89±2.07%, respectively; $p>0.05$), suggesting that the two promoters provided comparable levels of transgene expression. These results are consistent with previous observations reported by Li et al [12]. Furthermore, the minicircle showed more profound effects than

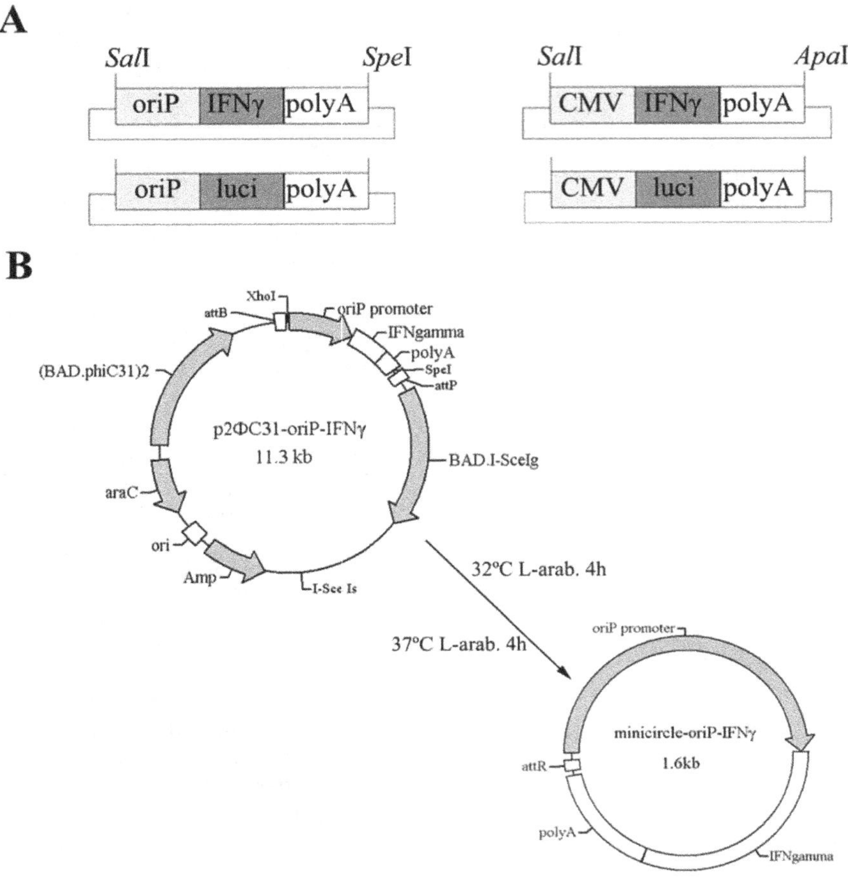

Figure 1. Schematic diagram of the construction of mc-oriP and control vectors and the generation of mc-oriP-IFNγ. (**A**) Diagram of the minicircle vectors carrying the IFNγ gene or firefly luciferase gene under the control of the oriP promoter (left) or CMV promoter (right). (**B**) Flow chart of ΦC31 integrase-mediated intramolecular recombination of p2ΦC31-oriP-IFNγ. The resulting product is minicircle-oriP-IFNγ. Amp, ampicillin resistance gene; BAD, araBAD promoter; araC, araC repressor; attB, bacterial attachment site; attP, phage attachment site; attR, right hybrid sequence; I-SceIg, I-SceI gene; I-SceIs, I-SceI cutting site; L-arab., L-arabinose.

the parent plasmid ($p<0.01$). In contrast to NPC cell lines, no growth inhibitory effect was observed in 293 and NP69 cells treated with *IFNγ* gene transfer ($p>0.05$).

The oriP-based promoter is responsive to EBNA1

Although endpoint PCR is at best only semi-quantitative, we observed a distinct increase in EBNA1 mRNA level following overexpression ($p<0.05$; Figure 4A) and a clear decrease following siRNA treatment ($p<0.05$; Figure 4B). To further verify whether the targeted gene expression of oriP promoter was regulated by EBNA1 and transient expression of EBNA1 was sufficient to enhance the luciferase activity of the mc-oriP-*luci* treatment group, the following experiments were performed. EBV-negative CNE-2 cells were pre-transfected with an EBNA1 expression plasmid, followed by a second round of transfection with mc-oriP-*luci* 48 hrs later. EBNA1 expression increased the luciferase activity in the mc-oriP-*luci* treatment group ($p<0.01$; Figure 4C) while had no effect on the luciferase activity in the mc-CMV-*luci* treatment group ($p>0.05$; Figure 4C). The EBV-positive C666-1 cells were treated with siRNA to down-regulate EBNA1 expression. EBNA1 silencing reduced the luciferase activity in the mc-oriP-*luci* treatment group ($p<0.0001$; Figure 4D) with no effect on the luciferase activity in the mc-CMV-*luci* treatment group ($p>0.05$; Figure 4D).

Targeted efficacy of mc-oriP-IFNγ on nasopharyngeal xenograft tumors

To determine whether the *in vitro* data of selective expression of the oriP-driven minicircle vector can be corroborated in a more complex *in vivo* model, CNE-2 (EBV-negative) and C666-1 (EBV-positive) tumors were treated with either mc-oriP-*IFNγ* or mc-CMV-*IFNγ*. Each mouse was treated with intratumoral injection of 100 μl plasmid-liposome complex containing 15 μg DNA and 60 μl lipofectamine 2000 once a week for 3 weeks (as shown in Table 1). The time-dependent evolution of tumor volume in mice inoculated with CNE-2 and C666-1 cells (Figure 5A and B) indicated that treatment with mc-oriP-*IFNγ* had minimal inhibitory effect on EBV-negative CNE-2 tumors compared with the control p2ΦC31 group (Figure 5A). In contrast, the tumor size of EBV-positive C666-1 xenografts treated with mc-oriP-*IFNγ* was significantly decreased compared with control groups ($p<0.05$; Figure 5B). Furthermore, mc-oriP-*IFNγ* treatment had similar effect on EBV-positive C666-1 tumors compared to mc-CMV-*IFNγ* treatment ($p>0.05$).

The inhibition rate of the treated group was determined according to tumor weight (Figure 5C and D), and the growth of tumors after mc-oriP-*IFNγ* or mc-CMV-*IFNγ* treatment was significantly slower than those of the control groups ($p<0.05$). In the CNE-2 cell-xenografted models, the inhibition rates of

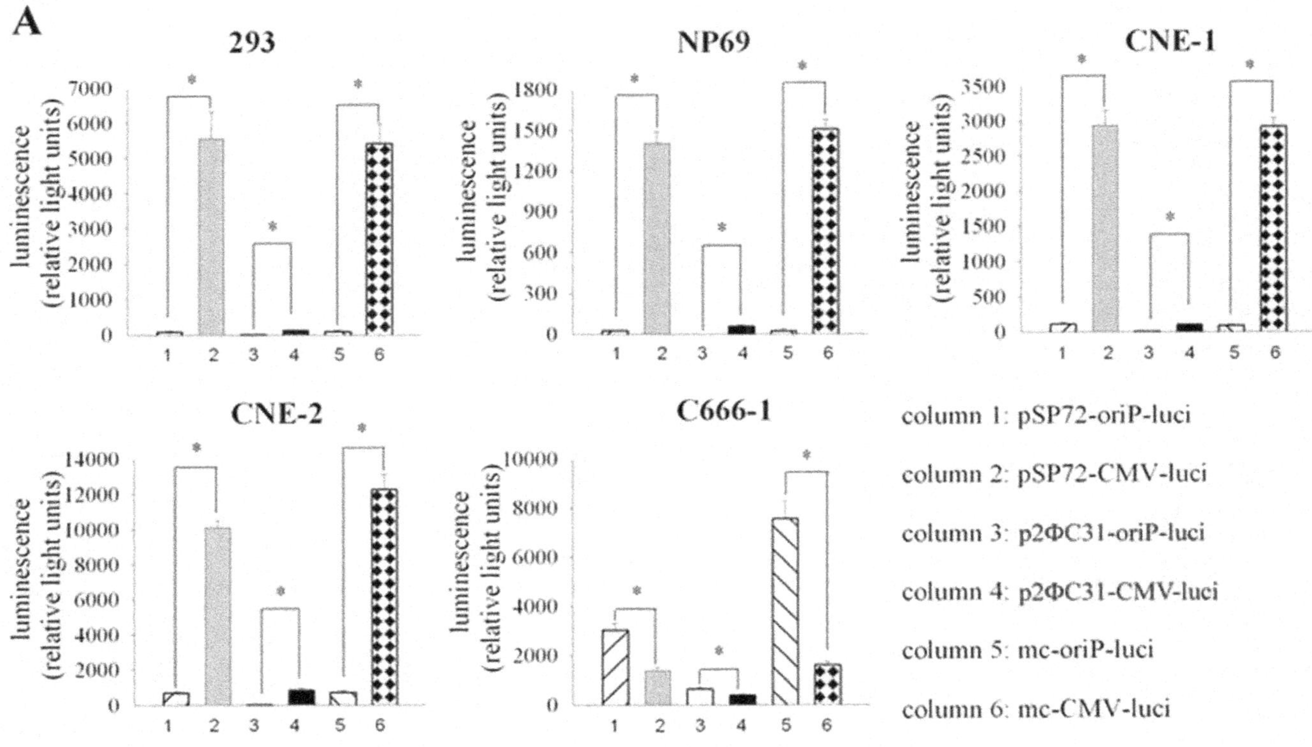

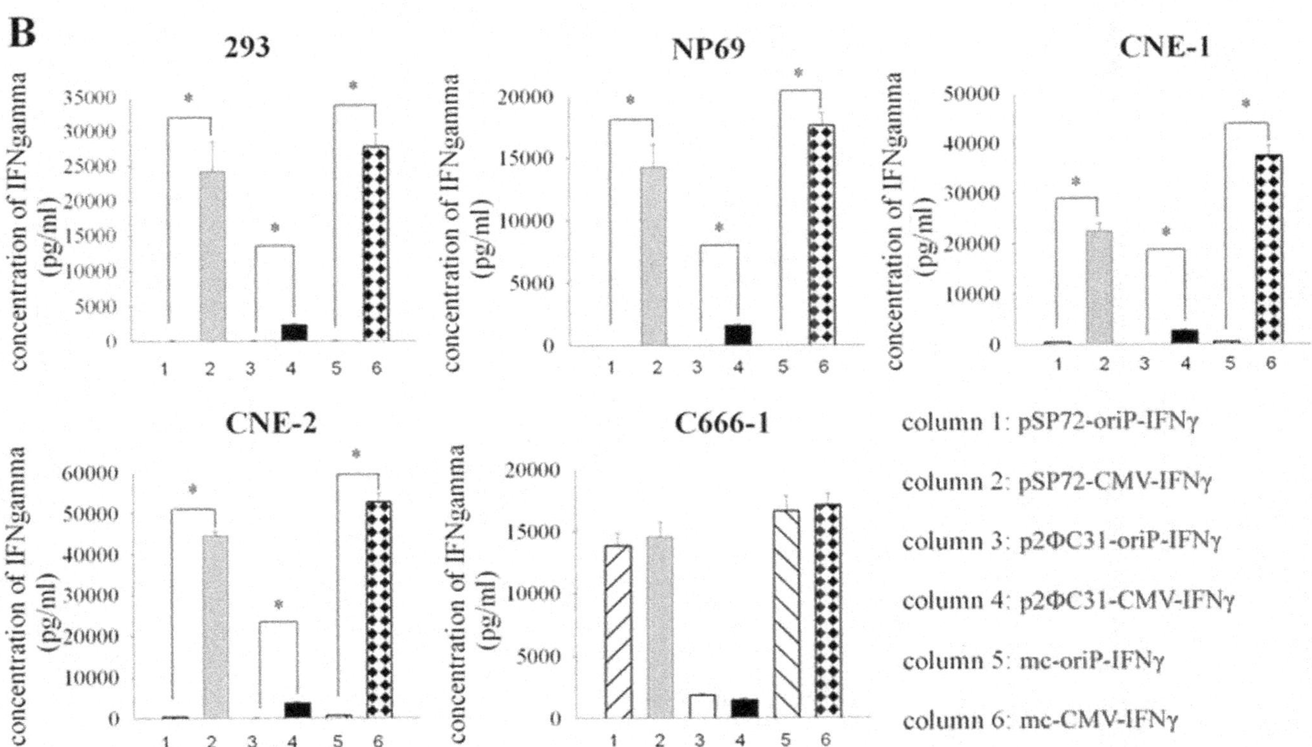

Figure 2. Selective expression of luciferase or IFNγ gene mediated by mc-oriP vector in EBV-positive cells. (**A**) Luciferase activities were assayed using the Dual-Luciferase Reporter Assay System for EBV-negative cell lines (293, NP69, CNE-1 and CNE-2) and the EBV-positive cell line (C666-1). (**B**) The expression level of IFNγ in the supernatant of different cells transfected with plasmids carrying the human IFNγ expression cassette as detected by an ELISA kit. Columns, mean of three independent experiments; bars, SD; *, $p<0.05$, gene expression under the control of oriP promoter compared with CMV promoter.

Table 1. Treatment regimens for *in vitro* and *in vivo* transfections.

Treatment regimen used for transfected cells (1 μg DNA +1 μl lipofectamine 2000/well) Group (*in vitro*)	Treatment regimen used for NPC-xenografted mice (15 μg DNA +60 μl lipofectamine 2000*/mouse) Group (*in vivo*)
pSP72-oriP-IFNγ/luci	p2ΦC31-oriP-IFNγ
pSP72-CMV-IFNγ/luci	p2ΦC31-CMV-IFNγ
p2ΦC31-oriP-IFNγ/luci	minicircle-oriP-IFNγ
p2ΦC31-CMV-IFNγ/luci	minicircle-CMV-IFNγ
minicircle-oriP-IFNγ/luci	p2ΦC31
minicircle-CMV-IFNγ/luci	
p2ΦC31	

*0.9% NaCl solution was added to adjust the total volume to 100 μl. Each mouse was treated with intratumoral injection of plasmid-liposome complex once a week for 3 weeks.

p2ΦC31-CMV-*IFNγ* and mc-CMV-*IFNγ* groups were 46.57% and 74.6%, respectively (Figure 5C). For the C666-1 cell-xenografted models, the inhibition rates in the p2ΦC31-oriP-*IFNγ*, p2ΦC31-CMV-*IFNγ*, mc-oriP-*IFNγ* and mc-CMV-*IFNγ* groups were 40.05%, 39.75%, 83.01%, and 82.05%, respectively (Figure 5D). In both models, the minicircle group showed more profound antitumor potential than the parent plasmid-treated group ($p<0.05$; Figure 5C and D).

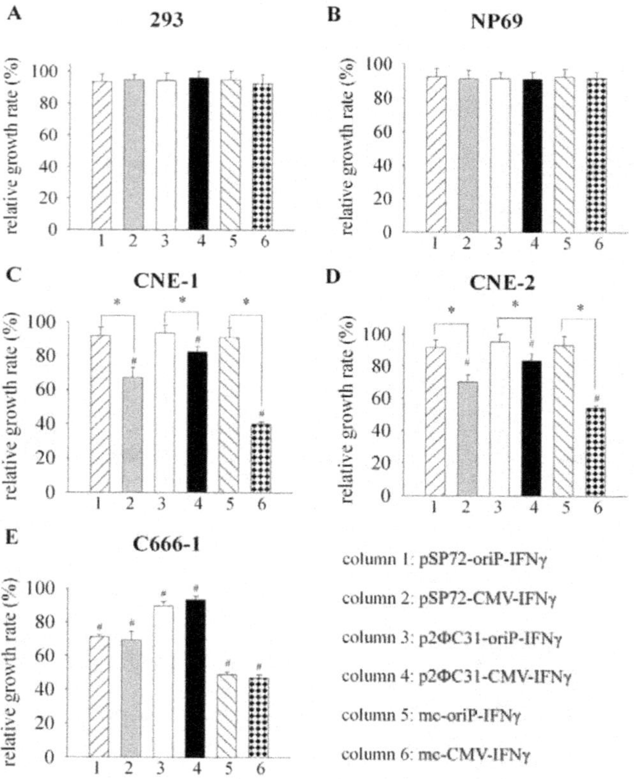

Figure 3. Minicircle-oriP-IFNγ selectively inhibits the growth of EBV-positive C666-1 cells *in vitro*. Cells were treated with minicircle-IFNγ or control plasmids for 48 hours (72 hours for C666-1). Cell viability was determined by WST assay. Data are given as relative growth rates compared with the p2ΦC31-treated group. Columns, mean of three independent experiments; bars, SD; #, $p<0.05$, compared with the p2ΦC31-treated group; *, $p<0.05$, gene expression under the control of oriP promoter compared with CMV promoter.

The long-term outcome of *IFNγ* gene transfer was evaluated by the survival rates of mice, using the protocol outlined in Table 1. There was no additional treatment after three weeks of treatment. For CNE-2 cell-xenografted mice, the median survival of the p2ΦC31, p2ΦC31-oriP-*IFNγ*, p2ΦC31-CMV-*IFNγ*, mc-oriP-*IFNγ* and mc-CMV-*IFNγ* groups was 33±2.828, 36±2.739, 47±2.828, 36±3.536, and 66±6.364 days, respectively (Figure 5E). For C666-1 cell-xenografted mice, the corresponding median survivals were 35±3.536, 45±4.243, 47±3.3, 63±6.364, and 63±4.243 days, respectively (Figure 5F). In both models, the minicircle group had a longer survival duration than the parent plasmid-treated group ($p<0.05$; Figure 5E and F).

Selective expression in EBV-positive C666-1 tumors mediated by mc-oriP vectors

To assay the targeted expression of mc-oriP-*IFNγ in vivo*, IFNγ protein levels were analyzed in tumor and liver using a human IFNγ ELISA kit. Intratumoral expression of mc-oriP-*IFNγ* was detected only in the EBV-positive C666-1 tumor, compared with mc-CMV-*IFNγ* treatment ($p>0.05$; Figure 6A and B). Systemic (liver) expression of mc-oriP-*IFNγ* was not detected in mice bearing either the EBV-negative CNE-2 tumor or the EBV-positive C666-1 tumor, compared with mc-CMV-*IFNγ* treatment ($p<0.01$). However, in mc-CMV-*IFNγ* treatment groups, mice bearing the CNE-2 tumor had much higher expression level of IFNγ in their livers than those bearing the C666-1 tumor (Figure 6A and B).

To further verify the above result of different expressions in liver mediated by the mc-CMV vector, we detected the expression of *luciferase* gene carried by minicircle in liver and tumor tissues through immunohistochemistry. Consistent with the above result, in mc-oriP-*luci* treatment groups, the staining of luciferase was observed only in the EBV-positive C666-1 tumor but neither in the EBV-negative CNE-2 tumor nor in all livers of mice tested. However, in mc-CMV-*luci* treatment groups, the staining of luciferase was observed both in the EBV-positive C666-1 tumor and in the EBV-negative CNE-2 tumor. Liver staining of mc-CMV-*luci* was observed mainly in the mice bearing the EBV-negative CNE-2 tumor (Figure S1). The result is similar to previous report [12].

Intratumoral injection of mc-oriP-IFNγ results in significant IRF-1, p21 and BAK staining only in the EBV-positive C666-1 tumor

We have demonstrated that IFNγ can effectively activate IRF-1 and lead to the inhibition of cell proliferation and the stimulation of cell apoptosis in NPC (unpublished data). IFNγ-induced G0/G1

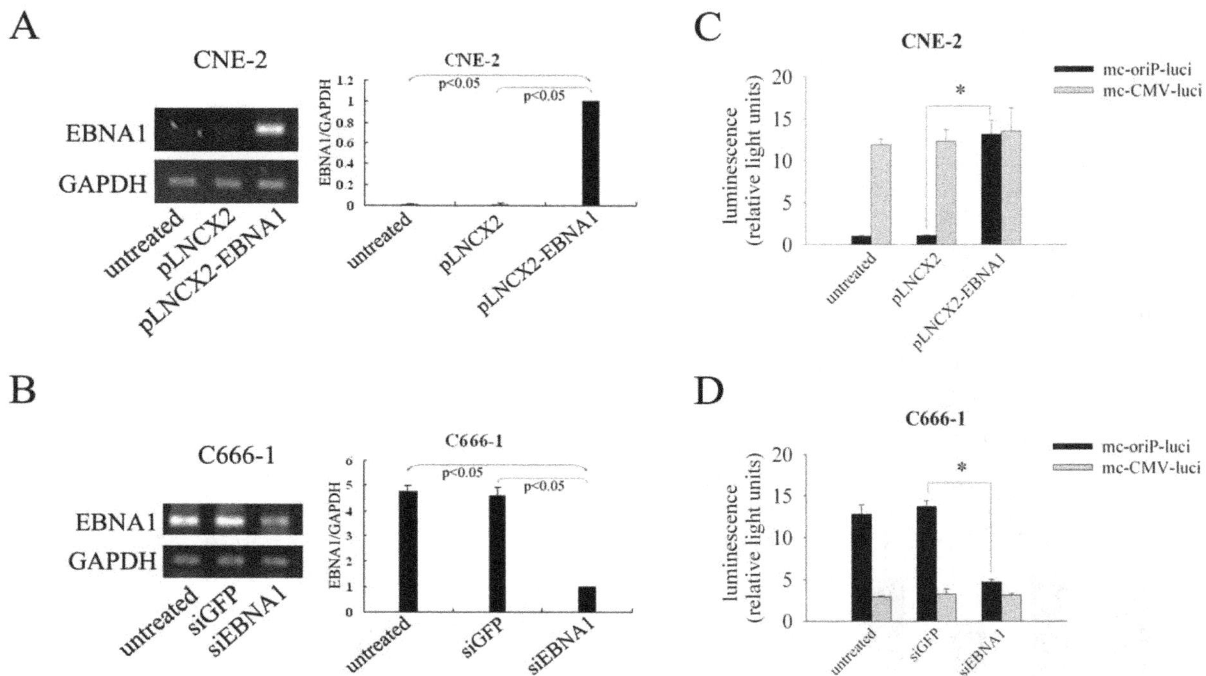

Figure 4. Transcriptional expression and function of EBNA1 in EBV-negative (CNE-2) and -positive (C666-1) NPC cell lines. (A, B) Reverse transcription-PCR analysis of EBNA1. A: CNE-2 cells were transiently transfected with plasmid expressing EBNA1 or control plasmid. For quantitative analysis, pLNCX2-EBNA1 group was normalized to 1; B: C666-1 cells were treated with siRNA against GFP (siGFP) or EBNA1 (siEBNA1). For quantitative analysis, siEBNA1 group was normalized to 1. **(C, D)** Luciferase activity was assayed in overexpressing EBNA1 (CNE-2) or silencing EBNA1 expression (C666-1) cell lines followed by transfection with mc-oriP-luci or mc-CMV-luci. Columns, mean of three independent experiments; bars, SD;*, $p<0.05$.

arrest and apoptosis has been associated with the induction of p21 and upregulation of Bak, respectively (unpublished data). Thus, immunohistochemistry was used to detect the expression of IRF-1, p21 and BAK. The intratumoral injection of mc-CMV-*IFNγ* resulted in significant IRF-1, p21 and BAK staining in both the EBV-negative CNE-2 and the EBV-positive C666-1 tumors, demonstrating that the expression of IFNγ mediated by the minicircle activated the downstream pathway of IFNγ (Figure 6C). In contrast, injection of mc-oriP-*IFNγ* resulted in obvious IRF-1, p21 and BAK staining only in the EBV-positive C666-1 tumor.

Minicircle mediates more robust antitumor effect than conventional plasmid

In order to compare the antitumor effects of minicircle and its derived plasmid pSP72 *in vivo*, C666-1 cell-xenografted mice were treated with mc-oriP-*IFNγ* and pSP72-oriP-*IFNγ*. Treatment regimen was conducted with the same protocol as shown in Table 1. Our results indicated that mc-oriP-*IFNγ* could mediate more robust antitumor effect than pSP72-oriP-*IFNγ* at days 16 and 21 ($p<0.05$) (Figure S2).

Discussion

Minicircle-mediated gene therapeutic techniques shown in previous studies were non-specific, which limited their application due to the potential systemic side effects. We report here for the first time both the non-viral minicircle vector used in targeted gene therapy and the combination of oriP promoter with minicircle system for NPC- targeted therapy. Our findings demonstrate that mc-oriP-*IFNγ* induces antiproliferation of EBV-positive tumor cells, represses tumor growth, and prolongs the mouse life span in a manner as effective as that of mc-CMV-*IFNγ* *in vitro* and *in vivo*. In addition, mc-oriP-*IFNγ* had minimal or no killing effects on EBV-negative tissues. Therefore, this study indicates the feasibility of mc-oriP-*IFNγ* as a safe and highly effective gene therapy system for NPC treatment.

Nasopharyngeal carcinoma has been shown to be the human tumor showing the most consistent association with EBV [8]. Utilization of molecules uniquely present within a tumor cell to elicit a cytotoxic response is an attractive strategy for the development of new approaches to the targeted therapy of neoplasia. The oriP promoter has been demonstrated to be very powerful in inducing targeted gene expression [12,17,18,19,20]. In previous studies, the oriP promoter was placed in adenovirus vectors, which achieved very high transduction efficiencies. Although viral-based systems have shown high transfection efficiencies *in vivo*, they have serious disadvantages such as immunogenicity and inflammatory responses [21].

Non-viral gene delivery strategies are usually based on plasmid DNA carrying the gene of interest. Conventional plasmid vectors include a bacterial backbone and a transcription unit. These sequences, however, may cause undesirable effects such as the production of antibodies against bacterial proteins expressed from cryptic upstream eukaryotic expression signals, changes in eukaryotic gene expression caused by antibiotic resistance markers, and immune responses to CpG sequences [22]. Compared to conventional plasmids, minicircle DNAs devoid of plasmid bacterial sequences are superior as non-viral DNA vector for multiple reasons: (*a*) relative safety due to the reduced numbers of inflammatory unmethylated CpG motifs; (*b*) more efficient

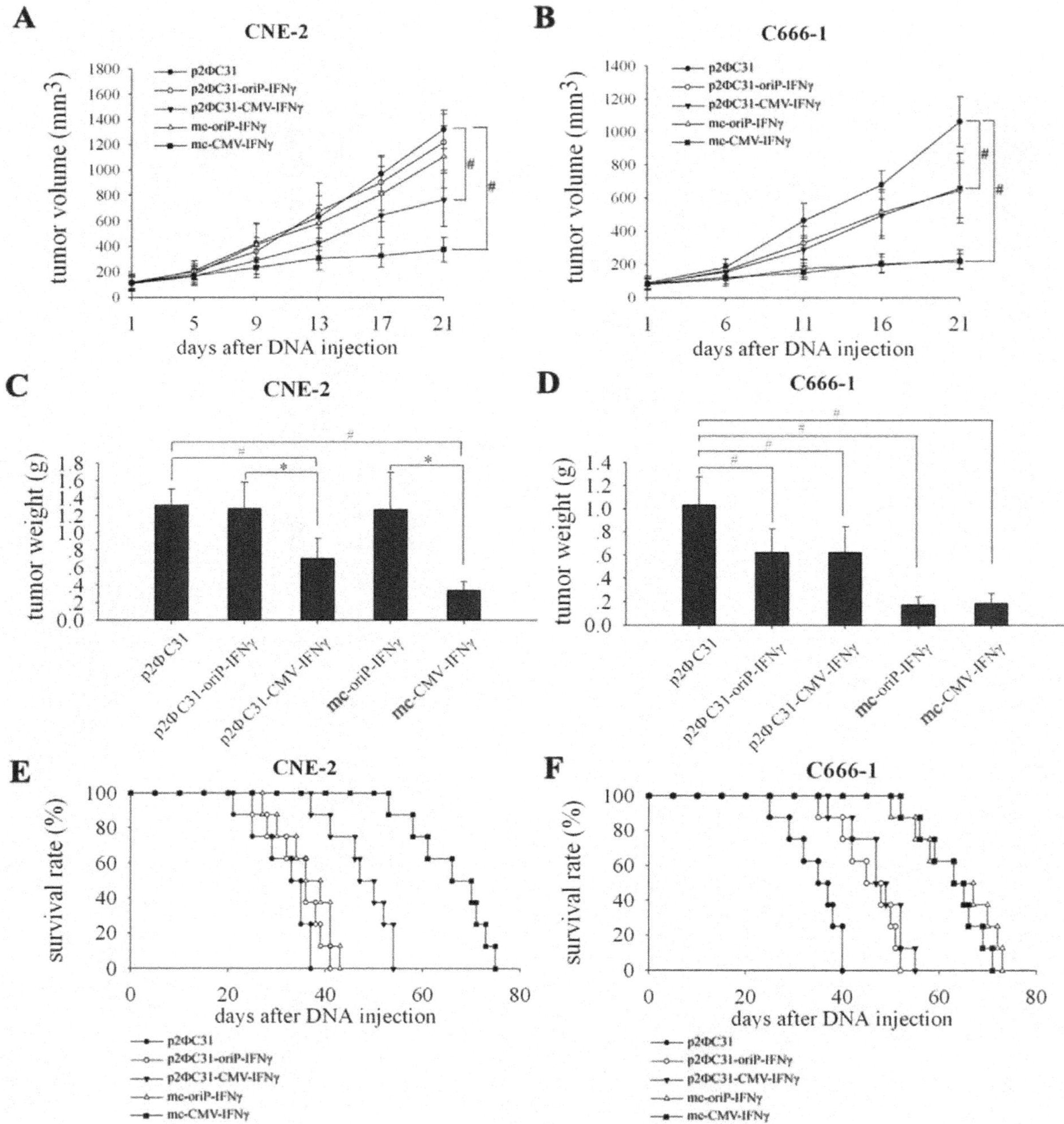

Figure 5. Selective antitumor effects of mc-oriP-IFNγ on the growth of NPC xenografts and survival analysis. (**A, B**) Time-dependent evolution of tumor volume in mice inoculated with the CNE-2 and C666-1 cell lines (n = 6, each group). For CNE-2 cell-xenografted mice, mc-oriP-IFNγ or p2ΦC31-oriP-IFNγ versus p2ΦC31, $p>0.05$; mc-CMV-IFNγ versus p2ΦC31, $p<0.05$ at days 9, 13, 17, and 21; p2ΦC31-CMV-IFNγ versus p2ΦC31, $p<0.05$ at days 13, 17, and 21. For C666-1 cell-xenografted mice, mc-oriP-IFNγ versus p2ΦC31, $p<0.05$ at days 11, 16, and 21; mc-CMV-IFNγ versus p2ΦC31, $p<0.05$ at days 11, 16, and 21; p2ΦC31-oriP-IFNγ versus p2ΦC31, $p<0.05$ at days 16, and 21; p2ΦC31-CMV-IFNγ versus p2ΦC31, $p<0.05$ at days 16 and 21; mc-oriP-IFNγ versus mc-CMV-IFNγ, $p>0.05$. (**C, D**) Specific antitumor effects of mc-oriP-IFNγ on C666-1 cell-xenografted nude mice (n = 6, each group). Mice were sacrificed after three weeks of treatment, and tumors were resected and weighted. Columns, mean of six mice; bars, SD; #, $p<0.05$, compared with p2ΦC31-treated group; *, $p<0.05$, gene expression under the control of oriP promoter compared with CMV promoter. (**E, F**) Effect of mc-oriP-IFNγ on survival (n = 8). For CNE-2 cell-xenografted mice, mc-oriP-IFNγ versus p2ΦC31, $p = 0.066$; mc-CMV-IFNγ versus p2ΦC31, $p<0.0001$. For C666-1 cell-xenografted mice, mc-oriP-IFNγ versus p2ΦC31, $p<0.0001$; mc-oriP-IFNγ versus mc-CMV-IFNγ, $p = 0.368$ (Kaplan-Meier).

transgene expression due to its reduced size; and (*c*) more robust and persistent transgene expression [16,23,24]. Previous studies have demonstrated that the use of minicircles may offer a promising avenue for safe and efficacious non-viral-based gene therapies [25,26,27,28]. Based on these superior attributes, we developed a recombinant minicircle vector carrying the human *IFNγ* gene that had antiproliferative and antitumor effects against NPC *in vitro* and *in vivo* and also demonstrated that the antiproliferative effects of *IFNγ* gene transfer on NPC cell lines could be attributed to G0-G1 arrest and apoptosis [13].

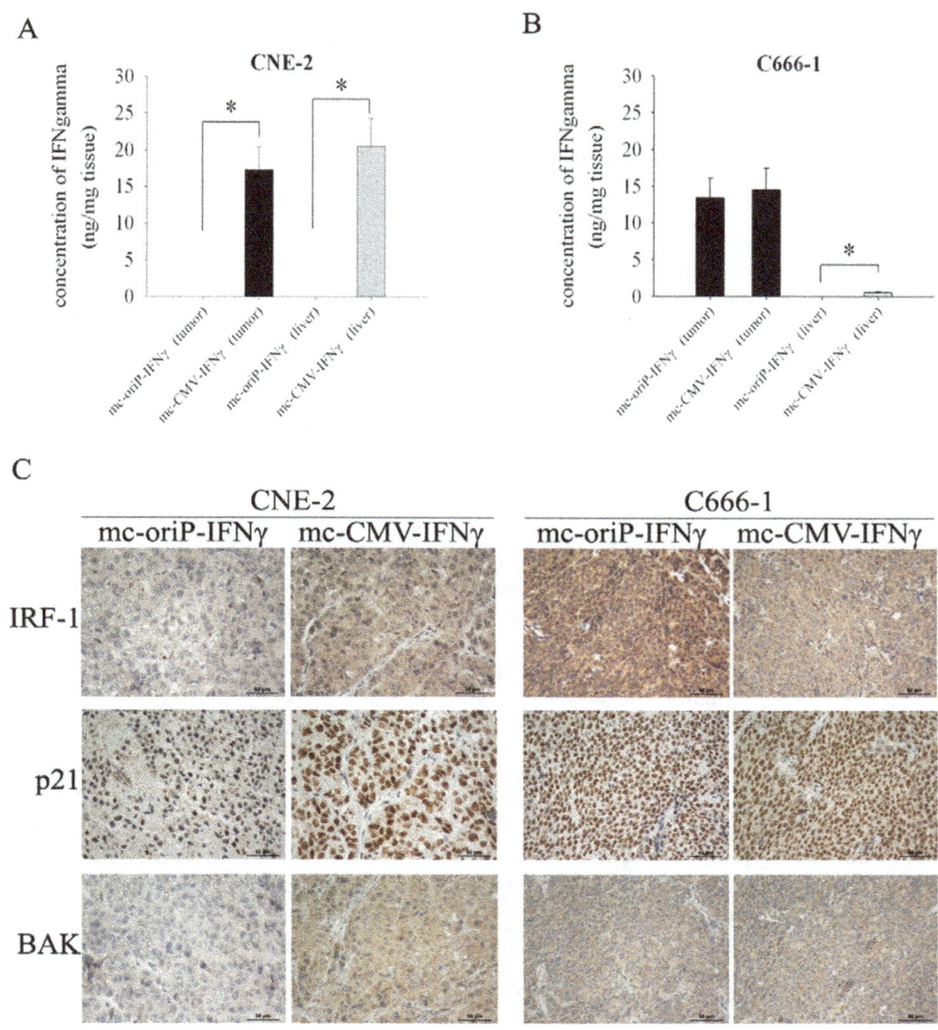

Figure 6. Tissue expression of IFNγ and immunohistochemical analysis. (**A, B**) Expression level of IFNγ in tumor and liver tissue. Results are given in ng/mg of tissue. Columns, mean of three mice; bars, SD. (**C**) Representative immunostaining of IRF-1, p21 and BAK in CNE-2 cell- and C666-1 cell-xenografted tumors treated with mc-oriP-IFNγ or mc-CMV-IFNγ, respectively. Mice were sacrificed after three weeks of treatment, and tumors were resected and frozen for immunohistochemistry assays. IRF-1 staining shows cytoplasmic and nuclear staining, p21 staining shows nuclear staining, and BAK staining shows cytoplasmic staining. In the mc-oriP-IFNγ-treated group, intense IRF-1, p21 and BAK staining were observed only in EBV-positive C666-1 tumors. Tissue sections are shown at ×400 magnification. Scale bar represents 50 μm.

Considering the need for selective NPC-specific expression, the minicircle vector used in the current study was constructed such that the CMV enhancer promoter was replaced with the oriP-CMV promoter. The new promoter provides significantly higher levels of luciferase reporter gene expression in EBV-positive NPC cells compared with CMV promoter ($p<0.05$; Figure 2A). Although the results of *IFNγ* gene expression are consistent with those of the reporter gene in EBV-negative cells, there was no significant difference between the mc-oriP-*IFNγ*-treated and the mc-CMV-*IFNγ*-treated groups in EBV-positive C666-1 cells, indicating approximately equivalent levels of *IFNγ* gene expression and cytotoxicity between the respective mc-oriP and mc-CMV vectors in the C666-1 cells ($p>0.05$; Figures 2B and 3). One explanation for these observations is that the expression of different genes is variable and consequently, the cell number for *IFNγ* gene expression was decreased after the cytotoxicity caused by IFNγ.

In the present study, the overexpression of the EBNA1 gene in CNE-2 cells resulted in an increase in luciferase activity in the mc-oriP-*luci* treatment group (Figure 4C). Inhibition of EBNA1 expression in C666-1 cells by EBNA1-specific siRNA subsequently reduced the luciferase activity in the mc-oriP-*luci* treatment group but had no effect on the mc-CMV-*luci* treatment group (Figure 4D). We and others have consistently demonstrated that the oriP-based promoter specifically responds to EBNA1 [12,18,19,20]. Therefore, the tumor-specific promoter oriP can be used for gene therapy in EBV-associated diseases, such as Burkitt's lymphoma (BL), Hodgkin's disease (HD), and post-transplant lymphoproliferative disorders (PTLD).

In addition to investigating the selective antiproliferation effects of mc-oriP-*IFNγ in vitro*, the targeted antitumor effects of mc-oriP-*IFNγ* were assessed in NPC-xenografts. The fact that the *in vitro* data could be replicated in *in vivo* tumor models is exciting. Our data show that the antitumor effects and survival rates were similar between the mc-oriP-*IFNγ*-treated and mc-CMV-*IFNγ*-treated groups in the C666-1 tumor model ($p>0.05$; Figure 5). However, the oriP promoter was much less active in the EBV-negative CNE-

2 tumor xenografts, resulting in very limited antitumor effect and a reduced survival rate ($p>0.05$; Figure 5). Again, the minicircle was much more efficient than the parent plasmid p2ΦC31 and conventional plasmid pSP72 ($p<0.05$; Figure 5 and Figure S2), this may be due to the fact that minicircle DNA does not contain extraneous plasmid backbone sequences that could cause transcriptional repression *in vivo* [23,29], which is consistent with previous studies [13,30,31].

Transgene expression can be detected in the host liver with extensive intratumoral injection of the mc-CMV-*IFNγ* (Figure 6A and B), which raises a concern about potential systemic cytotoxicity. Furthermore, there is a big difference in expression of mc-CMV-*IFNγ* in the livers of mice carrying different tumors. However, the reason for this unexpected result is unclear. A possible explanation is that the tissues of CNE-2 tumors that had higher amount of stroma are looser and softer than those of C666-1 tumors, which in turn may result in more minicircle DNAs in liver probably by the leakage. The underlying mechanism needs further to be elucidated. In addition, transgene expression in the mc-oriP-*IFNγ*-treated groups has not been detected in liver tissues (Figure 6A and B). These results provide support for the mc-oriP-*IFNγ* plasmid as a promising and NPC-specific vector for gene therapy. The minicircle vector is also a versatile tool to carry other tissue- or cancer-specific promoters for the development of promising therapeutics for other diseases.

Orthotopic models of many tumor types have been developed in which metastasis occurs in a similar manner as in patients [32]. Data on orthotopic human NPC models, however, are still limited. In one report investigating this issue, a fluorescent orthotopic NPC metastatic model was established in nude mice using stable and high GFP-expressing NPC cell lines. This model will be useful for understanding the biology of metastatic NPC and for discovering effective therapies for this disease [33]. The next step in developing the oriP-based minicircle system will be to investigate its antimetastatic effect on the orthotopic human NPC model in nude mice. This study will lay the foundation for targeted gene therapy of metastatic NPC by intravenous delivery of a therapeutic gene.

Materials and Methods

Cells and culture conditions

The cell lines used in this study were 293 (human embryonic kidney cell line, EBV negative), NP69 (immortalized human nasopharyngeal epithelial cell line, EBV negative), CNE-1 (well-differentiated NPC cell line, EBV negative), CNE-2 (poorly-differentiated NPC cell line, EBV negative), and C666-1 (undifferentiated and the only available EBV positive NPC cell line) [34,35]. CNE-1, CNE-2 and C666-1 cells were maintained in RPMI 1640 containing 100 units/mL penicillin, 100 μg/mL streptomycin, and 10% fetal bovine serum (Gibco, Paisley, United Kingdom) at 37°C in a 5% CO_2 humidified atmosphere. NP69 cells were maintained in Keratinocyte-SFM (Gibco, Invitrogen, Cat.10724), and the experiments were conducted when the cells were in an exponential growth phase. C666-1 is a kind gift from Dr. Saiwah Tsao (University of Hong Kong, Hong Kong, PR China). NP69 was kindly provided by Professor Musheng Zeng (State Key Laboratory of Oncology in South China, Cancer Center, Sun Yat-sen University, Guangzhou, PR China). 293, CNE-1, and CNE-2 cell lines were maintained by our lab [13].

Construction of recombinant parent plasmids

Plasmid p2ΦC31 (9.7 kb) was a kind gift from Dr. Zhiying Chen (Stanford University, Stanford, CA) [24]. Plasmid PDC312. oriP.luc (6 kb) carrying the oriP-CMV promoter was provided by Dr. FeiFei Liu (Department of Radiation Oncology, Princess Margaret Hospital University Health Network, Toronto, Ontario, Canada) [12]. pShuttle-*IFNγ* (4.6 kb) carrying the human *IFNγ* expression cassette was constructed by our lab. pSP72 (2462 bp) was obtained from Promega (Madison, WI). pcDNA3.1 (5428 bp) and the *E. coli* strains Top 10 were purchased from Invitrogen.

An 897-bp *Sal*I-*Hind*III fragment containing the EBV oriP-FR region and basal CMV IE promoter from plasmid PDC312•oriP•luc was subcloned into the *Sal*I-*Hind*III sites of the pSP72 plasmid to create pSP72-oriP. The polyA sequence was amplified by PCR from the pcDNA3.1 plasmid and subcloned into the downstream of the oriP promoter in pSP72-oriP plasmid to create pSP72-oriP-polyA. The *IFNγ* gene was amplified by PCR from the pShuttle-*IFNγ* plasmid and subcloned into the pSP72-oriP-polyA plasmid to create intermediate plasmid pSP72-oriP-*IFNγ*. Parent plasmid p2ΦC31-oriP-*IFNγ* (11.3 kb) (Figure 1B) was constructed by inserting the 1.6-kb *Sal*I-oriP-IFNγ-polyA-*Spe*I fragment from the above intermediate plasmid pSP72-oriP-*IFNγ* into the *Xho*I-*Spe*I sites of p2ΦC31 (*Sal*I and *Xho*I are isocaudamers).

Intermediate plasmid pSP72-oriP-*luci* was constructed by replacing *IFNγ* gene of pSP72-oriP-*IFNγ* with *luciferase* gene obtained from plasmid PDC312-oriP-luc. Then parent plasmid p2ΦC31-oriP-*luci* (12.5 kb) was constructed by inserting the 2.8-kb *Sal*I-oriP-luciferase-polyA-*Spe*I fragment from the above intermediate plasmid pSP72-oriP- *luci* into the *Xho*I-*Spe*I sites of p2ΦC31.

Intermediate plasmids pSP72-CMV-*IFNγ* and pSP72-CMV-*luci* were constructed by replacing oriP promoter of pSP72-oriP-*IFNγ* and pSP72-oriP-*luci* with CMV promoter amplified by PCR from the pcDNA3.1 plasmid, respectively. Then parent plasmids p2ΦC31-CMV-*IFNγ* (11.1 kb) and p2ΦC31-CMV-*luci* (12.3 kb) were constructed by inserting the 1.4-kb *Sal*I-CMV-IFNγ-polyA-*Apa*I fragment and 2.6-kb *Sal*I-CMV-luciferase-polyA-*Apa*I fragment from the above intermediate plasmids into the *Xho*I-*Apa*I sites of p2ΦC31, respectively. All constructs were confirmed by DNA sequencing (Figure 1).

Production and purification of minicircles

Minicircle-*IFNγ* and minicircle-*luciferase* were produced according to the methods described by Chen et al. [24] with minor modifications. Briefly, overnight bacterial growth from a single colony of parent plasmid-transformed E. coli Top 10 in Tris-borate medium was centrifuged at 20°C and 4,000 rpm for 20 minutes. The pellet was resuspended 4:1 (v/v) in fresh Luria-Bertani broth containing 1.5% L-arabinose. The bacteria were incubated at 32°C with constant shaking at 250 rpm for 4 hours. After adding one-half volume of fresh Luria-Bertani broth (pH 8.0) containing 1.0% L-arabinose, the incubation temperature was increased to 37°C, and the incubation was continued for an additional 4 hours. Episomal DNA circles were prepared from bacteria using plasmid purification kits from Qiagen (Chatsworth, CA).

Quantitative evaluation of mc-oriP-luciferase or mc-CMV-luciferase expression

To evaluate transgene expression from mc-oriP-*luciferase* or mc-CMV-*luciferase* in EBV-negative and -positive cells, luciferase activity was measured using the Dual-Luciferase Reporter Assay System (Promega). Cells were seeded in 24-well culture plates (5×10^4 cells/well for C666-1, and 3×10^4 cells/well for other cells). After one doubling, cells were cotransfected with mc-oriP-*luciferase* and pGL4.73 (Promega) simultaneously at a ratio of 50:1 (Table 1). Cell lysates were analyzed for luciferase activity using the Dual-Luciferase Reporter Assay System and a Luminometer (BERTHOLD Technologies, Centro LB-960) according to the manufacturers' protocols [12].

Quantitative evaluation of mc-oriP-IFNγ or mc-CMV-IFNγ expression

To evaluate transgene expression from mc-oriP-*IFNγ* or mc-CMV-*IFNγ* in EBV-negative and -positive cells, the concentration of IFNγ in the culture supernatant of transfected cell lines was measured with a human IFNγ ELISA kit (R&D Systems, Minneapolis, MN) according to the manufacturer's protocol. The culture supernatant of transfected cells treated with mc-*IFNγ* for 48 hours (C666-1 for 72 hours since its low growth rate) was collected and frozen (−70°C) for activity analysis [13]. The sensitivity of the kit was up to 16 pg/ml.

Effect of mc-oriP-IFNγ or mc-CMV-IFNγ on cell viability

To evaluate the effect of mc-oriP-*IFNγ* or mc-CMV-*IFNγ* treatment on viability, the WST assay was used as described previously [13,36]. WST assay was performed using Cell Counting Kit-8 which was nonradioactive, allowed sensitive colorimetric assays for the determination of the number of viable cells in cell proliferation and cytotoxicity assays. In brief, EBV-negative and -positive cell lines were transfected with mc-oriP-*IFNγ* and corresponding control plasmids (Table 1). After 48 hours (72 hours for C666-1), cell viability was measured with the Cell Counting Kit-8 (Dojindo Molecular Technologies, Inc., Gaithersburg, MD) according to the manufacturer's instructions.

Transfections and RNA interference

Transfections were conducted according to the manufacturer's instructions with minor modifications. Briefly, to generate CNE-2 cells expressing EBNA1 transiently, 2×10^5 cells were transfected with 5 μg of the EBNA1 expressing plasmid pLNCX$_2$/EBNA1 using 5 μL of lipofectamine 2000 (Invitrogen). For RNA interference experiments, 3×10^5 C666-1 cells were transfected with the indicated amounts of siRNA against GFP (GCAAGCUGACCCUGAAGUUCAU) or against EBNA1 (GGAGGUUCCAACCCGAAAU) using 5 μL of lipofectamine 2000 [37,38]. Twenty-four hours later, cells were split for either subsequent transfection or RT-PCR analysis.

RNA preparation and reverse transcription-PCR

Total RNA was prepared using the Micro-to-Midi Total RNA Purification System (Invitrogen) according to the manufacturer's instructions. RNA was submitted to DNase digestion and 1 μg aliquots were used for reverse transcription with the Reverse Transcription System (Promega). PCR reactions were performed using the following primers: human GAPDH, sense 5′-AGAAGGCTGGGGCTCATTTG-3′ and antisense 5′-AGGGGCCATCCACAGTCTTC-3′; and human EBNA1, sense 5′-AAGGAGGGTGGTTTGGAAAG-3′ and antisense 5′-TGGAATAGCAAGGGCAGTTC-3′. The PCR reaction for EBNA1 was carried out using the following conditions: denaturation—95°C (30 s), annealing—62°C (30 s), and extension—72°C (30 s), with 40 cycles [37]. For GAPDH, the following reaction conditions were used: denaturation—95°C (30 s), annealing—58°C (30 s), and extension—72°C (30 s), with 25 cycles. The sizes of the PCR products were 258 bp for *GAPDH* and 206 bp for *EBNA1*, respectively. ImageJ software was used for quantitative analysis of EBNA1/GAPDH from three independent experiments.

Antitumor activity of mc-oriP-IFNγ in a subcutaneous NPC tumor model

Care, use, and treatment of all animals in this study were in strict agreement with the institutionally approved protocol according to the USPHS Guide for the care and use of laboratory animals, as well as the guidelines set forth in the Care and Use of Laboratory Animals by the Sun Yat-sen University.

Female BALB/c nude mice (4–6 weeks old) were obtained from Shanghai Slike Experimental Animals Co. Ltd. (Shanghai, China; animal experimental license no. SCXKhu2007–0005). After 1 week of adaptation, the mice were inoculated s.c. in the scapular region with 2×10^6 CNE-2 cells or 1×10^7 C666-1 cells to generate tumors for the following experiments. Once the tumor dimension reached approximately 5–8 mm (100 mm^3), the animals were randomly assigned to groups. Each mouse was treated with intratumoral injection of 100 μl plasmid-liposome complex once a week for 3 weeks, according to the regimen shown in Table 1. For the antitumor experiments, a total of 30 mice were used for either xenograft model (6 mice per group, 5 groups). Tumor volume (V) was measured and calculated according to the following formula: $V = L\times W^2/2$ (L, length; W, width). Tumors were resected at the end point and frozen (−70°C) for analysis. For survival studies, there were eight mice in each group. Five treatment groups were included for either xenograft model. Animals were either found dead or sacrificed when tumors were observed by palpation to approach 10% of the body weight or when individual animals seemed to be stressed by weight loss, ruffled fur, and/or lethargy. All the animal experiments were conducted in accordance with the Guidelines for the Welfare of Animals in Experimental Neoplasia [13].

IFNγ production by minicircle-IFNγ transfected tumor tissues

Frozen samples were sonicated in 1×TBS (25 mmol/L Tris, 138 mmol/L NaCl, and 3 mmol/L KCl, pH 7.4) and centrifuged at 8,000×g for 1 minute. The resulting supernatants were used for analysis. IFNγ levels were determined using a human IFNγ ELISA kit (R&D Systems) according to the manufacturer's recommendations.

Antibodies and immunohistochemistry

The following commercial antibodies were used: IRF-1 (Beijing Biosynthesis Biotechnology Co., Ltd, China), p21 and BAK (Boster Biological Technology Ltd, Wuhan, China), Firefly Luciferase (Abcam Inc, UK). Sections of 5 μm from formalin-fixed and paraffin-embedded tumors were deparaffinized in two 5-min washes with xylene and rehydrated through a graded alcohol series to distilled water. The sections were then treated with 0.3% H_2O_2 in methanol for 15 min to block endogenous peroxidase activity. Before applying the primary antibody, sections were microwaved for antigen retrieval in 10 mmol/L citrate buffer (pH 6.0) for a total of 25 min, followed by equilibration in phosphate-buffered saline. Sections were treated first at room temperature for 30 minutes with goat serum blocking solution (Boster Biological Technology Ltd, Wuhan, China) in humidity chambers and then incubated with the respective primary antibody for 12–16 h at 4°C. After several washes, the sections were treated with the appropriate secondary antibody (Envison Kit; DAKO) for 30 min. The antigen-antibody complex was visualized by incubation with the DAB Kit (Envison Kit; DAKO). Finally, all sections were counterstained with hematoxylin. All immunostaining was first optimized in single tissue slides. Negative controls were obtained using the method as described above but without incubation with the appropriate primary antibody [39,40,41,42,43].

Statistical analysis

All results were evaluated using Student's *t* test with SPSS 11.0 software (SSPS, Inc., Chicago, IL). The survival results were evaluated using Kaplan-Meier curves. $p<0.05$ was considered statistically significant. Representative results from three independent experiments are shown, and the data were presented as mean ± SD.

Supporting Information

Figure S1 Immunohistochemical staining of tumor and liver cells expressing luciferase. CNE-2 or C666-1 s.c. tumors were intratumoral injected with 15 μg of either mc-oriP-*luci* or mc-CMV-*luci*. The mice were sacrificed 72 hours after treatment, and representative images of tumor and liver sections stained for luciferase were obtained. Tissue sections are shown at ×200 magnification. Scale bar represents 50 μm.

Figure S2 Antitumor effect of mc-oriP-IFNγ compared with conventional plasmid pSP72-oriP-IFNγ. pSP72-oriP-*IFNγ* versus p2ΦC31, $p < 0.05$ at days 11, 16, and 21; mc-oriP-*IFNγ* versus p2ΦC31, $p < 0.05$ at days 11, 16, and 21; pSP72-oriP-*IFNγ* versus mc-oriP-*IFNγ*, $p < 0.05$ at days 16 and 21. *, $p < 0.05$, pSP72-oriP-*IFNγ*-treated group compared with the mc-oriP-*IFNγ*-treated group.

Acknowledgments

We deeply appreciate Dr. Zhiying Chen (Stanford University, Stanford, CA) for his generous gift of p2ΦC31, Dr. Feifei Liu (University of Toronto, Ontario, Canada) for his kind supply of PDC312•oriP•Luci, and Dr. Musheng Zeng (Sun Yat-sen University, Guangzhou, PR China) for his critical suggestions and offer of pLNCX$_2$-EBNA1. We also thank Jiemin Chen and Shupeng Chen (Sun Yat-Sen University, Guangzhou, PR China) for their technical assistance.

Author Contributions

Conceived and designed the experiments: YZ JW WH. Performed the experiments: YZ ZX HY XM XY. Analyzed the data: YZ JW SY LT RL. Contributed reagents/materials/analysis tools: JW WH TK. Wrote the paper: YZ JW.

References

1. Hine CM, Seluanov A, Gorbunova V (2008) Use of the Rad51 promoter for targeted anti-cancer therapy. Proc Natl Acad Sci U S A 105: 20810–20815.
2. Dorer DE, Nettelbeck DM (2009) Targeting cancer by transcriptional control in cancer gene therapy and viral oncolysis. Adv Drug Deliv Rev 61: 554–571.
3. Chang DK, Lin CT, Wu CH, Wu HC (2009) A novel peptide enhances therapeutic efficacy of liposomal anti-cancer drugs in mice models of human lung cancer. PLoS One 4: e4171.
4. Glasgow JN, Mikheeva G, Krasnykh V, Curiel DT (2009) A strategy for adenovirus vector targeting with a secreted single chain antibody. PLoS One 4: e8355.
5. Wu L, Johnson M, Sato M (2003) Transcriptionally targeted gene therapy to detect and treat cancer. Trends Mol Med 9: 421–429.
6. Cohen JI (2000) Epstein-Barr virus infection. N Engl J Med 343: 481–492.
7. Bochkarev A, Barwell JA, Pfuetzner RA, Bochkareva E, Frappier L, et al. (1996) Crystal structure of the DNA-binding domain of the Epstein-Barr virus origin-binding protein, EBNA1, bound to DNA. Cell 84: 791–800.
8. Niedobitek G, Agathanggelou A, Nicholls JM (1996) Epstein-Barr virus infection and the pathogenesis of nasopharyngeal carcinoma: viral gene expression, tumour cell phenotype, and the role of the lymphoid stroma. Semin Cancer Biol 7: 165–174.
9. Altmann M, Pich D, Ruiss R, Wang J, Sugden B, et al. (2006) Transcriptional activation by EBV nuclear antigen 1 is essential for the expression of EBV's transforming genes. Proc Natl Acad Sci U S A 103: 14188–14193.
10. Leight ER, Sugden B (2000) EBNA-1: a protein pivotal to latent infection by Epstein-Barr virus. Rev Med Virol 10: 83–100.
11. Lindner SE, Sugden B (2007) The plasmid replicon of Epstein-Barr virus: mechanistic insights into efficient, licensed, extrachromosomal replication in human cells. Plasmid 58: 1–12.
12. Li JH, Chia M, Shi W, Ngo D, Strathdee CA, et al. (2002) Tumor-targeted gene therapy for nasopharyngeal carcinoma. Cancer Res 62: 171–178.
13. Wu J, Xiao X, Zhao P, Xue G, Zhu Y, et al. (2006) Minicircle-IFNgamma induces antiproliferative and antitumoral effects in human nasopharyngeal carcinoma. Clin Cancer Res 12: 4702–4713.
14. Wu J, Xiao X, Jia H, Chen J, Zhu Y, et al. (2009) Dynamic distribution and expression in vivo of the human interferon gamma gene delivered by adenoviral vector. BMC Cancer 9: 55.
15. Sher YP, Tzeng TF, Kan SF, Hsu J, Xie X, et al. (2009) Cancer targeted gene therapy of BikDD inhibits orthotopic lung cancer growth and improves long-term survival. Oncogene 28: 3286–3295.
16. Chen ZY, He CY, Ehrhardt A, Kay MA (2003) Minicircle DNA vectors devoid of bacterial DNA result in persistent and high-level transgene expression in vivo. Mol Ther 8: 495–500.
17. Judde JG, Spangler G, Magrath I, Bhatia K (1996) Use of Epstein-Barr virus nuclear antigen-1 in targeted therapy of EBV-associated neoplasia. Hum Gene Ther 7: 647–653.
18. Li JH, Shi W, Chia M, Sanchez-Sweatman O, Siatskas C, et al. (2003) Efficacy of targeted FasL in nasopharyngeal carcinoma. Mol Ther 8: 964–973.
19. Chia MC, Shi W, Li JH, Sanchez O, Strathdee CA, et al. (2004) A conditionally replicating adenovirus for nasopharyngeal carcinoma gene therapy. Mol Ther 9: 804–817.
20. Yip KW, Li A, Li JH, Shi W, Chia MC, et al. (2004) Potential utility of BimS as a novel apoptotic therapeutic molecule. Mol Ther 10: 533–544.
21. Marshall E (1999) Gene therapy death prompts review of adenovirus vector. Science 286: 2244–2245.
22. Jechlinger W (2006) Optimization and delivery of plasmid DNA for vaccination. Expert Rev Vaccines 5: 803–825.
23. Chen ZY, He CY, Meuse L, Kay MA (2004) Silencing of episomal transgene expression by plasmid bacterial DNA elements in vivo. Gene Ther 11: 856–864.
24. Chen ZY, He CY, Kay MA (2005) Improved production and purification of minicircle DNA vector free of plasmid bacterial sequences and capable of persistent transgene expression in vivo. Hum Gene Ther 16: 126–131.
25. Chang CW, Christensen LV, Lee M, Kim SW (2008) Efficient expression of vascular endothelial growth factor using minicircle DNA for angiogenic gene therapy. J Control Release 125: 155–163.
26. Zhang X, Epperly MW, Kay MA, Chen ZY, Dixon T, et al. (2008) Radioprotection in vitro and in vivo by minicircle plasmid carrying the human manganese superoxide dismutase transgene. Hum Gene Ther 19: 820–826.
27. Huang M, Chen Z, Hu S, Jia F, Li Z, et al. (2009) Novel minicircle vector for gene therapy in murine myocardial infarction. Circulation 120: S230–237.
28. Jia F, Wilson KD, Sun N, Gupta DM, Huang M, et al. (2010) A nonviral minicircle vector for deriving human iPS cells. Nat Methods 7: 197–199.
29. Chen ZY, Riu E, He CY, Xu H, Kay MA (2008) Silencing of episomal transgene expression in liver by plasmid bacterial backbone DNA is independent of CpG methylation. Mol Ther 16: 548–556.
30. Zhang C, Gao S, Jiang W, Lin S, Du F, et al. (2010) Targeted minicircle DNA delivery using folate-poly(ethylene glycol)-polyethylenimine as non-viral carrier. Biomaterials 31: 6075–6086.
31. Hu S, Huang M, Li Z, Jia F, Ghosh Z, et al. (2010) MicroRNA-210 as a novel therapy for treatment of ischemic heart disease. Circulation 122: S124–131.
32. Hoffman RM (1999) Orthotopic metastatic mouse models for anticancer drug discovery and evaluation: a bridge to the clinic. Invest New Drugs 17: 343–359.
33. Liu T, Ding Y, Xie W, Li Z, Bai X, et al. (2007) An imageable metastatic treatment model of nasopharyngeal carcinoma. Clin Cancer Res 13: 3960–3967.
34. Teng ZP, Ooka T, Huang DP, Zeng Y (1996) Detection of Epstein-Barr Virus DNA in well and poorly differentiated nasopharyngeal carcinoma cell lines. Virus Genes 13: 53–60.
35. Cheung ST, Huang DP, Hui AB, Lo KW, Ko CW, et al. (1999) Nasopharyngeal carcinoma cell line (C666-1) consistently harbouring Epstein-Barr virus. Int J Cancer 83: 121–126.
36. Friboulet L, Pioche-Durieu C, Rodriguez S, Valent A, Souquere S, et al. (2008) Recurrent overexpression of c-IAP2 in EBV-associated nasopharyngeal carcinomas: critical role in resistance to Toll-like receptor 3-mediated apoptosis. Neoplasia 10: 1183–1194.
37. Yin Q, Flemington EK (2006) siRNAs against the Epstein Barr virus latency replication factor, EBNA1, inhibit its function and growth of EBV-dependent tumor cells. Virology 346: 385–393.
38. Sivachandran N, Sarkari F, Frappier L (2008) Epstein-Barr nuclear antigen 1 contributes to nasopharyngeal carcinoma through disruption of PML nuclear bodies. PLoS Pathog 4: e1000170.
39. Fecker LF, Geilen CC, Tchernev G, Trefzer U, Assaf C, et al. (2006) Loss of proapoptotic Bcl-2-related multidomain proteins in primary melanomas is associated with poor prognosis. J Invest Dermatol 126: 1366–1371.

40. Zhu Y, Singh B, Hewitt S, Liu A, Gomez B, et al. (2006) Expression patterns among interferon regulatory factor-1, human X-box binding protein-1, nuclear factor kappa B, nucleophosmin, estrogen receptor-alpha and progesterone receptor proteins in breast cancer tissue microarrays. Int J Oncol 28: 67–76.
41. Wang Y, Liu DP, Chen PP, Koeffler HP, Tong XJ, et al. (2007) Involvement of IFN regulatory factor (IRF)-1 and IRF-2 in the formation and progression of human esophageal cancers. Cancer Res 67: 2535–2543.
42. Fauvet R, Poncelet C, Hugol D, Lavaur A, Feldmann G, et al. (2003) Expression of apoptosis-related proteins in endometriomas and benign and malignant ovarian tumours. Virchows Arch 443: 38–43.
43. Chen X, Larson CS, West J, Zhang X, Kaufman DB (2010) In vivo detection of extrapancreatic insulin gene expression in diabetic mice by bioluminescence imaging. PLoS One 5: e9397.

Establishment of an AAV Reverse Infection-Based Array

Xiaoyan Dong[1,2], Wenhong Tian[3], Gang Wang[3], Zheyue Dong[2], Wei Shen[2], Gang Zheng[2], Xiaobing Wu[3], Jinglun Xue[1], Yue Wang[3]*, Jinzhong Chen[1]*

1 State Key Laboratory of Genetic Engineering, Institute of Genetics, School of Life Science, Fudan University, Shanghai, China, **2** Beijing FivePlus Molecular Medicine Institute, Beijing, China, **3** State Key Laboratory for Molecular Virology and Genetic Engineering, National Institute for Viral Disease Control and Prevention, Chinese Center for Disease Control and Prevention, Beijing, China

Abstract

Background: The development of a convenient high-throughput gene transduction approach is critical for biological screening. Adeno-associated virus (AAV) vectors are broadly used in gene therapy studies, yet their applications in *in vitro* high-throughput gene transduction are limited.

Principal Findings: We established an AAV reverse infection (RI)-based method in which cells were transduced by quantified recombinant AAVs (rAAVs) pre-coated onto 96-well plates. The number of pre-coated rAAV particles and number of cells loaded per well, as well as the temperature stability of the rAAVs on the plates, were evaluated. As the first application of this method, six serotypes or hybrid serotypes of rAAVs (AAV1, AAV2, AAV5/5, AAV8, AAV25 m, AAV28 m) were compared for their transduction efficiencies using various cell lines, including BHK21, HEK293, BEAS-2BS, HeLaS3, Huh7, Hepa1-6, and A549. AAV2 and AAV1 displayed high transduction efficiency; thus, they were deemed to be suitable candidate vectors for the RI-based array. We next evaluated the impact of sodium butyrate (NaB) treatment on rAAV vector-mediated reporter gene expression and found it was significantly enhanced, suggesting that our system reflected the biological response of target cells to specific treatments.

Conclusions/Significance: Our study provides a novel method for establishing a highly efficient gene transduction array that may be developed into a platform for cell biological assays.

Editor: Robert E. Means, Yale Medical School, United States of America

Funding: This study was supported by the Research Programs of State Key Laboratory for Molecular Virology and Genetic Engineering of China (No. 2008-s-0008), and Beijing FivePlus Molecular Medicine Institute. The funders had no role in study design, data collection and analysis, decision to publish, or preparation of the manuscript.

Competing Interests: The authors have declared that no competing interests exist.

* E-mail: euy-tokyo@umin.ac.jp (YW); kingbellchen@fudan.edu.cn (JC)

These authors contributed equally to this work.

Introduction

High-throughput gene transduction methods are needed for gene function studies and drug discovery. Recently, reverse transfection or reverse infection (RI) approaches have been established by several groups [1,2,3], which appear to be promising for the large-scale analysis of gene function. Different from conventional transfection or infection of living cells using DNA (or RNA) or a viral vector, reverse transfection or infection requires immobilization of the DNA (RNA) or viral vector on a solid support. Transduction is achieved by adding cells to the immobilized DNA or vector, which can save time and labor and reduce readout variation. Although encouraging, improvements are needed before these methods are widely applied. In reverse transfection approaches, the transfection conditions may need to be modified when different cell lines are used. For RI, only a lentiviral vector has been tested [3], which may not be the best choice considering its stability. In this report, we describe an RI protocol based on another frequently used viral vector, an adeno-associated virus (AAV).

AAV is a 20-nm replication-defective virus that infects humans and other primates, yet does not cause any known disease [4]. Vectors derived from AAV are attractive for gene therapy because they transduce both dividing and non-dividing cells and have the ability to mediate long-term transgene expression *in vivo* [5]. To date, at least 11 serotypes (AAV1-11) have been described [6]. Among them, AAV1, AAV2, AAV5, and AAV8 are used more frequently than others in gene therapy studies because of their unique *in vivo* transduction profiles. AAV1 has the highest transduction efficiency in muscle [7], AAV2 has a broad tissue tropism, including muscle, liver, and the retina [8], AAV5 has the highest transduction efficiency in respiratory ducts [9], and AAV8 shows strong liver tropism [10]. AAVs with mosaic capsids represent one strategy for creating new tropisms [11]. These AAV serotypes or variants also display different transduction profiles *in vitro*.

As a non-enveloped icosahedron particle, AAV has distinct characteristics, including considerable resistance to heat, organic solvents, and pH extremes [12]. Moreover, AAV infection causes little cellular toxicity, which is a common consequence of other vectors [13]. It is these advantages that prompted us to attempt to expand the *in vitro* applications of AAVs.

In this study, we established an AAV array in which quantified recombinant AAVs (rAAVs) were coated on the wells of 96-well plates. The medium was then allowed to evaporate, and the coated plates were stored until use. Cells were then added to the prepared plates to achieve gene transduction. Our study provides a convenient high-throughput approach to gene transduction for biological research.

Results

The AAV plasmid, genomic structure of the helper virus used for rAAV packaging, and electron microscopic assessment.

AAV vectors harboring reporter genes were constructed by inserting the genes encoding *Gaussia* luciferase (Gluc) or enhanced green fluorescent protein (EGFP) between the cytomegalovirus (CMV) promoter and bovine growth hormone polyA (BGH polyA) in pAAV2neo (Fig. 1A) or pAAV5neo [14]. rAAVs were produced by infecting the AAV vector cell lines with recombinant herpes simplex virus carrying the AAV rep and cap genes (Fig. 1B); purification was achieved as described previously [15]. The purified rAAV particles were somewhat round (20–24 nm in diameter; Fig. 1C). The viral titers of the rAAVs were measured by dot blotting, as described in the Materials and Methods, and diluted to equal titers for coating the plates.

Optimization of rAAV RI

To determine the optimal amount of rAAV per well, 5×10^4, 5×10^5, 5×10^6, 5×10^7, and 5×10^8 viral genomes of rAAV2-Gluc were applied to each well. After drying, 4×10^4 BHK21 cells were applied to each well. Then, 24 h later, Gluc activity was measured. As shown in Figure 2A, Gluc activity was positively correlated with viral load; as the viral load increased, more Gluc activity was observed. Considering the different infectivity of AAV for different cells, we chose to coat each well with 5×10^8 viral genomes in each of the remaining experiments.

To determine the optimal number of cells per well, various numbers of BHK21 cells were applied to the wells coated with the same quantity of viral genomes. Then, 48 h later, EGFP fluorescence was assayed using an EnVision Multilabel Plate Reader (Perkin Elmer, Waltham, MA). As shown in Figure 2B, with the exception of AAV8, the highest level of EGFP intensity was achieved by adding either 2.5×10^4 or 1.25×10^4 cells per well; thus, 20,000–40,000 was taken as the optimal virus/cell ratio to obtain the highest transduction efficiency. Because the highest level of expression for most AAV serotypes was seen in the wells with 2.5×10^4 cells, we used this cell density in all subsequent experiments.

To assess the temperature stability of the rAAV2-coated plates, we placed the 96-well plates in incubators set at 37, 42, and 56°C for 24 h before application of the BHK21 cells. A plate stored at 4°C was used as a control. As shown in Figure 2C, no difference in Gluc activity was observed between the control plate stored at 4°C and the plate incubated at 37°C. The level of Gluc activity in the plates incubated at 42 and 56°C showed a 31–33% decrease. However, the total level of Gluc activity was still high, suggesting that the coated rAAVs were resistant to temperatures as high as 56°C for at least 24 h. Taken together, these data demonstrate that rAAV-coated 96-well plates can be used for RI, and that the rAAVs had not lost any infectivity when stored at 37°C for at least 24 h.

Transduction efficiency of the rAAVs in different cell lines

It has been reported that different rAAV serotypes displayed different transduction efficiencies; thus, we next evaluated the transduction efficiency of the rAAVs rAAV1, rAAV2, rAAV5/5, and rAAV8 using multiple cell lines and the above protocol. Hybrid vectors between AAV2 and 5 (designated rAAV25 m), and AAV2 and AAV8 (designated rAAV28 m) were also included in the test. The cell lines were then applied to each viral line, as shown in Figure 3A. rAAV5/5, rAAV8, rAAV25 m, and rAAV28 m showed low transduction efficiency in these cell lines; conversely, rAAV1 and, especially, rAAV2 showed high transduction efficiency in many cell lines, as assessed by fluorescence microscopy (Fig. 3B). rAAV2 was able to infect HEK293, BHK21, BEAS-2BS, and Huh7 cells with high efficiency, whereas rAAV1 was able to infect HEK293,

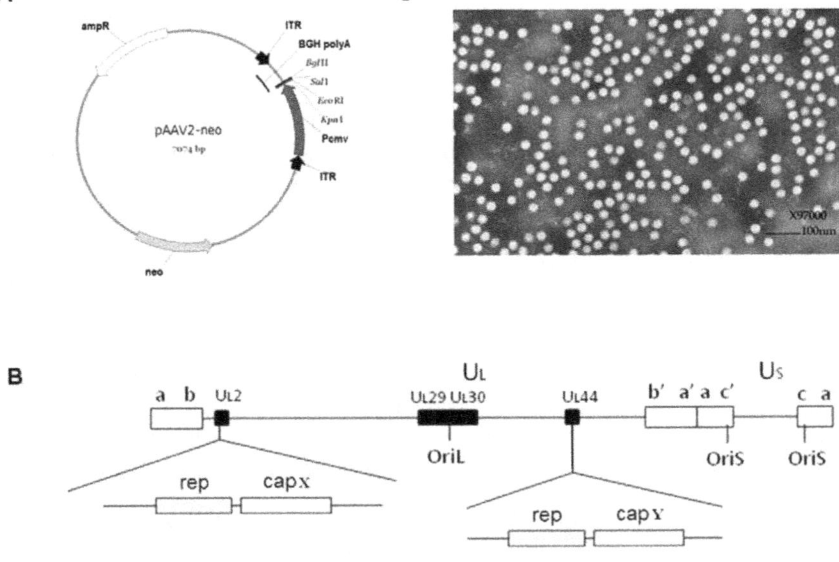

Figure 1. The AAV plasmid, genomic structure of the helper virus used for rAAV packaging, and electron microscopic assessment. A. Map of the AAV plasmid, showing the reporter gene; Gluc or EGFP was inserted between the CMV promoter and polyA region. B. Helper viruses used for packaging of the rAAV with different capsids. UL2 and UL44 were both used for repcap insertion. capX and capY represent capsid genes from the different AAV serotypes. C. Electron microscopic image of rAAV2-Gluc.

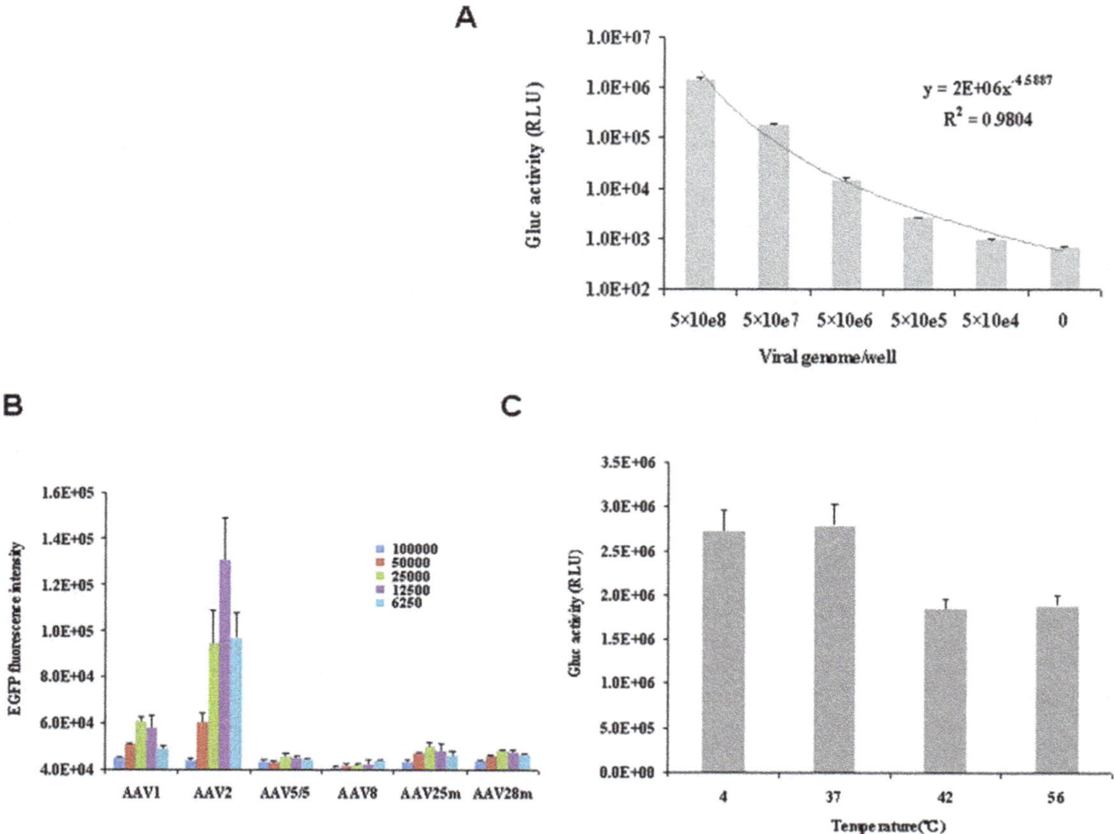

Figure 2. Optimization of rAAV RI. A. Transduction efficiency of different quantities of rAAV2-Gluc using 4×10^4 BHK21 cells; the transduction efficiency is represented by Gluc activity. B. Optimization of the virus/cell ratio. Different numbers of BHK21 cells were applied to a 96-well plate pre-coated with 5×10^8 viral genomes/well. The transduction efficiency is represented by the EGFP intensity. C. Temperature stability assessment of rAAV2-Gluc. In total, 5×10^8 viral genomes of rAAV were applied to each well. The plates were then treated at 4, 37, 42, or 56°C for 24 h, followed by the application of 4×10^4 BHK21 cells per well. Gluc activity was measured 24 h later.

BHK21, BEAS-2BS, HelaS3, and Huh7 cells with considerable efficiency (Fig. 3B). Among these cell lines, BHK21 was the most susceptible to the rAAVs (Fig. 3B). To quantify our fluorescence microscopic observations, the level of EGFP intensity in each plate was measured using an EnVision Multilabel Plate Reader (Perkin Elmer). As shown in Figure 3C, the data were consistent with those produced by fluorescence microscopy. In conclusion, we found that rAAV2 and rAAV1 were suitable for RI as part of a high-throughput array strategy.

Response to treatment with sodium butyrate (NaB)

We next evaluated the responses of the rAAV-transduced cell lines to NaB, which was used as an interfering factor. NaB is known to enhance gene expression [16]. Cells were applied to wells coated with rAAV1 or rAAV2 in the presence or absence of 10 mM NaB. Then, 24 h later, Gluc activity in the supernatant was measured. Gluc activity in the cells transduced by rAAV1 (Fig. 4A) or rAAV2 (Fig. 4B) was increased significantly, especially for HEK293 and BHK21. Of rAAV2, Gluc activity in BHK21 increased from 3×10^5 to 1.6×10^6 relative light units (RLU; Fig. 4B). Of rAAV1, Gluc activity in the BHK21 cells increased, from 1.5×10^5 to 4×10^5 RLU (Fig. 4A). In conclusion, our data show that our system can be used to monitor the response to a modulating factor with substantial sensitivity.

Discussion

Current *in vitro* gene transfer approaches, based on liposomes and cationic polymers, are both efficient and convenient. However, they sometimes show relatively low reproducibility due to various factors in the transfection procedure. To reduce readout variation, the order of addition of DNA and adherent cells has been reversed relative to conventional transfection methods (i.e., the DNA is printed on a glass slide before addition of the adherent cells). The advantages of reverse transfection [17] procedures, compared with conventional transfection methods, include reduced labor, the use of fewer materials, and the ability to perform high-throughput screening. However, the efficiency of reverse transfection varies depending on the cell type being used, and this, in turn, limits its use in high-throughput screening. The retroviral microarray-based platform created by Carbone et al. [3] showed an enabling tool for functional genomics and drug discovery. In the present study, we developed a novel gene transduction approach by pre-coating rAAVs on a cell culture plate and allowing them to dry until use. Our data show that the rAAVs were resistant to temperature changes. Furthermore, rAAVs coated on plates have been stored at 4°C for more than half a year without an apparent loss of infectivity (data not shown).

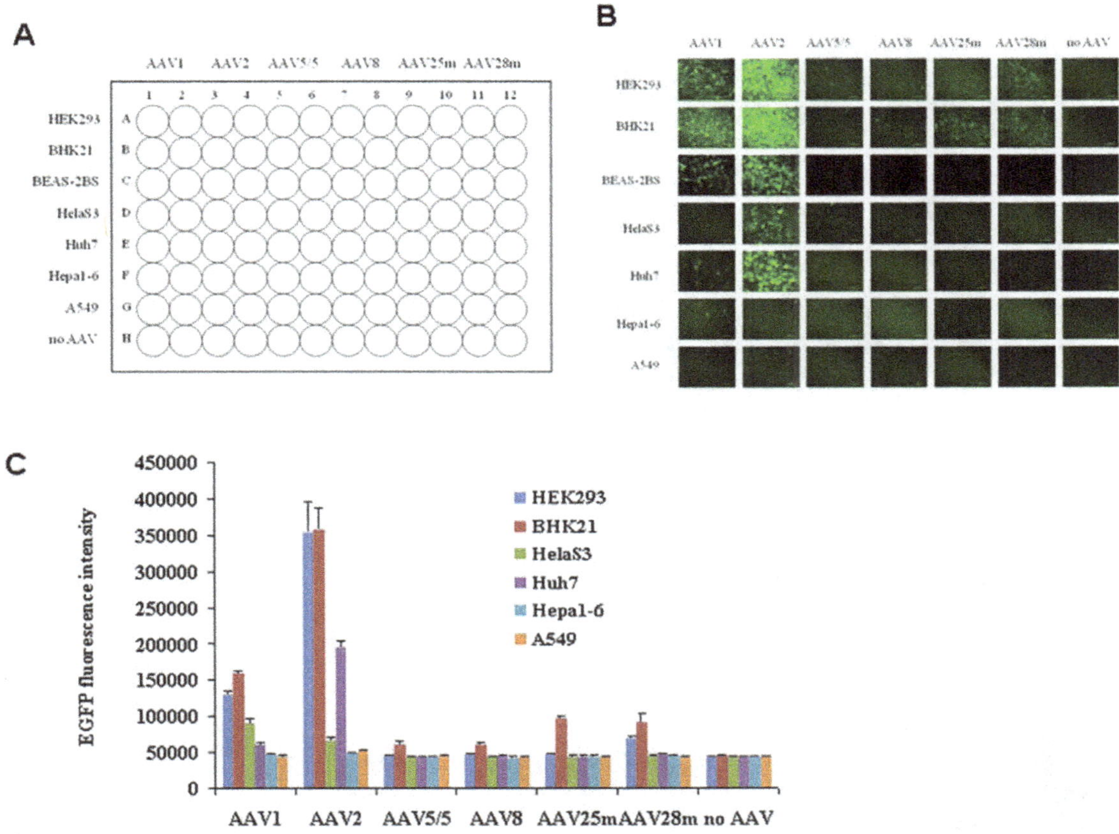

Figure 3. Description of the rAAV RI-based array plate. A. Schematic view of the AAV-based RI array plate. Six types of rAAVs were applied to 96-well plates in two columns, allowing seven types of cells (and a control) to be applied simultaneously to the assay plate. B. Fluorescence microscopic assessment of the infectivity of the rAAVs. C. EGFP intensity summary of Figure 2B.

AAV vectors have been broadly used in gene therapy studies, yet their application to *in vitro* high-throughput transduction is limited. In the present study, the transduction efficiency of different rAAV serotypes or variants was evaluated in HEK293, BHK21, BEAS-2BS, HelaS3, Huh7, Hepa1-6, and A549 cells. Among the AAV vectors tested, rAAV1 and rAAV2 displayed the most promising results when used for RI.

To our knowledge, this is the first report describing the RI of AAV vectors. The data in the present study suggest that our AAV RI method can be used to create "infection-ready" AAV arrays for high-throughput biological assays. This type of array can be used to test the response of cells to certain interfering factors, as exemplified in this study. RNAi screening can also be achieved if an AAV-based shRNA library is applied to the array. Additionally, microRNA profiles of cell lines can be established if microRNA target sequences linked with reporter genes are applied; this may become an alternative and supplemental tool for microarray analysis.

Materials and Methods

Cell culture

BHK21, HEK293, BEAS-2BS, HeLaS3, Huh7, Hepa1-6, and A549 cells were maintained as monolayer cultures in Dulbecco's Modified Eagle's Medium (DMEM) containing 10% fetal calf serum, 100 μg/mL penicillin, and 100 U/mL streptomycin, as recommended by the manufacturer (GIBCO, Gaithersburg, MD).

Plasmid construction

pAAV2neo was constructed by inserting a fragment containing two inverted terminal repeats (ITRs) from AAV2, the CMV promoter, multi-cloning sites, and BGH polyA into pSV2neo [18]. pAAV2neo-Gluc and pAAV2neo-EGFP were constructed by inserting the genes encoding Gluc and EGFP between the CMV promoter and BGH polyA. pAAV5neo has a similar structure to pAAV2neo, except that it carries ITRs from AAV5 rather than from AAV2. pAAV5neo-EGFP was constructed by inserting EGFP between the CMV promoter and BGH polyA in pAAV5neo.

rAAV vector cell lines

rAAV vector cell lines were obtained by transfecting pAAV2-neo-Gluc, pAAV2neo-EGFP, or pAAV5neo-EGFP [14] into BHK21 cells, which were then cultured in the presence of 800 μg/mL G418 for 2 weeks.

Preparation of competent helper virus

Recombinant herpes simplex virus type 1 carrying the AAV rep and cap genes (HSV1-RC) was used to provide helper functions for AAV vector packaging. rHSV1-UL2/rep2cap1, rHSV1-UL2/rep2-cap2, and rHSV1-UL2/rep2cap8 were used to package the rAAV1, rAAV2, and rAAV8 (containing the ITR of serotype 2 and corresponding capsid of serotypes 1, 2, and 8) vectors, respectively; rHSV1-UL2/rep5cap5 was used for rAAV5/5 (containing the ITR of serotype 5 and capsid of serotype 5). rHSV1-UL2/rep2cap2-UL44/rep5cap5 and rHSV1-UL2/rep2cap2-UL44/rep2cap8 were

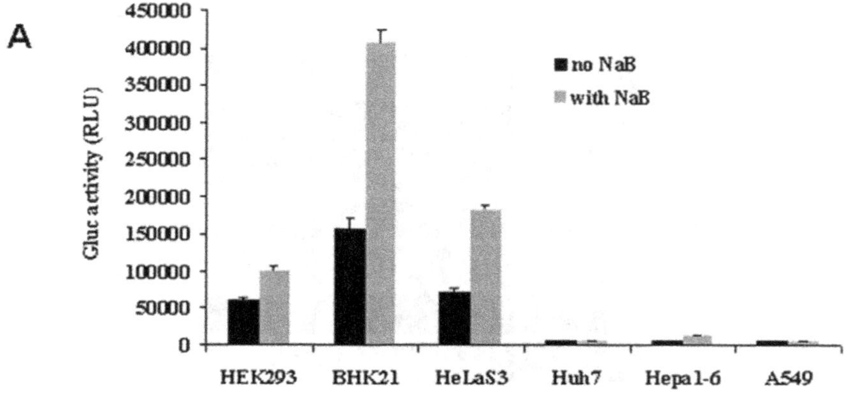

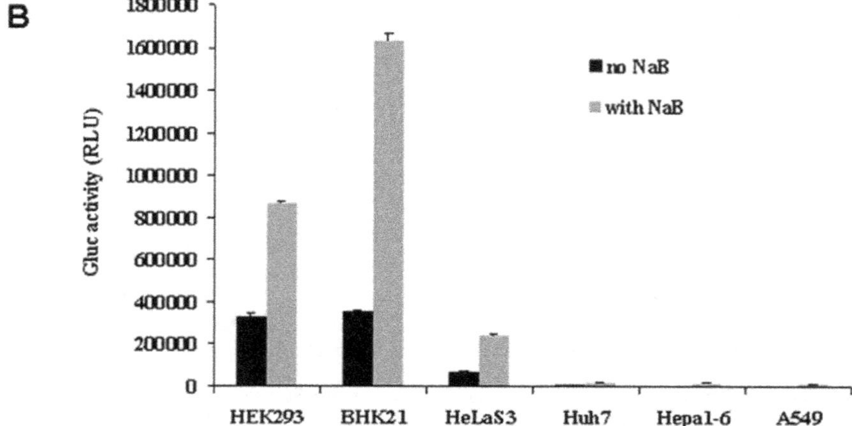

Figure 4. Response to NaB. Black bar, without NaB; gray bar, with NaB. A. AAV1 RI-based assay. B. AAV2 RI-based assay.

used for rAAV25 m (containing the ITR of serotype 2 and mosaic capsid of serotypes 2 and 5) and rAAV28 m (containing the ITR of serotype 2 and mosaic capsid of serotypes 2 and 8), respectively.

rAAV production

rAAVs were produced by infecting the AAV vector cell lines with HSV1-RC at an MOI of 1–5. After 48–72 h, the infected cells were harvested and purified, as described previously [15,19]. The rAAV titer was determined by dot blotting using a digoxin-labeled CMV promoter fragment as the probe.

Transmission electron microscopy

Purified rAAVs were observed by transmission electron microscopy (TECNAI 12, FEI, Blackwood, NJ) with an acceleration voltage of 80 kV, as reported by Chen et al. [20].

Preparation of the rAAV-coated plates

To prepare rAAV-coated plates, 20 μL/well of rAAVs with defined titers were added to a 96-well plate and placed under airflow overnight in a tissue culture hood to evaporate all liquid. The plate was stored at 4°C until use.

RI protocol

Cells were digested with 0.25% trypsin (Invitrogen, Carlsbad, CA) to create a single-cell suspension. An equal volume of the suspension (200 μL/well) was applied to the rAAV-coated plates and cultured at 37°C in an incubator under 5% CO_2 for 24–48 h.

Gluc activity assay

The Gluc activity level was measured as described in the *Gaussia* luciferase assay kit (New England Biolabs, Ipswich, MA) by adding 50 μL of substrate solution to 20 μL of the supernatant or cell lysate, followed by determination of the RLU using a luminometer.

Analysis of EGFP expression

EGFP expression was assayed by fluorescence microscopy (Olympus DP70, BH2-RFL-T3). The EGFP intensities in the 96-well plates were measured using an EnVision Multilabel Plate Reader (Perkin Elmer).

Acknowledgments

We thank Dr. Zhijian Wu (Ocular Gene Therapy Laboratory, Neurobiology-Neurodegeneration and Repair Laboratory, National Eye Institute, National Institutes of Health, Bethesda, Maryland 20892, USA) for helpful discussions and manuscript edition.

Author Contributions

Conceived and designed the experiments: XD XW. Performed the experiments: XD WT GW ZD WS GZ XW. Analyzed the data: XD WT XW YW JC. Contributed reagents/materials/analysis tools: XD XW JX JC. Wrote the paper: XW YW.

References

1. Webb BL, Díaz B, Martin GS, Lai F (2003) A reporter system for reverse transfection cell arrays. J Biomol Screen 8: 620–623.
2. Okazaki A, Jo J, Tabata Y (2007) A reverse transfection technology to genetically engineer adult stem cells. Tissue Eng 13: 245–251.
3. Carbone R, Giorgetti L, Zanardi A, Marangi I, Chierici E, et al. (2007) Retroviral microarray-based platform on nanostructured TiO2 for functional genomics and drug discovery. Biomaterials 28: 2244–2253.
4. Knipe DM, Howley PM (2007) Fields Virology. Lippincott Williams & Wilkins Immunology. pp 2438–2477.
5. Bartlett JS, Samulski RJ (1995) Genetics and biology of adeno-associated virus. In: Kaplitt MG, Loewy AD, eds. Viral Vectors: Gene therapy and neuroscience applications. San Diego: Academic Press. pp 55–73.
6. Choi VW, McCarty DM, Samulski RJ (2005) AAV hybrid serotypes: improved vectors for gene delivery. Curr Gene Ther 5: 299–310.
7. Rivière C, Danos O, Douar AM (2006) Long-term expression and repeated administration of AAV type 1, 2 and 5 vectors in skeletal muscle of immunocompetent adult mice. Gene Ther 13: 1300–1308.
8. Hueffer K, Parrish CR (2003) Parvovirus host range, cell tropism and evolution. Curr Opin Microbiol 6: 392–398.
9. Zabner J, Seiler M, Walters R, Kotin RM, Fulgeras W, et al. (2000) Adeno-associated virus type 5 (AAV5) but AAV2 binds to the apical surfaces of airway epithelia and facilitates gene transfer. J Virol 74: 3852–3858.
10. Pañeda A, Vanrell L, Mauleon I, Crettaz JS, Berraondo P, et al. (2009) Effect of adeno-associated virus serotype and genomic structure on liver transduction and biodistribution in mice of both genders. Hum Gene Ther 20: 908–917.
11. Rabinowiz JE, Bowles DE, Faust SM, Ledford JG, Cunningham SE, et al. (2004) Cross-dressing the virion: the transcapsidstion of adneo-associated virus serotypes functionally defines subgroups. J Virol 78: 4421–4432.
12. Hoggan MD, Blacklow NR, Rowe WP (1966) Studies of small DNA viruses found in various adenovirus preparations: physical, biological and immunological characteristics. Proc Natl Acad Sci USA 55: 1467–1474.
13. Samulski RJ, Sally M, Muzyczka N (1999) Adeno-associated viral vectors. In: Friedmann T, ed. Development of human gene therapy. Cold Spring Harbor: Cold Spring Harbor Laboratory Press. pp 131–172.
14. Dong X, Tian W, Yuan Z, Tan S, Wu X (2010) A novel packaging system of recombinant AAV5/5 vector. Chin J Biotech 26: 679–686.
15. Wu X, Dong X, Wu Z, Cao H, Niu D, et al. (2001) A novel method for purification of recombinant adeno-associated virus vectors on a large scale. Chin Sci Bull 46: 485–489.
16. Chen W, Bailey E, McCune S, Dong J, Townes T (1997) Reactivation of silenced, virally transduced genes by inhibitors of histone deacetylase. Proc Natl Acad Sci USA 94: 5798–5803.
17. Erfle H, Neumann B, Liebel U, Rogers P, Held M, et al. (2007) Reverse transfection on cell arrays for high cotent screening microscopy. Nat Protoc 2: 392–399.
18. Southern P, Berg P (1982) Transformation of mammalian cells to antibiotic resistance with a bacterial gene under control of the SV40 early region promoter. J Mol Appl Genet 1: 327–341.
19. Wu ZJ, Wu XB, Hou YD (1999) Construction of a recombinant herpes simplex virus which can provide packaging function for recombinant adeno-associated virus. Chin Sci Bull 44: 715–719.
20. Chen H (2007) Comparative observation of the recombinant adeno-associated virus 2 using transmission electron microscopy and atomic force microscopy. Microsc Microanal 13: 384–389.

15

Treatment of Mouse Limb Ischemia with an Integrative Hypoxia-Responsive Vector Expressing the Vascular Endothelial Growth Factor Gene

Eduardo Gallatti Yasumura, Roberta Sessa Stilhano, Vívian Yochiko Samoto, Priscila Keiko Matsumoto, Leonardo Pinto de Carvalho, Valderez Bastos Valero Lapchik, Sang Won Han*

Research Center for Gene Therapy, Department of Biophysics, Universidade Federal de São Paulo, São Paulo, São Paulo, Brazil

Abstract

Constitutive vascular endothelial growth factor (VEGF) gene expression systems have been extensively used to treat peripheral arterial diseases, but most of the results have not been satisfactory. In this study, we designed a plasmid vector with a hypoxia-responsive element sequence incorporated into it with the phiC31 integrative system (pVHAVI) to allow long-term VEGF gene expression and to be activated under hypoxia. Repeated activations of VEGF gene expression under hypoxia were confirmed in HEK293 and C2C12 cells transfected with pVHAVI. In limb ischemic mice, the local administration of pVHAVI promoted gastrocnemius mass and force recovery and ameliorated limb necrosis much better than the group treated with hypoxia-insensitive vector, even this last group had produced more VEGF in muscle. Histological analyses carried out after four weeks of gene therapy showed increased capillary density and matured vessels, and reduced number of necrotic cells and fibrosis in pVHAVI treated group. By our study, we demonstrate that the presence of high concentration of VEGF in ischemic tissue is not beneficial or is less beneficial than maintaining a lower but sufficient and long-term concentration of VEGF locally.

Editor: Holger K. Eltzschig, University of Colorado Denver, United States of America

Funding: This work was supported by Fundação de Amparo à Pesquisa do Estado de São Paulo (FAPESP) 2006/59630-0 and 2011/00859-6. EGY was a recipient of FAPESP scholarship 08/52381-0. The funders had no role in study design, data collection and analysis, decision to publish, or preparation of the manuscript.

Competing Interests: The authors have declared that no competing interests exist.

* E-mail: sang.han@unifesp.br

Introduction

Peripheral arterial disease (PAD) is characterized by arterial narrowing that reduces oxygen supply to the extremities resulting in severe pain, non-healing ulcers and possible loss of the affected limb. The incidence of PAD is high at about 1000 affected per million individuals, and this incidence increases in individuals over 70 years of age and in diabetics [1]. According to the Transatlantic Inter-Society Consensus, approximately 25% of patients with advanced PAD will suffer amputation because conventional medical and revascularization treatments are not feasible. The prognosis for these patients is bad; after one year, about 25% of them will die, and 20% will still have PAD [1]. Therefore, it is necessary to continue the search for new therapies.

The main cause of PAD is atherosclerosis, which leads to narrowing and malfunctioning of arteries, *i.e.*, ischemia. Consequently, current therapies promote new vessel formation by administering growth factors, which can be provided in protein or gene form or even as cells that produce these factors naturally or after genetic modification [2–4]. Among several growth factors used for angiogenic therapy, vascular endothelial growth factor (VEGF) has been the most extensively studied because it is a potent mitogenic factor that also has anti-apoptotic and vessel dilation activities [5,6]. This factor acts primarily on endothelial cells through the VEGFR1 and VEGFR2 receptors, but it also promotes chemotaxis of smooth muscle cells, monocytes and bone marrow progenitor cells [6–8]. In animal studies, VEGF has been shown to improve perfusion and to increase capillary density in ischemic limbs [9–15]. Many of these studies have advanced to clinical trials, but most of the results have not been satisfactory.

To date, all clinical trials on limb ischemia treatment have used plasmid or adenoviral vectors designed to express transiently and locally [2–4], and muscle has been the favorite target tissue. Transgene expression is transient because the genes are not integrated into the host genome. In clinical trials, these vectors are injected directly into the muscle at high enough doses to express high levels of angiogenic factors due to the characteristics of these vectors. As the angiogenic factor concentration required in loco to induce a therapeutically beneficial amount of angiogenesis is variable depending on the degree of ischemia, angiogenic gene therapy in some tissues can induce hemangioma due to the exaggerated production of growth factors [16,17], and in other tissues, it cannot ameliorate ischemia due to insufficient production of the angiogenic factor. Thus, the ideal vector system should have a mechanism to allow for the long-term production of angiogenic factors according to the local degree of ischemia.

To obtain a vector that is responsive to ischemia and is capable of long-term VEGF expression, we designed an integrative plasmid vector based on the ΦC31 integrase system that contains an HRE (hypoxia-responsive element) sequence. The HRE consensus sequence, isolated from the 3′ end of the erythropoietin (Epo) gene, is present in many genes involved in erythropoiesis, angiogenesis and glycolysis [18] that are activated during hypoxia. Cells and tissues exposed to hypoxia trigger an adaptive response driven by hypoxia induced factor 1 (HIF-1), which binds to the HRE sequence located in the enhancer regions of these genes. It has been demonstrated that vectors constructed with an HRE sequence provide enhanced transgene expression under hypoxic conditions through HIF-1 binding to the HRE [18,19]. In addition, to allow for integration of the vector, the attB sequence from phage ΦC31 was included. The integrase from ΦC31 recognizes plasmids with the attB sequence and inserts them into genomic regions containing pseudo-attP sequences [20], which are present in mammalian genomes. Because the integration process is unidirectional, once the plasmid is inserted into the genome, it is maintained stably [21]. In our study, we found that limb ischemic mice treated with our integrative vector that is responsive to variations in oxygen concentration had a better therapeutic response than mice treated with other delivery vectors.

Materials and Methods

Vector construction

The commercially available pVAX vector (Invitrogen, Carlsbad, EUA) was cut with HincII enzyme, and a cassette containing 9 copies of the HRE sequence (CCGGGTAGCTGGCG-TACGTGCTGCAG) from the AAV-H9-lacZ vector (kindly provided by Dr Hua Su, The Cardiovascular Research Institute, University of California, USA [22], which was obtained by digesting with EcoRI and BglII and treating with Klenow polymerase, was ligated to make pVAX-HRE. This vector was digested with NruI and was ligated with the attB sequence from the pTA-attB vector (kindly provided by Dr Michele P. Calos, Genetics department of Stanford University, USA [20]), which was previously digested with BamHI and EcoRV and treated with Klenow polymerase, to make pVAX-HRE-attB. Finally, to insert the human VEGF165 sequence into pVAX-HRE-attB, both it and the uP-VEGF vector [23], which expresses human VEGF165, were digested with HindIII and ApaI and ligated together to make pVAX-HRE-attB-VEGF. The integrase expression vector uP-INT was constructed by inserting the ΦC31 integrase gene into the uP vector. The p-INT vector has a construction similar to uP-INT, but it does not have a CMV promoter; therefore, it does not express integrase (Fig. 1).

Cell culture under normoxia and hypoxia

The human embryonic kidney cell line HEK293T [24] was maintained in DMEM supplemented with 10% fetal bovine serum (DMEM+). For transfection, in a 6-well plate 1×10^5 HEK 293 cells were seeded. Twenty-four hours later, 2.5 µg of the donor plasmid containing $hVEGF_{165}$ and 2.5 µg of pVAX or p-INT or uP-INT plasmids were mixed for transfection by the calcium-phosphate co-precipitation method. After 24 h, the medium was replaced with a fresh one, and at the indicated time, the supernatant was collected to determine VEGF levels by ELISA.

To establish hypoxic condition in vitro, the cells were cultured with DMEM+ containing 100 µM cobalt chloride [25]. To test the toxicity of the cobalt, HEK293 cells were cultured with 0, 200 or 400 µM cobalt chloride, and cell viability was assessed using the Trypan blue method.

The mouse myoblast cell line (C2C12) was also maintained in DMEM+, but for transfection the Amaxa NHDF Nucleofector kit and Nucleofector Amaxa (Lonza, Basel, Switzerland) were used following the provided protocol.

Ischemic hind limb model and muscular transfection

All procedures involving animals were approved by the Research Ethics Committee of the Federal University of São Paulo, Brazil (Approval number: CEP 0729/08). Initially, 10–12 week-old Balb/c male mice were anesthetized with an intraperitoneal injection of ketamine (40 mg/kg) and xylazine (20 mg/kg). Hind limb ischemia was induced surgically as previously described [26,27]. Briefly, the femoral artery was excised from its origin at the external iliac artery branch to its bifurcation into the saphenous and popliteal arteries without damaging the femoralis vein or nerves. Branches including the circumflex artery were also obstructed completely to avoid retrograde flow. Gene therapy was performed by injecting 50 µg of each vector in 100 µl of phosphate-buffered saline (PBS) into the middle of the quadriceps muscle soon after ischemic surgery. After plasmid injection, 3 electric pulses of 80 V/cm and 20 ms in duration were applied using needle electrodes (Electroporator T820; BTX Genetronics, San Diego, USA). After gene therapy, the animals were kept under analgesia with daily peritoneal injections of 5 mg/kg carprofen. In our study, the following groups were included with 7–10 animals per group: normal, ischemic and ischemic treated with vector.

Visual assessment of necrosis

Limb ischemia was visually evaluated 30 days after treatment. The following four grades were used to measure the degree of limb necrosis: grade 0, absence of necrosis; grade 1, necrosis limited to the toes; grade 2, necrosis extending to the dorsum pedis; grade 3, necrosis extending to the crus [26].

Muscle force determination

Isometric gastrocnemius muscle contraction was performed 30 days after treatment based on a previous study [28]. The animals

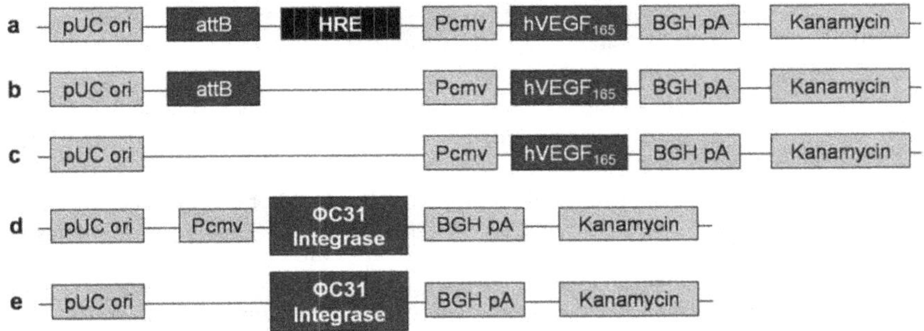

Figure 1. Schematic vector diagrams. (A) pVAX-HRE-attB-hVEGF165; (B) pVAX-attB-hVEGF165; (C) pVAX-hVEGF165; (D) uP-INT; (E) p-INT. pUC ori: replication origin. Pcmv: human cytomegalovirus promoter. BGHpA: polyadenylation signal of the bovine growth hormone. Kanamycin: kanamycin resistance gene.

were anesthetized and maintained at 37°C on a temperature-controlled plate. The leg and knee were fixed on the plate with the gastrocnemius muscle exposed. The Achilles tendon was cut and attached to a wire connected to a force transducer (MLT 1030/D - ADInstruments, Bella Vista NSW, Australia). The lateral gastrocnemius and soleus muscles were removed; the vascular and nerve systems were kept intact. Medial gastrocnemius muscles were left free from the surrounding tissue to minimize effects from the contraction of other muscles. The sciatic nerve was isolated and placed in contact with a bipolar silver electrode for electrostimulation. One stimulus of 5 volts at a frequency of 60 Hz was applied for 10 ms with a 1 minute interval between stimulations. The isometric contractions were measured as the highest force stretching the wire. All collected data were recorded and analyzed using the PowerLab 8/30 system and LabChart Pro software (ADInstruments, Bella Vista NSW, Australia). After force determination, the animals were subjected to euthanasia, and their medial gastrocnemius muscles were then removed for mass measurement and histological analysis.

Determination of $hVEGF_{165}$ by ELISA

Supernatant from cultured cells was collected periodically to determine the concentration of $hVEGF_{165}$ using a DuoSet ELISA kit (R&D Systems Inc., Minneapolis, USA) following the manufacturer's instructions. To determine $hVEGF_{165}$ levels in muscle, the quadriceps muscle was removed after muscle force measurement. The middle part of the gastrocnemius muscle was mechanically homogenized using lysis buffer (25 mM Tris-HCl, pH 7.4, 50 mM NaCl, 0.5% Na-deoxycholate, 2% NP-40, 0.2% sodium dodecyl sulfate, 1 mM phenylmethylsulphonyl fluoride). The homogenized tissue was centrifuged at 4500× g for 10 min at 4°C, and the supernatant was recovered. Total protein and $hVEGF_{165}$ concentrations were determined using the Bio-Rad Protein Assay (BioRad, California, USA) and a DuoSet ELISA Kit, respectively.

Gene expression analysis by quantitative reverse transcription polymerase chain reaction (qRT-PCR)

Total RNA from C2C12 or HEK293 cells was extracted with Trizol reagent (Invitrogen, Carlsbad, CA, USA) and treated with DNAse I (Invitrogen). cDNA was synthetized using High Capacity cDNA Reverse Transcription kit (Invitrogen) and qRT-PCR was conducted using QuantiFast SYBR Green RT-PCR Kit (Qiagen, Hilden, Germany) in the Rotor Gene-Q (Qiagen). The following primers were used to quantify mouse HIF1- α (m HIF1- α), human HIF1- α (h HIF1- α) and human VEGF (hVEGF): mHIF1-α_F (gca gca gga att gga acat t), mHIF1-α_R (gcat gct aaa tcg gag ggta), hHIF1-α_F (caa gaa cct act gct aat gc), hHIF1-α_R (tta tgt atg tgg gta gga gat g), hVEGF_F (ttc tgc tgt ctt ggg tgc att gg), hVEGF_R (gaa gat gtc cac cag ggt ctc g). Relative gene expression was calculated by $2^{-\Delta CT}$. The changes in mRNA expression were expressed as fold-changes relative to control, which was the RNA from C2C12 or HEK293 cells without cobalt and transfection. As normalizer of qRT-PCR, the ribosomal gene hRPS29 was used with primers hRPS29_F (gag cca ccc gcg aaa at) and hRPS29_R (ccg tgc cgg ttt gaa cag) for HEK 293 and the murine β-actin gene with primers mβ-actin_F (gct cct cct gac cgc aag) and mβ-actin_R (cat ctg ctg gaa ggt gga ca) for C2C12. Each reaction was carried out in duplicate and all experiments were carried more than three times. Values were expressed in the mean ± standard error of the mean. One way ANOVA with Bonferronis's multiple comparison was used to statistical analysis.

Vector integration analysis by PCR

Genomic DNA was extracted from quadriceps muscles or from transfected HEK293 cells using the QIAMP DNA Mini Kit (QIAGEN Inc., Valencia, USA). To check for vector integration into the host genome, a PCR reaction was carried out using a pair of primers, CMV reverse 5′-TCATTATTGACGTCAA TGGGC-3′ and attB sense 5′-CTCCACCTCACCCATCT-3′, at a final concentration of 0.5 μM. The PCR reaction was performed by programming a thermocycler to 94°C for 1 min and 35 cycles of 94°C/1 min, 52°C/1.5 min and 72°C/1 min. After the final cycle, the reaction continued for 7 min at 72°C, and the tubes were then maintained at 4°C. As an internal control for the PCR, the glyceraldehyde-3-phosphate dehydrogenase (GAPDH) housekeeping gene was used with GAPDH sense (5′-ACCA-CAGTCCATGCCATCAC-3′) and GAPDH antisense (5′-TCCACCACCCTGTTGCTGTA-3′) primers. The PCR products were analyzed by 1% agarose gel electrophoresis with ethidium bromide staining.

Histological analysis

Muscle samples were fixed in 10% formaldehyde, dehydrated and embedded in paraffin. Four micrometer sections were obtained and stained with hematoxylin-eosin (HE) and picrosirius. The extent of necrosis, muscle regeneration and fibrosis were analyzed from 20 fields and quantified using Image Pro Plus software (Media Cybernetics, Inc., Bethesda, USA). Other sections were collected in poly L-lysine coated slides and submitted for immunohistochemistry with biotinylated Griffonia (bandeiraea) simplicifolia lectin I (1:100) (Vector Laboratories, Peterborough, UK) or anti-alpha smooth muscle actin antibody (1:50) (Vector Laboratories, Peterborough, UK) followed by incubation with streptavidin conjugated peroxidase (Sigma-Aldrich, Saint Louis, USA) and detection with diaminobenzidine chromogen. Vessel and capillary densities were quantified from 20 random fields per slide. The results were expressed as the average number per square millimeter.

Statistical analysis

The results were expressed as mean ± standard error of the mean. Analysis of variance (ANOVA) was performed using a Bonferroni correction for multiple comparisons or a Mann-Whitney test for a comparison of two groups. Visual assessment of necrosis was analyzed by the one way ANOVA with Tukey's multiple comparison tests. Only $P<0.05$ was considered significant.

Results

In vitro evaluation of VEGF gene expression

To assess the functionality of the constructed vectors (Fig. 1), HEK293T cells were transfected with these vectors, and VEGF gene expression was monitored for more than 90 days (Fig. 2). The calcium co-precipitation method was used to transfect HEK293T cells because this method achieves more than 90% transfection efficiency in this cell line (data not shown). To induce hypoxia, $CoCl_2$ was added to the medium at a final concentration of 100 μM, which is a concentration commonly used to mimic hypoxia [24]. HEK293T cells incubated with 100 μM $CoCl_2$ for nine days retained about 90% cell viability (data not shown).

Under normoxia conditions, all groups showed a peak of VEGF gene expression at 48 hours post-transfection, which is a well-known transient gene expression pattern, but by the 14th day, VEGF expression in all groups had returned to basal levels (Fig. 2). Cells transfected with the integrative vectors pVAVI and pVHAVI

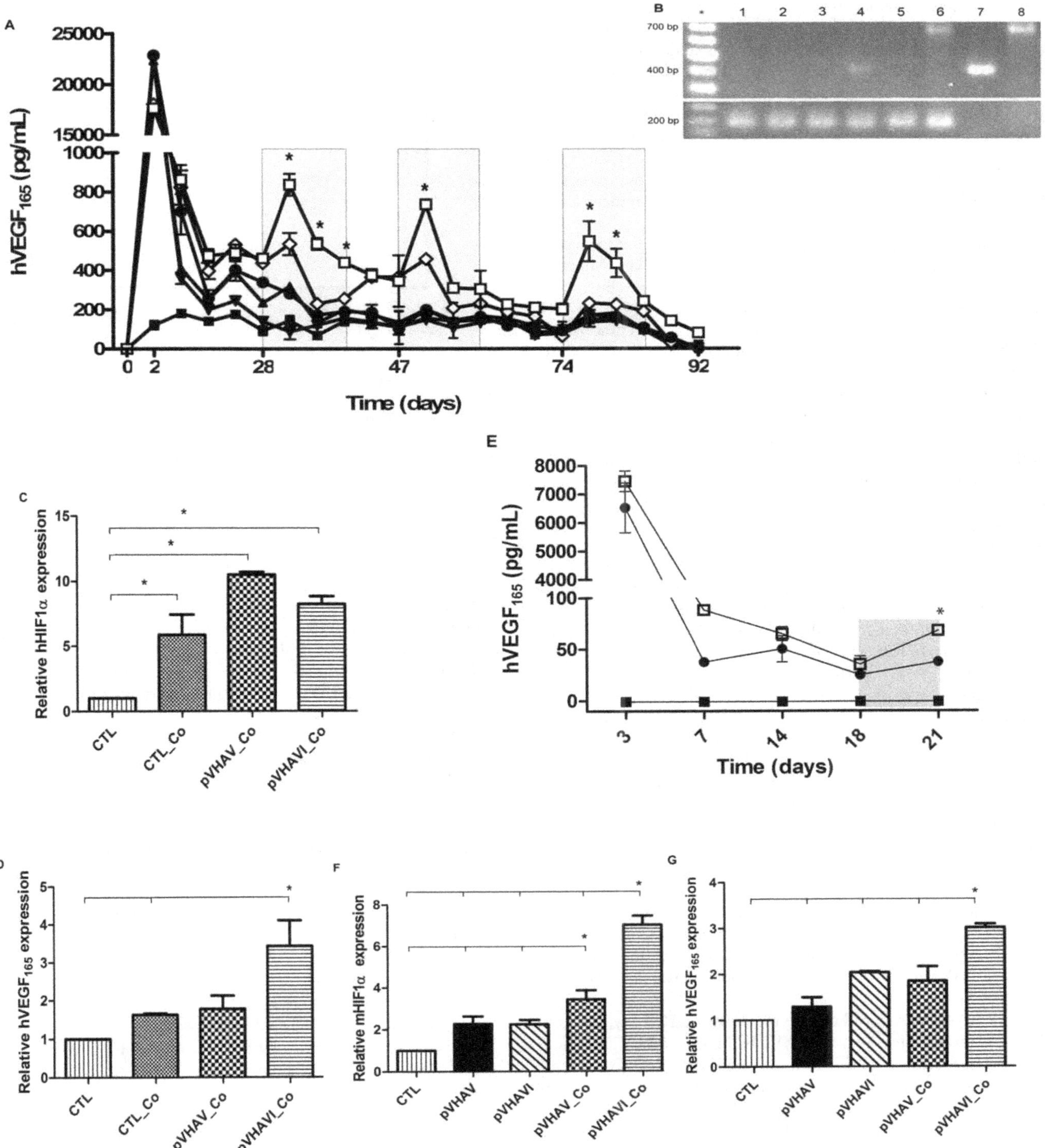

Figure 2. Assessment of VEGF expression vectors. (A) $hVEGF_{165}$ production under hypoxia and normoxia in HEK293 cells. On days 28, 47 and 74, $CoCl_2$ was added to a final concentration of 100 μM, and the medium was replaced every 3 days with fresh medium containing $CoCl_2$ for 9 days (gray bars). -■- no transfection; -▲- pVV; -▼- pVAV; -◇- pVAVI; -●- pVHAV; -□- pVHAVI. * $p<0.001$, pVHAVI in comparison to all groups. (B) Genomic DNA PCR after 4 weeks of transfection. 1: no transfection; 2: pVV; 3: pVAV; 4: pVAVI; 5: pVHAV; 6: pVHAVI; 7: pVAX-attB-$hVEGF_{165}$ (432 bp); 8: pVAX-HRE-attB-$hVEGF_{165}$ (725 bp). The 200 bp band is from GAPDH. * 100 bp ladder. pVV: pVAX-$hVEGF_{165}$ + pVAX; pVAV: pVAX-attB-$hVEGF_{165}$ + p-INT; pVAVI: pVAX-attB-$hVEGF_{165}$ + uP-INT; pVHAV: pVAX-HRE-attB-$hVEGF_{165}$ + p-INT pVHAVI: pVAX-HRE-attB-$hVEGF_{165}$ + uP-INT (C) HIF1α and (D) $hVEGF_{165}$ expression in HEK293 cells. On day 15 the HEK293 cells from the experiment (A) were collected for analysis by qRT-PCR. CTL: control; Co: $CoCl_2$; * $p<0.05$. (E) $hVEGF_{165}$ production under hypoxia and normoxia in C2C12 cells. On day 18 $CoCl_2$ was added to a final concentration of 100 μM and 3 days later the medium was collected for VEGF quantification by ELISA. -■- no transfection; -●- pVHAV; -□- pVHAVI. * $p<0.05$. (F) HIF1α and (G) $hVEGF_{165}$ expression in C2C12 cells. On day 15 the C2C12 cells from the experiment (C) were collected for analysis by qRT-PCR. CTL: control; Co: $CoCl_2$; * $p<0.05$ of pVHAVI_Co group versus all other groups.

still maintained about 500 pg/ml VEGF expression, whereas those transfected with non-integrative vectors expressed about half of this value. On the 28th day, $CoCl_2$ was added to the culture medium and maintained for 9 days. Three days after $CoCl_2$ addition, VEGF production was found to be enhanced only in the pVHAVI transfected cells; it reached about 900 pg/ml but returned to basal levels later. The pVAVI group did not show any increase in VEGF levels during the first 3 days, and these levels diminished even more in subsequent days. Upon removing $CoCl_2$, VEGF gene expression levels returned to their initial status.

Activation of VEGF gene expression by $CoCl_2$ was repeated on the 47th and 74th days and resulted in a very similar pattern of gene expression. After the third stimulation, the experiment was stopped because most of the cells became unviable. Long-term cell culturing with $CoCl_2$ seems to affect cell viability. These results clearly demonstrate that the vectors functioned correctly, particularly the pVHAVI system, which is the only system that is expected to be hypoxia-responsive.

To verify genomic integration of the pVHAVI and pVAVI vectors, genomic DNA was extracted 30 days after transfection, and a known region of the vectors was amplified by PCR. Fig. 2B shows the amplification of 735 bp and 432 bp products, which correspond to the pVAX-HRE-attB-$hVEGF_{165}$ and pVAX-attB-$hVEGF_{165}$ vectors, respectively. DNA from the other vectors was not amplified by PCR.

To demonstrate the activation of HIF1α by $CoCl_2$, the expression of HIF1α and hVEGF genes was evaluated by qRT-PCR at the 15th day. Irrespective of the presence or not of vectors, the presence of $CoCl_2$ in the medium elevated HIF1α gene expression 7 to 11 folds in relation to cells without $CoCl_2$ (Fig. 2C); however, only those cells transfected with pVHAVI had elevated VEGF gene expression in the presence of $CoCl_2$ (Fig. 2D), indicating the correct functioning of the pVHAVI system.

To strengthen these findings, we tested pVHAVI system in the murine myoblast cell line C2C12, which is the main cell type present in skeletal muscles. To transfect this cell line we chose nucleofection method, because we had very low level of transfection with calcium phosphate co-precipitation method (not shown). Even using nucleofection the VEGF gene expression levels were lower than HEK293 cells, but the profile of gene expression over 21 days was very similar (Fig. 2E). At the 3rd day after transfection, VEGF gene expression reached about 7,000 pg/ml by both pVHAVI and pVHAV systems, but in a week it dropped to basal level and, at 14th day, there was no significant difference of gene expression between these two systems.

$CoCl_2$ was added to cell culture media at the 18th day, but only those cells transfected with pVHAVI had increased hVEGF gene expression, meanwhile the cells transfected with pVHAV or non-transfected ones did not have any significant alterations. Activation of HIF1α by $CoCl_2$ was also seen in C2C12 cells (Fig. 2F), which was about 7 and 4 folds higher than control group by pVHAVI and pVHAV systems, respectively, but only pVHAVI transfected cells had increased hVEGF gene expression (Fig. 2G).

Visual, functional and molecular analyses of muscles after gene therapy

Visual assessment is an easy method to carry out and provides consistent and relevant information. To make this type of assessment quantitative, the degree of necrosis was scored as described in the "Materials and Methods" section. All animals in the ischemic group without gene therapy presented grade 1 or 2 necrosis. Two animals from the pVV group presented no necrosis,

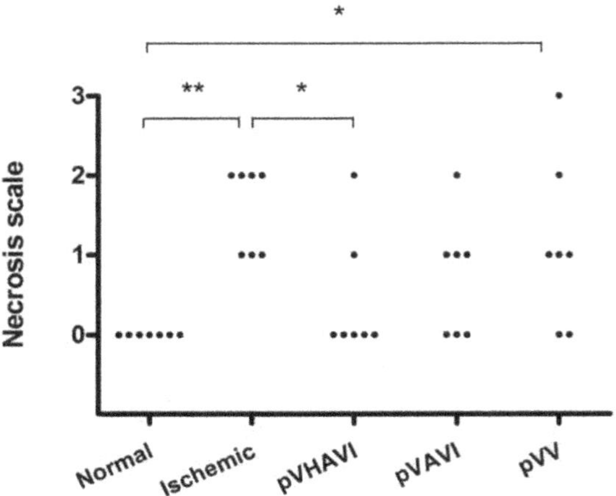

Figure 3. Visual assessment of ischemic limbs after gene therapy. Four weeks after gene therapy, limbs were evaluated according to the following necrosis scale: grade 0: absence of necrosis; grade I: necrosis limited to the toes; grade II: necrosis extending to the dorsum pedis, grade III: necrosis extending to the crus. * $P<0.05$; ** $P<0.005$.

demonstrating the therapeutic effect of the treatment, but the rest of group still showed some degree of necrosis. The pVAVI-treated animals had a better outcome than the pVV group because about half of them had no necrosis. However, the best result was obtained with pVHAVI treatment, which resulted in no visual necrosis in any animals in the group (Fig. 3).

To assess muscle functioning, the gastrocnemius muscle force was determined after 4 weeks of gene therapy. Ischemic limbs showed a drastically reduced force from 1.04 N to 0.12 N, but pVHAVI-treated animals exhibited a force of about 0.46 N, which is equivalent to a 400% improvement. pVV- and pVAVI-treated animals reached an intermediate score of 0.3 N (Fig. 4A). The weight of the gastrocnemius muscle varied among the groups in a pattern similar to that of the muscle force variation. In the pVHAVI-treated animals, this weight was about 50% that of the non-ischemic animals, whereas in the other groups, it was only about 36% (Fig. 4B). It is important to note that the untreated ischemic animals had a similar muscle weight compared to those treated with pVV or pVAVI, but in terms of muscle force, the untreated ischemic group had a much lower value. Muscle force depends on the number and volume of correctly functioning muscle fibers, whereas muscle mass encompasses the mass of all tissues including non-contractile fibrotic tissues, the amount of which varies with disease evolution. Therefore, a minor variation between muscle mass and force after 4 weeks of ischemia is expected.

The pVAVI and pVHAVI vectors are integrative systems, and consequently, gene delivery using these vectors is expected to result in long-term gene expression. To validate the correct functioning of these vectors, VEGF gene expression was evaluated in both serum and muscle tissue. In serum, VEGF was not detected at any time in any group. Muscle extracts obtained after 30 days from the pVHAVI and pVAVI groups had about 3.3 and 4.2 pg/mg of VEGF, respectively, and the ischemic and pVV-treated groups had less than 1.5 pg/mg (Fig. 5A). As 1.5 pg/mg is at the limit of VEGF detection by ELISA, we considered this to be a null value.

To check for vector integration in host cells, PCR was performed using genomic DNA obtained from muscles as a

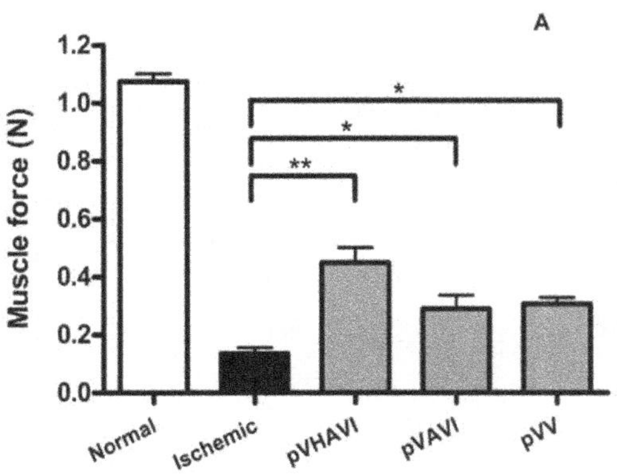

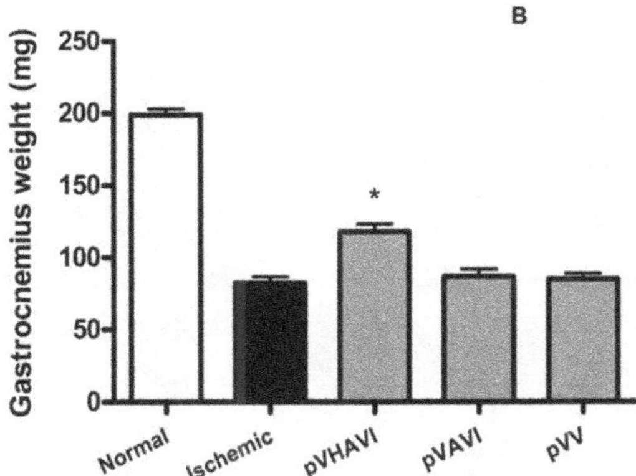

Figure 4. Determination of the mass and force of the gastrocnemius muscle. Muscle force (A) and mass (B) were measured 4 weeks after gene therapy. For each group, seven mice were used. The sham-operated and non-ischemic groups showed no difference in their results and are denoted here as normal. (A) * $P<0.05$; ** $P<0.005$. (B) * $P<0.05$, pVHAVI in comparison to each group.

template. DNA bands of 735 bp and 432 bp were detected in the pVHAVI and pVAVI groups, respectively, and these correspond to the pVAX-HRE-attB-hVEGF$_{165}$ and pVAX-attB-hVEGF$_{165}$ vectors, respectively (Fig. 5B). Other groups showed no amplification, indicating that no vector integration had occurred after 30 days.

Histological analyses

Gastrocnemius muscles were stained with HE, and the numbers of necrotic, normal and regenerative cells were quantified (Fig. 6A and 6B). The ischemic group showed about 15 cells/mm^2 of necrotic cells, and this was reduced to 5 cells/mm^2 in the pVHAVI-treated group. Moreover, the normal cell count increased from 5 cells/mm^2 in the untreated ischemic group to almost 20 cells/mm^2 in the pVHAVI-treated group. The groups treated with the other vectors showed intermediate values. In terms of regenerative cell count, the pVHAVI group (12 cells/mm^2) had a smaller count than the pVAVI group (18 cells/mm^2) but a much higher count than the ischemic group (4 cells/mm^2).

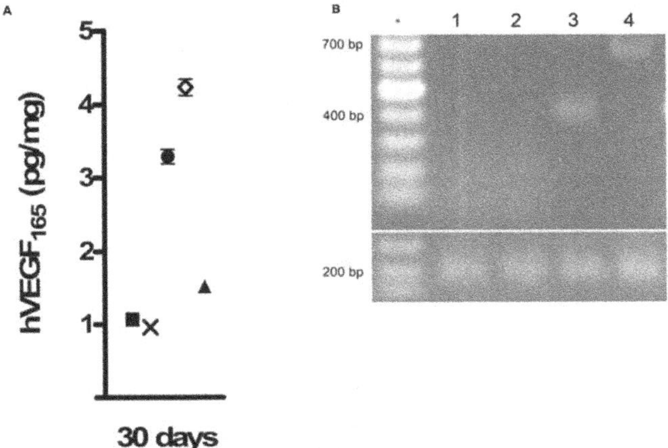

Figure 5. Assessment of VEGF expression vectors after gene therapy. (A) Concentration of hVEGF$_{165}$ in the quadriceps muscle: -x- Ischemic; -■- Normal; -▲- pVV; -●- pVHAVI; - ◇ - pVAVI. (B) Genomic DNA PCR after four weeks of gene therapy. 1: normal; 2: pVV; 3: pVAVI (432 bp); 4: pVHAVI (725 bp). The 200 bp band is from GAPDH. * 100 bp ladder.

A similar order of fibrotic area was seen after staining with Picrossirus (Fig. 6C): ischemic>pVV>pVAVI>pVHAVI>normal. These findings corroborate the previously obtained results demonstrating that the therapeutic effect of pVHAVI is better than that of either the non-integrative pVV system or the integrative and constitutive pVAVI system.

To evaluate angiogenic activity promoted by VEGF, vessels were stained with lectin Griffonia, which recognizes endothelial vessels and macrophages. This staining system was chosen over staining with an anti-CD31 antibody to allow both vessels and infiltrated macrophages to be visualized in the same section. Macrophages and endothelial cells can be differentiated easily by optical microscopy using high magnification. In addition, the anti-alpha-actin antibody was used to localize mature and larger vessels. The number of vessels stained with the two systems was similar (Fig. 6D and 6E). The pVHAVI-treated group had the highest number of vessels followed by the pVAVI and the pVV groups. Even though the difference between the pVHAVI and pVAVI groups was not statistically significant, the pVHAVI treatment tended to be superior.

Discussion

Since the first clinical trial of gene therapy for the treatment of ischemic limbs (which used a plasmid vector expressing the VEGF gene) by Jeffrey Isner in 1996 [29], more than 150 gene therapy trials have been initiated, and about half of them are still opened (http://www.wiley.co.uk/genetherapy/clinical/). The VEGF gene has been widely used in preclinical and clinical assays to treat ischemic diseases because it is a pleiotropic factor involved in many cellular activities, most of which are closely related to angiogenesis. In most of the animal studies, vectors expressing VEGF have been injected directly into the ischemic tissue, and this was found to improve blood flux and transiently augment vessel density [2]. However, we and other groups have demonstrated that long periods of high expression of this gene in ischemic tissue can lead to deleterious effects, such as a decrease in capillary density, the loss of muscle mass and force and the augmentation of limb necrosis [27,30,31]. It is likely that the high concentration of VEGF provided by the ischemic tissues together with the transfected cells promotes fast endothelial cell proliferation and vessel formation, which are not followed by adequate vessel maturation. These premature vessels in muscles can be easily disassembled by muscular movements, potentially leading to

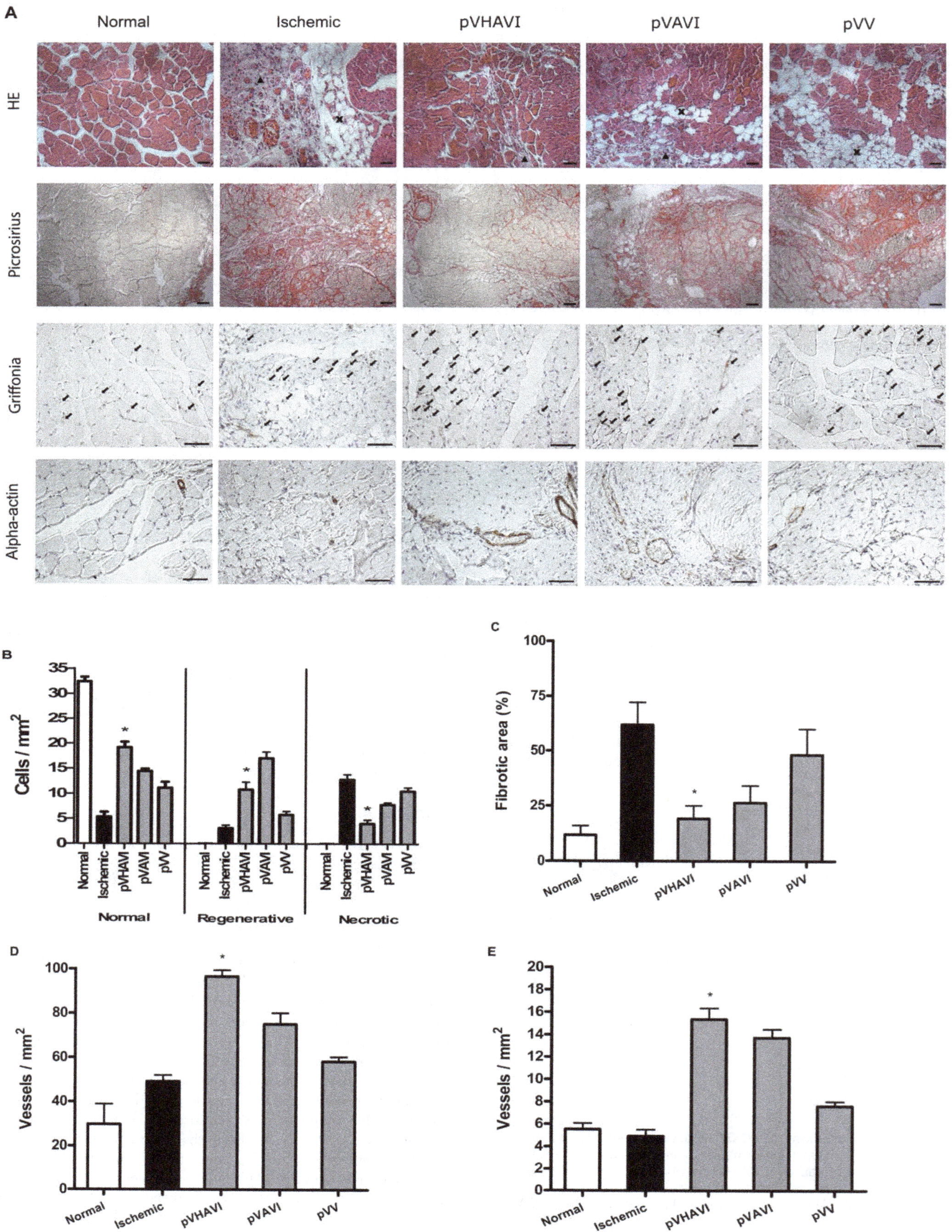
A
Normal
Ischemic
pVHAVI
pVAVI
pVV
HE
Picrosirius
Griffonia
Alpha-actin
B
Cells / mm²
Normal
Regenerative
Necrotic
C
Fibrotic area (%)
D
Vessels / mm²
E
Vessels / mm²
Normal
Ischemic
pVHAVI
pVAVI
pVV

Figure 6. Morphometric analysis of limb muscles. The gastrocnemius muscle was collected from mice after four weeks of gene therapy. Tissue samples were stained with HE (A) and used to quantify necrotic, regenerative and normal areas (B). The sham-operated and non-ischemic groups showed no difference in their results and are denoted here as normal. Fibrotic area, capillary density and mature vessel density were determined after staining with Picrosirius (C), Griffonia (D) and alpha-actin antibody (E), respectively. Bar = 50 μm. * $p<0.05$. ▲, Infiltrated mononuclear cells; X, adipocytes; →, capillary; In the figure B, pVHAVI was different statistically in comparison to all groups.

edema and cell death. Using VEGF together with either the stem cell mobilizing factor G-CSF (granulocyte colony stimulating factor) or the arteriogenic and vasculogenic factor GM-CSF (granulocyte macrophage-colony stimulating factor) to treat mouse ischemic limbs has resulted in much better outcomes than treatment with VEGF alone [26,27]. Our interpretation of these results is that, to make a stable and functional vessel, it is necessary to recruit more growth factors and cells in an adequate time frame and at adequate concentrations, as happens physiologically.

In angiogenic gene therapy assays, plasmid and adenoviral vectors are primarily used because they provide efficient gene transfer to muscles in vivo and express transgenes transiently. Most (if not all) of these vectors are designed to express transgenes highly and continuously using strong constitutive promoters, with the expectation that the secreted angiogenic factors will be spread around the whole ischemic area. However, most angiogenic factors like VEGF contain a heparin-binding domain in their structure [32–34], which causes these factors to be retained around the production area. Consequently, an area with cells transfected with VEGF produces this factor continuously irrespective of the local production due to ischemia, making the local concentration higher than necessary after a certain period of time. Such a condition usually leads to the formation of unstable, immature and hypofunctional vessels [16,35]. The best way of expressing VEGF for therapy is ideally by using vectors that respond to the requirements of the local tissue, *i.e.*, vectors that are regulated by the local degree of ischemia, as normal cells are.

Physiological VEGF gene expression is modulated by the local oxygen concentration. In ischemic tissue, the oxygen supply is limited, and oxygen distribution occurs mostly by passive diffusion from arteries to tissues [36]. This is one of the reasons that limbs distant from the obstructed artery are more affected than proximal limbs. Therefore, it is expected that the degree of ischemia, or the degree of oxygenation, will be variable in different parts of ischemic tissue. In this manner, VEGF production should correlate with either the degree of ischemia or the oxygen concentration. In humans, to overcome the ischemic condition, the ischemic tissues naturally express angiogenic factors based on the local oxygen concentration, such as VEGF, which is monitored by HIF-1 [37]. HIF-1α translocates to the nucleus during hypoxia, where it associates with HIF-1β to make a dimer, which in turn activates genes containing HRE (hypoxia responsive element) sequences. Genes involved in survival under hypoxic conditions, such as those that regulate angiogenesis, vessel dilation, erythropoiesis and glycolysis, are regulated by the binding of HIF to the HRE [19,37].

To make a VEGF-expressing vector responsive to hypoxia, we used nine repeats of the HRE sequence, which is responsive to HIF. A vector with nine repeats was used because it functioned better than vectors with fewer repeats [38]. In addition, with the goal of making an integrative vector capable of providing long-term VEGF expression, the phiC31 integrase system was used. This system allows integration of the vector in one direction, *i.e.*, once the vector is integrated into the host genome it cannot be removed enzymatically [20,21]. Using this system, our expectation was that one treatment of an ischemic limb with the vector (pVHAVI) would be sufficient for a long period, and VEGF gene expression would be regulated by the vector itself.

To demonstrate that the pVHAVI system was functioning correctly, these vectors were tested *in vitro* using HEK293T cells and myoblast cell line C2C12 and *in vivo* using a mouse ischemic limb model. In our *in vitro* study, HEK293T cells were transfected with several vectors (Fig. 1), and VEGF gene expression was followed for more than 90 days. The pVHAVI system was the only one that responded to hypoxia, which was induced by $CoCl_2$ to stabilize HIF1α from degradation. It is important to note that hypoxia was induced at three different times and the cells modified with pVHAVI responded precisely to the hypoxic signal each time. A very similar result was also seen in C2C12 cell line. These results demonstrate clearly that VEGF expression can be activated at any moment by hypoxia, as we predicted.

Correct functioning of the pVHAVI system, as indicated by the induction of VEGF gene expression by hypoxia, was observed for a month. In this study, we opted to use the limb ischemia model rather than administration of $CoCl_2$ because the first model is much more similar to human ischemic disease, and it is a well-established animal model [26,27,39]. Additionally, we have not found a method for using $CoCl_2$ to induce ischemia in vivo or any other method that can induce limb ischemia repeatedly without significantly affecting the animal's physiology. As a result, we could not induce hypoxia repeatedly in animals to evaluate the functioning of the pVHAVI system over a long period as we could for the in vitro model. Consequently, we chose to evaluate the system indirectly after gene therapy by examining therapeutic parameters such as alterations in muscle mass, force and histology and by visually assessing muscle necrosis. For in vivo gene transference, electroporation was used because in our previous studies, we demonstrated that this method is reproducible and results in high levels of transfection [26,27].

The first important step in our in vivo study was to demonstrate that the pVHAVI and pVAVI systems were integrated into muscle cells by phiC31 integrase after one month, and this was proven by PCR (Fig. 5B). It is also very important to note that both systems produced VEGF at a similar level (Fig. 5A), but the physiological response was quite different between them, as follows: 1) most of the animals treated with pVHAVI showed no necrosis, whereas half of those treated with pVAVI had some degree of necrosis (Fig. 3); 2) muscle weight and force were higher in animals treated with the pVHAVI system (Fig. 4A and 4B) and 3) the degree of angiogenesis and fibrosis was better with the pVHAVI system than the pVAVI system (Fig. 6).

Even though the VEGF concentration in muscles was similar in both systems, it is important to note that this concentration was determined from the whole muscle only once, at the 4th week, due to limitations of the method. Therefore, whether any variation in VEGF gene expression occurred in different parts of the muscle after transfection with either vector system during the 4 weeks is unknown. However, it is reasonable to assume that the pVHAVI system, which mainly expresses VEGF during hypoxia, acted differently than the pVAVI system, which expresses VEGF constitutively. We have no direct evidence to support this assumption, but the in vitro data and the improvement of animals treated with the pVHAVI system allow us to make this interpretation.

In this study, the viral CMV promoter was used to construct pVHAVI, which promoted hVEGF expression for three months in vitro and one month in vivo, at least. However, it is a well-known phenomenon that viral promoters, used to express mammalian genes, are frequently silenced during long-term studies. The use of muscle specific promoters like MCK (muscle creatine kinase) in construction of pVHAVI can bring better benefit to PAD patients in long-term treatment.

In conclusion, we demonstrated that a plasmid vector with an HRE sequence incorporated into it provides hypoxia-inducible VEGF expression. This vector, produced with the phiC31 integrative system, allowed for long-term VEGF gene expression, which was only activated under hypoxic conditions. For the treatment of mouse limb ischemia, the hypoxia-sensitive vector pVHAVI ameliorated the symptoms much better than the hypoxia-insensitive vector pVAVI. This last result corroborates the idea that the presence of high concentrations of VEGF in ischemic tissue is not beneficial or is less beneficial than maintaining a lower but sufficient and long-term concentration of VEGF locally.

Author Contributions

Conceived and designed the experiments: SWH. Performed the experiments: EGY RSS VYS PKM LPC VBVL. Analyzed the data: EGY RSS VYS PKM LPC VBVL SWH. Contributed reagents/materials/analysis tools: VBVL SWH. Wrote the paper: EGY SWH.

References

1. Norgren L, Hiatt WR, Dormandy JA, Nehler MR, Harris KA, et al. (2007) Inter-Society Consensus for the Management of Peripheral Arterial Disease (TASC II). Eur J Vasc Endovasc Surg 33 Suppl 1: S1–75.
2. Hammond HK, McKirnan MD (2001) Angiogenic gene therapy for heart disease: a review of animal studies and clinical trials. Cardiovasc Res 49: 561–567.
3. Gupta R, Tongers J, Losordo DW (2009) Human studies of angiogenic gene therapy. Circ Res 105: 724–736.
4. Rissanen TT, Yla-Herttuala S (2007) Current status of cardiovascular gene therapy. Mol Ther 15: 1233–1247.
5. Carmeliet P, Collen D (2000) Molecular basis of angiogenesis. Role of VEGF and VE-cadherin. Ann N Y Acad Sci 902: 249–262; discussion 262–244.
6. Ferrara N, Gerber HP, LeCouter J (2003) The biology of VEGF and its receptors. Nat Med 9: 669–676.
7. Grosskreutz CL, Anand-Apte B, Duplaa C, Quinn TP, Terman BI, et al. (1999) Vascular endothelial growth factor-induced migration of vascular smooth muscle cells in vitro. Microvasc Res 58: 128–136.
8. Barleon B, Sozzani S, Zhou D, Weich HA, Mantovani A, et al. (1996) Migration of human monocytes in response to vascular endothelial growth factor (VEGF) is mediated via the VEGF receptor flt-1. Blood 87: 3336–3343.
9. Bauters C, Asahara T, Zheng LP, Takeshita S, Bunting S, et al. (1995) Site-specific therapeutic angiogenesis after systemic administration of vascular endothelial growth factor. J Vasc Surg 21: 324–315.
10. Becit N, Ceviz M, Kocak H, Yekeler I, Unlu Y, et al. (2001) The effect of vascular endothelial growth factor on angiogenesis: an experimental study. Eur J Vasc Endovasc Surg 22: 310–316.
11. Takeshita S, Rossow ST, Kearney M, Zheng LP, Bauters C, et al. (1995) Time course of increased cellular proliferation in collateral arteries after administration of vascular endothelial growth factor in a rabbit model of lower limb vascular insufficiency. Am J Pathol 147: 1649–1660.
12. Takeshita S, Weir L, Chen D, Zheng LP, Riessen R, et al. (1996) Therapeutic angiogenesis following arterial gene transfer of vascular endothelial growth factor in a rabbit model of hindlimb ischemia. Biochem Biophys Res Commun 227: 628–635.
13. Takeshita S, Zheng LP, Brogi E, Kearney M, Pu LQ, et al. (1994) Therapeutic angiogenesis. A single intraarterial bolus of vascular endothelial growth factor augments revascularization in a rabbit ischemic hind limb model. J Clin Invest 93: 662–670.
14. Tsurumi Y, Takeshita S, Chen D, Kearney M, Rossow ST, et al. (1996) Direct intramuscular gene transfer of naked DNA encoding vascular endothelial growth factor augments collateral development and tissue perfusion. Circulation 94: 3281–3290.
15. van Weel V, Deckers MM, Grimbergen JM, van Leuven KJ, Lardenoye JH, et al. (2004) Vascular endothelial growth factor overexpression in ischemic skeletal muscle enhances myoglobin expression in vivo. Circ Res95: 58–66.
16. Schwarz ER, Speakman MT, Patterson M, Hale SS, Isner JM, et al. (2000) Evaluation of the effects of intramyocardial injection of DNA expressing vascular endothelial growth factor (VEGF) in a myocardial infarction model in the rat–angiogenesis and angioma formation. J Am Coll Cardiol 35: 1323–1330.
17. Lee RJ, Springer ML, Blanco-Bose WE, Shaw R, Ursell PC, et al. (2000) VEGF gene delivery to myocardium: deleterious effects of unregulated expression. Circulation 102: 898–901.
18. Semenza GL (1999) Perspectives on oxygen sensing. Cell 98: 281–284.
19. Semenza GL (2004) Hydroxylation of HIF-1: oxygen sensing at the molecular level. Physiology (Bethesda) 19: 176–182.
20. Calos MP (2006) The phiC31 integrase system for gene therapy. Curr Gene Ther 6: 633–645.
21. Chalberg TW, Portlock JL, Olivares EC, Thyagarajan B, Kirby PJ, et al. (2006) Integration specificity of phage phiC31 integrase in the human genome. J Mol Biol 357: 28–48.
22. Su H, Arakawa-Hoyt J, Kan YW (2002) Adeno-associated viral vector-mediated hypoxia response element-regulated gene expression in mouse ischemic heart model. Proc Natl Acad Sci U S A America 99: 9480–9485.
23. Sacramento CB, Moraes JZ, Denapolis PM, Han SW (2010) Gene expression promoted by the SV40 DNA targeting sequence and the hypoxia-responsive element under normoxia and hypoxia. Braz J Med Biol Res 43: 722–727.
24. DuBridge RB, Tang P, Hsia HC, Leong PM, Miller JH, et al. (1987) Analysis of mutation in human cells by using an Epstein-Barr virus shuttle system. Mol Cell Biol 7: 379–387.
25. Yuan Y, Hilliard G, Ferguson T, Millhorn DE (2003) Cobalt inhibits the interaction between hypoxia-inducible factor-alpha and von Hippel-Lindau protein by direct binding to hypoxia-inducible factor-alpha. J Biol Chem 278: 15911–15916.
26. Sacramento CB, Cantagalli VD, Grings M, Carvalho LP, Baptista-Silva JC, et al. (2009) Granulocyte-macrophage colony-stimulating factor gene based therapy for acute limb ischemia in a mouse model. J Gene Med 11: 345–353.
27. Sacramento CB, da Silva FH, Nardi NB, Yasumura EG, Baptista-Silva JC, et al. (2010) Synergistic effect of vascular endothelial growth factor and granulocyte colony-stimulating factor double gene therapy in mouse limb ischemia. J Gene Med 12: 310–319.
28. Hourde C, Vignaud A, Beurdy I, Martelly I, Keller A, et al. (2006) Sustained peripheral arterial insufficiency durably impairs normal and regenerating skeletal muscle function. J Physiol Sci 56: 361–367.
29. Isner JM, Pieczek A, Schainfeld R, Blair R, Haley L, et al. (1996) Clinical evidence of angiogenesis after arterial gene transfer of phVEGF165 in patient with ischaemic limb. Lancet 348: 370–374.
30. Masaki I, Yonemitsu Y, Yamashita A, Sata S, Tanii M, et al. (2002) Angiogenic gene therapy for experimental critical limb ischemia: acceleration of limb loss by overexpression of vascular endothelial growth factor 165 but not of fibroblast growth factor-2. Circ Res 90: 966–973.
31. Ozawa CR, Banfi A, Glazer NL, Thurston G, Springer ML, et al. (2004) Microenvironmental VEGF concentration, not total dose, determines a threshold between normal and aberrant angiogenesis. J Clin Invest 113: 516–527.
32. Nugent MA, Edelman ER (1992) Kinetics of basic fibroblast growth factor binding to its receptor and heparan sulfate proteoglycan: a mechanism for cooperactivity. Biochemistry 31: 8876–8883.
33. Maciag T, Mehlman T, Friesel R, Schreiber AB (1984) Heparin binds endothelial cell growth factor, the principal endothelial cell mitogen in bovine brain. Science 225: 932–935.
34. McCaffrey TA, Falcone DJ, Du B (1992) Transforming growth factor-beta 1 is a heparin-binding protein: identification of putative heparin-binding regions and isolation of heparins with varying affinity for TGF-beta 1. J Cell Physiol 152: 430–440.
35. von Degenfeld G, Banfi A, Springer ML, Wagner RA, Jacobi J, et al. (2006) Microenvironmental VEGF distribution is critical for stable and functional vessel growth in ischemia. FASEB J 20: 2657–2659.
36. Wittenberg BA, Wittenberg JB (1989) Transport of oxygen in muscle. Annu Rev Physiol 51: 857–878.
37. Wang GL, Semenza GL (1993) General involvement of hypoxia-inducible factor 1 in transcriptional response to hypoxia. Proc Natl Acad Sci U S A 90: 4304–4308.
38. Ruan H, Su H, Hu L, Lamborn KR, Kan YW, et al. (2001) A hypoxia-regulated adeno-associated virus vector for cancer-specific gene therapy. Neoplasia 3: 255–263.
39. Goto T, Fukuyama N, Aki A, Kanabuchi K, Kimura K, et al. (2006) Search for appropriate experimental methods to create stable hind-limb ischemia in mouse. Tokai J Exp Clin Med 31: 128–132.

16

In Vivo Electroporation Mediated Gene Delivery to the Beating Heart

Erick L. Ayuni[1], Amiq Gazdhar[2], Marie Noelle Giraud[1], Alexander Kadner[1], Mathias Gugger[3], Marco Cecchini[4], Thierry Caus[1], Thierry P. Carrel[1], Ralph A. Schmid[2]*, Hendrik T. Tevaearai[1]

1 Department of Cardiovascular Surgery, University Hospital of Berne, Berne, Switzerland, **2** Division of General Thoracic Surgery, University Hospital of Berne, Berne, Switzerland, **3** Department of Pathology, University of Berne, Berne, Switzerland, **4** Department of Urology, University Hospital of Berne, Berne, Switzerland

Abstract

Gene therapy may represent a promising alternative strategy for cardiac muscle regeneration. *In vivo* electroporation, a physical method of gene transfer, has recently evolved as an efficient method for gene transfer. In the current study, we investigated the efficiency and safety of a protocol involving *in vivo* electroporation for gene transfer to the beating heart. Adult male rats were anesthetised and the heart exposed through a left thoracotomy. Naked plasmid DNA was injected retrograde into the transiently occluded coronary sinus before the electric pulses were applied. Animals were sacrificed at specific time points and gene expression was detected. Results were compared to the group of animals where no electric pulses were applied. No post-procedure arrhythmia was observed. Left ventricular function was temporarily altered only in the group were high pulses were applied; CK-MB (Creatine kinase) and TNT (Troponin T) were also altered only in this group. Histology showed no signs of toxicity. Gene expression was highest at day one. Our results provide evidence that *in vivo* electroporation with an optimized protocol is a safe and effective tool for nonviral gene delivery to the beating heart. This method may be promising for clinical settings especially for perioperative gene delivery.

Editor: Pieter H. Reitsma, Leiden University Medical Center, Netherlands

Funding: This work was supported by a grant from the Olga Mayenfisch Foundation, Zurich Switzerland and by two grants from the Swiss National Science Foundation (3200-068304- 2006 to RAS and 310000-118270-2007 to AK).The funders had no role in study design, data collection and analysis, decision to publish, or preparation of the manuscript.

Competing Interests: The authors have declared that no competing interests exist.

* E-mail: ralph.schmid@insel.ch

Introduction

Coronary artery disease continues to be a major cause of morbidity and mortality worldwide. Currently, the medical treatment and/or myocardial revascularization procedure, either by percutaneous angioplasty or by coronary bypass surgery (CABG) remains the standard therapy [1]. Regeneration of the infracted myocardium, however, is the major challenge and its lack remains the predominant cause of death. New therapeutic modalities which may yield better and consistent results have to be evaluated. Gene therapy, the transfer of nucleic acids to achieve therapeutic benefits is one promising approach. However, progress towards effective human gene therapy in cardiovascular diseases has been hindered by a number of problems including vector toxicity, poor targeting of diseased tissues, and host immune and inflammatory activity [2,3,4]. Hence, safe and reproducible methods have to be established. Electroporation a physical method of gene transfer is one such promising technique.

It is based on the application of strong electric pulses for a very short duration to enhance transfer of macromolecules like DNA and proteins through cell membranes. Even though a number of hypothesis regarding the cell membrane permeabilization have been suggested [5,6], the exact mechanism remains unclear. Nevertheless, electroporation has been shown to be one of the most efficient gene transfer strategies in vivo [7,8] and was tested in a broad range of target tissues and organs [9,10,11,12,13,14]. *Ex vivo* electroporation to the heart in experimental models has also been reported [15,16] and showed a 100 to 1000 folds increase in transgene expression as compared to direct DNA injection. Consequently, the use of *in vivo* electroporation mediated transfer may represent a promising method to overcome the common limitations of gene therapy protocols using other types of vectors. Regarding cardiac gene delivery more specifically, direct injection into the cardiac muscle is the most common approach. Gene therapy protocols also involve antegrade coronary injection after aortic cross clamping, however, both approaches do not result in global vector distribution in the heart. Furthermore, the antegrade approach is also limited by heterogeneous and inefficient distribution in the presence of coronary stenosis or occlusion. To overcome this problem we present a retrograde approach by injection via the coronary veins after transient occlusion of the coronary sinus, to study the efficiency and the effect of *in vivo* electroporation mediated gene transfer to the beating heart.

Materials and Methods

Plasmid

The plasmids pCiKlux expresses firefly luciferase from the CMV immediate early promoter/enhancer as described before [13,17]. EGFP plasmid was from Add gene (USA). The endotoxin-free plasmids were produced in large scale at Plasmid Factory GmbH & Co (Bielefeld, Germany). For electroporation, plasmids were suspended in endotoxin-free water.

Animals

Inbreed male Wistar rats (200–220 g) (Janvier, France) were used and maintained on rodent feed and water in a air and temperature controlled room. The experiments were performed in compliance with the standards of the European convention of animal care. The study protocols permission numbers 32/03 and 21/06, were approved by the University of Berne Animal Studies Committee.

Gene Transfer technique

Adult male rats were anesthetized by inhalation of 4% isoflurane in a glass chamber before being intubated and ventilated via a 14GA catheter (Insyte, Madrid, Spain) with FIO2 = 1.0 and 1.5% isoflurane to maintain anesthesia, a breathing frequency of 100/min, and a tidal volume of 10 ml/kg body weight with a rodent ventilator (model 683 Harvard Apparatus, South Natick MA).

A left thoracotomy in the 4th intercostal space was performed and the heart was immobilized, the apex was lifted using an apical 7-0 prolene suture (Ethicon) and a 6-0 tourniquet was placed around the distal coronary vein to allow temporary coronary sinus occlusion (Figure 1a), immediately followed by the retrograde injection of plasmid solution in a volume of 150 µl (plasmid concentration 1 mg/ml). Animals in all groups below were injected with equal volume of plasmid. Plate electrodes (2 cm×1 cm) were placed on each side of the heart followed by the application of 8 pulses of 20 ms and 200 V/cm,1 Hz using the pulse generator (Inovio, San Diego) (Figure 1b). The distance between the two plates of electrode was 1.2 mm. The tourniquet was then immediately released. After the procedure, the heart was observed for 2 minutes before a small chest drain was inserted into the left hemithorax and the thoracotomy was closed with four layers of continuous sutures (4/0 prolene). The drain was removed after the animals restored spontaneous breathing, followed by extubation.

Experimental design

Three sets of experiments were performed.

First, to establish the safety of *in vivo* electroporation as method of gene transfer to the beating heart. The animals underwent gene transfer as described, with different pulsing parameters of 8, 16 and 32 pulses. Animals were evaluated for different parameters of toxicity at different time points.

Second, to establish *in vivo* electroporation as a method of gene transfer to the beating heart. Two groups were studied (n = 5). All animals underwent gene transfer as described. In the control group, the entire procedure was identical with the exception that the animals were not exposed to the electric pulses. Firefly luciferase under control of CMV immediate early promoter/enhancer was used and the animals were sacrificed 1 day after gene transfer. One animal was injected with 150 µl EGFP expression plasmid and electroporated as described above to localize the gene expression.

Third, to evaluate transgene expression over time. All animals underwent gene transfer as described and subgroups were sacrificed at day 1, 3, 5 and 7 after gene transfer (n = 4 per subgroup).As reporter gene firefly luciferase under control of CMV immediate early promoter/enhancer was used.

Analysis of Toxicity

Haemodynamic Measurements. Rats were anaesthetized with isoflurane. The right carotid artery was exposed and a 1.4-French pressure micro-catheter (Millar®, Mikro-Tip®, Millar Instruments, Houston, TX, USA) was inserted into the left ventricle (LV). LV pressure curves were recorded and analyzed (PowerLab system and its Chart 5.2 software, AD Instruments, Spechbach, Germany). Data were recorded before the electroporation procedure (basal), then continuously over a 60 minutes period. Thereafter, in a subgroup of animals, (n = 4) data were measured 6 hours following the electroporation.

Cardiac Enzyme measurements. Two early cardiac specific biomarkers, CK-MB (Creatine kinase) and TnT (Troponin T) were used as indicators of myocardial injury. Blood samples were collected 6 hours following the electroporation, centrifuged and the serum was frozen at −20°C. Serum TnT and CK-MB were measured using commercial kits (respectively Roche Diagnostics, Basel Switzerland and Meia, Abbott, Baar, Switzerland) according to manufacturer's instructions.

Histological analysis at each time point. Immediately following euthanasia, the heart was placed in a container with 4%

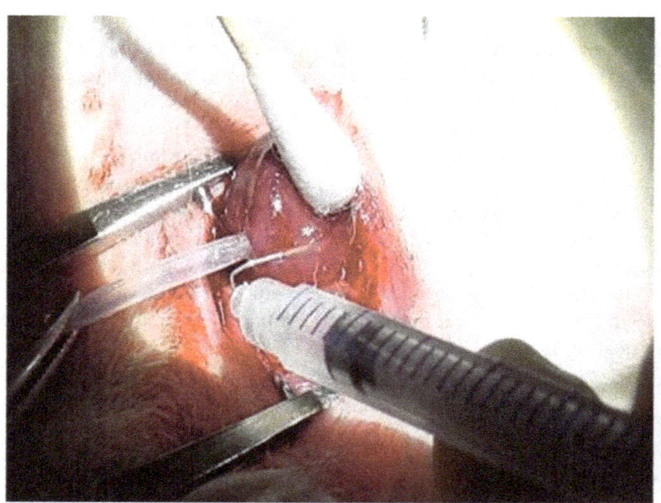

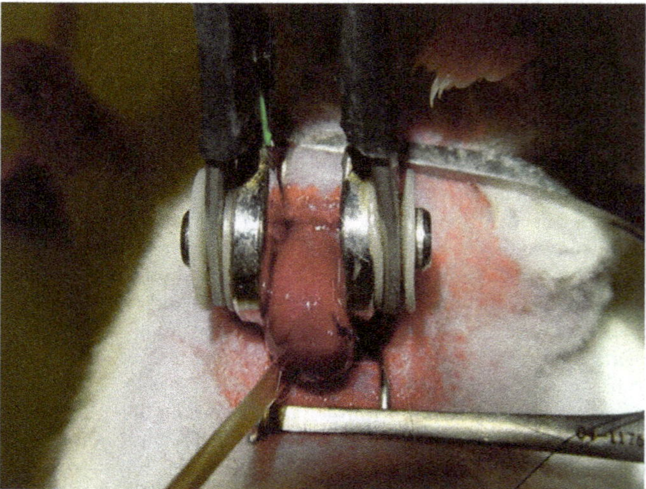

Figure 1. The *in vivo* electroporation mediated gene transfer to the heart is a two step procedure. (a) First, the coronary sinus is occluded with a 6-0 prolene tourniquet and the plasmid is injected into the coronary vein. (b) The heart is then positioned between the plate electrodes and the electric field is applied.

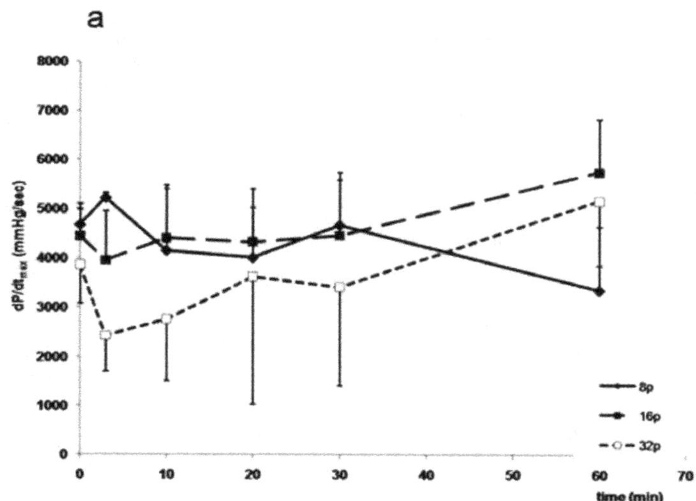
a
8000
7000
6000
5000
4000
3000
2000
1000
0
dP/dt$_{max}$ (mmHg/sec)
0
10
20
30
40
50
60
70
time (min)
8p
16p
32p

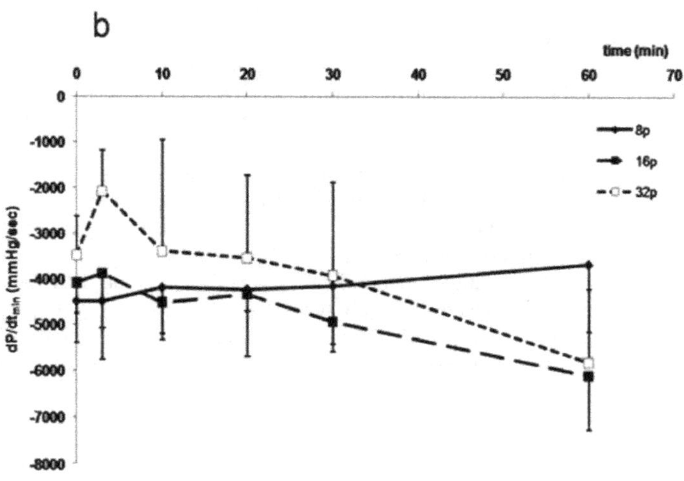
b
time (min)
0
10
20
30
40
50
60
70
0
-1000
-2000
-3000
-4000
-5000
-6000
-7000
-8000
dP/dt$_{min}$ (mmHg/sec)
8p
16p
32p

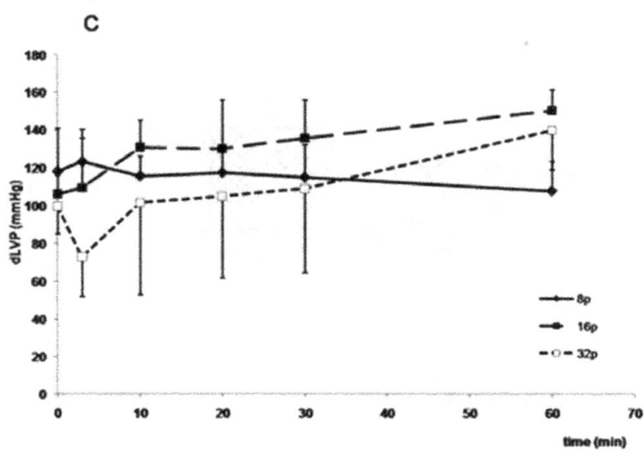
c
180
160
140
120
100
80
60
40
20
0
dLVP (mmHg)
0
10
20
30
40
50
60
70
time (min)
8p
16p
32p

Figure 2. Left ventricular contractile function of heart following electroporation mediated gene transfer using 8, 16 and 32 pulses protocols (n = 5 each group). Indices of contractility and relaxation determined respectively by the maximum (dP/dt max) (a) and the minimum (dP/dt min) (b) and developed LVP (dLVP) (c) of the first derivative of ventricular pressure with respect to time. These parameters remained unchanged before (time 0) and after electroporation except for the 32 pulses group where the values are transiently altered. A complete normalization of the values occurred within 10–20 minutes. No abnormality was detected in the group in which invivo electroporation was not performed.

formalin for 12 hrs. After paraffin embedding the sections where cut and routine haematoxylin and eosin staining was performed. The sections were blinded and reviewed by an experienced pathologist. Gene expression was analyzed at day 1, 3, 5, and 7 following the *in vivo* electroporation procedure.

Bioluminescent reporter imaging (BLI). The animals were anesthetized with thiopental (50 mg/kg Penthotal, Abbot AG, Baar, Switzerland). Monosodium luciferin (750 µl of an 80 mg/ml solution, Molecular Probes, The Netherlands) was injected i.p, 15 min before the heart was removed and imaged in an intensified charge-coupled device (CCD) camera (C2400-32, Hamamatsu), fitted with a 50 mm Nikkor lens (Nikon, Japan) and an image processor (Argus 20, Hamamatsu). An imaging system similar to that described by Contag et al [18] was employed for these studies as previously described [19].

Quantification of the Bioluminescent Signal. The luciferase activity was measured by counting the photon emission in the defined region of interest (ROI) with the aid of the open lab software (Improvision, Coventry, UK) [19].

Measurement of reporter gene expression. Slices of the hearts were frozen in liquid nitrogen immediately after imaging. The tissue was grinded and suspended in 1 ml of lysis buffer (Promega, Madison, WI, USA) and homogenized immediately. Samples were thawed at room temperature and vortexed for 30 sec. Subsequently they were refrozen in liquid nitrogen. Three freeze-thaw cycles were performed by alternating between liquid nitrogen and room temperature water bath. Debris was removed by centrifugation. Luciferase activity was then measured and expressed as RLU/mg protein, using the slow glow assay system (Promega, Madison WI) in MiniLumat LB 9506 luminometer (Berthold Technologies, Switzerland).

EGFP reporter gene expression and confocal microscopy. At day one after electroporation mediated gene transfer, the animal was sacrificed and the heart was fixed in O.C.T compound, the cryosections were made at the 10 µm thickness and sections were observed under LSM 510 exciter confocal microscope from Carl Zeiss (Germany).

Statistics. Data are presented as mean±SEM. The non parametric Mann Whitney U test was performed to compare the groups using GraphPad Prism version 4.00 for Windows, GraphPad Prism version 4.00 for Windows, GraphPad Software, San Diego California USA, www.graphpad.com. $p<0.05$ was taken as the level of significance.

Results

Electroporation mediated gene transfer to the beating heart is safe

Electroporation mediated gene transfer to the beating heart is safe Fifty-eight animals were used in the entire study. Overall mortality was 3.4% (2/58), due to bleeding from the coronary vein. Therefore, mortality was never related to the electroporation procedure itself. Especially, mortality remained null among the two groups of animals treated with the higher electroporation doses of 16 and 32 pulses.

Nevertheless, a very transient asystole followed the electroporation in 2/8 animals in the 32 pulses protocol. The asystole resumed spontaneously within 5 seconds. No fibrillation or other rhythm alteration was recorded.

LV contractility function was analyzed over the first hour following the electroporation procedure. Contractility (LVdp/dt max) and relaxation (LVdP/dt min) as well as the developed LVP (dLVP) were altered after the electroporation procedure only in the group of animals with the maximum pulses regimen of 32 pulses (Figure 2); However, these functional alterations were rapidly reversible and complete normalization occurred within

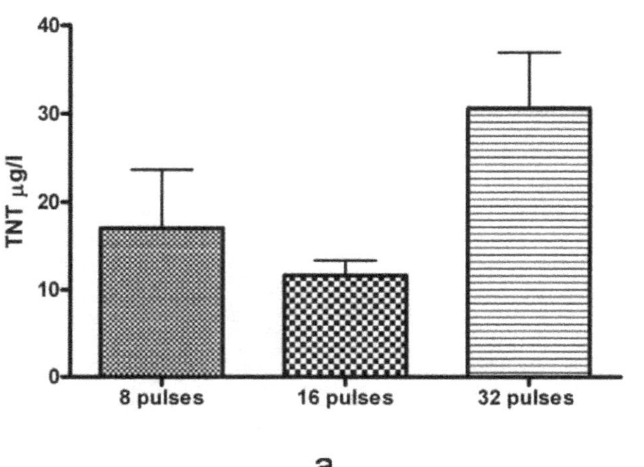

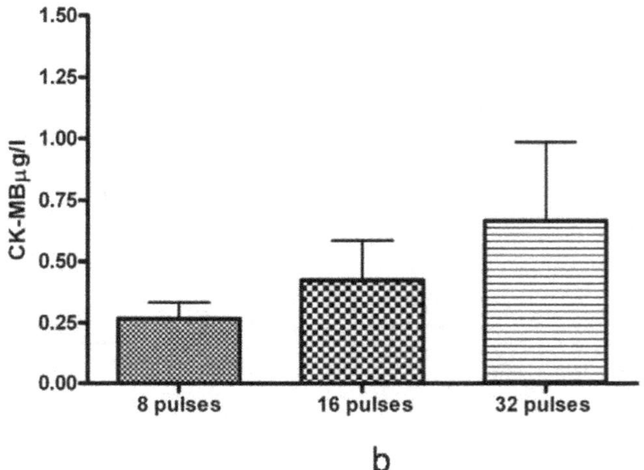

Figure 3. The two early cardiac enzymes for injury TnT and CK-MB were measured; both enzymes remained within normal range after *in vivo* electroporation mediated gene transfer with 8 and 16 pulses, but the values were altered with the 32 pulses protocol. (a) TnT levels (b) CK-MB levels. The levels were below detection levels in the group in which invivo electroporation was not performed.

10–20 minutes and persisted thereafter. Conversely, contractile function remained within a normal range in animals' electroporated with either 8 or 16 pulses.

Six hours post-electroporation TNT (Figure 3a) and CK-MB (Figure 3b) values also remained in the normal range in animals treated with 8 and 16 pulses; Values were altered only when a 32 pulses regimen was tested (30.6±6.3 µg/l for TnT, and 0.66±0.318 µg/l for CK-MB). The levels in the control group without electroporation, were below detection value. Histological analysis performed at each time point, revealed no signs of fibrosis or necrosis however very moderate blood stasis, and very few interstitial lymphocytes, were observed after 8 pulses. For 16 pulses and 32 pulses slightly more blood stasis was observed with some interstitial and perivascular lymphocytes, but no signs of necrosis or fibrosis was seen (Figure 4).

In vivo electroporation mediated gene transfer to the heart increases gene expression

When 150 µl of plasmid DNA pCiklux was injected without electroporation very low transgene expression was detected by BLI imaging (Figure 5 d). In contrast, when field strength of 200 V/cm and 8 pulses was applied after injection of 150 µg of plasmid pCiklux the mean lux activity was easily detected with BLI imaging at day 1 (Figure 5a). The luciferase activity was measured by counting the photon emission in the defined region of interest (ROI), RLU measured were 16479±4338 RLU for electroporated heart vs. 3539±1555 RLU for non electroporated heart ($p = 0.018$) (Figure 5b). These findings were further confirmed with conventional luciferase assay in the same samples. Luciferase activity observed on day 1 after electroporation mediated gene transfer was highest; 6594±1806 RLU/mg for electroporated heart vs 1684±760 RLU/mg of total protein for non electroporated heart ($p = 0.011$) (Figure 5c); however, the activity showed a gradual decrease, and at day 7 no transgene expression was seen (Figure 6). The confocal images showed the expression of the EGFP on the cell surface after *invivo* electroporation mediated gene transfer of the EGFP plasmid (Figure 5 e).

Discussion

Regenerative medicine is a rapidly evolving field and efficient and reliable methods are needed to expedite the process of regeneration and healing. Current study demonstrates that *in vivo* electroporation mediated gene transfer to the beating heart is a feasible novel approach; it is also safe, quick, efficient and reproducible. After retrograde injection of plasmid DNA into the transiently occluded coronary sinus and immediate local application of a series of 8 electric pulses, a high gene expression can be achieved with no obvious adverse effect.

With the shortcomings of viral vectors and the inefficiency of the other non-viral vectors, the physical method of electroporation mediated gene transfer has emerged as a promising tool. Recently the use of this technique *in vivo* has gained increasing acceptance and has been used successfully in many tissues and organs [8,11,20], under various conditions [12,14,21,22]. Even though interest has been shown towards this promising approach, yet its use in the cardiac muscles is limited. Few prior investigations reported the use of electroporation mediated gene transfer to cardiac tissue ex-vivo. Harrisson *et al* [15] electroporated chick embryonic hearts *ex vivo* by placing the heart in a bath containing the plasmid DNA, and showed high GFP and luciferase expression after 48 hrs. Similarly in the mice heterotopic heart transplant model Wang *et al* [16] demonstrated that *ex vivo* electroporation mediated gene transfer of the graft before its implantation, allowed significant gene expression. Very recently this technique was also applied on the pig heart [23]. Therefore, it was with no doubt that electroporation would enhance gene expression in the cardiac muscle. In the current study, however we demonstrate the applicability of this technique with ease and safety on beating hearts of normal rats.

Various routes of administration of the plasmids in the heart have been reported, but none of the protocols could achieve satisfactory global distribution in the heart, especially not in animals with heart failure. Some studies have evaluated the easy direct injection of plasmid into the heart muscles as an efficient method. It is however limited by local needle injury and time consuming electromechanical mapping techniques [24]. The epicardial delivery is another approach where the natural cavity formed by the pericardial pouch was thought to be an advantage. The higher permeability of the pericardium as compared to the epicardium, lets the injected solution diffuse more eccentrically than concentrically [25]. Most recently the percutaneous transluminal approach gathered a lot of attention as specially designed ventricular catheters allow direct injection within the myocardium [26], however, the problem of local needle injury and adequate distribution still remains. In laboratory experiments the coronary delivery approach has been largely used by cross clamping of the ascending aorta and immediate injection of the gene solution to the left ventricular cavity, the solution being delivered to perfuse both coronaries [27]. Unfortunately limitations of this technique involve an acute elevation of the afterload that will further reduce LV function following aortic cross clamping. In the present study we evaluated a retrograde approach where the coronary sinus is clamped transiently before the plasmid solution is injected

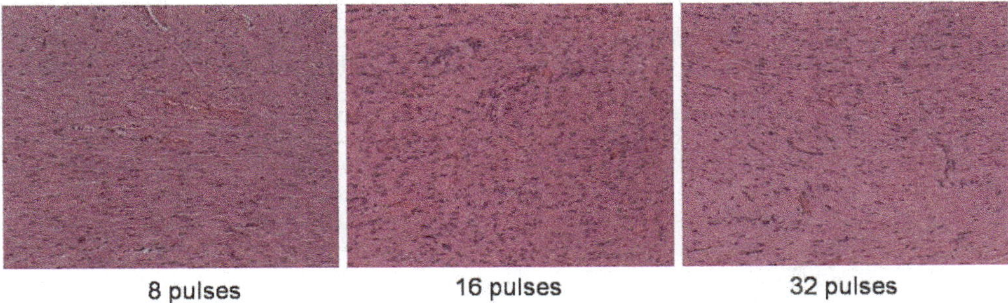

Figure 4. For histological analysis the hearts were evaluated at 24 hrs post gene transfer. The following criteria were considered: vascular congestion, infiltration and polymorphonuclear infiltrates. No haemorrhage or infiltration was noticed with any pulsing protocol. (a) 8 pulses (b) 16 pulses (c) 32 pulses (Magnification = ×200).

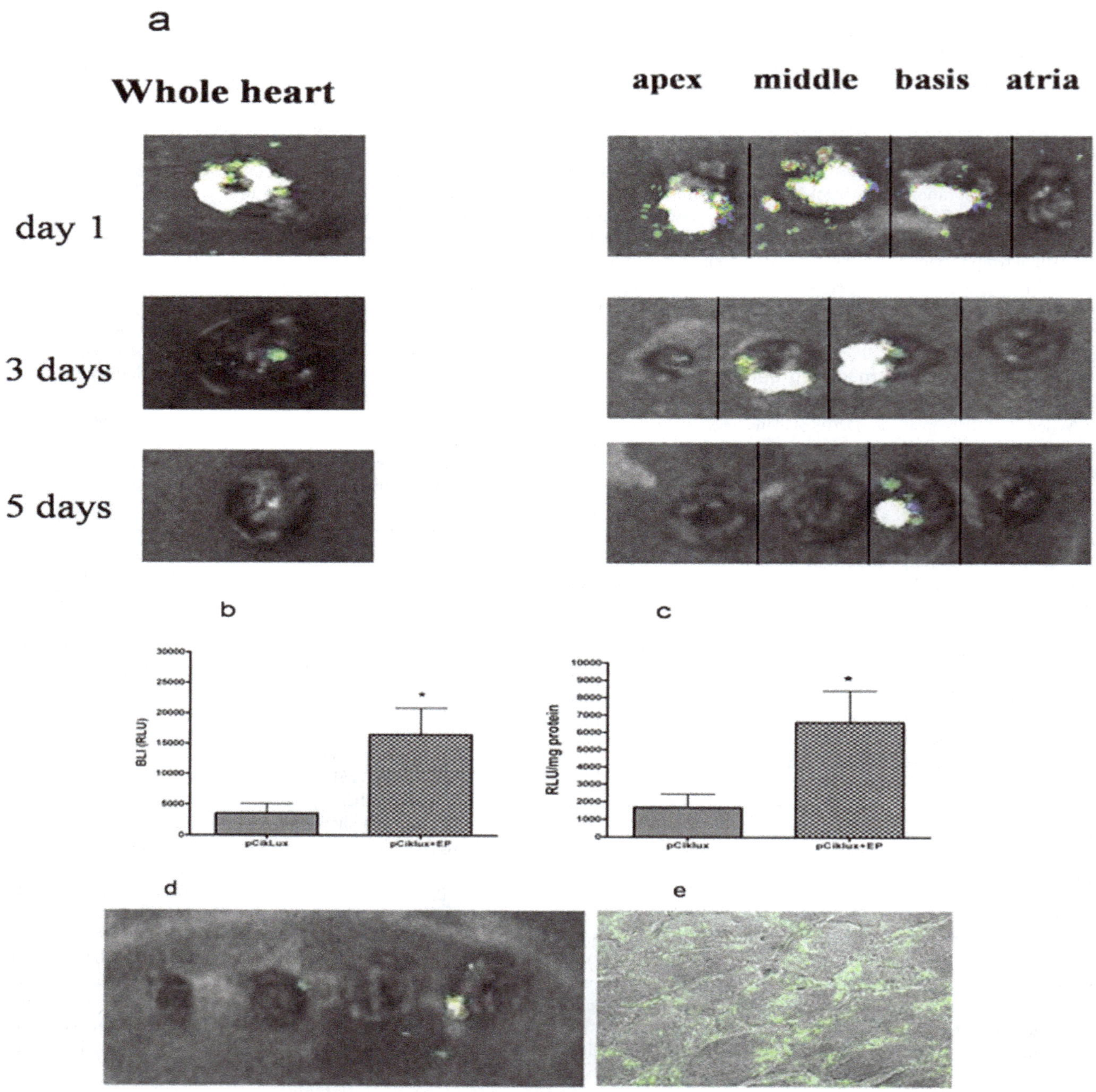

Figure 5. ***In vivo*** **electroporation mediated gene transfer to the beating heart.** (a) BLI images at day 1, 3 and 5 after *in vivo* electroporation mediated gene transfer to the normal heart. Graphical representation of the quantification of the luciferase activity, with electroporated compared to non-electroporated hearts; (b) BLI measurements, the photon counts per heart field are expressed in relative light units (RLU) 16479±4338 RLU for electroporated heart vs. 3539±1555 RLU for non electroporated heart ($p = 0.018$) at day 1. (c) Luciferase assay, RLU per milligram (mg) of protein was measured using a luminometer in the same sample 6594±1806 RLU/mg for electroporated heart vs 1684±760 RLU/mg of total protein for non electroporated heart ($p = 0.011$) at day 1. (d) Control heart, plasmid was injected but not elecroporated. (e) Expression of EGFP was found on the cell surface.

retrograde into the coronary veins. Using this approach, we were able to achieve global transgene expression in the heart, hence opening new ways of delivering genes to failing hearts.

Since application of direct defibrillation to the heart is almost a routine procedure at the end of cardiac surgery procedures, hence *in vivo* electroporation mediated gene transfer to the beating heart could easily be applied intraoperatively in routine clinical practice. Numerous studies of myocardial damage caused by electrical currents have been performed [28] and experiments have been conducted to evaluate the toxic effect of electroporation mediated gene transfer to the myocardium [29,30]. It has been shown recently that electroporation induces only very transient phenotypic

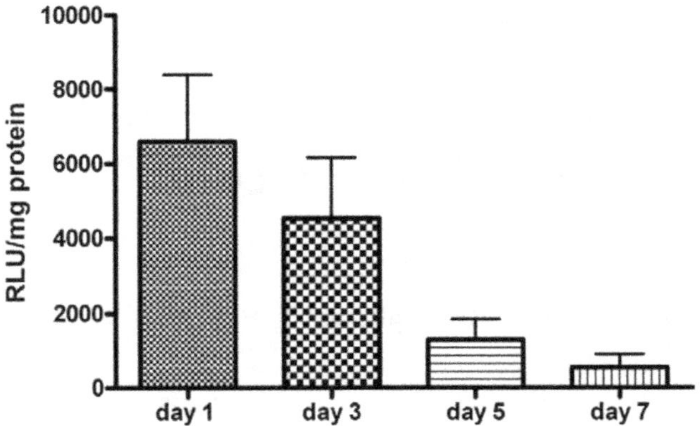

Figure 6. Graphical representation of transgene expression measured over time. After electroporation mediated gene transfer the animals were sacrificed at different time points.

and morphological alterations of skeletal muscle fibres [31]. In our current study, we also systematically analyzed the possible side effects of *in vivo* electroporation on the cardiac muscle including biochemical, functional and histological parameters. In the group treated with 8 and 16 pulses, no alteration in LV function was observed; transient asystole and reduced contractile function as well as slightly elevated levels of TNT and CK-MB were observed only when 32 pulses were administered. Histological assessment revealed no signs of injury, haemorrhage or infiltration.

Although the results are very promising, the technique has a few limitations. Electroporation is a novel approach and needs practice; indeed, the injection has to be performed very diligently since the coronary vein is fragile. There may be concern about the homogenous distribution with retrograde injection, as compared to the antegrade approach. However, the retrograde approach offers the major advantage that it can perfuse ischemic areas whereas the antegrade delivery is limited by coronary stenosis and/or occlusion. For effective gene therapy of chronic disease, persistent transgene expression is needed. In this present study we have used the CMV early promoter enhancer which allows early and transient expression; undergoing transcriptional inactivation [32,33]. Further studies are needed with more advanced promoter systems which could provide prolonged transgene expression [13] and also this technique should be tested in infracted heart.

In conclusion, this initial study demonstrates that *in vivo* electroporation mediated gene transfer to the beating heart is feasible and safe. A high gene expression can be achieved in normal hearts. These observations make *in vivo* electroporation an attractive alternative to commonly used delivery techniques for gene therapy for heart disease. However, further evaluations including the use of functional genes are required to further evaluate this technique before clinical applications.

Author Contributions

Conceived and designed the experiments: RAS HTT. Performed the experiments: ELA AG. Analyzed the data: AG MNG AK MG MC. Contributed reagents/materials/analysis tools: MC RAS. Wrote the paper: TC TPC RAS HTT. Corresponding author.

References

1. Freedman SB, Isner JM (2002) Therapeutic angiogenesis for coronary artery disease. Ann Intern Med 136: 54–71.
2. Byrnes AP, Rusby JE, Wood MJ, Charlton HM (1995) Adenovirus gene transfer causes inflammation in the brain. Neuroscience 66: 1015–1024.
3. Marshall E (1999) CLINICAL TRIALS: Gene Therapy Death Prompts Review of Adenovirus Vector 10.1126/science.286.5448.2244. Science 286: 2244–2245.
4. Mitani K, Kubo S (2002) Adenovirus as an integrating vector. Curr Gene Ther 2: 135–144.
5. Neumann ES, Sowers AE, Jordan CA (1989) Electroporation and Electrofusion in Cell Biology. New York: Plenum Press.
6. Gehl J, Sorensen TH, Nielsen K, Raskmark P, Nielsen SL, et al. (1999) In vivo electroporation of skeletal muscle: threshold, efficacy and relation to electric field distribution. Biochim Biophys Acta 1428: 233–240.
7. Mathiesen I (1999) Electropermeabilization of skeletal muscle enhances gene transfer in vivo. Gene Ther 6: 508–514.
8. Mir LM, Bureau MF, Gehl J, Rangara R, Rouy D, et al. (1999) High-efficiency gene transfer into skeletal muscle mediated by electric pulses. Proc Natl Acad Sci U S A 96: 4262–4267.
9. Aihara H, Miyazaki J (1998) Gene transfer into muscle by electroporation in vivo. Nat Biotechnol 16: 867–870.
10. Blair-Parks K, Weston BC, Dean DA (2002) High-level gene transfer to the cornea using electroporation. J Gene Med 4: 92–100.
11. Heller R, Jaroszeski M, Atkin A, Moradpour D, Gilbert R, et al. (1996) In vivo gene electroinjection and expression in rat liver. FEBS Lett 389: 225–228.
12. Nunamaker EA, Zhang HY, Shirasawa Y, Benoit JN, Dean DA (2003) Electroporation-mediated delivery of catalytic oligodeoxynucleotides for manipulation of vascular gene expression. Am J Physiol Heart Circ Physiol 285: H2240–2247.
13. Gazdhar A, Bilici M, Pierog J, Ayuni EL, Gugger M, et al. (2006) In vivo electroporation and ubiquitin promoter—a protocol for sustained gene expression in the lung. J Gene Med 8: 910–918.
14. Tavakoli R, Gazdhar A, Pierog J, Bogdanova A, Gugger M, et al. (2006) Electroporation-mediated interleukin-10 overexpression in skeletal muscle reduces acute rejection in rat cardiac allografts. J Gene Med 8: 242–248.
15. Harrison RL, Byrne BJ, Tung L (1998) Electroporation-mediated gene transfer in cardiac tissue. FEBS Lett 435: 1–5.
16. Wang Y, Bai Y, Price C, Boros P, Qin L, et al. (2001) Combination of electroporation and DNA/dendrimer complexes enhances gene transfer into murine cardiac transplants. Am J Transplant 1: 334–338.
17. Gill DR, Smyth SE, Goddard CA, Pringle IA, Higgins CF, et al. (2001) Increased persistence of lung gene expression using plasmids containing the ubiquitin C or elongation factor 1alpha promoter. Gene Ther 8: 1539–1546.
18. Contag CH, Spilman SD, Contag PR, Oshiro M, Eames B, et al. (1997) Visualizing gene expression in living mammals using a bioluminescent reporter. Photochem Photobiol 66: 523–531.
19. Wetterwald A, van der Pluijm G, Que I, Sijmons B, Buijs J, et al. (2002) Optical Imaging of Cancer Metastasis to Bone Marrow: A Mouse Model of Minimal Residual Disease. Am J Pathol 160: 1143–1153.
20. Lin CR, Tai MH, Cheng JT, Chou AK, Wang JJ, et al. (2002) Electroporation for direct spinal gene transfer in rats. Neurosci Lett 317: 1–4.
21. Lin CR, Yang LC, Lee TH, Lee CT, Huang HT, et al. (2002) Electroporation-mediated pain-killer gene therapy for mononeuropathic rats. Gene Ther 9: 1247–1253.
22. Gothelf A, Mir LM, Gehl J (2003) Electrochemotherapy: results of cancer treatment using enhanced delivery of bleomycin by electroporation. Cancer Treat Rev 29: 371–387.
23. Marshall WG, Jr., Boone BA, Burgos JD, Gografe SI, Baldwin MK, et al. Electroporation-mediated delivery of a naked DNA plasmid expressing VEGF to the porcine heart enhances protein expression. Gene Ther 17: 419–423.
24. Vale PR, Losordo DW, Milliken CE, Maysky M, Esakof DD, et al. (2000) Left ventricular electromechanical mapping to assess efficacy of phVEGF(165) gene transfer for therapeutic angiogenesis in chronic myocardial ischemia. Circulation 102: 965–974.
25. Fromes Y, Salmon A, Wang X, Collin H, Rouche A, et al. (1999) Gene delivery to the myocardium by intrapericardial injection. Gene Ther 6: 683–688.
26. Parsa CJ, Reed RC, Walton GB, Pascal LS, Thompson RB, et al. (2005) Catheter-mediated subselective intracoronary gene delivery to the rabbit heart: introduction of a novel method. J Gene Med 7: 595–603.
27. Wright MJ, Wightman LM, Latchman DS, Marber MS (2001) In vivo myocardial gene transfer: optimization and evaluation of intracoronary gene delivery in vivo. Gene Ther 8: 1833–1839.
28. Nikolski VP, Efimov IR (2005) Electroporation of the heart. Europace 7 Suppl 2: 146–154.
29. Bonnafous P, Vernhes M, Teissie J, Gabriel B (1999) The generation of reactive-oxygen species associated with long-lasting pulse-induced electropermeabilisation of mammalian cells is based on a non-destructive alteration of the plasma membrane. Biochim Biophys Acta 1461: 123–134.
30. Rubenstrunk A, Mahfoudi A, Scherman D (2004) Delivery of electric pulses for DNA electrotransfer to mouse muscle does not induce the expression of stress related genes. Cell Biol Toxicol 20: 25–31.
31. Bertrand A, Ngo-Muller V, Hentzen D, Concordet JP, Daegelen D, et al. (2003) Muscle electrotransfer as a tool for studying muscle fiber-specific and nerve-dependent activity of promoters. Am J Physiol Cell Physiol 285: C1071–1081.

17

Transcellular Targeting of Fiber- and Hexon-Modified Adenovirus Vectors across the Brain Microvascular Endothelial Cells *In Vitro*

Johanna P. Laakkonen[1], Tatjana Engler[1], Ignacio A. Romero[2¤a], Babette Weksler[2¤b], Pierre-Olivier Couraud[2,3,4], Florian Kreppel[1], Stefan Kochanek[1]*

1 Department of Gene Therapy, University of Ulm, Ulm, Germany, **2** Inserm, U1016, Cochin Institute, Paris, France, **3** CNRS, UMR8104, Paris, France, **4** University Paris Descartes, Paris, France

Abstract

In central nervous system (CNS)-directed gene therapy, efficient targeting of brain parenchyma through the vascular route is prevented by the endothelium and the epithelium of the blood-brain and the blood-cerebrospinal fluid barriers, respectively. In this study, we evaluated the feasibility of the combined genetic and chemical adenovirus capsid modification technology to enable transcellular delivery of targeted adenovirus (Ad) vectors across the blood-brain barrier (BBB) *in vitro* models. As a proof-of-principle ligand, maleimide-activated full-length human transferrin (hTf) was covalently attached to cysteine-modified Ad serotype 5 vectors either to its fiber or hexon protein. In transcytosis experiments, hTf-coupled vectors were shown to be redirected across the BBB models, the transcytosis activity of the vectors being dependent on the location of the capsid modification and the *in vitro* model used. The transduction efficiency of hTf-targeted vectors decreased significantly in confluent, polarized cells, indicating that the intracellular route of the vectors differed between unpolarized and polarized cells. After transcellular delivery the majority of the hTf-modified vectors remained intact and partly capable of gene transfer. Altogether, our results demonstrate that i) covalent attachment of a ligand to Ad capsid can mediate transcellular targeting across the cerebral endothelium *in vitro*, ii) the attachment site of the ligand influences its transcytosis efficiency and iii) combined genetic/chemical modification of Ad vector can be used as a versatile platform for the development of Ad vectors for transcellular targeting.

Editor: Eric J. Kremer, French National Centre for Scientific Research, France

Funding: This work was supported by Academy of Finland (130242), Finnish Cultural Foundation (00107022) and the EU (NoE Clinigene - LSHB-CT-2006-018933). The funders had no role in study design, data collection and analysis, decision to publish, or preparation of the manuscript.

Competing Interests: The authors have declared that no competing interests exist.

* E-mail: stefan.kochanek@uni-ulm.de

¤a Current address: Department of Life Sciences, The Open University, Milton Keynes, United Kingdom
¤b Current address: Cornell University, New York, United States of America

Introduction

The endothelial cells of the blood-brain barrier (BBB), lining the inner surface of the brain capillary endothelium, form the major barrier to the passage of macromolecules, circulating cells and pharmaceutical drugs from blood to brain parenchyma. To develop treatments for central nervous system (CNS) disorders such as Multiple Sclerosis, Alzheimer's or Parkinson's disease, numerous studies have attempted to enhance drug or vector delivery across the BBB by targeting receptor molecules residing on the luminal side of the brain microvascular endothelial cells known to be involved in transcytosis [1,2]. Previously, various *in vitro* BBB models have been used as valuable tools to estimate the potency of the drugs or vectors to cross the brain endothelium [3]. *In vivo*, receptor-mediated transcytosis across the BBB has been suggested with molecules such as iron-transferrin, melanotransferrin, insulin, TNF-alpha and leptin [1,2,4] and absorptive or fluid-phase transcytosis with molecules such as albumin, immunoglobulin G, wheat germ agglutinin and avidin [5]. The transcellular delivery and internalization of vectors based on viruses, antibodies, protein carriers, liposomes, or nanoparticles has been shown to be dependent on various parameters such as their solubility, size, charge and receptor-ligand interactions [2,6].

Human adenovirus serotype 5 vectors (Ad5) are among the most efficient gene transfer vectors available for CNS-directed gene therapy into non-dividing cells [7–9]. In brain tissue, long-term Ad-mediated gene expression [10] and transcriptional targeting by tissue specific promoters [11,12] have previously been demonstrated after intracranial injection. Besides inflammatory responses upon vector administration into the brain [11,13,14], small injection volumes in stereotactic delivery as well as poor spreading of the Ad vectors in brain parenchyma have limited the development of gene therapy strategies for neurological disorders. While many studies have shown successful transduction of peripheral endothelial cells and unpolarized cerebral endothelial cells by tropism-modified Ad vectors [15,16], Ad-mediated gene delivery in or across confluent, polarized cerebral endothelial cells has received less attention. Recently, for the first time, tropism-modified Ad vectors were shown to be targeted across bovine brain microvascular endothelium by LRP-receptor mediated transcytosis [17], showing that the size of Ad vectors did not inhibit the transcellular delivery *in vitro*. To date, no *in vitro* studies of targeted Ad delivery across human brain microvascular endothelium by transcytosis have been presented.

Previously, we demonstrated genetic introduction of cysteine residues into the Ad fiber, hexon or pIX proteins enabling covalent attachment of maleimide-activated ligands to defined sites of the Ad vector capsid [18–20]. In this study, we utilized the cysteine-based targeting platform of Ad vectors to analyze whether Ad5 vectors could be targeted across polarized brain microvascular endothelium *in vitro* by using a known transcytotic ligand, human transferrin. Despite of transductional targeting of the Ad vectors to non-polarized brain microcapillary endothelial cells by transferrin receptor (TfR) -targeted peptide motifs (Xia et al. 2000), no previous studies have been performed in polarized BBB cell models, which have unique receptor patterns on their apical/basolateral side, restricted paracellular passage and transcellular delivery mechanisms. In the present study, we demonstrate that i) transductional targeting of Ad vectors in the cerebral endothelial cells is dependent on the cellular integrity of the polarized brain microvascular endothelium, ii) Ad vectors do not disrupt the brain microvascular endothelium integrity, iii) transferrin-receptor targeted Ad vectors can be delivered across the endothelial cell barrier *in vitro*, and that iv) majority of the targeted vectors remain intact after their transcellular delivery. In summary, we demonstrate that combined genetic/chemical modification of Ad vectors may be used as a platform for development of Ad vectors with improved transcytosis activity.

Results

Unpolarized Human Brain Microvascular Endothelial Cells are Highly Susceptible to Transferrin-Coupled Ad Vectors

Previously, we demonstrated the successful production and transductional targeting of cysteine modified Ad vectors [18–20]. In this study, transferrin coupled cysteine-bearing Ad vectors were utilized for transcellular targeting across the brain microvascular endothelium *in vitro*. To chemically couple human transferrin (hTf) to cysteine-modified Ad vectors, maleimide activation of hTf was performed with a heterobifunctional crosslinker, followed by coupling of activated hTf to thiol groups of the fiber HI loop (AdFiberCys) or the hypervariable region 5 of hexon (AdHexonCys, Fig. 1A). Successful coupling was confirmed by western blot analysis and chemiluminescence detection by Ad fiber or hexon antibodies (data not shown) as previously presented [19,20].

To detect the transductional targeting of hTf-coupled Ad vectors, vector-mediated EGFP expression was analyzed by flow cytometry in the immortalized human brain microvascular endothelial cells (hCMEC/D3) and in the non-endothelial human hematopoietic (K562) cell line, known to express the human transferrin receptor (hTfR) on their surface [21,22]. Flow cytometry experiments at 24 hrs post transduction (p.t.) in semiconfluent, unpolarized hCMEC/D3 cells showed that hTfR-targeted fiber-modified vectors had a 1.3 and 1.8-fold higher transduction efficiency than the untargeted control vectors at pMOIs of 200 and 5000 (expression percentages 33.8% and 75.4%, Fig. 1C, $P<0.01$), resulting in increased transgene expression in 62.9%±0.92 and 94.3%±0.31 of cells, respectively (Fig. 1C, $P<0.01$). In contrast, hTf-coupled hexon-modified vectors had a 1.5-fold and 2.4-fold lower transduction efficiency (19.5% and 80.9%) than corresponding untargeted control vectors (48.6% and 94.3%, Figs. 1C, $P<0.01$). In line with our previous studies (Kreppel et al. 2005), EGFP transgene expression of hTfR-targeted fiber-modified vectors increased up to 12-fold in K562 cells (41.3% and 94.9%, Fig. 1B) in comparison to AdFiberCys transduced cells (9.58% and 55.8%). The transduction efficiency of hTfR-targeted hexon-modified vectors instead decreased by 12 to 20-fold (1.2% and 19.0%, Fig. 1B) compared with their corresponding untargeted control vectors (17.9% and 68.0%).

Since the transduction efficiency of unpolarized hCMEC/D3 cells with hTfR-targeted hexon-modified Ad vectors was significantly higher than in K562 cells (pMOIs 1000–5000), we hypothesized that unspecific fluid-phase endocytosis could be involved in the uptake of the vectors in hCMEC/D3 cells. Therefore, the activity of unspecific fluid-phase endocytosis in the absence or presence of Ad vectors was determined by flow cytometry using 70 kDa FITC-dextran. After 1 hr uptake, untransduced hCMEC/D3 cells were detected to have 10-fold more active internalization of dextran than the corresponding untransduced K562 cells (Fig. 1D). However, no significant change of dextran uptake was detected in the presence of untargeted Ad vectors at pMOIs of 200 and 5000, respectively ($P>0.1$, Fig. 1D, pMOI 5000; pMOI 200, data not shown). In addition to dextran uptake, expression of hCAR, the primary receptor of Ad5, was determined in unpolarized hCMEC/D3 cells by immunolabeling experiments. By flow cytometry, hCAR expression was detected in 34.4%±2.34% of hCMEC/D3 cells (data not shown), whereas expression has been shown to be nearly non-existent in K562 cells [23]. Altogether, these data suggest that in unpolarized hCMEC/D3 cells the uptake of fiber-modified Ad vector is in part mediated by the transferrin receptor. However, regardless of the TfR-targeting, fluid-phase endocytosis may also contribute to the uptake of all the vectors in hCMEC/D3 cells but is not further enhanced by high vector doses. Additionally, hCAR-mediated entry of hexon-modified vectors may increase their uptake into hCMEC/D3 cells. Since both vector types expressed their transgenes efficiently in hCMEC/D3 at high pMOIs, the decreased transduction efficiencies of hexon-modified vectors in K562 cells (pMOIs 200–5000) is likely due to aberrant intracellular trafficking of the vectors [24,25].

Transduction Efficiency of Brain Microvascular Endothelial Cells is Dependent on the Cellular Integrity of the Polarized Endothelium

To study the transductional and transcellular targeting into/across the endothelium barrier *in vitro*, two-compartment endothelial cellular models are required. Here, hCMEC/D3 cells cultured on collagen-coated Transwell-filters were used to determine the targeting ability of hTf-coupled Ad vectors. Previously, hCMEC/D3 cells have shown to retain many characteristics of primary brain capillary endothelial cells and to form a highly restrictive endothelium barrier [26]. In this study, for transcytosis and transduction experiments in polarized cells, hCMEC/D3 cells were grown for 6–7 days on a Transwell system with an apical chamber containing a collagen-coated insert (pore size 0.4 µm, apical side) and a bottom, basolateral chamber (Fig. 2A). Prior to experiments with virus vectors, the cell monolayer integrity was analyzed by measuring the passage of small ions i.e. transendothelial electrical resistance (TEER) or diffusion of fluorescent markers across the endothelium. TEER was measured from each well as a triplicate with Endohm Millicell device. In hCMEC/D3 endothelial monolayers, all transcytosis experiments were performed at TEER values 50–75 Ω/cm^2 (Fig. 2B). In addition, permeability coefficient for lucifer yellow (LY) and 70 kDa FITC-Dextran was determined. All obtained permeability values were shown to be in the range

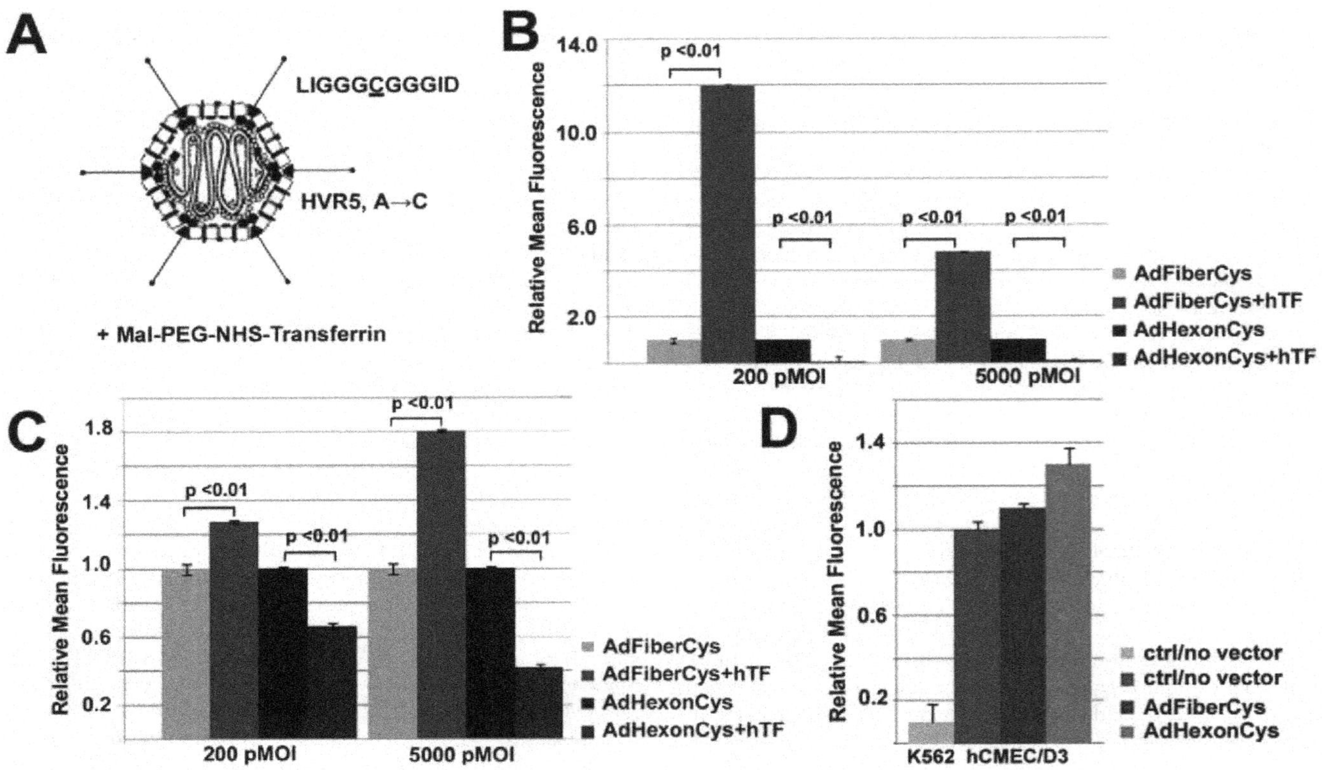

Figure 1. Covalent attachment of maleimide-activated human transferrin to cysteine-modified Ad vectors and their transduction efficiency in hTfR-positive human brain microvascular endothelial cells. A) Schematic illustration of Ad vector particles containing a solvent-exposed cysteine either on fiber (LIGGGCGGGID) or hexon (HRV5, alanine to cysteine substitution), to which maleimide-activated transferrin is covalently attached (for details see materials and methods). B–C) Relative transduction efficiency of fiber (AdFiberCys) and hexon-modified (AdHexonCys) vectors with or without covalently attached transferrin in K562 (B) and hCMEC/D3 (C) cells at 24 hrs p.t. by flow cytometry (multiplicities of infection based on particles (pMOIs) 200 and 5000). Relative mean fluorescence and standard deviations are shown (n = 3, 10.000 cells/sample). D) Cellular uptake of the fluid-phase endocytosis marker 70 kDa FITC-Dextran in untransduced K562 and hCMEC/D3 and transduced hCMEC/D3 cells (pMOI 5000) after 1 hr uptake at 37°C determined by flow cytometry. Relative mean fluorescence normalized to untransduced hCMEC/D3 cells, as well as standard deviations are shown (n = 3, 10.000 cells/sample).

of published permeability index values (Poller et al. 2008) i.e. 0.81×10^{-3} cm/min for LY and 0.05×10^{-3} cm/min for FITC-Dextran (n = 3 monolayers), resembling the tight characteristics of the monolayers. To detect the impact of Ad vectors on the hCMEC/D3 barrier integrity and functionality, TEER was measured before and after transcytosis experiments. The resistances of the monolayers were unchanged during the 4 hr-experiments with all vector types and particle amounts (Fig. 2C, *P*-values >0.1).

To assess the vector transduction efficiency in polarized brain endothelium, known to express TfR only on their apical side, hCMEC/D3 cells were cultured on Transwell filters to confluency for 6–7 days (TEER >50 Ω/cm^2) and transduced for 24 hrs with Ad vectors. By fluorescence microscopy, the percentage of cells expressing EGFP was visibly lower with all the vectors than in unpolarized hCMEC/D3 cells without the barrier properties (data not shown). By further analysis with fluorimetry, uncoupled fiber-modified Ad vectors were shown to transduce polarized endothelium more efficiently than the corresponding hTf-coupled vectors (Fig. 2D, *P*<0.01). This suggests that in polarized cells hTf-coupled Ad vectors had a limited accessibility to TfRs or that the vectors were redirected to a different cellular route than in non-polarized endothelial cells.

Transferrin-Receptor Targeted Ad Vectors are Delivered Across the Brain Endothelial Barrier

To determine the ability of hTf-targeted Ad vectors to be transported across the endothelium barrier, the experiments were performed in the hCMEC/D3 Transwell cell model. Unmodified or modified Ad vectors (2×10^8, 1×10^9 or 5×10^9 VPs) were added to Transwell plates for 4 hrs and the medium from the basolateral side was collected. To validate the copy numbers of transcytosed viral particles, real-time quantitative PCR (qPCR) for the Ad fiber or E4 gene was performed. The cellular barrier integrity was monitored by measuring TEER before and after incubation with Ad vectors to confirm that vector delivery to the basolateral side was not due to leakage of the endothelial barrier.

With hTf-coupled fiber-modified vectors, 2.4-fold increase in transport across the polarized hCMEC/D3 cells was observed in comparison to untargeted control vectors (Fig. 3A, 3C, p<0.05, 1×10^9 VPs, 2.57%; n = 6 monolayers). The copy numbers of vectors detected on the basolateral side increased with higher vector dose. Interestingly, with a lower vector dose (2×10^8 VPs), more untargeted vector (AdFiberCys) was detected on the basolateral side than with TfR-targeted vectors (*P*<0.01, n = 3 monolayers), implying that the vector uptake, recycling to apical side or delivery mechanisms across the cell monolayer differed between the targeted and untargeted vectors. Notably, no

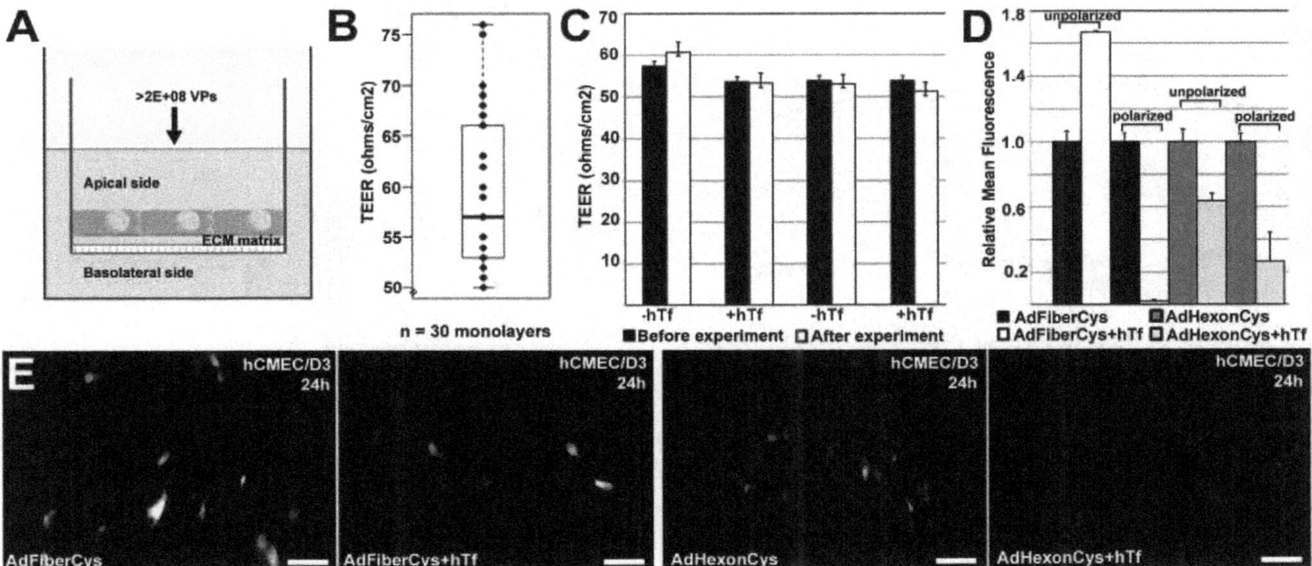

Figure 2. Integrity of hcmec/d3 endothelium in the presence of Ad vectors and their transduction efficiencies in polarized cells. A) Schematic illustration of the *in vitro* hCMEC/D3 endothelium model on collagen-coated 0.4 µm-Transwell filters. Cells are grown to confluency for 6–7 days in EBM-2 media, after which the barrier properties of the endothelium are measured by voltohmeter and permeability assays with fluorescent markers. Extracellular matrix (ECM), filter, and apical and basolateral sides of the Transwell chamber are shown. B) Transendothelial electrical resistance (TEER) values of hCMEC/D3 monolayers after 6 days in culture ($59.4 \pm 1.5\ \Omega/cm^2$; mean±S.E., n = 30 monolayers). Boxplot data is shown, containing median (bar), quartile range (box) and minimum and maximum values (whiskers). C) Representative TEER values of hCMEC/D3 monolayers before and after 4 hrs incubation with hexon (AdHexonCys, 5×10^9 VPs/monolayer) or fiber-modified (AdFiberCys, 1×10^9 VPs/monolayer) vectors with or without human transferrin (n = 3–4 monolayers/vector). In all experiments, TEER measurements were performed as triplicates with Milli-Cell ERS equipment (mean $\Omega/cm^2 \pm$SD, $P>0.1$). D–E) Transduction efficiencies of fiber or hexon-modified vectors with or without transferrin in unpolarized or transwell-cultured, polarized hCMEC/D3 cells at 24 hrs p.t. detected by fluorimetry (D; n = 3 monolayers, TEER $>60\ \Omega/cm^2$) or fluorescence microscopy (E; polarized cells). Relative mean fluorescence and standard deviation is calculated from the obtained mean fluorescence values. Scale bars in the images, 50 µm.

significant changes in TEER values were detected between 0 to 4 hrs after adding the Ad vectors, indicating that the hCMEC/D3 cells maintained a functional barrier (data not shown).

With hexon-modified vectors, re-targeting of hTf-coupled vectors was also detected at higher vector dose (Fig. 3B, $P<0.05$, 1×10^9 VPs, n = 6 monolayers). However, overall percentage of the targeted transcytosed vectors remained low (0.63%, Fig. 3C). No targeting with lower vector dose was detected (2×10^8 VPs, n = 3 monolayers). To analyze the transcytosis capability of hTf-modified Ad vectors further and determine their ability to be used in CNS-directed targeting in general, another BBB cell model based on primary porcine brain capillary endothelial cells (PBCEC) was used. The PBCEC model is known to have one of the highest TEER values *in vitro* and a very low cell monolayer permeability [27–29]. Here, all experiments in PBCEC cells were performed as TEER reached >600 ohms/cm^2. With hTf-targeted fiber-modified vectors, no reliable vector copy amounts were detected by qPCR either with E4 or fiber primers, due to the extremely low vector presence in the basolateral media (data not shown, n = 3 monolayers). However, a 3.7-fold increase of hTf-targeted AdHexonCys delivery across the cell monolayer was detected (Fig. 3C, 0.21%, 5×10^9 VPs, n = 2–3 monolayers).

Part of the Re-targeted Ad Vectors Remains Capable of Gene Transfer after Transcellular Targeting

To test whether transferrin-modified vectors remained intact and DNAse resistant after delivery, transcytosed vectors were treated with heat and/or DNAse prior to virus DNA extraction and analysis by qPCR. In comparison to non-treated transcytosed vectors, the majority of heat and DNAse treated transcytosed vectors were degraded (Fig. 4A), whereas DNAse treatment alone decreased the transcytosed viral DNA detection by only 1.3 to 1.5-fold. The data therefore indicated that the majority of the vector DNA remained encapsulated and DNAse resistant after the transcellular delivery.

Previously, cellular uptake of hTf across the BBB has been shown to occur by receptor-mediated endocytosis, followed by the release of iron-transferrin to brain parenchyma [30]. To determine whether transcytosis and endosomal delivery also affected the gene transfer capability of transcytosed Ad vectors, transduction studies in hTfR positive 293 cells were performed using the basolateral media collected from the Transwell chambers after transcytosis. By fluorescence microscopy vector-mediated EGFP expression was detected at 16 hrs p.t., showing that some of the transcytosed Ad vectors remained functional and the cellular processes did not harm the integrity of the vectors (Fig. 4B–C). hTf-coupled fiber-modified vectors were shown to have approximately an 1.5-fold increase in their transgene expression compared to unmodified control vectors after their transcellular delivery (Fig. 4B, n = 500 cells). No transgene expression was detected in the corresponding experiments with the PBCEC cells (data not shown). With the hexon-modified vectors hTf-coupling led to a 2.3-fold decrease in EGFP transgene expression after their transcellular delivery across hCMEC/D3 (Figs. 4B–C, n = 400–500 cells) and 4.1-fold decrease in PBCEC cells, respectively (data not shown).

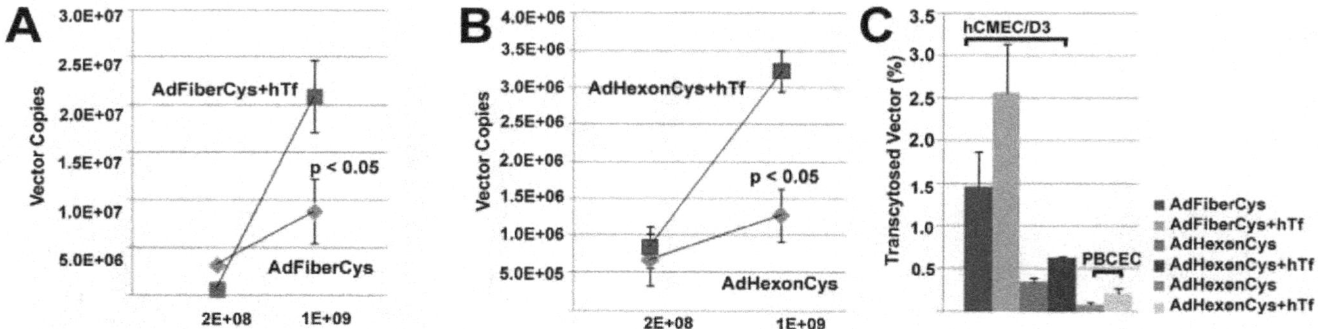

Figure 3. Delivery of transferrin-coupled fiber-modified Ad vectors across the endothelium barrier. A, B) After transcytosis experiments in Transwell plates, qPCR was performed from the basolateral media using Ad fiber and E4 primers. The corresponding Ad copy number was determined by the standard curve of linearized pGS66 plasmid. The detected vector copy numbers of fiber- (A) and hexon-modified vectors (B) are shown (2×10^8, n = 2–3 monolayers; and 1×10^9 VPs, $P<0.05$, n = 6 monolayers; mean ± S.E.). C) Transcytosis percentages of the vectors after transcellular delivery detected by qPCR across hCMEC/D3 and PBCEC cells (1×10^9 and 5×10^9 VPs). The percentages were calculated by comparing the detected copy numbers of the input vector to the copy numbers on the basolateral side.

Discussion

In brain disorders, inefficient cellular targeting and distribution of therapeutic macromolecules have been restricting the development of brain-related gene therapy strategies. Since only <2% of small drug molecules are able to cross the BBB after systemic administration and large molecules are believed not to pass the BBB at all [31], CNS-directed gene therapy has mainly been based on intracranial injections [9]. Besides the invasive surgical procedures, numerous localized injections are typically needed for sufficient gene delivery. Since most of the CNS diseases are currently poorly or not treatable with small molecule therapies [32], development of gene therapy vectors suitable for overcoming the BBB non-invasively upon systemic administration has been suggested [17,33]. In the present study, we evaluated the feasibility of combined genetic and chemical Ad capsid modification to target Ad vectors across the BBB *in vitro* by transcytosis. As a proof-of-principle ligand we used human transferrin, a well characterized transcytotic ligand which has been shown to bind TfR on the luminal side of the brain endothelial cells and to be delivered to brain parenchyma after receptor-mediated uptake [1,30]. In this paper, we showed that transferrin led to enhanced transcellular delivery of fiber- and hexon-modified Ad vectors across the polarized brain endothelium *in vitro*, the transport being approximately 2 to 4-fold higher than that of untargeted control vector. Importantly, the targeted vectors stayed largely intact and partly functional after transcytosis, showing the potential of the combined genetic and chemical modification of Ad vectors in successful transcellular targeting.

In vitro cerebral endothelium models have been shown to be valuable tools for development of pharmacological drug delivery and gene therapy, being solely based on primary or immortalized brain microvascular endothelial cells or cocultures of astrocytes and/or pericytes. In this study, we used two *in vitro* BBB models, immortalized hCMEC/D3 and primary PBCEC cells, which have been shown to form highly restrictive endothelium barriers and to have similar permeability characteristics than primary human brain microvascular endothelial cells [21,26–28,34]. Similarly as in previous studies with the bovine brain endothelium with untargeted Ad5 [35] or melanotransferrin-targeted Ad5 vectors [17,35], no significant changes of TEER were observed in the presence of Ad vectors with or without transferrin, thus implying that the Ad vectors did not alter the interendothelial integrity of the cerebral endothelium. Interestingly, despite of the high TfR expression on the apical side of polarized hCMEC/D3 cells [21] and transgene expression in unpolarized hCMEC/D3 cells (20–60% efficiencies, 200 pMOI), poor transduction efficiencies of iron-transferrin targeted Ad vectors were detected in polarized hCMEC/D3 cells. This strongly indicated that in polarized brain endothelium, the majority of iron-transferrin targeted Ad vectors were redirected to another cellular entry route leading either to recycling of vectors back to the apical side, lysosomal degradation or transcellular delivery of the vectors across the endothelium.

For gene therapy purposes, virus vectors need to stay intact and capable of gene transfer after their transcellular delivery. Recently, systemic administration of rAAV9 was shown to lead to transduction of astrocytes in adult mice (Foust et al. 2009). Additionally, *in vitro* transcellular delivery of HIV-1 (0.01–0.77% at 24 hrs p.t), AAV4, AAV5 or BAAV (3–15% at 3 hrs p.t) and melanotransferrin-targeted Ad5 (5% at 6 hrs p.t.) have been detected to cross the BBB *in vitro* models, simultaneously retaining their infectivity or capability for gene transfer [35,36]. In this study, targeting of Ad5 by iron-transferrin led to enhanced transcytosis of fiber- and hexon-modified vectors. The targeting across the endothelium was shown to be dose-dependent, being characteristics of receptor-mediated uptake. With hexon-modified Ad vectors, transcytosis percentage remained modest (0.6% at 4 hrs p.t.), whereas 2.6% of fiber-modified vectors were able to cross the human *in vitro* BBB model. The experiments in primary porcine cerebral endothelium showed transport of 0.2% of the hexon-modified Ad vectors across the cells and no transcellular targeting of the fiber-modified vectors, implying that the mode and activity of transcellular delivery vary between immortalized and primary brain microvascular endothelial cells. Similar to studies with untargeted AAV viruses [35] the majority of the TfR-targeted Ad vectors were shown to remain intact after their transcellular delivery. Additionally, transcytosed vectors were able to mediate transgene expression. The delivery of the vectors across the brain endothelium in transcellular vesicles thus did not seem to impair the majority of the capsids. Notably, as in previous Ad vector studies [17] non-specific crossing of the endothelium by untargeted vectors was observed, probably due to undetected paracellular leakage. In our study, human brain microvascular endothelium seemed to be more permeable to human Ad5 vectors than primary porcine cells were, which might be due to species specific differences between the human and non-human brain endothe-

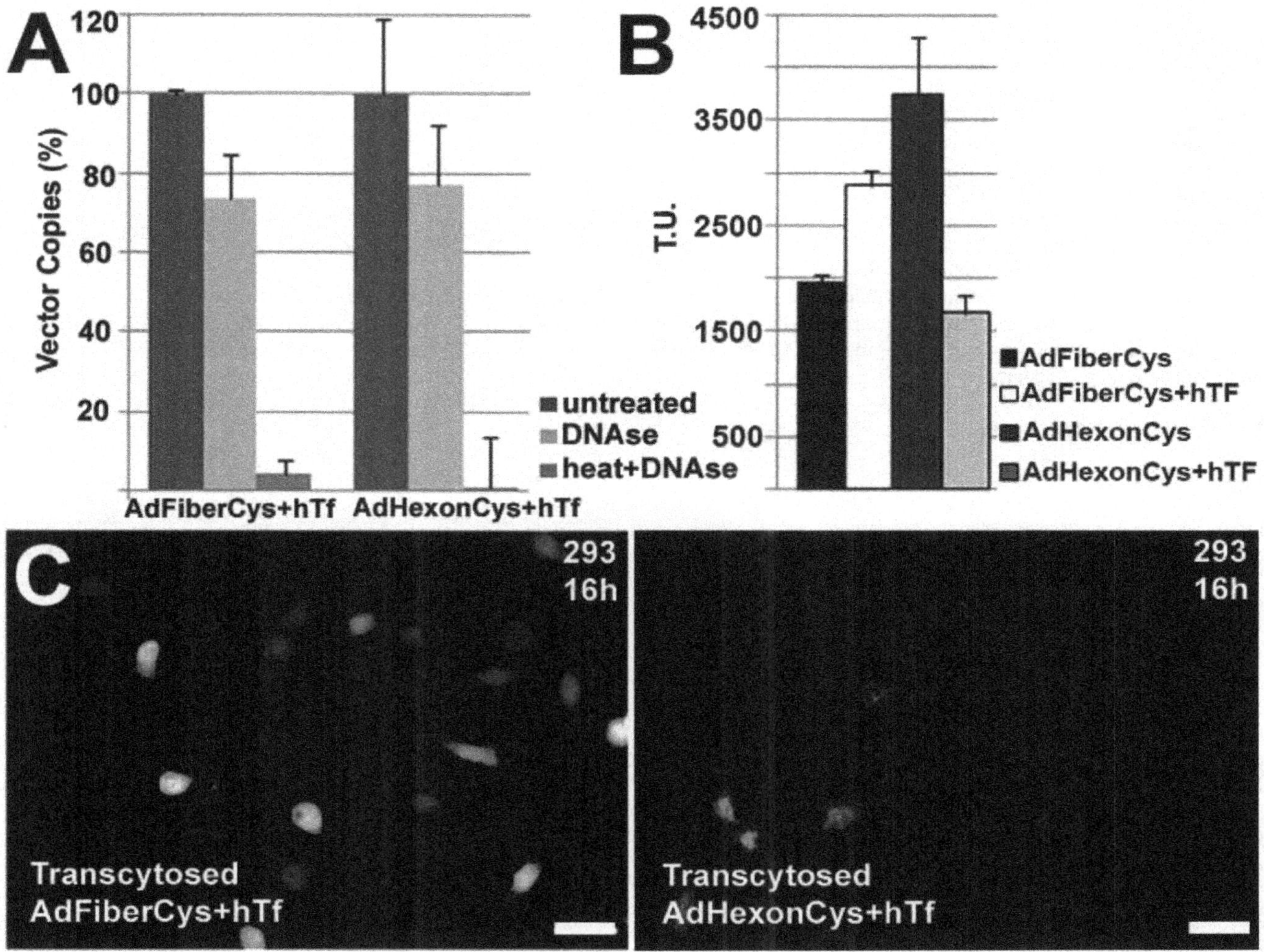

Figure 4. Delivery of transferrin-coupled hexon-modified Ad vectors across the endothelium barrier. A) qPCR detection of the transcytosed hTf-coupled vectors after DNAse treatment and viral DNA isolation. Heat and DNAse treated vectors, as well as untreated vectors were used as controls. The percentages were calculated by comparing the detected copy numbers of the untreated vector to the copy numbers of the transcytosed vector. B–C) Gene transfer efficiency of transcytosed hTf-coupled vectors in 293 cells at 16 hrs p.t. as determined by fluorescence microscopy. For quantification, six to eight random areas were imaged and the cells were counted with the help of ImageJ Cell Counter. Transduction units (T.U.) presented were counted from the total sample volume obtained on the basolateral side of the hCMEC/D3 cells (n = 500 cells, mean ± S.E.). Scale bars in all images, 20 µm.

lium or differences between immortalized and primary brain microvascular endothelial cells, such as tightness of the cell monolayer, variations in receptor expression patterns or differences in the mode and activity of transcellular delivery mechanisms. However, as Ad vectors were clearly targeted by iron-transferrin across the human brain microvascular endothelium without affecting the TEER, we can conclude that hCMEC/D3 cell model is suitable for screening ligands for Ad vector mediated transcellular targeting.

In order to circumvent the BBB and to deliver therapeutic macromolecules to brain parenchyma, multiple delivery approaches have been attempted, e.g. intrathecal injection to the cerebrospinal fluid, intracisternal administration to ventricles, intranasal delivery and intracarotid infusion of hyperosmolar solutions or vasoactive drugs. Restricted diffusion of the vector and cerebral edema due to the disrupted BBB has been the limiting factors of these approaches. Numerous factors have also been shown to affect the vectors targeted to cross the BBB by receptor-mediated transcytosis after intravenous administration, such as competitive receptor binding with endogenous ligands, irreversible antibody-antigen binding, species-specific differences between receptor expression patterns, charge of the target ligand, high expression of target receptors in the peripheral capillaries and immune reactions against the vectors [1,6]. So far very little has been known about the transcellular targeting of large particles such as gene therapy vectors across the human microvascular brain endothelial cells. While our data demonstrate the general feasibility of Ad targeting *in vitro*, our model ligand is likely to be suboptimal for *in vivo* purposes due to competition of receptor binding by the endogenous transferrin and Ad vector targeting to liver after intravenous administration. Therefore, our Ad capsid modification technology will be used to study the transcellular targeting of novel transcytotic ligands derived from bacteria or viruses, which have been suggested to be involved in the transcellular delivery of large pathogens across the BBB *in vivo* [37]. In regard to *in vivo* transcellular targeting of Ad5 vectors, hexon based PEGylation combined with coupling of transcytotic ligands to the Ad fiber may be an option to enhance Ad5 vector targeting across anatomical barriers, as polymer coating may decrease capsid interaction with cellular or non-cellular compartments.

To conclude, our data indicate that i) virus vectors can be targeted across the brain microvascular endothelial cells *in vitro* by chemically attaching transcytotic ligands on their capsid surface, ii) full-length protein attached to the Ad vector surface is capable of mediating transcellular targeting *in vitro* and that iii) attachment site of the ligand on Ad capsid affects to the transcytosis efficiency of the vectors. This study also suggests that combined genetic/chemical modification of Ad vector with targeting ligands can be used as a versatile platform for the development of Ad vectors with improved transcytosis activity.

Materials and Methods

Cells and Cell Barrier Models

Human embryonic kidney cells (293, ATCC CRL-1573) and lung carcinoma epithelial cells (A549, ATCC CCL-185) were cultured in MEM, the human erythroleukemia cell line K562 (ATCC CCL-243) in RPMI-1640 and human N52.E6 cells (Schiedner et al. 2000) in α-MEM (Invitrogen, Eugene, OR). All cell lines were supplemented with 10% fetal calf serum (FCS) and 1% penicillin/streptomycin (Invitrogen) and subcultured twice a week.

The human BBB *in vitro* model based on immortalized human brain capillary endothelial cells (hCMEC/D3) has been described previously [26]. Briefly, hCMEC/D3 cell line was generated by isolating brain microvascular endothelial cells from the human brain tissue, followed by immortalization with catalytic subunit of human telomerase and SV40-T antigen. hCMEC/D3 cells used in the experiments of this report were between passages 25 to 35, and were routinely cultured on plates coated with rat-tail collagen type I (0.15 mg/ml; Cultrex, R&D Systems Inc., Minneapolis, MN) at a cell density of 27.000 cells/cm^2. The cells were grown in the endothelial basal medium (EBM-2; Clonetics, Cambrex BioScience, Wokingham, UK) supplemented with human basic fibroblast growth factor (bFGF, 1 ng/ml), hydrocortisone (1.4 μM), ascorbic acid (5 μg/ml; Sigma-Aldrich, St. Louis, MO), penicillin-streptomycin (1%), chemically defined lipid concentrate (1%; Invitrogen) and FBS Gold (5%; PAA Laboratories GmbH, Pasching, Austria). For transwell assays, hCMEC/D3 cells were cultured at a density of 10.000 cells/mm^2 on collagen-coated, 0.4 μm PTFE Transwells (Corning Inc., Corning, NY) for 6–7 days.

Integrity and functionality of the cultured cell monolayers were analyzed by measuring the transendothelial electrical resistance (TEER) using a volt/ohm meter (World Precision Instruments, Sarasota, FL/Millipore, Bedford, MA). The resistance of the collagen-coated inserts without cells was substracted from the resistance generated by the cell monolayers. Transcytosis assays were performed as TEER reached >50 ohms/cm^2 [26]. TEER was measured routinely before and after the experiments with Ad vectors. Permeability assays based on the diffusion of lucifer yellow (LY; MW 457.25, Sigma-Aldrich) and 70 kDa dextran-FITC (De-FITC, Invitrogen) were performed as previously described [38]. Permeability coefficients were calculated according to published algorithms and compared to known permeability index of hCMEC/D3 cells (LY$<1.33\times10^{-3}$ cm/min, De-FITC$<0.06\times10^{-3}$ cm/min; [21].

Primary porcine brain capillary endothelial cells (PBCEC) were obtained or isolated according to established protocols [27–29]. Prior to transcytosis experiments the transwell inserts were coated with rat tail collagen (133 μg/ml, Sigma-Aldrich; 0.4 μm pore size polycarbonate filters, Corning Inc.) for 4 hrs and thawed cells were cultured at a density of 250.000 cells/filter for 5 days. Integrity of PBCEC monolayers were analyzed by measuring TEER using a voltohmeter in an electrode chamber. The cells were grown in serum-free DMEM/Hams F12 medium (Biochrom), supplemented with hydrocortisone (0.55 μM), L-glutamine (4.1 mM, Biochrom), penicillin-streptomycin (1%) and gentamycin (1%; Sigma-Aldrich). Transcytosis assays were performed in PBCEC cells as TEER reached >600 ohms/cm^2.

Ad Vector Production and Titration

Ad5-based E1-deleted first generation vectors were used, expressing EGFP under control of the hCMV promoter. AdFiberCys contains the peptide motif LIGGGCGGGID inserted in the fiber HI loop after amino acid 543 of the fiber protein sequence (size ~110 nm; [19]. In AdHexonCys an alanine residue (amino acid position 273 in GenBank:AAQ19298.1) in the hypervariable region 5 of hexon was exchanged for a cysteine residue by mutating the corresponding alanine codon GCC (nt position 19658 in GenBank:AY339865.1) to TGC ([20]. All vectors were produced in E1-transcomplementing N52.E6 cells [39], followed by subsequent purification by CsCl gradients (step and isopycnic) and desalting by gel filtration (PD-10; Amersham, Buckinghamshire, UK). Cysteine-bearing vectors were purified under reducing conditions as described previously [19]. Vectors were stored at −80°C in PBS supplemented with 10% glycerol. Viral titers were determined by DNA-based slot blot procedure in A549 cells [19,20].

Covalent Chemical Coupling of Transferrin to Ad Vectors

Human apotransferrin was kindly provided by Prof. E. Wagner (Dept. of Pharmacy, Center for Drug Research, Ludwig-Maximilians-Universität Munich, Munich, Germany) and chemically coupled to Ad vectors as previously described [19,20]. Briefly, to modify a surface amino group of apotransferrin with a thiol-reactive compound, apotransferrin was first incubated with NHS-PEG(3 kDa)-Mal crosslinker (Nektar Therapeutics, San Carlos, CA, PBS pH 7.3, molar ratio 1:1, 4 hrs, RT), followed by purification with size exclusion chromatography (Äkta Purifier, Amersham). To couple the maleimide-activated apotransferrin molecules covalently to the cysteine-bearing Ad vectors, 10^{11} vector particles were incubated with the maleimide-modified proteins overnight at RT in an argon atmosphere (molar ratio vector surface cysteine:maleimide, 1:30). Prior to all transduction or transcytosis experiments, iron was added to the cell culture media in order to enable the formation of iron-transferrin (hTf). For SDS-polyacrylamide gel electrophoresis and western blot analysis, transferrin was detected by horseradish peroxidase–labeled transferrin Ab (Bethyl Laboratories, Montgomery, TX). Virus proteins were identified by Ad5-fiber MAb (Ms IgG2a, DM3002; Acris GmbH, Hiddenhausen, Germany) or Ad5-hexon MAb (65H6, Ab Frontier, Seoul, Korea) using a horseradish peroxidase–labeled secondary Ab and the ECL kit (Thermo Fisher Scientific, Waltham, MA) for detection.

Flow Cytometry Assays

K562 or hCMEC/D3 cells were seeded into 24-well-plates with or without the collagen coating (100.000–150.000 cells/well). After 24 hrs, 200–5000 physical vector particles per cell (pMOI) were added to medium (300–500 μl) for 3 hrs. The medium was filled up to 1 ml and incubated up to 24 hrs. hCMEC/D3 cells were washed with PBS and detached with PBS containing 50 mM EDTA. Both cell lines were centrifuged (350–500 g, 5 min), followed by resuspension in PBS/2%FCS/20 mM EDTA. For dextran uptake assays in K562 or hCMEC/D3 cells, 1 mg/ml of 70 kDa FITC-Dextran was incubated with the cells for 1 h at 37°C or 4°C followed by extensive washes with PBS. For hCAR cell surface labeling experiments, hCMEC/D3 cells were first detached by trypsin and incubated with hCAR MAb (Acris GmbH) for 30 min on ice, followed by subsequent washing and incubation with goat anti-mouse Alexa-488 (30 min, dark). To confirm that trypsin treatment did not impair hCAR antibody recognition, similar experiment was performed in A549 cells, known to have a high hCAR expression.

Flow cytometric analysis of virus-mediated EGFP expression, dextran uptake or hCAR expression was performed with a Becton-Dickinson FACSCalibur without gating (Becton-Dickinson, Franklin Lakes, NJ). For virus expression experiments, relative transduction efficiencies were calculated from the mean fluorescence intensity. For dextran uptake assays, fluorescence values obtained from samples on ice were substracted from those obtained at 37°C.

Transwell Assays

Transcytosis assays were performed in Transwell-filter cultured hCMEC/D3 and PBCEC cells as TEER reached >50 ohms/cm^2 or >600 ohms/cm^2, respectively. Unmodified and modified Ad vectors (2×10^8, 1×10^9 or 5×10^9 viral particles/filter/300 µl of full medium) were added to the apical side of the Transwells and incubated for 4 hrs at 37°C, 5% CO_2. The medium from the basolateral side of the Transwell (800 µl) was collected, frozen (−80°C) and tested for the presence of transcytosed Ad particles by qPCR. To determine the intactness of the Ad particles, 20 µl of transcytosed vectors were diluted 10-fold to Tris-buffer (50 mM Tris, 1 mM $MgCl_2$, pH 8), followed by treatment with DNAse (Sigma-Aldrich, 100 U/ml, 15 min, 37°C). Untreated vectors or heat (10 min, 95°C) and DNAse treated vectors were used as controls. Virus DNA was isolated with virus spin kit (Qiagen, Hilden, Germany) and analyzed by qPCR. For gene delivery studies, transcytosed vectors were immediately used to transduce 293 cells in order to avoid unnecessary freeze-thawing of the vectors. For transgene expression experiments in polarized hCMEC/D3 cells, after collecting the basolateral media, the cells were transferred to new plates and incubated further up to 24 hrs at 37°C, 5% CO_2. The transduction efficiency was detected by fluorescence microscopy or fluorimetry (Twinkle LB970, Berthold Technologies, Bad Wildbad, Germany) after detaching the cells by scraping and diluting them to PBS-EDTA.

Quantitative Real-Time PCR

To determine the number of transcytosed vector particles, qPCR was performed from basolateral media using either Ad fiber or E4 primers and appropriate standards (fiber primers, AdFiberCys/AdHexonCys vectors: sense 5-GCTACAGTTT-CAGTTTTGGCTG-3, reverse 5-GTTGTGGCCAGAC-CAGTCCC-3, amplicon length 386 bp; E4 primers, AdFiberCys; sense 5-TAGACGATCCCTACTGTACG-3, reverse 5-CCGGACGTAGTCATATTTCC-3, amplicon length 96 bp). The corresponding Ad copy number was determined by standard curve of linearized plasmid pGS66 (r^2>0.995, E = >98%), containing the Ad vector genome (Schiedner et al., 2000). Five to ten microliters of virus spin kit isolated viral DNA (Qiagen) was added to a total of 25 µl reaction mixture consisting of primers (10 pmol) and 10 µl of 2x SYBR Green Master Mix (Stratagene, Agilent Technologies, Santa Clara, CA). Amplification was detected by MxPro3005p on 96-well plates (Stratagene, Agilent Technologies). Following denaturation at 95°C for 10 min, cycling conditions were 95°C for 30s, 60°C for 30s, 72°C for 30s for 40 cycles. The formation of primer dimers was monitored by gel electrophoresis of the PCR products and by the melting curves with MxPro3005p software. Total copy numbers of input vectors detected were between 60–90%. Data presented is shown either as copy numbers of the detected fiber or E4 gene or as the percentage of transcytosed virus from the applied input virus.

Gene Transfer Assay for Transcytosed Vectors

The functional integrity of the transcytosed vector particles was tested by examining their gene transfer efficiency in hTf-receptor positive 293 cells. For each experiment, 100–150 µl of collected basolateral media was used to transduce 293 cells for 16 hrs. Untransduced control cells were used to substract the autofluorescence and set-up the imaging settings. By fluorescence microscopy (Zeiss Axiovert 25, 20x/0.4 objective, Carl Zeiss AG, Oberkochen, Germany) and ImageJ [40] EGFP expressing cells were counted from six to eight random areas and compared to total amount of the cells in the same areas (n = 400–500 cells). Transduction units (t.u.) were calculated from the total sample volumes.

Statistical Analysis

The significance of the data was determined by Student's t-test or Wilcoxon-Mann-Whitney U-test (SPSS). Box plot data was done by R software (R Development Core Team, Vienna, Austria).

Acknowledgments

We thank Prof. Hans-Joachim Galla and Sabine Hüwel for introduction into and teaching of the PBCEC BBB model, for cells and advice.

Author Contributions

Conceived and designed the experiments: JPL FK SK. Performed the experiments: JPL TE. Analyzed the data: JPL. Contributed reagents/materials/analysis tools: IAR BW POC SK. Wrote the paper: JPL FK SK.

References

1. Lichota J, Skjorringe T, Thomsen LB, Moos T (2010) Macromolecular drug transport into the brain using targeted therapy. J Neurochem 113: 1–13.
2. Tuma PL, Hubbard AL (2003) Transcytosis: crossing cellular barriers. Physiol Rev 83: 871–932.
3. Cecchelli R, Berezowski V, Lundquist S, Culot M, Renftel M, et al. (2007) Modelling of the blood-brain barrier in drug discovery and development. Nat Rev Drug Discov 6: 650–661.
4. Jones AR, Shusta EV (2007) Blood-brain barrier transport of therapeutics via receptor-mediation. Pharm Res 24: 1759–1771.
5. Herve F, Ghinea N, Scherrmann JM (2008) CNS delivery via adsorptive transcytosis. Aaps J 10: 455–472.
6. Georgieva JV, Kalicharan D, Couraud PO, Romero IA, Weksler B, et al. (2010) Surface characteristics of nanoparticles determine their intracellular fate in and processing by human blood-brain barrier endothelial cells in vitro. Mol Ther 19: 318–325.
7. Glasgow JN, Everts M, Curiel DT (2006) Transductional targeting of adenovirus vectors for gene therapy. Cancer Gene Ther 13: 830–844.
8. Thomas CE, Ehrhardt A, Kay MA (2003) Progress and problems with the use of viral vectors for gene therapy. Nat Rev Genet 4: 346–358.
9. Manfredsson FP, Mandel RJ (2010) Development of gene therapy for neurological disorders. Discovery Medicine 9: 204–211.
10. Barcia C, Jimenez-Dalmaroni M, Kroeger KM, Puntel M, Rapaport AJ, et al (2007) One-year expression from high-capacity adenoviral vectors in the brains of animals with pre-existing anti-adenoviral immunity: clinical implications. Mol Ther 15: 2154–2163.
11. Smith-Arica JR, Morelli AE, Larregina AT, Smith J, Lowenstein PR, et al. (2000) Cell-type-specific and regulatable transgenesis in the adult brain: adenovirus-encoded combined transcriptional targeting and inducible transgene expression. Mol Ther 2: 579–587.

12. Miyoshi G, Fishell G (2006) Directing neuron-specific transgene expression in the mouse CNS. Curr Opin Neurobiol 16: 577–584.
13. Thomas CE, Edwards P, Wickham TJ, Castro MG, Lowenstein PR (2002) Adenovirus binding to the coxsackievirus and adenovirus receptor or integrins is not required to elicit brain inflammation but is necessary to transduce specific neural cell types. J Virol 76: 3452–3460.
14. Akli S, Caillaud C, Vigne E, Stratford-Perricaudet LD, Poenaru L, et al. (1993) Transfer of a foreign gene into the brain using adenovirus vectors. Nat Genet 3: 224–228.
15. Lindemann D, Schnittler H (2009) Genetic manipulation of endothelial cells by viral vectors. Thromb Haemost 102: 1135–1143.
16. Xia H, Anderson B, Mao Q, Davidson BL (2000) Recombinant human adenovirus: targeting to the human transferrin receptor improves gene transfer to brain microcapillary endothelium. J Virol 74: 11359–11366.
17. Tang Y, Han T, Everts M, Zhu ZB, Gillespie GY, et al. (2007) Directing adenovirus across the blood-brain barrier via melanotransferrin (P97) transcytosis pathway in an in vitro model. Gene Ther 14: 523–532.
18. Corjon S, Wortmann A, Engler T, van Rooijen N, Kochanek S, et al. (2008) Targeting of adenovirus vectors to the LRP receptor family with the high-affinity ligand RAP via combined genetic and chemical modification of the pIX capsomere. Mol Ther 16: 1813–1824.
19. Kreppel F, Gackowski J, Schmidt E, Kochanek S (2005) Combined genetic and chemical capsid modifications enable flexible and efficient de- and retargeting of adenovirus vectors. Mol Ther 12: 107–117.
20. Prill JM, Espenlaub S, Samen U, Engler T, Schmidt E, et al. (2010) Modifications of adenovirus hexon allow for either hepatocyte detargeting or targeting with potential evasion from Kupffer cells. Mol Ther 19: 83–92.
21. Poller B, Gutmann H, Krahenbuhl S, Weksler B, Romero I, et al. (2008) The human brain endothelial cell line hCMEC/D3 as a human blood-brain barrier model for drug transport studies. J Neurochem 107: 1358–1368.
22. Cudkowicz A, Klausner RD, Bridges KR (1984) Regulation of the transferrin receptor in K562 erythroleukemia cells. Prog Clin Biol Res 165: 509–519.
23. Goldsmith ME, Kitazono M, Fok P, Aikou T, Bates S, et al. (2003) The histone deacetylase inhibitor FK228 preferentially enhances adenovirus transgene expression in malignant cells. Clin Cancer Res 9: 5394–5401.
24. Espenlaub S, Corjon S, Engler T, Fella C, Ogris M, et al. (2010) Capsomer-specific fluorescent labeling of adenoviral vector particles allows for detailed analysis of intracellular particle trafficking and the performance of bioresponsive bonds for vector capsid modifications. Hum Gene Ther 21: 1155–1167.
25. Campos SK, Barry MA (2006) Comparison of adenovirus fiber, protein IX, and hexon capsomeres as scaffolds for vector purification and cell targeting. Virology 349: 453–462.
26. Weksler BB, Subileau EA, Perriere N, Charneau P, Holloway K, et al. (2005) Blood-brain barrier-specific properties of a human adult brain endothelial cell line. Faseb J 19: 1872–1874.
27. Franke H, Galla H, Beuckmann CT (2000) Primary cultures of brain microvessel endothelial cells: a valid and flexible model to study drug transport through the blood-brain barrier in vitro. Brain Res Brain Res Protoc 5: 248–256.
28. Franke H, Galla HJ, Beuckmann CT (1999) An improved low-permeability in vitro-model of the blood-brain barrier: transport studies on retinoids, sucrose, haloperidol, caffeine and mannitol. Brain Res 818: 65–71.
29. Nitz T, Eisenblatter T, Psathaki K, Galla HJ (2003) Serum-derived factors weaken the barrier properties of cultured porcine brain capillary endothelial cells in vitro. Brain Res 981: 30–40.
30. Moos T, Rosengren Nielsen T, Skjorringe T, Morgan EH (2007) Iron trafficking inside the brain. J Neurochem 103: 1730–1740.
31. Pardridge WM (1998) CNS drug design based on principles of blood-brain barrier transport. Journal Neurochem 70: 1781–1792.
32. Pardridge WM (2002) Drug and gene targeting to the brain with molecular Trojan horses. Nat Rev Drug Discov 1: 131–139.
33. Foust KD, Nurre E, Montgomery CL, Hernandez A, Chan CM, et al (2009) Intravascular AAV9 preferentially targets neonatal neurons and adult astrocytes. Nat Biotechnol 27: 59–65.
34. Batista L, Miller F, Clave C, Arfi A, Douillard-Guilloux G, et al. (2010) Induced secretion of beta-hexosaminidase by human brain endothelial cells: a novel approach in Sandhoff disease? Neurobiol Dis 37: 656–660.
35. Di Pasquale G, Chiorini JA (2006) AAV transcytosis through barrier epithelia and endothelium. Mol Ther 13: 506–516.
36. Hocini H, Becquart P, Bouhlal H, Chomont N, Ancuta P, et al. (2001) Active and selective transcytosis of cell-free human immunodeficiency virus through a tight polarized monolayer of human endometrial cells. J Virol 75: 5370–5374.
37. Pulzova L, Bhide MR, Andrej K (2009) Pathogen translocation across the blood-brain barrier. FEMS Immunol Med Microbiol 57: 203–213.
38. Dehouck MP, Jolliet-Riant P, Bree F, Fruchart JC, Cecchelli R, et al. (1992) Drug transfer across the blood-brain barrier: correlation between in vitro and in vivo models. J Neurochem 58: 1790–1797.
39. Schiedner G, Hertel S, Kochanek S (2000) Efficient transformation of primary human amniocytes by E1 functions of Ad5: generation of new cell lines for adenoviral vector production. Hum Gene Ther 11: 2105–2116.
40. Abramoff MD, Magelhaes PJ, Ram SJ (2004) Image processing with ImageJ. Biophotonics Int. 11: 36.

18

Chitosan-Graft-Polyethylenimine/DNA Nanoparticles as Novel Non-Viral Gene Delivery Vectors Targeting Osteoarthritis

Huading Lu*⁹, Yuhu Dai⁹, Lulu Lv, Huiqing Zhao

Department of Orthopedics, Third Affiliated Hospital of Sun Yat-sen University, Guangzhou, P. R. China

Abstract

The development of safe and efficient gene carriers is the key to the clinical success of gene therapy. The present study was designed to develop and evaluate the chitosan-graft-polyethylenimine (CP)/DNA nanoparticles as novel non-viral gene vectors for gene therapy of osteoarthritis. The CP/DNA nanoparticles were produced through a complex coacervation of the cationic polymers with pEGFP after grafting chitosan (CS) with a low molecular weight (Mw) PEI (Mw = 1.8 kDa). Particle size and zeta potential were related to the weight ratio of CP:DNA, where decreases in nanoparticle size and increases in surface charge were observed as CP content increased. The buffering capacity of CP was significantly greater than that of CS. The transfection efficiency of CP/DNA nanoparticles was similar with that of the Lipofectamine^{TM} 2000, and significantly higher than that of CS/DNA and PEI (25 kDa)/DNA nanoparticles. The transfection efficiency of the CP/DNA nanoparticles was dependent on the weight ratio of CP:DNA (w/w). The average cell viability after the treatment with CP/DNA nanoparticles was over 90% in both chondrocytes and synoviocytes, which was much higher than that of PEI (25 kDa)/DNA nanoparticles. The CP copolymers efficiently carried the pDNA inside chondrocytes and synoviocytes, and the pDNA was detected entering into nucleus. These results suggest that CP/DNA nanoparticles with improved transfection efficiency and low cytotoxicity might be a safe and efficient non-viral vector for gene delivery to both chondrocytes and synoviocytes.

Editor: Xiaoming He, The Ohio State University, United States of America

Funding: This study was supported by the National Natural Science Foundation of China (No. 81272040; 30600632), the Natural Science Foundation of Guangdong Province, P. R. China (No. S2011010004808), and the Science and Technology Projects of Guangdong Province, P. R. China (No. 2012B031800451). The funders had no role in study design, data collection and analysis, decision to publish, or preparation of the manuscript.

Competing Interests: The authors have declared that no competing interests exist.

* E-mail: johnniehuading@163.com

⁹ These authors contributed equally to this work.

Introduction

Osteoarthritis (OA) is one of the greatest challenges for clinical therapy due to avascularity and the lack innervation of cartilage. Current therapy shows little effects because of the rapid clearance of therapeutic agents by the synovium and the difficulty of infiltrating into the dense extracellular matrix (ECM) [1]. Gene therapy represents a promising technology for OA treatment by targeting specific disease-relevant mechanisms, and thus by treating the causes of OA rather than the symptoms [2]. The development of an efficient and safe gene transfer system is one of the most important factors for a successful gene therapy with practical use in the clinic. Although most gene therapy protocols in clinical trials actually employ viral vectors due to their high transfection efficiency, their fatal drawbacks, such as immunogenicity, potential infectivity, complicated production, and oncogenic effects, may prevent their further use in the clinic [3–6]. On the other hand, non-viral vectors have attracted much attention because of their potential advantages, such as ease of synthesis and modification, efficient cell/tissue targeting, low immune response, and unrestricted plasmid size, among others [4–9].

Among various non-viral vectors, chitosan (CS) is considered to be an excellent candidate, because of its biocompatibility, biodegradability, lower toxicity, and higher cationic potential properties [10–12]. CS/DNA complexes have been shown to be capable of transfecting chondrocytes under *in vitro* and *in vivo* conditions [2]. However, they also have low transfection efficiency, thus limiting its further application as a non-viral gene delivery vector [7,9,12–15]. There is an increasing interest in improving CS properties by various modifications. In our previous study [16], we designed hybrid hyaluronic acid (HA)/CS-plasmid nanoparticles as novel non-viral gene delivery vectors targeting OA. In this study, HA/CS-plasmid nanoparticles demonstrated significantly higher transfection efficiency towards chondrocytes compared to CS/DNA complexes. HA-containing nanoparticles gain facilitated access to target cells via receptor-mediated endocytosis pathway through HA-CD44 interaction, and this interaction also leads to a cellular signaling process, which could promote the success of the gene transfection [16]. However, the transfection efficiency of HA/CS-plasmid nanoparticles in synoviocytes has been demonstrated to be very poor (unpublished data), which may restrict their future clinical application. The unsatisfactory transfection efficiency of either CS or its derivatives is mainly a result from its poor endosomal escape due to lack of buffering amines [9,17], and also from the very strong binding with DNA resulting in inefficient unpackaging of genetic material in the cytoplasm [9,18].

As reported, the transfection efficiency CS vectors can be improved by combining CS with either cationic or anionic biopolymers, such as polyethylenimine (PEI) [8,9,19], prior to the addition of DNA. PEI is another promising cationic non-viral vector, thanks to its high buffering capacity. PEI can protect DNA from nuclease degradation and facilitate endosomal escape of PEI/DNA complexes [8,9,15,20,21]. However, the high toxicity *in vitro* and *in vivo* of this non-viral vector limits its application in gene therapy [5,6,8,9,21]. Fortunately, many pilot studies had proved that the combination of CS and PEI (CS/PEI blend or CS-graft-PEI -CP) can simultaneously enhance the transfection efficiency and decreasing the cytotoxicity [4,8,9,13–15]. However, most of these studies were carried out in tumor cells such as HeLa, A549, and HepG2 cells [8,9,13–15,22]. Consequently, it is unknown how the novel non-viral vector behaves in both chondrocytes and synoviocytes, which is important for us to determine its value in gene therapy for OA or other joint diseases. To address the limitations of HA/CS-plasmid nanoparticles and explore an effective non-viral gene vector focused on OA, we deliberately selected a low Mw PEI (1.8 kDa), which possesses an adequate buffering capacity with poor transfection efficiency. For its part, both PEI and CS are biodegradable [8].

Usually the gene therapy for OA select chondrocytes as target cells, which enables the function of gene expression products through autocrine and paracrine mechanisms [2]. However, since chondrocytes are wrapped around the dense cartilage matrix it is quite difficult for a non-viral gene vector to infiltrate into the dense ECM and thus to reach the deep cartilage. In addition to the destruction of articular cartilage and the formation of osteophytes, OA is accompanied with chronic inflammation of the synovium, which plays an important role in the occurrence and development of the disease [23,24]. Synovium is widely distributed in the intra-articular joint cavity, and directly contacts with the articular cartilage in some place; its secreted synovial fluid provides nutrition and exchange material with articular cartilage. Gene therapy towards synoviocytes enables gene expression products to reach the cartilage surface through synovial fluid, thus affecting the metabolism of the cartilage and reversing the OA progression. Therefore, gene therapy targeting the synoviocytes may be more effective than targeting other cell types for either OA or other joint diseases [25,26].

In the present study, a novel CS/DNA complex grafted with low Mw PEI was prepared as a new non-viral gene carrier for the OA-targeted intracellular delivery of therapeutic genes into chondrocytes and synoviocytes. We investigated the characteristics of CP/plasmid enhanced green fluorescent protein (pEGFP) nanoparticles and their cytotoxicity, the transfection efficiency in chondrocytes and synoviocytes, and their ability to carry nucleic acids into the nucleus of chondrocytes and synoviocytes. Our results will facilitate the assessment of CP/DNA nanoparticles feasibility as an efficient and safe non-viral vector to deliver therapeutic genes to chondrocytes and synoviocytes for the treatment of either OA or other joint diseases.

Materials and Methods

Materials

CS (Mw = 50 kDa and deacetylation degree = 90%), PEI (Mw = 1.8 kDa and 25 kDa), and 4', 6-diamidino-2-phenylindole (DAPI) were purchased in Sigma-Aldrich (St. Louis, MO, USA). Dulbecco's modified Eagle's medium (DMEM), D-Hanks, 0.25% trypsin/ethylenediaminetetraacetic acid (EDTA), penicillin, and streptomycin were obtained from Gibco-BRL (Gaithersberg, MD, USA). The fetal bovine serum (FBS) was obtained from HyClone (Logan, UT, USA). The Cell Counting Kit-8 (CCK-8) was purchased in Dojindo (Kumamoto, Japan). The 1,1′-carbonyldiimidazole (CDI) was obtained from Pierce (Rockford, IL, USA). The pReceiver-M29 vector carrying an EGFP, Lipofectamine^{TM} 2000, and LysoTracker Green DND-26 were purchased in Invitrogen (Carlsbad, CA, USA). The Cy3-labeled plasmid DNA (pDNA) was made by RiboBio (Guangzhou, P. R. China). The plasmid was propagated in *Escherichia coli* cells, isolated, and then purified.

Synthesis of Copolymer

Copolymer of CP was prepared according to the methods described by Gao *et al.* [8]. Briefly, 0.5 g CS was dissolved in 20 ml of a 0.5% acetic acid solution, which was then adjusted at pH 7.0, and the mixture was stirred overnight. CDI was then added at a molar ratio of CDI:CS amine = 2:1, followed by stirring for 1 h. The PEI (1.8 kDa) was added dropwise into the solution under stirring at a molar ratio of PEI:amine = 2:1. The polymerization was performed at room temperature (25°C) overnight. The resultant product was purified by dialysis in water for 48 h. Finally, the resultant CP powder was collected by lyophilization.

Characterization of Copolymer

The composition of the prepared CP copolymer was analyzed by proton nuclear magnetic resonance spectroscopy (^{1}H NMR). CS and CP were dissolved in the mixed solvent D_2O/CD_3COOD (V_{D2O}: $V_{CD3COOD}$ = 1:1). ^{1}H NMR spectra were recorded using a Bruker AV600 spectrometer (Advance TM 600, Bruker, Germany). The molecular weights and molecular weight distributions of CS and CP were measured by using a Gel permeation chromatography (GPC) system (Malvern, Viscotek GPC Max VE 2001, MA, UK) equipped with a Viscotek TDA 305 Triple detector array, a Malvern CLM 3021 A6000M column using 0.2 mol/l HAc/NaAc buffer as the eluent at a flow rate of 0.5 ml/min at 40°C. Polymer samples were dissolved in 0.2 mol/l of HAc/NaAc to form the 2.5 mg/ml solution and filtered through a 0.45-μm syringe filter, and 100 μl of polymer solution was injected into the GPC system. The molecular weights of the polymer samples were analyzed by using OmniSec 4.6.0 software.

Preparation of CP/DNA Complex

All CP/DNA nanoparticles were freshly prepared before use. The principle of nanoparticle formation was mutual attraction between positive and negative charges. The CP powder was dissolved in distilled water and filtered through a 0.22 μm membrane. Then, CP/DNA nanoparticles were prepared at various CP:DNA weight ratios (0.5, 1, 2, 3, 4, and 5) by gently dropwise adding the copolymer solution to equal volumes of DNA solution (1 μg/μl). The mixture was vortexed gently for 5 min and left at room temperature for 30 min to form CP/DNA nanoparticles solution. The charge ratio (N/P) of CP/DNA complexes are defined as the molar relation of amine groups in the cationic molecule of CP complex to phosphate groups in the DNA. For calculation of N/P ratios, 330 Da was used as an average mass per charge for DNA [8].

Scanning Electron Microscopy (SEM)

Nanoparticles in solution were dropped onto a silica surface, lyophilized using a JFD-310 (JEOL, Japan), then precoated with a thin layer of gold and palladium prior to analysis. Micrographs were obtained using a SEM (JSM-6360, Japan).

Particle Size and Zeta Potential Measurements

A Mastersizer 2000 laser diffractometer (Malvern Instruments, Worcestershire, UK) was used to measure the particle size and the surface charge (represented by the surface zeta potential) of the test nanoparticles prepared and analyzed in distilled water at 25°C. The volume of samples was 1 ml containing a final DNA concentration of 50 μg/ml.

Gel Retardation Assay

CP/DNA nanoparticles were evaluated by agarose gel electrophoresis (AGE). Nanoparticles were prepared at different weight ratios of CP:DNA of 1:2, 1:1, 2:1, 3:1, 4:1, 5:1, 6:1, and 7:1. The effect of CP on DNA condensations was investigated by electrophoresis on a 1% agarose gel containing ethidium bromide in Tris-borate EDTA buffer at pH 6.5. The samples were run on a gel at 100 V for 30 min. The resultant DNA migration pattern was revealed under a GDS-8000 (UVP, USA).

In order to determine whether the combination between CP and pDNA was affected by pH value, CP/DNA nanoparticles samples (e.g., CP:DNA weight ratios = 3) were evaluated under different pH conditions (5.5 to 8.0) by AGE as described above. Similarly, CS/DNA nanoparticles (e.g., CS:DNA weight ratios = 3) were evaluated and used as control under the same pH conditions.

Analysis of Buffering Capacity

The buffering capacity of different complexes (CS, PEI -25 kDa-, and CP) was compared by acid titration experiments, with the NaCl solution (0.1 N) as negative control. Briefly, CS, PEI (25 kDa), and CP copolymers were separately dissolved in 0.1 M NaCl to obtain the final concentration of 0.1 mg/ml, and the pH of each solution was adjusted to pH10 with 0.1 N NaOH. Then, 0.1 M HCl (~20 μl per drop) was added dropwise to sample solutions. Different pH values were measured using a pH meter. The slope of the line in the plot for pH against the amount of HCl consumed indicated the intrinsic buffering capacity of the system [27,28].

Animals and Cell Culture

All procedures involving animals in this study were reviewed and approved by the Institutional Animal Care and Use Committee at the Sun Yat-sen University (Guangzhou, P. R. China) (Approval ID: 2011-0905). Cartilage and synovial tissues were harvested under sterile conditions from knee joints of three-week-old New Zealand white rabbits (n = 6; Laboratory Animal Center of Sun Yat-Sen University, Guangzhou, P. R. China; Animal quality certificate numbers: SCXK 2008-0002).

Cartilage slices were treated at 37°C with 0.25% trypsin for 30 min, thoroughly washed with phosphate-buffered saline (PBS), and incubated with 0.2% (w/v) collagenase II (activity 277.0 units/mg; Gibco-BRL, Gaithersberg, MD, USA) at 37°C for 12 h. After digestion of tissues with trypsin and collagenase II, the cells were harvested every 2 h for a total of 4–6 times, and isolated chondrocytes were cultured in monolayer in DMEM supplemented with 10% FBS, 100 μg/ml of streptomycin and 100 U/ml of penicillin at 37°C and 5% CO_2.

Synoviocytes were isolated and cultured according to the method previously described [29]. Briefly, synovial tissues were minced aseptically into 1–2 mm^2, and then digested in DMEM containing 5% (v/v) FBS and 0.2% (w/v) collagenase II at 37°C and 5% CO_2 for 2 h. The adherent cells were discarded, and non-adherent tissues were digested in serum-free DMEM containing 0.25% trypsin for 30 min. Then, they were transferred through sterile 108 μm^2 nylon mesh into a sterile centrifuge tube, and centrifuged at 300×g for 10 min. Resulting cells were washed extensively with DMEM, and then cultured in DMEM supplemented with 10% (v/v) FBS, 100 U/ml penicillin, and 100 μg/ml streptomycin at 37°C and 5% CO_2. At confluence, adherent cells were trypsinized, split in a 1:3 ratio, and recultured in medium.

Cytotoxicity Assay

In vitro cytotoxicity tests were performed by the CCK-8 assay [16]. Chondrocytes and synoviocytes were seeded at a density of 5×10^4 cells per well in 100 μl of culture medium in 96-well plates, and incubated for 24 h to reach 80% confluence at treatment. Immediately after culture medium was removed, CP/DNA, CS/DNA, and PEI (25 kDa)/DNA nanoparticles (weight ratio = 3), at polymer concentrations ranging from 5 to 40 μg/ml in fresh culture medium without serum, were added to cells. In another group of cells, culture media were replaced by fresh serum-free media containing Lipofectamine™ 2000 (5 μg DNA/ml) as positive controls. A group of cells treated with only fresh culture medium was used as blank controls. Cells were incubated with various complexes for 4 h; various media were then removed and replaced with fresh culture media. Then, medium containing CCK-8 (10 μg per well) was added, and cells were maintained in an incubator at 37°C and 5% CO_2 for 3 h. Optical density was measured using a microplate reader (Bio-RAD, model 680) at a wavelength of 570 nm, using a blank control consisting of CCK-8 solution. Three replicates were performed for each sample and the mean value was reported as final results.

In vitro GFP Transfection Experiment

Chondrocytes and synoviocytes were seeded into 24-well plates at a density of 1×10^5 cells per well in 500 μl of culture medium, and incubated for 24 h. For the transfection assay, the medium was discarded and cells were washed once with PBS. Nanoparticles containing pEGFP (CP/DNA nanoparticles with CP:DNA weight ratio = 3 were used as example) were added to cells in FBS-free DMEM, which were then incubated for 4 h. The nanoparticles solution was removed and replaced with fresh culture medium supplemented with serum and antibiotics. After being cultured for 48 h, EGFP-positive cells were detected using a fluorescence microscope (Nikon-TE2000U, Tokyo, Japan).

Cells were collected and resuspended in PBS (pH 7.4), and transfection results were measured using a fluorescence-activated cell sorting (FACS) device (Calibur, BD, USA) through the first fluorescence channel. Cells which were exposed to naked pDNA, CS/DNA nanoparticles, or PEI (25 kDa)/DNA nanoparticles (weight ratio = 3) were analyzed using FACS as controls (at a pEGFP concentration of 4 μg/ml and incubated for 4 h in FBS-free DMEM, respectively). Lipofectamine™ 2000 was used as a positive control for transfection study, and was added to DMEM without serum or antibiotics, following manufacturer procedures. Then, Lipofectamine™ 2000 was incubated with 0.8 μg pEGFP per well for 4 h. Posteriorly, the medium was discarded and replaced with a complete medium containing serum and antibiotics for 48 h, according to instructions. All transfection experiments were performed in triplicate.

To evaluate the transfection efficiency of CP/DNA with different CP:DNA weight ratios, nanoparticles containing pEGFP (CP:DNA weight ratio range from 1:2, 1:1, 2:1, 4:1, 8:1 to 10:1) were added to cells (with a concentration of 2 μg DNA per well) in FBS-free DMEM, and incubated for 4 h at 37°C and 5% CO_2, as described above. The transfection efficiency was determined by fluorescent microscopy and FACS, as aforementioned.

Intracellular Trafficking

Prior to treatment, either chondrocytes or synoviocytes were seeded at a density of 1×10^5 cells/dish in a culture medium containing 10% FBS for 24 h. When cells were cultured at 70% confluence, the medium was removed and cells were washed twice with PBS. Before adding 300 µl treatment solution containing LysoTracker Green DND-26 (50 µM) (Invitrogen, Carlsbad, CA, USA) in FBS-free DMEM for the mixture the medium was incubated for 20 min to label lysosomes. After removal of the medium, the cells were washed with PBS twice. Subsequently, CP/DNA nanoparticles containing 2 µg Cy3-labeled pDNA (RiboBio, P. R. China) were diluted in 200 µl of serum-free DMEM medium, and were gently added into dishes. At specified intervals (30 min and 1, 2, and 4 h), the treatment medium was removed and cells were washed twice with PBS, and fixed with 4% paraformaldehyde (PFA) solution for 10 min at 37°C. Fixed cells were counter-stained with a blue nuclear dye, DAPI, for 30 min at room temperature, and washed with PBS thrice. Coverclips were mounted on microslides, and cells were analyzed with a confocal laser scanning microscope (Zeiss LSM710, Jena, Germany).

Statistical Analysis

All of the measurement data were displayed as means±standard deviation of the mean ($\overline{x}\pm s$). The statistical significance was determined by ANOVA and, when needed, by LSD-*t* test, by using the statistical software SPSS package v13.0. Differences were considered to be significant when $P<0.05$.

Results and Discussion

Synthesis and Characterization of Copolymer

The chitosan-graft-polyethylenimine (CP) was synthesized by reaction between CS and PEI with the presence of CDI (Figure S1). During the synthesis of CP, we used excessive PEI, low reactive temperature, and relative slow reaction rate to avoid gelation. Composition of synthesized copolymer was analyzed by ^{1}H NMR. As shown in Figure 1, the proton peaks area of CS appeared at 4.94 ppm (H-1 of glucosamine ring), 3.26 ppm (H-2 of glucosamine ring), 3.52–4.31 ppm (H-3, H-4, H-5, H-6 of glucosamine ring). Compared with CS, there were the characteristic chemical shifts of PEI (2.72–3.38 ppm) on the ^{1}H NMR spectra of CP, indicating that PEI was grafted to the CS chain [30]. The degree of grafted (DG) of PEI onto CS was calculated by the following formula:

$$DG=\frac{M_{(CH_2CH_2NH)}\left[I_{CP(H2,\,H3\sim H6,\,NCH_2CH_2)}-I_{CS(H2,\,H3\sim H6)}\right]}{4I_{(H1)}M_{PEI}}\times 100\%$$

Where $\boldsymbol{M}_{PEI}$ and $\boldsymbol{M}_{CH2CH2NH}$ represents the molecular weight of PEI and -CH_2CH_2NH- respectively, $I_{CP(H2,\ H3\sim H6,\ NCH2CH2)}$ represents the sum of the integral value of correspondent peaks (-CH_2CH_2NH-, H-2, H-3, H-4, H-5, H-6 of glucosamine ring on CS chain on CP chain), $I_{CS\ (H2,\ H3\sim H6)}$ represents the integration values of correspondent peaks (H-2, H-3, H-4, H-5, H-6 of glucosamine ring on CS chain), I_{H1} represents the integration values of H-1, which was defined as 1 during the process of calculation. The DG of PEI was calculated as 7.4% as shown in Table 1. Molecular weights of CS and CS-*g*-PEI (CP) were traced by gel permeation chromatography (GPC). The molecular weight distribution of CP shifted into the shorter retention time, indicating an increase in the molecular weight after grafting PEI onto CS as compared with nascent CS (Figure 2). From the results of GPC (Table 1), the molecular weights (M_n) of CS and CP were 1.98×10^4 and 4.55×10^4, respectively, and the DG of PEI onto CS were calculated by the following equation:

$$DG=\frac{(M_{n,\,CP}-M_{n,\,CS})M_{\text{unit of CS}}}{M_{PEI}M_{n,\,CS}}\times 100\%$$

M_{PEI} is 1800, and $M_{\text{unit of CS}}=M_{C6H11O4}\times90\%+M_{C8H13O5}\times10\%=151.2$. The DG of PEI calculated as 10.9% from GPC was different from that calculated as 7.4% from ^{1}H NMR, which may result from different measure and calculation methods.

Physiochemical Characteristics of CP/DNA Nanoparticles

The CP/DNA nanoparticles formation and the CP with DNA condensation capability were evaluated by AGE. Figure 3(a) demonstrates that the DNA migration was completely retarded when CP:DNA weight ratios were around three, indicating DNA bound to CP tightly and completely with little free DNA existing. Figure 3(b) shows that the CP with DNA nanoparticles' condensation capability at CP:DNA weight ratio = 3 was not affected by pH levels. Figure 3(c) demonstrates that some pDNA escaped from CS/DNA nanoparticles when pH value increased to ≥7.0, indicating that the interaction between pDNA phosphate groups and CS amino groups was dependent on pH level to a certain degree. This is because CS contains primary amine group

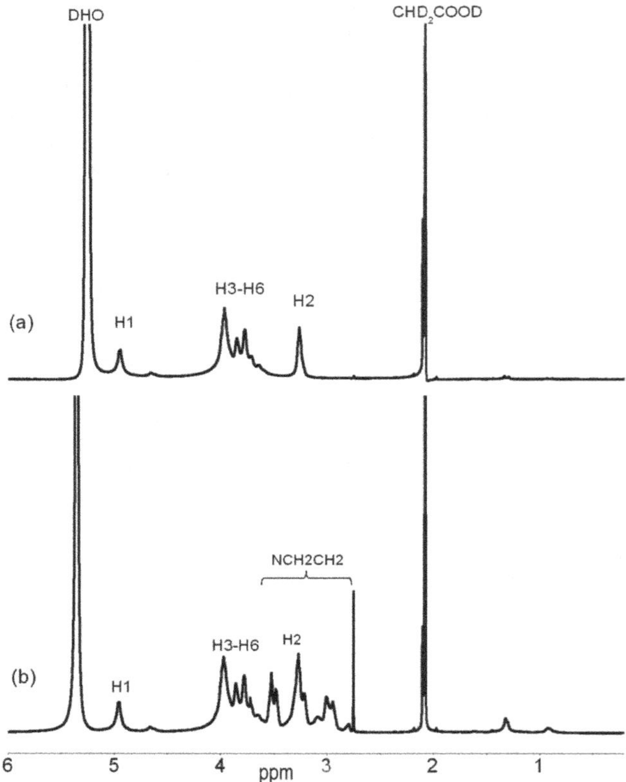

Figure 1. Representative ^{1}H NMR spectra of chitosan (CS) and CS-*g*-PEI (CP) in a mixture solution (D_2O/CD_3COOD (V_{D2O}: $V_{CD3COOD}$ = 1:1) at 40°C.

Table 1. Characteristic of prepared CS-g-PEI (CP).

M_n of CS	M_n of CS-*g*-PEI	DG[a] (mol %)	DG[b](mol %)
1.98×10^4	4.55×10^4	10.9%	7.4%

[a]calculated from GPC.
[b]calculated from ^{1}H NMR.

with a pKa value of about 6.5, at acidic pH<pKa, primary amines in CS backbone become positively charged, and this protonated amine enables CS to bind to negatively charged DNA via an electrostatic interaction. The interaction between the positively charged CS and negatively DNA leads to the nanoparticles formation in the aqueous milieu, preventing pDNA to be released from complexes. However, under either neutral or alkaline condition, where CS is slightly charged, CS cannot completely encapsulate all pDNA [12]. This is quite different from above results with CP as shown in Figure 3(b).

The CP/DNA nanoparticles formation was also monitored by observation of the morphology and their particle size and zeta potential changes as a function of the CP:DNA (w/w) ratio. Figure 4(a) shows a representative SEM image of a CP/DNA complex consisting of spherical particles with diameters of approximately 100–300 nm. Surface properties are important factors that influence the complex uptake by cells. Generally, small particle size and positive surface charge would lead to higher internalization rates [8]. As shown in Figure 4(b), the particle size and zeta potential of nanoparticles were highly dependent on the CP:DNA (w/w) ratio. When the CP:DNA (w/w) ratio was 0.5, the complex size was 583.7±123.0 nm; however, at a ratio of 4, the complex size declined to 152.3±9.1 nm. This could be explained by the fact that the formation of polymer complexes with DNA is through ionic interactions [8,14,31]. Additionally, at high CP:DNA (w/w) ratios, can be observed net electrostatic repulsive forces to prevent aggregation among complexes. The relatively homogenous size distributions of nanoparticles, measured by dynamic light scattering, are shown in Figure 4(c). As shown in Figure 4(b), the zeta potential became more positive as the CP amount within the polyelectrolyte complex increased. The zeta potential was negative when CP:DNA (w/w) ratio = 0.5, but with the increasing of the CP:DNA (w/w) ratio the zeta potential rapidly increased to positive values. These results, together with those obtained from gel retardation experiments, suggested that CP/DNA complexes could form positive potential nanoparticles when CP:DNA (w/w) ratio >2. These properties are necessary for CP/DNA nanoparticles to obtain successful gene transfection as the positive surface charge and the small complex size are vital parameters to determine their cellular uptake and interactability with the cell membrane [14,32].

Figure 4(d) shows the buffering capacity of different polymers in the pH range of 10 to 2.6. It demonstrated that the amount of 0.1 N HCl required in bringing the pH from 10 to 2.6 increased from NaCl, CS, and CP to PEI, showing the maximum buffering capacity of PEI. The endosomal DNA nanoplexes release into the cytoplasm is one of the most important parameters that depend on the intrinsic buffering capacity of the vector. It is interesting to note that CP copolymers exhibits considerable buffering capacity, which would help in release of pDNA from endosomes/lysosomes (proton-sponge effect) [27,33].

Cell Viability

In this study, the cytotoxicity of various nanoparticles (CP/DNA, CS/DNA, and PEI/DNA) was determined by the MTT assay. As the concentration of the CP/DNA nanoparticles increased to 20 μg/ml, it showed a slight increase in cytotoxicity. However, the average cell viability was >90% for both chondrocytes and synoviocytes. Such viability was much higher than that of either PEI (25 kDa)/DNA nanoparticles or Lipofectamine™ 2000, which showed a viability <70% at 5 μg/ml, and even decreased to <40% viability for PEI/DNA nanoparticles at 20 μg/ml (Figure 5). For CP/DNA nanoparticles, when the concentration increased to 40 μg/ml, it showed a slight increase in cytotoxicity, with the cell viabilities being >85% for both chondrocytes and synoviocytes. However, the cell viability was still significantly higher than that of either PEI/DNA nanoparticles (5 μg/ml) or Lipofectamine™ 2000 (5 μg/ml). For cell viability assay on chondrocytes, one-way ANOVA showed statistical significance (F= 24.11, P<0.01); further analysis with LSD-t test revealed that the cell viability of CP/DNA group in 40 μg/ml was significantly higher than that of other two groups (P<0.01). Similarly, for cell viability assay on synoviocytes, One-way ANOVA indicated statistical significance (F= 19.99, P<0.01);

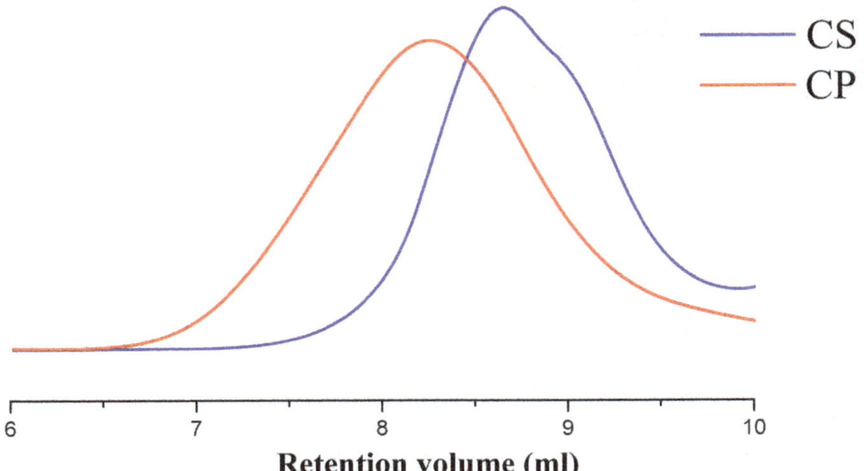

Figure 2. GPC Curves of chitosan (CS) and CS-g-PEI (CP).

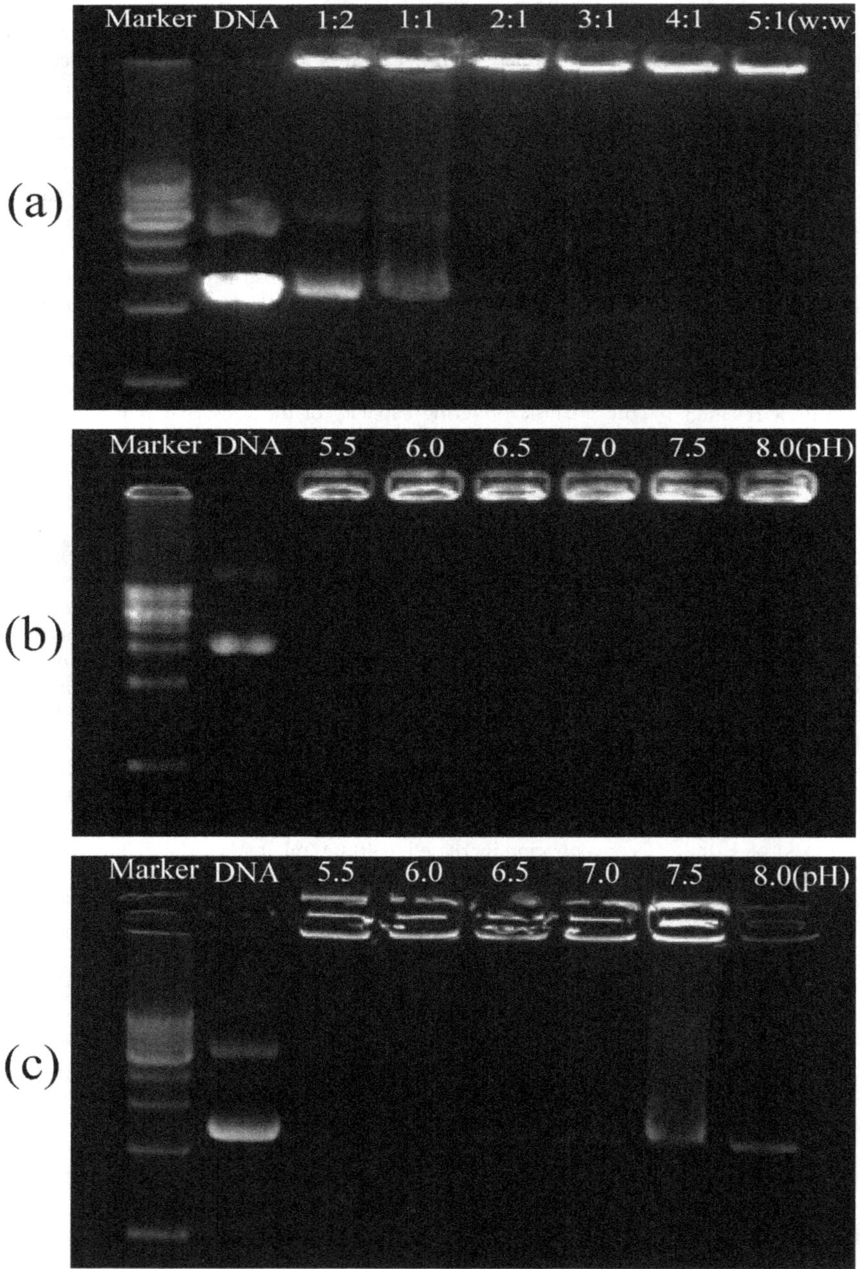

Figure 3. Gel retarding analysis of CP/DNA nanoparticles. Lane 1: DNA marker. Lane 2: naked DNA control. Lane 3–8: CP/DNA nanoparticles prepared at CP:DNA weight ratios of 1:2, 1:1, 2:1, 3:1, 4:1, and 5:1 (a); electrophoresis photo of CP/DNA nanoparticles prepared with CP:DNA weight ratio = 3 at different pH levels (b); electrophoresis of CS/DNA nanoparticles prepared with the CS:DNA weight ratio = 3 at different pH levels (c).

further analysis with LSD-*t* test revealed that the cell viability of CP/DNA group in 40 μg/ml were also significantly higher than that of other two groups ($P<0.01$). These results may be related to that low Mw PEI is less toxic, and CS has good biocompatibility and biodegradability [8–12]. These cytotoxicity results indicate that CP/DNA nanoparticles should be a safer carrier than PEI/DNA nanoparticles and Lipofectamine^{TM} 2000, and specify a safe range for the CP/DNA nanoparticles (5–20 μg/ml) application to joint tissue/chondrocytes or synoviocytes.

CP/DNA Complex Transfection Efficiency

In the present study, we compared the transfection efficiency of CP/DNA nanoparticles with that of CS/DNA nanoparticles, naked pDNA, PEI (25 kDa)/DNA nanoparticles, and Lipofectamine^{TM} 2000. Figures 6 and 7(a) show that the transfection efficiency of CP/DNA complex was similar to that of the Lipofectamine^{TM} 2000 at CP:DNA (w/w) ratio = 3, and significantly higher than that of CS/DNA nanoparticles, PEI (25 kDa)/DNA nanoparticles, and naked pDNA [Figs. 7(a) and S2], which is consistent with some previous studies [14,34]. The transfection efficiency of different groups were analyzed by one-way ANOVA,

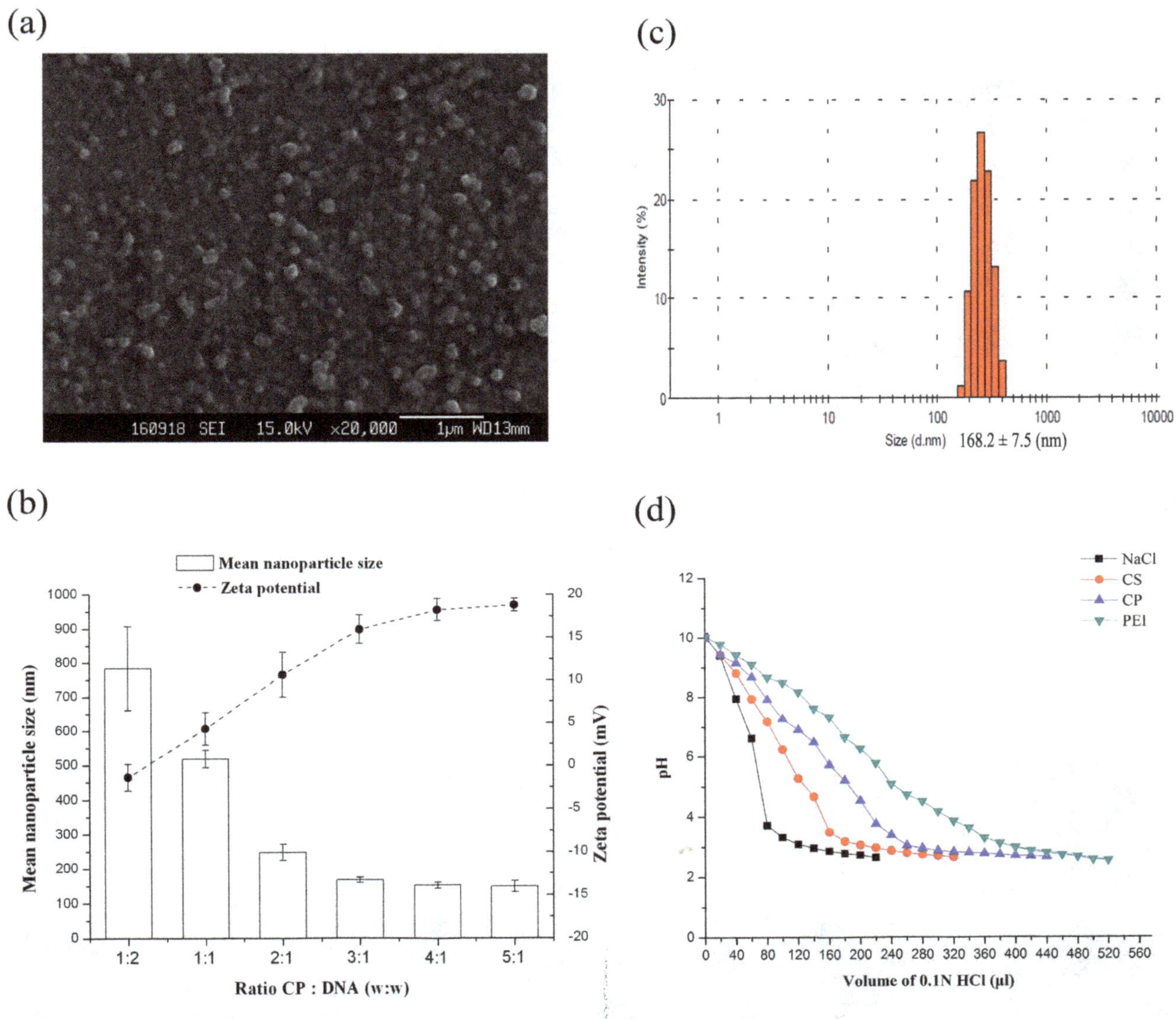

Figure 4. Physiochemical property of CP and CP/DNA nanoparticles. (a) SEM images of CP/DNA nanoparticles at CP:DNA weight ratio = 3; (b) the effect of CP:DNA weight ratios on the particle size and the zeta potential of resulting nanoparticles (n = 3; error bars represent standard deviation); (c) size distribution of CP/DNA complexes prepared at the CP:DNA weight ratio = 3 measured by Mastersizer 2000 laser diffractometer; (d) buffering capacities of PEI (25 kDa), CS, and CP copolymers.

which demonstrated statistical significance for chondrocytes ($F = 21.88$, $P < 0.01$); further analysis with LSD-t test revealed that the transfection efficiency of CP/DNA nanoparticles was significantly higher than that of the naked plasmid, PEI (25 kDa)/DNA, and CS/DNA nanoparticles ($P < 0.01$). However, there were no significant differences between CP/DNA nanoparticles and Lipofectamine^{TM} 2000 ($P > 0.05$). Similarly, for synoviocytes, one-way ANOVA demonstrated statistical significance ($F = 152.825$, $P < 0.01$); further analysis with LSD-t test revealed that the transfection efficiency of CP/DNA nanoparticles was higher than that of the naked plasmid, PEI (25 kDa)/DNA and CS/DNA nanoparticles ($P < 0.01$). However, there were no significant differences between CP/DNA nanoparticles and Lipofectamine^{TM} 2000 ($P > 0.05$). Jiang *et al.* [14] reported that the transfection efficiency of CP/DNA copolymer is cell-type dependent. However, in the present study no significant differences were observed between chondrocytes and synoviocytes, situation that was also quite different from either CS/DNA nanoparticles or HA-modified CS/DNA nanoparticles in our previous study [16]. It is known that a key cellular barrier impeding the transfection efficiency of non-viral gene vectors is the inefficiency release of endosomally trapped DNA into the cell cytosol [4,5,8,9]. PEI is known to possess a very good buffering capacity [21], which has also been confirmed in the present study, and could escape from endosome through the proton-sponge mechanism, thus facilitating gene entry into the nucleus [8,9]. However, PEI also exhibits Mw-dependent transfection efficiency: PEIs with high Mw have better gene transfer capability, but suffer from charge associated toxicity. PEIs with low Mw are non-toxic, but have poor transfection efficiency [9,20,34]. In the present study, we deliberately choose low Mw of PEI graft with CS to form CP complexes. The total amount of amine content in complex is close to PEI (25 kDa), which allows complexes easily to escape from endosome due to a higher buffering capacity, and

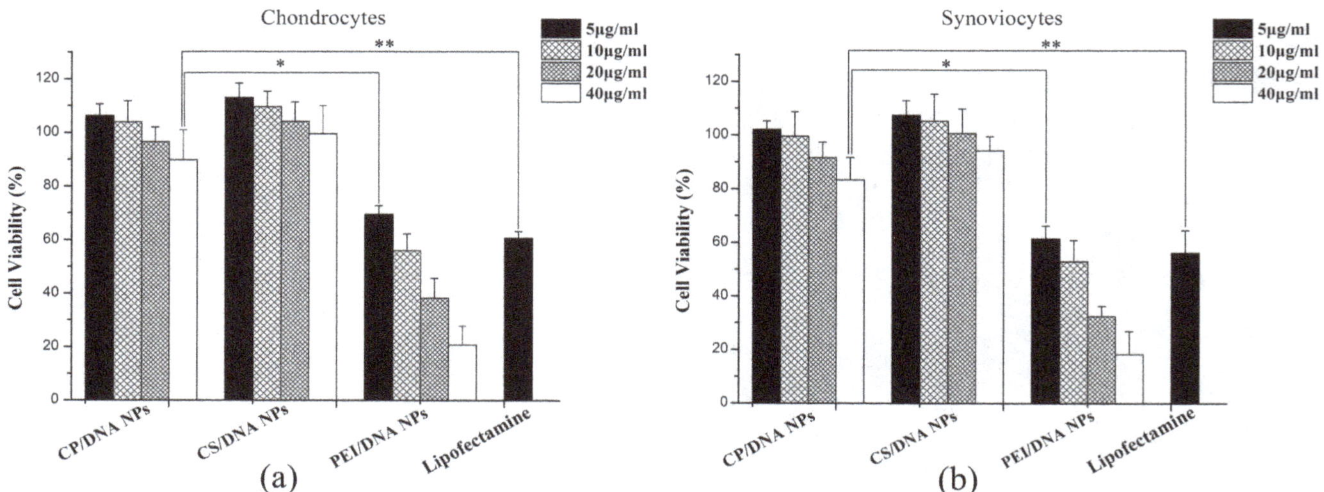

Figure 5. Cell viabilities of CP/DNA nanoparticles, CS/DNA nanoparticles, PEI/DNA nanoparticles, and Lipofectamine™ 2000 in primary chondrocytes (a) and synoviocytes (b). *$P<0.01$ compared to PEI/DNA nanoparticles; **$P<0.01$ compared to Lipofectamine™ 2000.

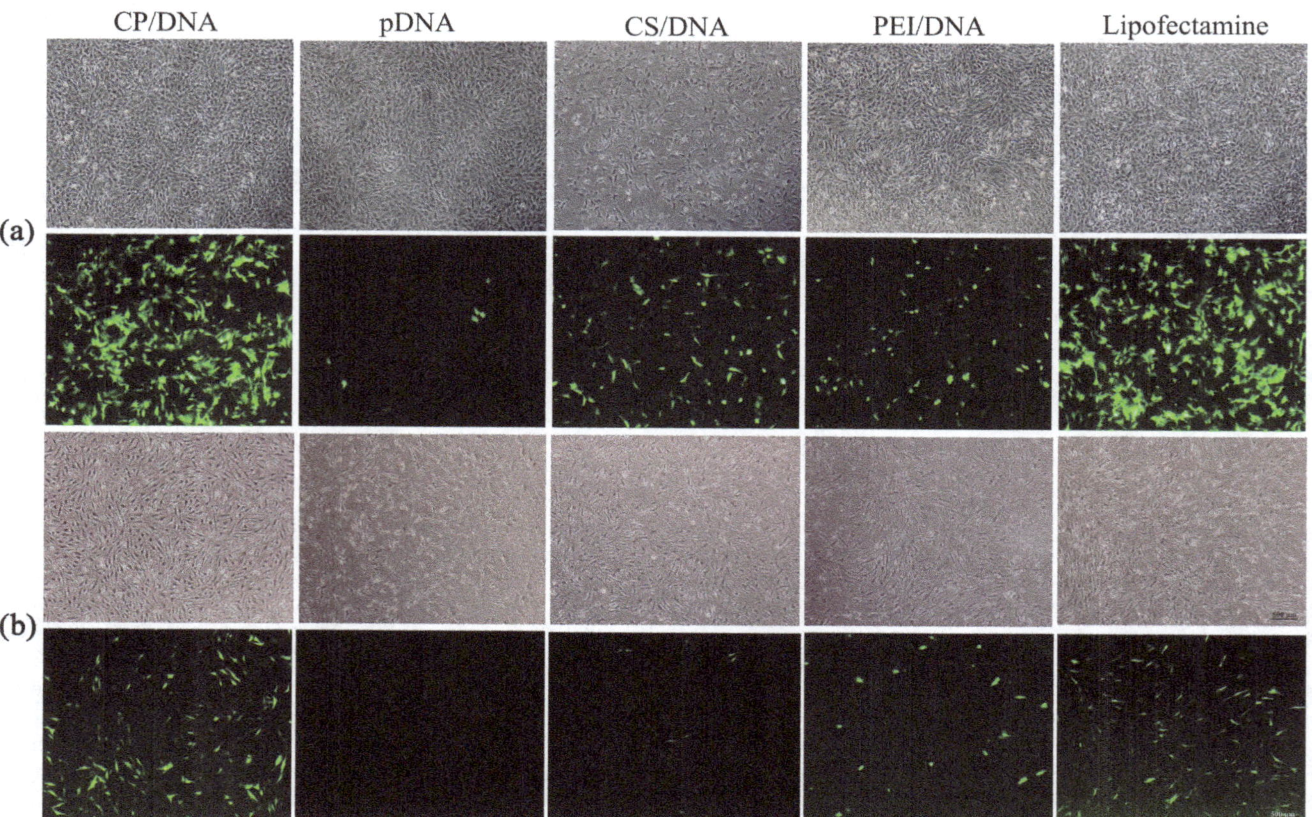

Figure 6. Images of chondrocytes (a) or synoviocytes (b) transfected with CP/DNA nanoparticles, naked pDNA, CS/DNA nanoparticles, PEI (25 kDa)/DNA nanoparticles, and Lipofectamine™ 2000 as observed under fluorescence microscope or inverted phase contrast microscope. (40× magnification for upper panel under inverted phase contrast microscope, and 40× magnification for lower panel under fluorescence microscope).

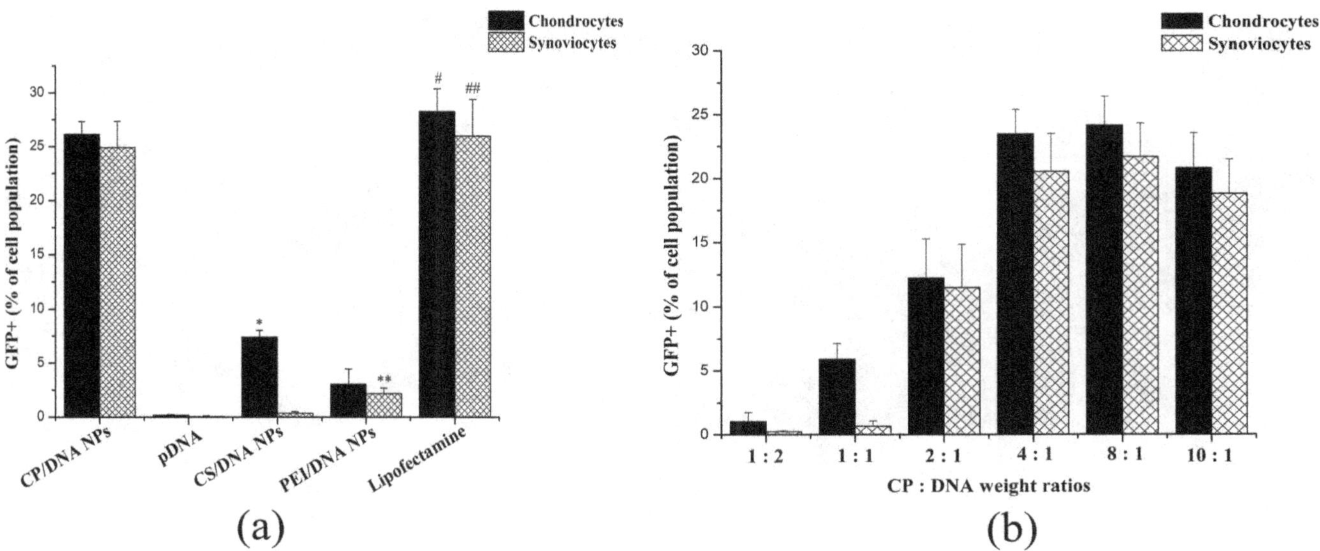

Figure 7. *In vitro* transfection efficiency of CP/DNA nanoparticles. (a) *In vitro* transfection efficiency of CP/DNA nanoparticles in both chondrocytes and synoviocytes compared to that of naked pDNA, CS/DNA nanoparticles, PEI (25 kDa)/DNA nanoparticles, and Lipofectamine™ 2000 (n = 3; 48 h post-transfection; error bars represent standard deviation). **P*<0.01 when CP/DNA nanoparticles compared to CS/DNA nanoparticles transfected towards chondrocytes (n = 3); ***P*<0.01 when CP/DNA nanoparticles compared to PEI (25 kDa)/DNA nanoparticles transfected towards synoviocytes (n = 3); # or ## *P*>0.05 when CP/DNA nanoparticles compared to Lipofectamine™ 2000 transfected towards chondrocytes or synoviocytes (n = 3). (b) Percentage of chondrocytes or synoviocytes transfected *in vitro* using CP/DNA nanoparticles as measured by flow cytometry 48 h post-transfection. The influence of CP:DNA weight ratios on the transfection efficiency was assessed 48 h post-transfection (n = 3; error bars represent standard deviation).

simultaneously to achieve high transfection efficiency due to its low cytotoxicity.

Another prerequisite to achieve successful transfection is that the bound pDNA must release from complexes: the unpacking of DNA from the polymeric vector is an important and crucial step in the transfection mediated by polymers [35]. CS has been reported to interact with pDNA via either strong electrostatic/hydrogen bonding or hydrophobic interactions [36]. High Mw PEIs also show high binding capacity with pDNA [37]. The binding ability has been found to be in the order CS>>>PEI (25 kDa)>CP>PEI (2.5 kDa) [9]. These crucial observations suggest that the CP copolymer binding capability is neither strong nor weak, which may be beneficial for improving transfection efficiency. CP/DNA nanoparticles' transfections showed a delayed EGFP expression, which was quite different from that of Lipofectamine™ 2000. At 24 h post-transfection, both CP/DNA and CS/DNA nanoparticles expressed weak EGFP. For its part, in cells transfected with naked pDNA, almost no expression of EGFP was observed. At 48 h, the EGFP-expression increased significantly in the CP/DNA nanoparticles group, and its fluorescence intensity also increased significantly compared to that of CS/DNA nanoparticles, PEI (25 kDa)/DNA nanoparticles, and naked pDNA [Figs. 6 and 7(a)]. The CS sustained-release property leads to relatively retardant release of pDNA from nanoparticles, which may explain why the expression of foreign transfected genes remained lower initially, the transfection efficiency increased after prolonged time, and the expression lasted much longer, which was different from that with Lipofectamine ™ 2000, associated with a rapid expression [16,38].

Figure 7(b) shows that the transfection efficiency of CP/DNA complex increased with the increasing of CP:DNA (w/w) ratio, and appeared a plateau after CP:DNA (w/w) ratio = 4. The transfection efficiencies of CP/DNA nanoparticles for chondrocytes of different CP:DNA (w/w) ratios were analyzed by one-way ANOVA, which demonstrated statistically significant difference ($F = 62.07$, $P < 0.01$); further analysis with LSD-*t* test revealed that, when the CP:DNA weight ratio reached 8, the transfection efficiency of CP/DNA nanoparticles was significantly higher than that when CP:DNA weight ratio was 0.5 to 2 ($P < 0.01$). Similar results were obtained for synoviocytes. With the increasing CP amount, the content of grafted PEI (1.8 kDa) helped complex to escape from endosome more easily, and it will not cause cytotoxicity to either chondrocytes or synoviocytes. On the other hand, as the CP:DNA (w/w) ratio increased, the copolymer size became smaller, and surface charge became more positive, thus leading to higher complexes internalization rates. This also would facilitate the higher transfection efficiency. However, when CP: DNA (w/w) ratio was greater than 8, it implies an considerable increase in the CP concentration in the complex, with too higher positive charge of the polyplexes yielding an overly stable complexes with anion DNA which leads to hard dissociation between CP and DNA, and as a consequence, the efficiency of plasmid release may decrease, thus showing reduced transfection [12,39,40]. In addition, with the CP concentration became too high, as shown in Figure 5, its cytotoxicity was also increased slightly, which would affect the transfection efficiency and even conversely lead to decreased gene transfection [14,41]. As a result, the transfection efficiency of CP/DNA complex appeared a plateau after CP:DNA (w/w) ratio = 4.

CP/DNA Complex Intracellular Trafficking

To investigate the cellular entry path, Cy3-labeled pDNA (red) CP/DNA was simultaneously added to both chondrocytes and synoviocytes, LysoTracker Green DND-26 was added to label lysosomes, and cells were fixed with PFA at specified intervals. We

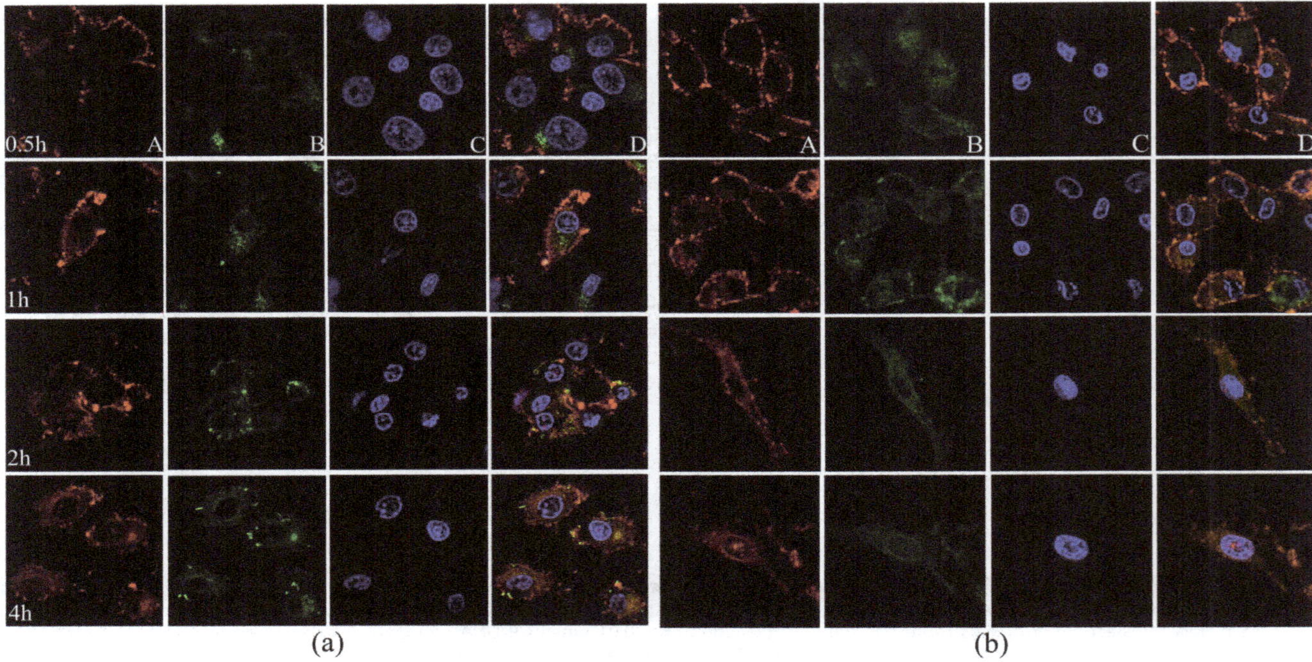

Figure 8. Intracellular distribution of Cy3-labeled pDNA/CP complexes was observed with a confocal fluorescence microscope in chondrocytes (a) and synoviocytes (b). (Panel 1) 0.5 h post-incubation; (Panel 2) 1 h post-incubation; (Panel 3) 2 h post-incubation; and (Panel 4) 4 h post-incubation. Row A shows the Cy3-labeled pDNA (red); row B shows the lysosomal (green); row C shows the nucleus (blue); and row D shows the overlap of A, B, and C rows content.

observed that CP was able to carry pDNA inside cells (cytoplasm) within 30 min to 1 h after the addition of nanoparticles to the cells. Further, pDNA could be observed inside the nucleus 2 h post addition of complexes, and a greater pDNA mount could be detected in nucleus after 4 h (Fig. 8). These observations clearly indicated that CP copolymers are capable of efficiently carrying the desired gene inside both chondrocytes and synoviocytes. In contrast, as Feng *et al.* [42] reported previously, PEI (25 kDa)/DNA nanoparticles could escape from endosome quickly, and the pDNA carried by nanoparticles detached from these and quickly localized in HeLa cells nuclei. However, the pDNA carried by CS was difficult to enter the nucleus even after 6 h of the CS/DNA complexes incubation [43], suggesting that it might take more time for CS-based polyplexes to escape from endosomes, and to undergo uncoupling of CS/DNA complexes than PEI polyplexes [12]. It has been suggested that, if polyplexes escape from the endosome too fast, it may lead to a large number of endosome ruptures in a short term, thus causing damage to the cell physiological environment and increasing the cytotoxicity [8]. In the present study, we have shown that the CP/DNA complex could escape from endosomes at a proper rate, simultaneously resulting in increased transfection efficiency and reduced cytotoxicity.

Conclusions

In the present study, CP/DNA nanoparticles were created as a novel, non-viral gene carrier targeted to OA and other joint diseases. The particle size and zeta potential of CP/DNA nanoparticles were related to the CP:DNA (w/w) ratio: there was a decrease in size and an increase in the surface charge with increasing of CP:DNA (w/w) ratio. The CP buffering capacity was found to be significantly enhanced compared to that of the CS. The transfection efficiency of CP/DNA nanoparticles was significantly higher than that of CS/DNA nanoparticles, PEI (25 kDa)/DNA nanoparticles and naked pDNA, and was similar to that of the Lipofectamine^{TM} 2000 towards articular chondrocytes and synoviocytes. The *in vitro* transfection efficiency of CP/DNA nanoparticles was found to be dependent on the CP:DNA (w/w) ratio. The average cell viability post-treatment with CP/DNA nanoparticles was >90% for both chondrocytes and synoviocytes, even when nanoparticles dose was increased to 20 μg/ml. This viability was much higher than that of PEI (25 kDa)/DNA nanoparticles. Intracellular trafficking studies found that CP copolymers were capable of efficiently carrying the pDNA inside both chondrocytes and synoviocytes, and the pDNA could be detected entering into the nucleus post 4 h incubation.

These results suggest that CP/DNA nanoparticles might be a safe and efficient non-viral vector for gene delivery to both chondrocytes and synoviocytes. Further studies should focus on evaluating the *in vivo* application of these novel CP/DNA nanoparticles in the treatment for joint diseases such as OA.

Acknowledgments

We thank the members of the Central Laboratory of Third Affiliated Hospital of Sun Yat-sen University for their excellent assistance in this study and to Medjaden Bioscience Limited for assisting in the preparation of this manuscript.

Author Contributions

Conceived and designed the experiments: HDL. Performed the experiments: HDL YHD LLL HQZ. Analyzed the data: HDL YHD LLL. Contributed reagents/materials/analysis tools: HDL YHD LLL HQZ. Wrote the paper: HDL YHD.

References

1. Pi Y, Zhang X, Shi J, Zhu J, Chen W, et al. (2011) Targeted delivery of non-viral vectors to cartilage in vivo using a chondrocyte-homing peptide identified by phage display. Biomaterials 32: 6324–6332. doi:10.1016/j.biomaterials.2011.05.017. PMID: 21624651.
2. Zhang X, Yu C, Xushi, Zhang C, Tang T, et al. (2006) Direct chitosan-mediated gene delivery to the rabbit knee joints in vitro and in vivo. Biochem Biophys Res Commun 341: 202–208. doi: 10.1016/j.bbrc.2005.12.171. PMID: 16413501.
3. Simon RH, Engelhardt JF, Yang Y, Zepeda M, Weber-Pendleton S, et al. (1993) Adenovirus-mediated transfer of the CFTR gene to lung of nonhuman primates: toxicity study. Hum Gene Ther 4: 771–780. doi:10.1089/hum.1993.4.6-771. PMID: 7514446.
4. Jiang HL, Kim TH, Kim YK, Park IY, Cho MH, et al. (2008) Efficient gene delivery using chitosan-polyethylenimine hybrid systems. Biomed Mater 3: 025013. doi: 10.1088/1748-6041/3/2/025013. PMID: 18477817.
5. Rekha MR, Sharma CP (2012) Polymers for gene delivery: current status and future perspectives. Recent Pat DNA Gene Seq 6: 98–107. doi:10.2174/187221512801327389. PMID: 22670610.
6. Tiera MJ, Shi Q, Winnik FM, Fernandes JC (2011) Polycation-based gene therapy: current knowledge and new perspectives. Curr Gene Ther 11: 288–306. doi: 10.2174/156652311796150408. PMID: 21453278.
7. Gao Y, Xu Z, Chen S, Gu W, Chen L, et al. (2008) Arginine-chitosan/DNA self-assemble nanoparticles for gene delivery: In vitro characteristics and transfection efficiency. Int J Pharm 359: 241–246. doi:10.1016/j.ijpharm.2008.03.037. PMID: 18479851.
8. Gao JQ, Zhao QQ, Lv TF, Shuai WP, Zhou J, et al. (2010) Gene-carried chitosan-linked-PEI induced high gene transfection efficiency with low toxicity and significant tumor-suppressive activity. Int J Pharm 387: 286–294. doi:10.1016/j.ijpharm.2009.12.033. PMID: 20035848.
9. Tripathi SK, Goyal R, Kumar P, Gupta KC (2012) Linear polyethylenimine-graft-chitosan copolymers as efficient DNA/siRNA delivery vectors in vitro and in vivo. Nanomedicine 8: 337–345. doi: 10.1016/j.nano.2011.06.022. PMID: 21756861.
10. Hejazi R, Amiji M (2003) Chitosan-based gastrointestinal delivery systems. J Control Release 89: 151–165. doi:10.1016/S0168-3659(03)00126-3. PMID: 12711440.
11. Li Z, Zhang M (2005) Chitosan-alginate as scaffolding material for cartilage tissue engineering. J Biomed Mater Res A 75: 485–493. doi:10.1002/jbm.a.30449. PMID: 16092113.
12. Mao S, Sun W, Kissel T (2010) Chitosan-based formulations for delivery of DNA and siRNA. Adv Drug Deliv Rev 62: 12–27. doi:10.1016/j.addr.2009.08.004. PMID: 19796660.
13. Kim TH, Kim SI, Akaike T, Cho CS (2005) Synergistic effect of poly(ethylenimine) on the transfection efficiency of galactosylated chitosan/DNA complexes. J Control Release 105: 354–366. doi:10.1016/j.jconrel.2005.03.024. PMID: 15949861.
14. Jiang HL, Kim YK, Arote R, Nah JW, Cho MH, et al. (2007) Chitosan-graft-polyethylenimine as a gene carrier. J Control Release 117: 273–280. doi:10.1016/j.jconrel.2006.10.025. PMID: 17166614.
15. Zhao QQ, Chen JL, Han M, Liang WQ, Tabata Y, et al. (2008) Combination of poly(ethylenimine) and chitosan induces high gene transfection efficiency and low cytotoxicity. J Biosci Bioeng 105: 65–68. doi:10.1263/jbb.105.65. PMID: 18295723.
16. Lu HD, Zhao HQ, Wang K, Lv LL (2011) Novel hyaluronic acid-chitosan nanoparticles as non-viral gene delivery vectors targeting osteoarthritis. Int J Pharm 420: 358–365. doi:10.1016/j.ijpharm.2011.08.046. PMID: 21911044.
17. Wong K, Sun G, Zhang X, Dai H, Liu Y, et al. (2006) PEI-g-chitosan, a novel gene delivery system with transfection efficiency comparable to polyethylenimine in vitro and after liver administration in vivo. Bioconjug Chem 17: 152–158. doi:10.1021/bc0501597. PMID: 16417264.
18. Lavertu M, Méthot S, Tran-Khanh N, Buschmann MD (2006) High efficiency gene transfer using chitosan/DNA nanoparticles with specific combinations of molecular weight and degree of deacetylation. Biomaterials 27: 4815–4824. doi:10.1016/j.biomaterials.2006.04.029. PMID: 16725196.
19. Zhao QQ, Chen JL, Lv TF, He CX, Tang GP, et al. (2009) N/P ratio significantly influences the transfection efficiency and cytotoxicity of a polyethylenimine/chitosan/DNA complex. Biol Pharm Bull 32: 706–710. doi:10.1248/bpb.32.706. PMID: 19336909.
20. Kichler A, Leborgne C, Danos O (2005) Dilution of reporter gene with stuffer DNA does not alter the transfection efficiency of polyethylenimines. J Gene Med 7: 1459–1467. doi:10.1002/jgm.805. PMID: 16041686.
21. Lungwitz U, Breunig M, Blunk T, Göpferich A (2005) Polyethylenimine-based non-viral gene delivery systems. Eur J Pharm Biopharm 60: 247–266. doi: 10.1016/j.ejpb.2004.11.011. PMID: 15939236.
22. Jere D, Jiang HL, Kim YK, Arote R, Choi YJ, et al. (2009) Chitosan-graft-polyethylenimine for Akt1 siRNA delivery to lung cancer cells. Int J Pharm. 378: 194–200. doi:10.1016/j.ijpharm.2009.05.046. PMID: 19501140.
23. de Lange-Brokaar BJ, Ioan-Facsinay A, van Osch GJ, Zuurmond AM, Schoones J, et al. (2012) Synovial inflammation, immune cells and their cytokines in osteoarthritis: a review. Osteoarthritis Cartilage 20: 1484–1499. doi: 10.1016/j.joca.2012.08.027. PMID: 22960092.
24. Berenbaum F (2013) Osteoarthritis as an inflammatory disease (osteoarthritis is not osteoarthrosis!). Osteoarthritis Cartilage 21: 16–21. doi:10.1016/j.joca.2012.11.012. PMID: 23194896.
25. Huang MJ, Wang L, Zheng XC, Zhang ZM, Yan B, et al. (2012) Intra-articular lentivirus-mediated insertion of the fat-1 gene ameliorates osteoarthritis. Med Hypotheses 79: 614–616. doi:10.1016/j.mehy.2012.07.035. PMID: 22939867.
26. Honjo K, Takahashi KA, Mazda O, Kishida T, Shinya M, et al. (2010) MDR1a/1b gene silencing enhances drug sensitivity in rat fibroblast-like synoviocytes. J Gene Med 12: 219–227. doi: 10.1002/jgm.1378. PMID:19950109.
27. Goyal R, Tripathi SK, Tyagi S, Sharma A, Ram KR, et al. (2012) Linear PEI nanoparticles: efficient pDNA/siRNA carriers in vitro and in vivo. Nanomedicine 8: 167–175. doi:10.1016/j.nano.2011.06.001. PMID:21703995.
28. Tseng WC, Tang CH, Fang TY (2004) The role of dextran conjugation in transfection mediated by dextran-grafted polyethylenimine. J Gene Med 6: 895–905. doi:10.1002/jgm.572. PMID:15293348.
29. Chang Y, Wei W, Zhang L, Xu HM (2009) Effects and mechanisms of total glucosides of paeony on synoviocytes activities in rat collagen-induced arthritis. J Ethnopharmacol 121: 43–48. doi: 10.1016/j.jep.2008.09.028. PMID:18977427.
30. Petersen H, Kunath K, Martin AL, Stolnik S, Roberts CJ, et al. (2002) Star-shaped poly(ethylene glycol)-block-polyethylenimine copolymers enhance DNA condensation of low molecular weight polyethylenimines. Biomacromolecules 3: 926–936. doi: 10.1021/bm025539z. PMID: 12217037.
31. Kubota N, Tatsumoto N, Sano T, Toya K (2000) A simple preparation of half N-acetylated chitosan highly soluble in water and aqueous organic solvents. Carbohydr Res 324: 268–274. doi:10.1016/S0008-6215(99)00263-3. PMID: 10744335.
32. Kunath K, von Harpe A, Fischer D, Petersen H, Bickel U, et al. (2003) Low-molecular-weight polyethylenimine as a non-viral vector for DNA delivery: comparison of physicochemical properties, transfection efficiency and in vivo distribution with high-molecular-weight polyethylenimine. J Control Release 89: 113–125. doi:10.1016/S0168-3659(03)00076-2. PMID: 12695067.
33. Jeong JH, Song SH, Lim DW, Lee H, Park TG (2001) DNA transfection using linear poly(ethylenimine) prepared by controlled acid hydrolysis of poly(2-ethyl-2-oxazoline). J Control Release 73: 391–399. doi:10.1016/S0168-3659(01)00310-8. PMID: 11516514.
34. Sun X, Zhang N (2010) Cationic polymer optimization for efficient gene delivery. Mini Rev Med Chem 10: 108–125. doi:10.2174/138955710791185109. PMID: 20408796.
35. Kircheis R, Wightman L, Wagner E (2001) Design and gene delivery activity of modified polyethylenimines. Adv Drug Deliv Rev 53: 341–358. doi:10.1016/S0169-409X(01)00202-2. PMID: 11744176.
36. Chang KL, Higuchi Y, Kawakami S, Yamashita F, Hashida M (2010) Efficient gene transfection by histidine-modified chitosan through enhancement of endosomal escape. Bioconjug Chem 21: 1087–1095. doi:10.1021/bc1000609. PMID: 20499901.
37. Choi S, Lee KD (2008) Enhanced gene delivery using disulfide-crosslinked low molecular weight polyethylenimine with listeriolysin o-polyethylenimine disulfide conjugate. J Control Release 131: 70–76. doi:10.1016/j.jconrel.2008.07.007. PMID: 18692533.
38. Sezer AD, Akbuğa J (2009) Comparison on in vitro characterization of fucospheres and chitosan microspheres encapsulated plasmid DNA (pGM-CSF): formulation design and release characteristics. AAPS PharmSciTech 10: 1193–1199. doi:10.1208/s12249-009-9324-0. PMID: 19859814.
39. Köping-Höggård M, Tubulekas I, Guan H, Edwards K, Nilsson M, et al. (2001) Chitosan as a nonviral gene delivery system. Structure-property relationships and characteristics compared with polyethylenimine in vitro and after lung administration in vivo. Gene Ther 8: 1108–1121. doi:10.1038/sj.gt.3301492. PMID: 11526458.
40. Köping-Höggård M, Mel'nikova YS, Vårum KM, Lindman B, Artursson P (2003) Relationship between the physical shape and the efficiency of oligomeric chitosan as a gene delivery system in vitro and in vivo. J Gene Med 5: 130–141. doi: 10.1002/jgm.327. PMID: 12539151.

41. Gao Y, Zhang Z, Chen L, Gu W, Li Y (2009) Chitosan N-betainates/DNA self-assembly nanoparticles for gene delivery: in vitro uptake and transfection efficiency. Int J Pharm 371: 156–162. doi: 10.1016/j.ijpharm.2008.12.012. PMID: 19135139.
42. Feng M, Lee D, Li P (2006) Intracellular uptake and release of poly(ethyleneimine)-co-poly(methyl methacrylate) nanoparticle/pDNA complexes for gene delivery. Int J Pharm 311: 209–214. doi:10.1016/j.ijpharm.2005.12.035. PMID: 16442245.
43. Hashimoto M, Morimoto M, Saimoto H, Shigemasa Y, Sato T (2006) Lactosylated chitosan for DNA delivery into hepatocytes: the effect of lactosylation on the physicochemical properties and intracellular trafficking of pDNA/chitosan complexes. Bioconjug Chem 17: 309–316. doi:10.1021/bc050228h. PMID: 16536460.

19

Porcine Model of Hemophilia A

Yuji Kashiwakura[1]🙰, Jun Mimuro[1*]🙰, Akira Onishi[2]🙰, Masaki Iwamoto[2,3]🙰, Seiji Madoiwa[1], Daiichiro Fuchimoto[2], Shunichi Suzuki[2], Misae Suzuki[2], Shoichiro Sembon[2], Akira Ishiwata[1], Atsushi Yasumoto[1], Asuka Sakata[1], Tsukasa Ohmori[1], Michiko Hashimoto[3], Satoko Yazaki[3], Yoichi Sakata[1]

1 Research Division of Cell and Molecular Medicine, Center for Molecular Medicine, Jichi Medical University, Shimotsuke, Tochigi-ken, Japan, **2** Transgenic Animal Research Center, National Institute of Agrobiological Sciences, Tsukuba, Ibaraki-ken, Japan, **3** Advanced Technology Development Team, Prime Tech Ltd., Tsuchiura, Ibaraki-ken, Japan

Abstract

Hemophilia A is a common X chromosome-linked genetic bleeding disorder caused by abnormalities in the coagulation factor VIII gene (*F8*). Hemophilia A patients suffer from a bleeding diathesis, such as life-threatening bleeding in the brain and harmful bleeding in joints and muscles. Because it could potentially be cured by gene therapy, subhuman animal models have been sought. Current mouse hemophilia A models generated by gene targeting of the *F8* have difficulties to extrapolate human disease due to differences in the coagulation and immune systems between mice and humans. Here, we generated a porcine model of hemophilia A by nuclear transfer cloning from *F8*-targeted fibroblasts. The hemophilia A pigs showed a severe bleeding tendency upon birth, similar to human severe hemophiliacs, but in contrast to hemophilia A mice which rarely bleed under standard breed conditions. Infusion of human factor VIII was effective in stopping bleeding and reducing the bleeding frequency of a hemophilia A piglet but was blocked by the inhibitor against human factor VIII. These data suggest that the hemophilia A pig is a severe hemophilia A animal model for studying not only hemophilia A gene therapy but also the next generation recombinant coagulation factors, such as recombinant factor VIII variants with a slower clearance rate.

Editor: Christopher B. Doering, Emory University School of Medicine, United States of America

Funding: This study was supported by Grants-in-Aid for Scientific Research (20591155, 21591249 and 21790920) and the Support Program for Strategic Research Infrastructure from the Japanese Ministry of Education, Culture, Sports, Science and Technology; and Health, Labour and Science Research Grants for Research on HIV/AIDS and Research on Intractable Diseases from the Japanese Ministry of Health, Labour and Welfare. The funders had no role in study design, data collection and analysis, decision to publish, or preparation of the manuscript.

Competing Interests: MI, MH, and SY are employees of Prim Tech Ltd., the developer of Piezo micromanipulators for nuclear transfer, and are collaborative with National Institute of Agrobiological Sciences and Jichi Meidical University for basic research. Other authors declare no conflict of interest.

* E-mail: mimuro-j@jichi.ac.jp

🙰 These authors contributed equally to this work.

Introduction

Hemophilia A is an inherited X-linked bleeding disorder caused by abnormalities in the coagulation factor VIII (FVIII) gene (*F8*). The genetic abnormalities result in FVIII deficiency, which in turn creates a bleeding diathesis, such as life-threatening bleeding in the brain and harmful bleeding in joints and muscles. The morbidity of hemophilia A is one in 5,000 male live births [1]. The current standard therapy for hemophilia A is intravenous injection of recombinant FVIII or monoclonal antibody-purified FVIII from plasma. Prophylactic administration of FVIII is effective in preventing harmful bleeding; however, hemophilia A patients are still not free from the risks of life-threatening intracranial and other harmful bleeding [1] [2]. In addition, severe hemophilia A patients develop antibody against FVIII (inhibitor) upon infusion of FVIII frequently [1].

Gene therapy, that enables sustained elevation of coagulation factor levels, will provide the next-generation therapy for hemophilia [1,3,4]. In fact, gene and cell therapy for hemophilia clinical trials were conducted. Compared with clinical trials of the gene therapy for hemophilia B [5,6], gene and cell therapies for hemophilia A have had limited successes [7,8]. Upcoming therapeutic alternatives for hemophilia A are FVIII variants with a slower clearance rate. Therapeutic factors, such as recombinant activated factor VII and plasma-derived activated prothrombin complex, are used for the treatment of hemophilia A patients with inhibitors, and the second generation therapeutic factors for hemophilia A patients with inhibitors are also currently under development. For studying next-generation therapeutics, good animal models are required. Hemophilia A mice generated by targeted ablation of mouse *F8* [9] have been the mainstay for assessment of hemophilia A gene therapy and evaluation of FVIII variants. However, there are significant species differences between mice and humans. For example, the half-life of human FVIII in the mouse circulation is very short, making it difficult to analyze the efficacy of human FVIII-expressing vectors for gene therapy or novel FVIII variants. As alternatives, there are natural hemophilia A dogs and hemophilia A sheep. Hemophilia A dogs have been used for gene therapy studies [10,11,12]. Hemophilia A sheep would be an alternative model [13]. There may be interspecies differences, such as body size, physiology, disease progression and chromosome structure homology, between these animal models and humans.

Pigs are excellent biomedical models of human diseases [14,15]. The porcine blood coagulation system is very similar to that in humans, because of the high homology between the coagulation factor amino acid sequences [16,17,18]. In addition, porcine FVIII has been used to treat hemophilia A patients with FVIII inhibitors [19,20,21]. Therefore, the hemophilia A pig could be a good animal model to study the next-generation therapeutics for hemophilia A. Moreover, a miniature pig strain exists, and thus, cloned pigs could be downsized to an adequate size, approximately 20–30 kg in weight. For these reasons, we decided to generate hemophilia A pigs by cloning technology.

Results

Firstly, we constructed a *F8* targeting vector (Figure 1**A**) and targeted *F8* in male porcine embryonic fibroblasts (PEF) with the *F8*-targeting vector as shown in Figure 1. The DNA fragment amplified from the non-transfected PEF DNA migrated at 6.5 kb on agarose gel electrophoresis, whereas two DNA fragments, migrating at 6.5 kb and 8.3 kb, were amplified from PEF colony 134. The 8.3 kb DNA was not amplified from genomic DNA of PEF colonies 135–137. The 8.3 kb fragment PCR-amplified from PEF colony 134 was cleaved into a 2.4-kb fragment and a 5.9-kb fragment by *Stu* I, whereas the PCR-amplified 6.5-kb DNA fragment was not susceptible to *Stu* I digestion. This supports that the PCR-amplified 8.3-kb fragment is derived from the *F8*-targeted genome because a *Stu* I recognition sequence present in the neo-resistant gene but not in the PCR amplified DNA fragment from the wild-type *F8*. The expected DNA fragments were amplified by PCR with Neo primers from genomic DNA from PEF colony 134, but not from wild-type genomic DNA (WT). PCR analysis of genomic DNA with three primer sets revealed a recombination event in *F8* of a colony, 134 (PEF-134). PEF-134 nuclei were then injected into enucleated oocytes. After an electrical pulse, the oocytes were transplanted into the oviduct of a female pig [22,23]. Transplantation of nucleus-transferred oocytes to the oviducts of female pigs was repeated four times. Three months later, a fetus was obtained by induced abortion. Dermal fibroblasts from this PEF-134-derived fetus (134-fetus) were isolated and cultured, and genomic DNA was isolated for analysis by PCR and by Southern blotting (Figure 2). The PCR amplified wild-type (WT) *F8* exon 14–18 fragment migrated at 6.5 kb, whereas the 8.3-kb targeted DNA fragment was amplified solely from 134-fetus fibroblast DNA. PCR-amplified DNA fragments using an *F8* exonic primer and a Neo primer were obtained only from 134-fetus DNA. The PCRs demonstrated insertion of the neomycin-resistance gene in *F8* (Figure 2**A**). Southern blotting showed that the 5′ probe hybridized with the 8.1 kb DNA fragment of Sac I-digested wild-type DNA while the 5′ probe hybridized with 9.9 kb DNA fragment of Sac I-digested 134-fetus DNA. Southern blotting with the 3′ probe confirmed recombination in the *F8* gene in the 134-fetus genome because a Sph I recognition sequence and a Xba I recognition sequence located in the 3′ end of the Neo resistant gene of the targeted allele (Figure 2**B**). Therefore, five transfers of fetal fibroblast nuclei to oocytes followed by oocyte transplantation were performed. Four females became pregnant and each produced a full-term delivery.

Four live offspring were obtained and PCR analysis and Southern blotting were carried out. As shown in Figure 3**A**, the 8.3 kb DNA fragments were PCR amplified from piglets DNA as same as that of 134-fetus (Figure 2). Similarly, Southern blotting of Sac I-treated and *Sac* I and *Stu* I-treated DNA of the piglets with

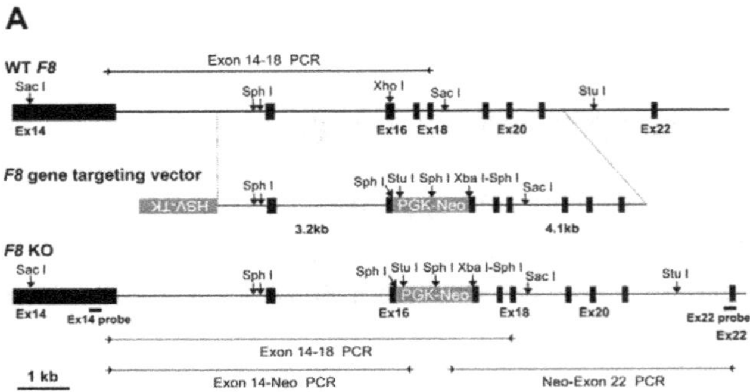

B Exon14-18 PCR

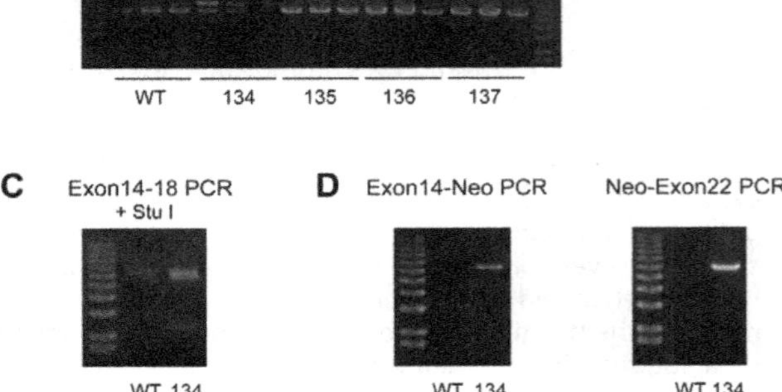

Figure 1. *F8* targeting of porcine fetal fibroblasts (PEF). (A) Schematic diagram of part of porcine *F8*, the positions of the restriction endonuclease sites, the *F8* targeting vector structure, and the targeted *F8* (*F8* KO) allele are shown. The neomycin-resistance gene (PGK-neo) was inserted in the exon 16 DNA fragment with deletion of a part of exon 16 and was flanked by two *F8* DNA fragments (5′ arm: 3.2 kb; 3′ arm: 4.1 kb) in *F8* targeting vector. The positions of PCR primers (arrowheads), expected amplified DNA fragments (bars), and restriction endonuclease sites used for the Southern blot analysis are indicated in the schema for *F8* KO. (**B**) *F8* exon 14–18 PCR on genomic DNA from non-transfected PEF (WT), PEF colony 134 (134), and three other PEF colonies (135–137) was shown. (**C**) The *F8* exon 14–18 PCR products were treated with *Stu* I and analyzed by agarose gel electrophoresis. (**D**) PCR analyses with two sets of primer pairs for exon 14 and the neomycin resistance gene and for the neomycin resistance gene and exon 22 were shown.

the 5′ probe confirmed the recombination of F8 of piglets and showed that each piglet had a single copy of the targeted *F8* (Figure 3, **A** & **B**). RT-PCR analysis revealed that FVIII mRNA was not detected in the liver of piglet #3 (Figure 3**C**). Analysis of the blood of piglets #3 and #4 confirmed that the FVIII level was severely decreased to less than 1%, using an activated partial thromboplastin time (APTT)-based coagulation assay for human FVIII (Table 1). Other coagulation factors were moderately decreased (Table 1). The levels of albumin and cholinesterase of these piglet blood were also measured as the references to study whether the decreased level of coagulation factors II, V, VII, IX, and X were specific or not. The albumin levels of piglet #3 and #4 were decreased significantly compared with the wild type piglets. However, the cholinesterase activities of piglets #3 and #4 were not decreased. The data suggested that synthesis of some proteins in the liver of the cloned piglets was altered. The precise mechanism of the moderately decreased levels of coagulation factors II, V, VII, IX, and X, and albumin was not elucidated in this study.

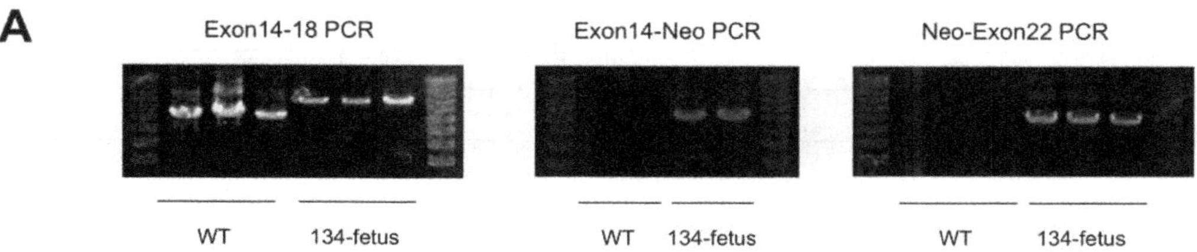

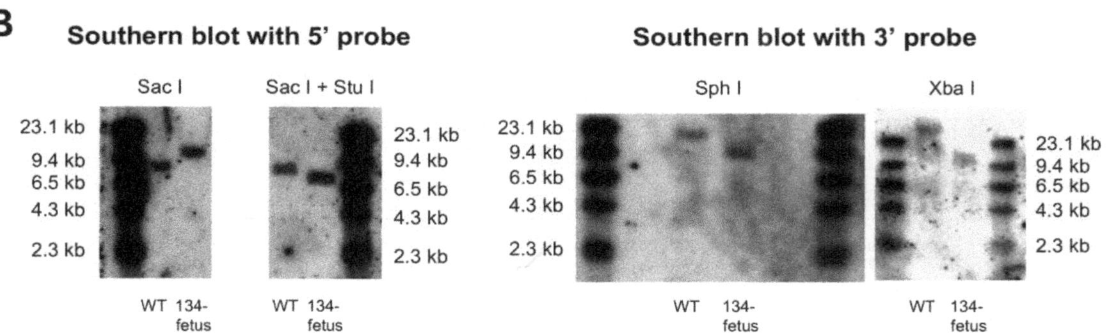

Figure 2. *F8* targeting and genetic analysis of the colony 134-derived fetus. PCR analysis of genomic DNA of 134-fetus was shown. (**A**) Two or three independent PCR reactions were carried out for detection of recombination in *F8* of 134-fetus. (**B**) Southern blotting with a 5′ exon 14 probe (on *Sac* I− or *Sac* I + *Stu* I-digested DNA) and with a 3′ exon 22 probe (on *Sph* I− or *Xba* I-digested DNA) showed correct targeting of the *F8* in 134-fetus.

Two of the piglets (#1 and #2) found dead the next day (day 2) after delivery. The cause of death of these two piglets was not certain. Early deaths of cloned piglets after birth are not uncommon as described [24,25]. Accidental bleeding might affect the condition of piglet #1 since large hematomas were observed in piglet #1 (Figure 4). Massive traumatic intramuscular bleeding was thought to affect the death of piglet #3 on day 3 because the general condition of piglet #3 became severe immediately after the bleeding took place and piglet #3 died. Piglet #4 was born with bleeding in the left forelimb, thus, human FVIII concentrate (150 U/kg) was injected intravenously on day 2 after delivery, which cured the bleeding in the limb (Figure 4). However, because this piglet still showed a bleeding in the limbs and the tongue, which was cured with human FVIII infusion, it was given a prophylactic infusion of human FVIII (150 U/kg) twice a week, which was effective in reducing the bleeding frequency. The human FVIII activity at 12.1% (average of two points; day 10 and day 23 after birth) was detected in the piglet #4 plasma obtained two days after the injection. However, spontaneous bleeding still occurred in piglet #4, in particular repeated bleeding in the left forelimb, causing limping (Figure 4 and video S1). Piglet #4 died due to gastric bleeding from a gastric ulcer on day 38 after birth. Inhibitor (856 BU/mL) against human FVIII was detected in the plasma obtained on the day when piglet #4 died. The development of inhibitor might explain why human FVIII injected two days before was not effective to reduce bleeding from the gastric ulcer.

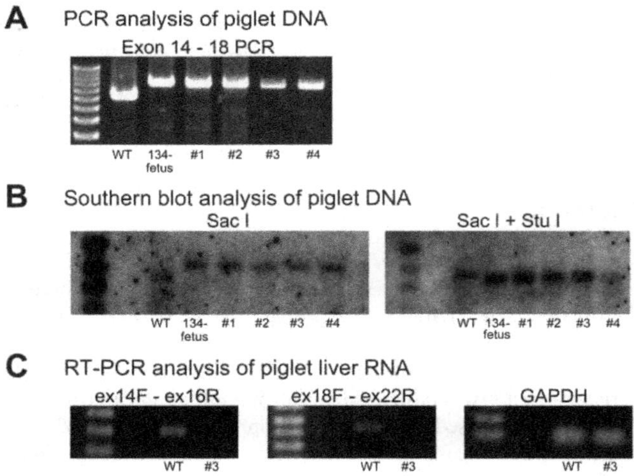

Figure 3. Analysis of the *F8* in cloned piglets. (**A**) PCR analysis of genomic DNA of piglet DNA was shown. Genomic DNA of wild-type, 134-fetus, piglet #1, piglet #2, piglet #3, and piglet #4 was subjected to PCR analysis with primers Exon 14 sF and Exon 18 sR as in Figure 1. The 8.3 kb exon 14–18 band was amplified from the 134-fetus DNA and the cloned piglet DNA. (**B**) Southern blotting with a 5′ exon 14 probe (on *Sac* I− or *Sac* I + *Stu* I-digested DNA) showed the same mobility shifts of the bands as those in Figure 2**B** and confirmed the insertion of the Neo resistant gene in *F8* of the cloned piglets. (**C**) RT-PCR analysis of piglet liver RNA was shown. Two independent PCRs (exons 14–16 and exons 18–22) revealed the absence of FVIII mRNA from the liver of cloned piglet #3. Control GAPDH mRNA was detected in the liver RNA of piglet #3 as in the wild type (WT).

Discussion

Advances in cloning technology have allowed us to generate genetically modified animals [22,26,27]. Among these, a few gene-targeted pigs have been reported, such as cystic fibrosis pigs [28] and heterozygous fumarylacetoacetate hydrolase deficient pigs [29]as a disease model, and α1, 3-galactosyltransferase gene-knockout (KO) pigs [30] for organ transplantation [30,31]. Considering the limitations in studying human disease in murine models, gene-targeted pigs are thought to be preferred for studying

Table 1. Coagulation factor activity of piglets #3 and #4.

Coagulation factor	Wild type (n = 4)	Piglet #3	Piglet #4
Fibrinogen (μmol/L)	2.67±1.39	1.56	ND
Factor II (%)	75.7±3.9	53	47
Factor V (%)	>200	118	168
Factor VII (%)	68.5±3.4	19	19
Factor VIII (%)	>200	1>	1>
Factor IX (%)	>200	96	69
Factor X (%)	134±7.0	72	64
	Wild type (n = 4)	**Piglet #3**	**Piglet #4**
von Willebrand Factor (%)	174.7±25.9	124	251
Albumin (g/dL)	2.8±0.08	1.0	1.9
Cholinesterase (IU/L)	3.75±1.50	15	3

The coagulation factor levels of piglet #3 and #4 are shown with the control coagulation factor levels of wild-type piglets. Each coagulation factor activity was calculated from the standard curve generated with normal human plasma and expressed as the percentage of the respective coagulation factor activity in normal human plasma.
ND: not determined.

human diseases and for translational research. We explore the possibility of *F8* KO pigs (hemophilia A pigs) for studying the next generation therapy for hemophilia A in the current study. The genotype of cloned pigs showed the proper recombination in the *F8* of the pigs and the blood coagulation factor levels of cloned pigs confirmed severe FVIII deficiency. The precise mechanism of moderately decreased other coagulation factor levels in piglets #3 and #4 was not elucidated yet, these changes may not be specific to the coagulation factors since the level of albumin was decreased but the cholinesterase level was not decreased (both albumin and cholinesterase are synthesized in the liver). One possible mechanism of the changes could be the epigenetic effect genome DNA methylation and histone acetylation, which alter gene expression in cloned pigs [24,32,33,34]. Hemophilia A pigs generated by the nuclear transfer technology did show a severe bleeding phenotype that is in contrast to *F8* KO mice that rarely exhibit spontaneous bleeding into the muscles and joints under standard breed conditions [9]. Therefore, hemophilia A pig can be used to evaluate an efficacy of novel therapy such as gene therapy for hemophilia A in a standard breed condition. Moreover, prophylactic infusion of human FVIII was effective in reducing bleeding in *F8* KO piglet #4 thought its therapeutic effect was not perfect. This suggests that the *F8* KO pig is a subhuman animal model of severe hemophilia A for the study of upcoming therapeutic factors, such novel FVIII variants. Piglet #4 died because of bleeding from a gastric ulcer. Since inhibitor against human FVIII was detected in the plasma sample obtained on the day when piglet #4 died, the therapeutic effect of human FVIII no longer existed at the time, resulting in severe bleeding from the gastric ulcer. It is possible that *F8* KO pigs might develop antibodies against porcine FVIII as against human FVIII. The possibility of the use of *F8* KO pigs as a model for studying immune tolerance induction therapy for FVIII inhibitor remains to be studied.

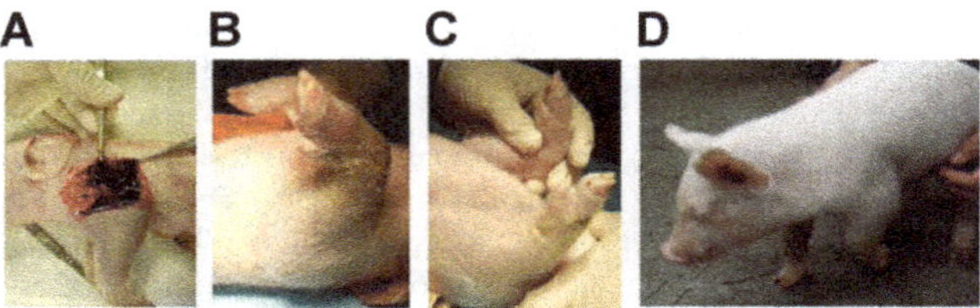

Figure 4. The bleeding phenotype of cloned *F8* KO piglets. (**A**) A part of macroscopic picture of cloned piglet #1, which died by day 2 after birth is shown. Ecchymosis was seen in the cheek, the forelimb, and the hind limb (not shown). Pathological examination revealed hematomas in these areas of piglet #1. (**B**) Forelimb of cloned piglet #4 on day 1 after delivery was shown. Ecchymosis had been seen in the left forelimb of cloned piglet #4 since delivery. (**C**) On day 5 after administration of human FVIII (150 U/kg), the bleeding in the left forelimb was not observed. Macroscopic picture of cloned piglet #4 on day 28 after birth showed that the left forelimb was swollen because of the repeated bleeding (**D**), causing the piglet to limp (also see video 1).

Methods

Construction of the F8 targeting vector

Porcine genomic DNA was isolated from porcine embryonic fibroblasts (LW; Landrace – Large White, ED65). The *F8* targeting vector was constructed by inserting two genomic DNA fragments into the plasmid vector pHSV-TK/PGK-Neo. The *F8* targeting vector was designed by referring to the *F8* exon 16 gene-targeting vector used to generate hemophilia A mice [9]. *F8* DNA fragments from exons 14–22 were isolated by PCR using primers (Table S1) based on the *Sus scrofa* coagulation factor VIII mRNA sequence (accession number: NM_214167) and sequenced. The two homologous arms of the gene-targeting vector were generated by reference to this sequence. The 5′ DNA fragment spanning intron 15 to exon 21 of *F8* was PCR-amplified, digested with *Xho* I to generate an 11-nucleotide deletion of exon 16, and inserted into pHSV-TK/PGK-Neo. The 3′ DNA fragment was PCR-amplified from exon 16 to intron 21, and cloned into pHSV-TK/PGK-Neo containing the 5′ *F8* DNA fragment. The herpes simplex virus thymidine kinase gene was located in the opposite orientation on the 5′ end of the 5′ arm. The targeting vector was linearized with *Not* I before transfection.

Isolation of porcine embryonic fibroblasts and isolation of F8-targeted cells

Porcine embryonic fibroblasts (PEF) were isolated from a male fetus of the LW strain as described [22]. PEFs (1×10^7 cells) were transfected with the *F8* targeting vector by electroporation (Gene Pulser II; Bio-Rad, Hercules, CA) at 278 V and 950 µF. After transfection, cells were cultured in Dulbecco's modified Eagle's medium with low-glucose (Invitrogen, Carlsbad, CA) containing 10% fetal bovine serum. After 48 h incubation, cells were selected with 800 µg/ml G418 (Nacalai Tesque, Inc., Kyoto, Japan) and 2 µM gancyclovir (Tanabe-Mitsubishi Pharma, Tokyo, Japan). On the eighth day following selection, G418-resistant colonies had grown. Cells from these colonies were grown in 24-well plates (Corning) in medium containing 4 ng/ml bFGF, and expanded for genomic DNA extraction and storage. DNA isolated from three wells of each colony was analyzed by three independent PCR reactions for recombination in the porcine *F8* (Table S1).

Southern blotting

Southern blotting for the *F8* recombination was performed by the standard procedure. Digoxigenin (DIG)-labeled 5′ and 3′ probes were generated by PCR (497 bp from exon 14 and 469 bp from exon 22, respectively) (Table S1). Signals were visualized using a DIG detection module (anti-DIG-alkaline phosphatase and a CSPD) (Roche Diagnostics GmbH., Mannheim, Germany).

RT-PCR of porcine FVIII mRNA

Total RNA was isolated from piglet liver using an RNeasy Mini kit (Invitrogen), converted to cDNA and PCR amplified using the SuperScript One-Step RT-PCR System (Invitrogen) with primer pairs specific for FVIII mRNA (Table S1) [35,36].

Nuclear transfer and transplantation of manipulated embryos to recipients

Production of clone piglets by nuclear transfer was performed as described previously [22,23]. In brief, metaphase II oocytes were enucleated by gentle aspiration of the first polar body and adjacent cytoplasm using a beveled pipette (25 to 30 µm) in PZM3 medium containing 5.0 µg/ml cytochalasin B. Enucleated oocytes were washed in PZM3 medium lacking cytochalasin B and nuclei of the *F8*-targeted cells introduced by direct intracytoplasmic injection using a piezo-actuated micromanipulator (Prime Tech., Tsuchiura, Japan). Oocytes were then stimulated with a direct current pulse of 1.5 kV/cm for 100 µS using a somatic hybridizer (SSH-10, Shimadzu, Kyoto, Japan) and transferred to PZM3 supplemented with cytochalasin B to prevent extrusion of a pseudo-second polar body. The nuclear transferred oocytes were then cultured in PZM3 medium in an atmosphere of 5% CO_2, 5% O_2 and 90% air at 38.5°C for 2 days until reaching the two-to-eight-cell stage. Cleaved embryos were transferred to the oviducts (200 embryos per recipient) of an anesthetized pseudopregnant surrogate mother (matured LWD; a Landrace×Large White× Duroc triple cross). Following embryo transfer, mother pigs were observed daily to confirm pregnancy by checking estrus. Farrowing was synchronized by injection of the prostaglandin F2α analog, (1)-cloprostenol (Planate, Osaka, Japan) on day 113–116 of gestation.

Coagulation factor activity measurement

Activities of porcine coagulation factors were measured at a clinical laboratory (SRL, Tokyo, Japan) by the standard clotting time method with respective coagulation factor-deficient human plasma. Normal human plasma was used as the standard for each test. The coagulation factor activity in piglet plasma was expressed as the percentage of the coagulation factor activity in normal pooled plasma, except for fibrinogen. The fibrinogen concentration was determined by the thrombin time method. von Willebrand factor levels in pig plasma were measured with an enzyme immunoassay with latex particle conjugated antibody (performed at SRL, Tokyo, Japan) since the von Willebrand factor activity (Ristocetin cofactor activity) in pig plasma was unable to be measured with human platelets. The von Willebrand factor antigen levels in pig plasma were expressed as percentages of the normal human plasma. An inhibitor assay for human FVIII was performed as described [36].

Blood chemistry analysis

The levels of albumin and choline esterase of piglet blood were measured at the Nagahama Life-science Laboratory of Oriental East Co. Ltd (Hagahama, Shiga-ken, Japan). Choline esterase activities of blood samples were measured with p-hydroxy benzoyl choline iodide as the substrate [37].

Animal experiments

All the animal experiments and surgical procedures were carried out in accordance with guidelines approved by the Institutional Animal Care and Concern Committees of Jichi Medical University and the National Institute of Agrobiological Sciences. Protocols for the use of animals in this study were approved by the review boards of Animal Care Committees of Jichi Medical University and the National Institute of Agrobiological Sciences. Wild type pigs used in this study were bred under a standard condition according to the institutional guideline of Animal Care Committee of National Institute of Agrobiological Sciences. After delivery, cloned F8KO pigs were separated from mother pigs and each cloned F8KO pig was bred by artificial suckling in a cage with protection of soft buffers to avoid traumas. All the experimental procedures including injection of FVIII were carried out under inhalation anesthesia with isoflurane and monitoring of body temperature. The endpoint of this study was to generate F8KO pigs and analyze the genotype and the phenotype of the F8KO pig precisely to investigate whether the F8KO pig can be a subhuman model of severe hemophilia A.

Author Contributions

Wrote the paper: JM. Senior investigator and supervised this study: YS. Acted as a senior investigator, planned, generated constructs for F8 gene targeting, and conducted the study: JM. Postdoctoral fellow, conducted most of the F8 targeting work and injected human FVIII into a cloned piglet: YK. Performed nuclear transfer of targeted cells to oocytes and transplantation of the oocytes, and managed care of cloned pigs: AO MI. Injected human FVIII into a cloned piglet on day 1 after birth: SM. Cared for cloned piglets and did pathological examination of cloned piglets: DF SS MS SS MH SY. Performed cell culture experiments: AI AY AS TO.

References

1. Mannucci PM, Tuddenham EG (2001) The hemophilias–from royal genes to gene therapy. N Engl J Med 344: 1773–1779.
2. Manco-Johnson MJ, Abshire TC, Shapiro AD, Riske B, Hacker MR, et al. (2007) Prophylaxis versus episodic treatment to prevent joint disease in boys with severe hemophilia. N Engl J Med 357: 535–544.
3. Hasbrouck NC, High KA (2008) AAV-mediated gene transfer for the treatment of hemophilia B: problems and prospects. Gene Ther 15: 870–875.
4. VandenDriessche T, Collen D, Chuah MK (2003) Gene therapy for the hemophilias. J Thromb Haemost 1: 1550–1558.
5. Manno CS, Pierce GF, Arruda VR, Glader B, Ragni M, et al. (2006) Successful transduction of liver in hemophilia by AAV-Factor IX and limitations imposed by the host immune response. Nat Med 12: 342–347.
6. Nathwani AC, Tuddenham EG, Rangarajan S, Rosales C, McIntosh J, et al. (2011) Adenovirus-associated virus vector-mediated gene transfer in hemophilia B. N Engl J Med 365: 2357–2365.
7. Roth DA, Tawa NE Jr, O'Brien JM, Treco DA, Selden RF (2001) Nonviral transfer of the gene encoding coagulation factor VIII in patients with severe hemophilia A. N Engl J Med 344: 1735–1742.
8. Powell JS, Ragni MV, White GC 2nd, Lusher JM, Hillman-Wiseman C, et al. (2003) Phase 1 trial of FVIII gene transfer for severe hemophilia A using a retroviral construct administered by peripheral intravenous infusion. Blood 102: 2038–2045.
9. Bi L, Lawler AM, Antonarakis SE, High KA, Gearhart JD, et al. (1995) Targeted disruption of the mouse factor VIII gene produces a model of haemophilia A. Nat Genet 10: 119–121.
10. Brown BD, Shi CX, Powell S, Hurlbut D, Graham FL, et al. (2004) Helper-dependent adenoviral vectors mediate therapeutic factor VIII expression for several months with minimal accompanying toxicity in a canine model of severe hemophilia A. Blood 103: 804–810.
11. Finn JD, Ozelo MC, Sabatino DE, Franck HW, Merricks EP, et al. (2010) Eradication of neutralizing antibodies to factor VIII in canine hemophilia A after liver gene therapy. Blood 116: 5842–5848.
12. Sabatino DE, Freguia CF, Toso R, Santos A, Merricks EP, et al. (2009) Recombinant canine B-domain-deleted FVIII exhibits high specific activity and is safe in the canine hemophilia A model. Blood 114: 4562–4565.
13. Porada CD, Sanada C, Long CR, Wood JA, Desai J, et al. (2010) Clinical and molecular characterization of a re-established line of sheep exhibiting hemophilia A. J Thromb Haemost 8: 276–285.
14. Lunney JK (2007) Advances in swine biomedical model genomics. Int J Biol Sci 3: 179–184.
15. Bendixen E, Danielsen M, Larsen K, Bendixen C (2010) Advances in porcine genomics and proteomics–a toolbox for developing the pig as a model organism for molecular biomedical research. Brief Funct Genomics 9: 208–219.
16. Massicotte P, Mitchell L, Andrew M (1986) A comparative study of coagulation systems in newborn animals. Pediatr Res 20: 961–965.
17. Reverdiau-Moalic P, Watier H, Vallee I, Lebranchu Y, Bardos P, et al. (1996) Comparative study of porcine and human blood coagulation systems: possible relevance in xenotransplantation. Transplant Proc 28: 643–644.
18. Chen Y, Qiao J, Tan W, Lu Y, Qin S, et al. (2009) Characterization of porcine factor VII, X and comparison with human factor VII, X. Blood Cells Mol Dis 43: 111–118.
19. Morrison AE, Ludlam CA (1991) The use of porcine factor VIII in the treatment of patients with acquired hemophilia: the United Kingdom experience. Am J Med 91: 23S–26S.
20. Toschi V (2010) OBI-1, porcine recombinant Factor VIII for the potential treatment of patients with congenital hemophilia A and alloantibodies against human Factor VIII. Curr Opin Mol Ther 12: 617–625.
21. Barrow RT, Lollar P (2006) Neutralization of antifactor VIII inhibitors by recombinant porcine factor VIII. J Thromb Haemost 4: 2223–2229.
22. Onishi A, Iwamoto M, Akita T, Mikawa S, Takeda K, et al. (2000) Pig cloning by microinjection of fetal fibroblast nuclei. Science 289: 1188–1190.
23. Suzuki S, Iwamoto M, Saito Y, Fuchimoto D, Sembon S, et al. (2012) Il2rg gene-targeted severe combined immunodeficiency pigs. Cell Stem Cell 10: 753–758.
24. Cho SK, Kim JH, Park JY, Choi YJ, Bang JI, et al. (2007) Serial cloning of pigs by somatic cell nuclear transfer: restoration of phenotypic normality during serial cloning. Dev Dyn 236: 3369–3382.
25. Umeyama K, Watanabe M, Saito H, Kurome M, Tohi S, et al. (2009) Dominant-negative mutant hepatocyte nuclear factor 1alpha induces diabetes in transgenic-cloned pigs. Transgenic Res 18: 697–706.
26. Chesne P, Adenot PG, Viglietta C, Baratte M, Boulanger L, et al. (2002) Cloned rabbits produced by nuclear transfer from adult somatic cells. Nat Biotechnol 20: 366–369.
27. Shin T, Kraemer D, Pryor J, Liu L, Rugila J, et al. (2002) A cat cloned by nuclear transplantation. Nature 415: 859.
28. Rogers CS, Stoltz DA, Meyerholz DK, Ostedgaard LS, Rokhlina T, et al. (2008) Disruption of the CFTR gene produces a model of cystic fibrosis in newborn pigs. Science 321: 1837–1841.
29. Hickey RD, Lillegard JB, Fisher JE, McKenzie TJ, Hofherr SE, et al. (2011) Efficient production of Fah-null heterozygote pigs by chimeric adeno-associated virus-mediated gene knockout and somatic cell nuclear transfer. Hepatology.
30. Lai L, Kolber-Simonds D, Park KW, Cheong HT, Greenstein JL, et al. (2002) Production of alpha-1,3-galactosyltransferase knockout pigs by nuclear transfer cloning. Science 295: 1089–1092.
31. Yamada K, Yazawa K, Shimizu A, Iwanaga T, Hisashi Y, et al. (2005) Marked prolongation of porcine renal xenograft survival in baboons through the use of alpha1,3-galactosyltransferase gene-knockout donors and the cotransplantation of vascularized thymic tissue. Nat Med 11: 32–34.
32. Tian XC, Park J, Bruno R, French R, Jiang L, et al. (2009) Altered gene expression in cloned piglets. Reprod Fertil Dev 21: 60–66.
33. Shen CJ, Cheng WT, Wu SC, Chen HL, Tsai TC, et al. (2012) Differential differences in methylation status of putative imprinted genes among cloned swine genomes. PLoS One 7: e32812.
34. Kim YJ, Ahn KS, Kim M, Shim H (2011) Comparison of potency between histone deacetylase inhibitors trichostatin A and valproic acid on enhancing in vitro development of porcine somatic cell nuclear transfer embryos. In Vitro Cell Dev Biol Anim 47: 283–289.
35. Ishiwata A, Mimuro J, Kashiwakura Y, Niimura M, Takano K, et al. (2006) Phenotype correction of hemophilia A mice with adeno-associated virus vectors carrying the B domain-deleted canine factor VIII gene. Thromb Res 118: 627–635.
36. Ishiwata A, Mimuro J, Mizukami H, Kashiwakura Y, Takano K, et al. (2009) Liver-restricted expression of the canine factor VIII gene facilitates prevention of inhibitor formation in factor VIII-deficient mice. J Gene Med 11: 1020–1029.
37. Tanaka H, Igarashi T, Lefor AT, Kobayashi E (2009) The effects of fasting and general anesthesia on serum chemistries in KCG miniature pigs. J Am Assoc Lab Anim Sci 48: 33–38.

High-Efficiency Transduction of Primary Human Hematopoietic Stem Cells and Erythroid Lineage-Restricted Expression by Optimized AAV6 Serotype Vectors *In Vitro* and in a Murine Xenograft Model *In Vivo*

Liujiang Song[1,2,3,4,5], Xiaomiao Li[3,4,5], Giridhara R. Jayandharan[3,4,5,6,7], Yuan Wang[8,9], George V. Aslanidi[3,4,5], Chen Ling[3,4,5], Li Zhong[3,4,5,10,11], Guangping Gao[10,12], Mervin C. Yoder[13,14], Changquan Ling[8,9], Mengqun Tan[1,2]*, Arun Srivastava[3,4,5,15,16]*

1 Experimental Hematology Laboratory, Department of Physiology, School of Basic Medical Sciences, Central South University, Changsha, China, **2** Shenzhen Institute of Xiangya Biomedicine, Shenzhen, China, **3** Division of Cellular and Molecular Therapy, Department of Pediatrics, University of Florida College of Medicine, Gainesville, Florida, United States of America, **4** Powell Gene Therapy Center, University of Florida College of Medicine, Gainesville, Florida, United States of America, **5** Genetics Institute, University of Florida College of Medicine, Gainesville, Florida, United States of America, **6** Department of Haematology, Christian Medical College, Vellore, Tamil Nadu, India, **7** Center for Stem Cell Research, Christian Medical College, Vellore, Tamil Nadu, India, **8** Department of Traditional Chinese Medicine, Changhai Hospital, Second Military Medical University, Shanghai, China, **9** Shanghai University of Traditional Chinese Medicine, Shanghai, China, **10** Gene Therapy Center, University of Massachusetts Medical School, Worcester, Massachusetts, United States of America, **11** Department of Pediatrics, University of Massachusetts Medical School, Worcester, Massachusetts, United States of America, **12** Department of Microbiology & Physiology Systems, University of Massachusetts Medical School, Worcester, Massachusetts, United States of America, **13** Herman B Well Center for Pediatric Research, Indiana University School of Medicine, Indianapolis, Indiana, United States of America, **14** Department of Pediatrics, Indiana University School of Medicine, Indianapolis, Indiana, United States of America, **15** Department of Molecular Genetics and Microbiology, University of Florida College of Medicine, Gainesville, Florida, United States of America, **16** Shands Cancer Center, University of Florida College of Medicine, Gainesville, Florida, United States of America

Abstract

We have observed that of the 10 AAV serotypes, AAV6 is the most efficient in transducing primary human hematopoietic stem cells (HSCs), and that the transduction efficiency can be further increased by specifically mutating single surface-exposed tyrosine (Y) residues on AAV6 capsids. In the present studies, we combined the two mutations to generate a tyrosine double-mutant (Y705+731F) AAV6 vector, with which >70% of $CD34^+$ cells could be transduced. With the long-term objective of developing recombinant AAV vectors for the potential gene therapy of human hemoglobinopathies, we generated the wild-type (WT) and tyrosine-mutant AAV6 vectors containing the following erythroid cell-specific promoters: β-globin promoter (βp) with the upstream hyper-sensitive site 2 (HS2) enhancer from the β-globin locus control region (HS2-βbp), and the human parvovirus B19 promoter at map unit 6 (B19p6). Transgene expression from the B19p6 was significantly higher than that from the HS2-βp, and increased up to 30-fold and up to 20-fold, respectively, following erythropoietin (Epo)-induced differentiation of $CD34^+$ cells *in vitro*. Transgene expression from the B19p6 or the HS2-βp was also evaluated in an immuno-deficient xenograft mouse model *in vivo*. Whereas low levels of expression were detected from the B19p6 in the WT AAV6 capsid, and that from the HS2-βp in the Y705+731F AAV6 capsid, transgene expression from the B19p6 promoter in the Y705+731F AAV6 capsid was significantly higher than that from the HS2-βp, and was detectable up to 12 weeks post-transplantation in primary recipients, and up to 6 additional weeks in secondary transplanted animals. These data demonstrate the feasibility of the use of the novel Y705+731F AAV6-B19p6 vectors for high-efficiency transduction of HSCs as well as expression of the b-globin gene in erythroid progenitor cells for the potential gene therapy of human hemoglobinopathies such as β-thalassemia and sickle cell disease.

Editor: Andrew C. Wilber, Southern Illinois University School of Medicine, United States of America

Funding: This research was supported in part by a grant from the Fanconi Anemia Research Fund, Inc. (to LZ), a Natural Science Foundation of China (NSFC) grant 30971299 (to MT), and Public Health Service grants R01 HL-065770, HL-076901, P01 DK-058327 (Project 1), and R01 HL-097088 from the National Institutes of Health (to AS). GRJ was supported in part by an Overseas Associate Fellowship-2006 from the Department of Biotechnology, Government of India. The funders had no role in study design, data collection and analysis, decision to publish, or preparation of the manuscript.

Competing Interests: The authors have declared that no competing interests exist.

* E-mail: mqtan26@163.com (MT); aruns@peds.ufl.edu (AS)

Introduction

Hemoglobinopathies, such as β-thalassemia and sickle cell disease, are by far the most common monogenic diseases that afflict humans worldwide, with an incidence rate of 1:600. These diseases are also the ideal targets for the potential gene therapy, if high-efficiency transduction of HSCs, and erythroid lineage-restricted expression of the human β-globin gene can be achieved.

Indeed, recombinant lentiviral vectors were recently shown to mediate β-globin gene transfer and transgene expression in an adult patient with severe β-thalassemia, which led to transfusion-independence [1]. Unfortunately, however, the observed therapeutic benefit was also compromised by transcriptional activation of a cellular proto-oncogene, HMGA2 and clonal expansion of myeloid cells. Thus, it is important to develop alternatives to lentiviral vectors. Recombinant vectors based on a non-pathogenic human virus, the adeno-associated virus 2 (AAV2) have been developed and shown to be safe and effective in a number of recent clinical trials [2,3]. Others and we have generated recombinant AAV2-globin vectors [4–8], but the transduction efficiency of these vectors in primary human HSCs has not been evaluated.

More recently, up to 12 additional AAV serotype vectors have become available [9–11], and we and others have documented that AAV6 is the most efficient serotype among AAV1 through AAV12 in transducing primary human $CD34^+$ cells [12–14]. We and others have also documented that site-directed mutagenesis of specific surface-exposed tyrosine (Y) residues on AAV serotype capsids leads to higher transduction efficiency both *in vitro* and in *vivo* in various cell types [15–20], and that Y705 and Y731 single-mutants are capable of transducing primary human $CD34^+$ cells more efficiently than their WT counterpart [14].

In the present studies, we combined both these mutations to generate a tyrosine double-mutant (Y705+731F) self-complementary (sc) AAV6 vector to evaluate whether the transduction efficiency in primary human $CD34^+$ cells could be further augmented. In addition, we also compared the transcriptional potential of the following two erythroid cell-specific promoters: (i) HS2-βbp [21,22], and (ii) B19p6 [23–28], both *in vitro* and in a murine xenograft model *in vivo*.

We report here that the transduction efficiency of the Y705+731F double-mutant scAAV6 vectors is significantly higher than that of the single-mutant or the WT scAAV6 vectors in $CD34^+$ cells *in vitro*. We also document that the transgene expression from the B19p6 is significantly higher than that from the HS2-βp, and can be further increased following erythroid-differentiation. Expression from the B19p6 in the Y705+731F double-mutant scAAV6 vectors is also significantly higher than that from the HS2-βp in human $CD34^+$ cells in a murine xenograft model *in vivo*. Transgene expression was detectable up to 12 weeks post-transplantation in primary recipients, and up to 6 additional weeks in secondary transplanted animals. These data suggest that the Y705+731F scAAV6-B19p6-βb-globin vectors might prove to be useful for the potential gene therapy of human hemoglobinopathies in general, and β-thalassemia and sickle cell disease in particular.

Materials and Methods

Cell Lines, Cells, and Cell Cultures

Human embryonic kidney 293 (HEK293) and erythroleukemia K562 cells were obtained from American Type Culture Collections (Manassas, VA) and maintained in Dulbecco's-modified Eagle's medium (DMEM; Lonza, Walkersville, MD), or Iscove's-modified Dulbecco's medium (IMDM; Irvine Scientific, Santa Ana, CA) supplemented with 10% fetal bovine serum (FBS; Sigma, St. Louis, MO), 100 μg/ml of penicillin and 100 U/ml of streptomycin (Invitrogen, Grand Island, NY). Human cord blood $CD34^+$ cells and $CD36^+$ cells were purchased from AllCells (AllCells Technologies, Emeryville, CA) and maintained in StemSpan^{TM} Serum-Free Expansion Medium (SFEM) (StemCell Technologies, Vancouver, BC, Canada) with 10 ng/ml of recombinant human interleukin 6 (rhIL6) (Peprotech), 10 ng/ml of Interleukin 3 (rhIL3) (Peprotech, Rocky Hill, NJ) and 10 ng/ml of recombinant human stem cell factor (rhSCF) (R&D Systems, Minneapolis, MN).

Plasmids

Plasmid pACGr2c6 and plasmid pscAAV2-CBAp-EGFP were a kind gifts from Drs. R. Jude Samulski and Xiao Xiao, University of North Carolina at Chapel Hill, Chapel Hill, NC. Plasmid pscAAV2-HS2-βp-EGFP plasmid was constructed by replacing the CBAp in plasmid pscAAV2-CBAp-EGFP with the HS2-βbp from plasmid pHPV37, generously provided by Dr. Philippe LeBoulch, Harvard Medical School, Boston, MA. Tyrosine double-mutant (DM) plasmid pAAV-Y705+731F was generated by using QuikChange® II Site-Directed Mutagenesis Kit (Stratagene, Santa Clara, CA) as described previously [15,17]. pscAAV-CBAp-GLuc containing Gaussia luciferase (Gluc) reporter gene was used to generate plasmid pscAAV-B19p6-Gluc, in which the CBA promoter was replaced by the B19p6 promoter from plasmid pscAAV-B19p6-Fluc by digesting with Mlu I and Age I restriction enzymes. Plasmid pscAAV-HS2-βp-Gluc was constructed using standard cloning methods. Briefly, the HS2-βp insert with Mlu I and Age I sites was first cloned by polymerase chain reaction (PCR) from plasmid pscAAV-HS2-βp-globin using following primers-pair: βp-Age I-F: 5′-GCGACCGGTGGTGTCTGTTT-GAGGTTGCTA-3′; and HS2-Mlu I-R: 5′-CGACGCGTTCA-GATCGATCTCTCCCCAGCAT-3′. The PCR product was cloned as an insert in plasmid vector pscAAV-CBAp-GLuc following digestion with Mlu I and Age I restriction enzymes and ligation.

Viral Vector Production

Viral vectors were packaged using a protocol described previously [15,17]. Briefly, HEK 293 cells were co-transfected with three plasmids using Polyethelenimine (PEI, linear, MW 25000, Polyscinces, Inc., Warrington, PA), and medium was replaced 4 hrs post-transfection. Cells were harvested 72 hrs post-transfection, subjected to 3 rounds of freeze-thaw and digested with Benzonase (Invitrogen, Grand Island, NY). Vectors were purified by iodixanol (Sigma, St. Louis, MO) gradient ultra-centrifugation followed by ion exchange chromatography using HiTrap Q HP (GE Healthcare, Piscataway, NJ), washed with phosphate-buffered saline (PBS) and concentrated by centrifugation using centrifugal spin concentrators with 150K molecular-weight cutoff (MWCO). Titers were determined by quantitative DNA slot blot using ^{32}P-labeled specific DNA probes as previously described [15].

Induction of Erythroid Differentiation and Evaluation of Gluc Expression *in vitro*

Epo is commonly used for $CD34^+$ cells erythroid introduction [29]. In the current study, $CD34^+$ cells (15,000 cell/well, 3 well/group) were cultured in SFEM containing IL-3 (10 ng/ml), IL-6 (10 ng/ml), SCF (10 ng/ml) and with or without Epo (3 U/ml). $CD34^+$ and $CD36^+$ cells were cultured in SFEM with 10 ng/ml of rhIL6, rhIL3, and 10 ng/ml of rhSCF with or without 3 U/ml of recombinant human Epo for up to 15 days. Surface glycophorin A (GPA) expression were determined by flow cytometry using PE conjugated anti-GPA antibodies. K562 cells were seeded at a density of 1×10^5 cells/ml in 6-well plates and cultured for 4 days in the presence or absence of 3 U/ml of Epo or 0.6 mM sodium butyrate or 400 μM hydroxyurea (HU). Benzidine staining was used to determine hemoglobin synthesis. Briefly, 100 μl of 0.2%

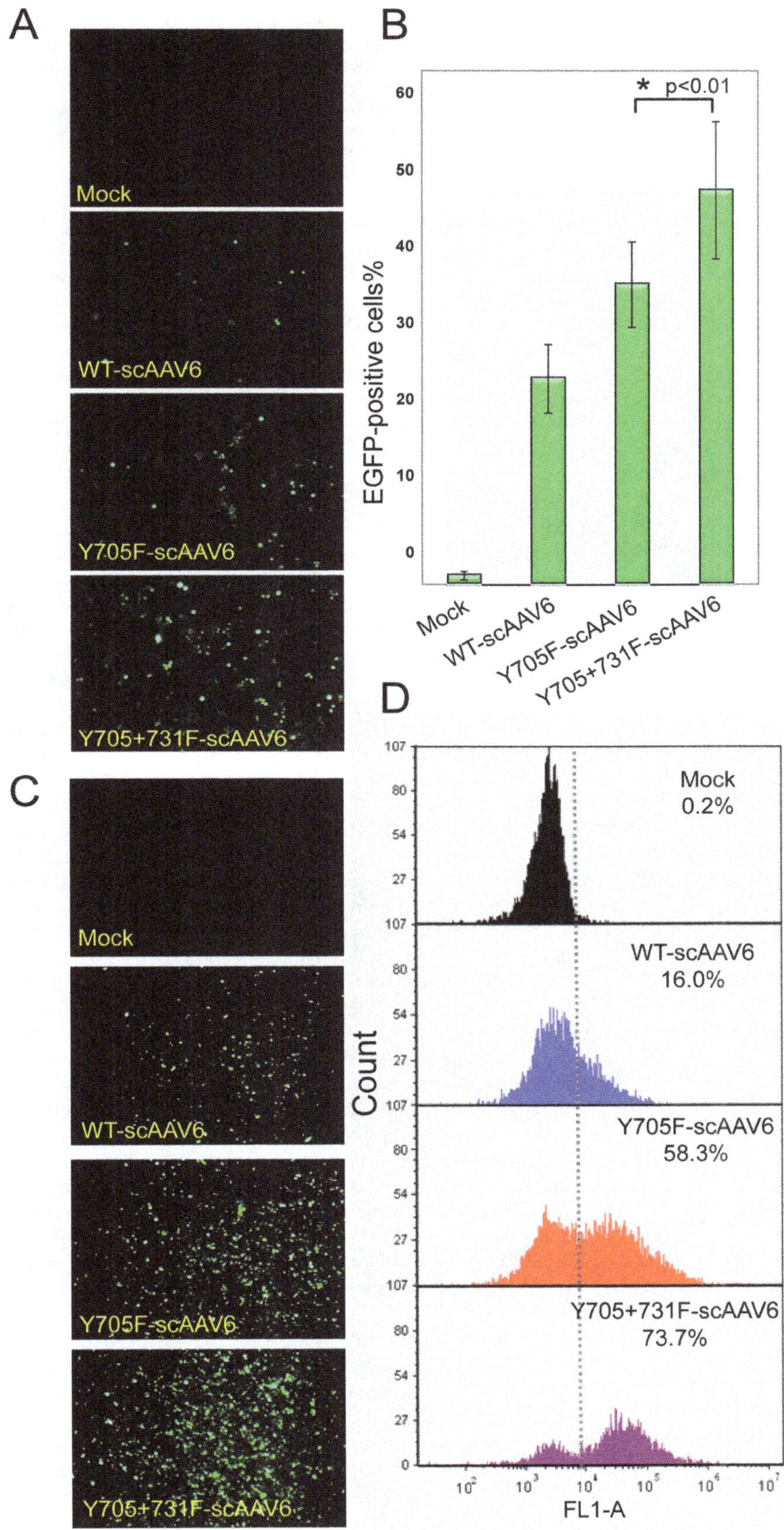
A
Mock
WT-scAAV6
Y705F-scAAV6
Y705+731F-scAAV6
B
* p<0.01
EGFP-positive cells%
Mock
WT-scAAV6
Y705F-scAAV6
Y705+731F-scAAV6
C
Mock
WT-scAAV6
Y705F-scAAV6
Y705+731F-scAAV6
D
Mock
0.2%
WT-scAAV6
16.0%
Y705F-scAAV6
58.3%
Y705+731F-scAAV6
73.7%
Count
FL1-A

Figure 1. Transduction efficiency of WT and tyrosine-mutant scAAV6 vectors in human hematopoietic cells. Approximately 5×10^3 K562 cells were either mock-infected, or infected with 5×10^3 vgs/cell of WT or various tyrosine-mutant scAAV6-CBAp-EGFP vectors, and transgene expression was determined 48 hrs post-infection using a Zeiss fluorescence microscope (Panel A), and Accuri C6 flow cytometer (Panel B) (Original magnification, x100) Approximately 1×10^4 primary human CD34$^+$ cells were either mock-infected, or infected with 2×10^4 vgs/cell of WT or various tyrosine-mutant scAAV6-CBAp-EGFP vectors under identical conditions, and transgene expression was determined 72 hrs post-infection by fluorescence microscopy (Panel C) (Original magnification, x200), and quantified by fluorescence-activated cell sorting (FACS) using a BD FACS Aria Flow Cytometer followed by processing with software FCS Express 4 (Panel D). *Y705+731F-scAAV6 vs. WT-scAAV6 vectors, $p<0.01$.

benzidine (Sigma, St. Louis, MO) staining buffer prepared in 0.5 M glacial acetic acid was added to 100 µl cells; and then 5 µl of 30% hydrogen peroxide (H_2O_2) was added to the mixture; after incubation at RT for 10 minutes, the proportion of benzidine-positive cells was quantified using a hemocytometer under a light microscope.

For Epo-induction, equivalent numbers of K562 cells, CD34$^+$, and CD36$^+$ cells were cultured as described above, and at indicated time-points, were either mock-infected, or infected with scAAV6-Gluc vectors under the control of CBAp, HS2-βp, or B19p6 promoters, respectively, for 2 hrs. Gluc activity in the medium was examined at 18 hrs post-infection using commercially available BioLux® Gaussia Luciferase Flex Assay Kits (New England Biolabs, Inc, Ipswich, MA) with an injector-equipped luminometer (BMG Labtech, FLUOstar Optima, Cary, NC).

Xenotransplantation

Equivalent numbers of human cord blood-derived CD34$^+$ cells were cultured in four round-bottom 15×75 mm Falcon tubes (BD Biosciences) and either mock-infected, or infected with 2×10^4 vgs/cell of WT-scAAV6-B19p6-Gluc, DM-scAAV6-HS2-βp-Gluc, or DM-scAAV6-B19p6-Gluc vectors for 2 hr at 37°C. Tubes were gently shaken every 15 min during infection. Cells were then washed and resuspended at a cell density of 5×10^6/ml in DPBS prior to transplantation.

Five to 12-week-old NOD.Cg-*Prkdc*^{scid} Il2rgtm1Wjl/SzJ (NSG) female recipient mice were used in the present study since female mice have been reported to be more efficient recipient than male mice for engraftment of human HSCs [30]. Mice were bred and kept in microisolator cages in the SPF facility at the University of Florida. Antibiotics were administrated by supplementing the drinking water with 0.2 mg/ml enrofloxacin (Bayer Healthcare, Shawnee Mission, KS) for 2 days before performing transplantation and 2 weeks post-transplantation to prevent infection. Mice were irradiated with a dose of 250 cGY from a Cesium-137 source at 4 hrs before injecting the mock- or AAV vector-transduced human cord blood-derived CD34$^+$ cells. Approximately 1×10^6 cells were injected into the lateral tail vein of each mouse. All animal experiments were approved by the University of Florida Institutional Animal Care and Use Committee. All procedures were carried out in accordance with the principles of the National Research Council's Guide for the Care and Use of Laboratory Animals. All efforts were made to minimize suffering.

Evaluation of Transgene Expression in Peripheral Blood

The method to evaluate Gluc activity was modified from the protocol described previously [31,32]. Coelenterazine free base, the Gluc substrate, was purchased from Nanolight Technology, Pinetop, AZ. To prepare the stock solution, one drop of concentrated HCl was added to 10 ml of methanol to make acidified methanol. The corresponding amount of acidified methanol (2 ml) was then added to coelenterazine (10 mg) in an amber vial to make 5 mg/ml (~12 mM) substrate solution. Stock solution was aliquoted and stored at −80°C. For *in vitro* blood Gluc activity assay, the stock solution was freshly diluted to 100 mM in PBS supplemented with 5 mM NaCl (pH 7.2). Mice were restrained with the tail exposed. The lateral tail vein was punctured using a 1 ml insulin needle; five to 20 µl of blood was collected using 20 µl tips. Samples were collected in anticoagulant tube in the presence of EDTA as an anticoagulant and placed on ice until all samples were collected. Blood samples were transferred to a 96-well plate, and the Gluc activity was measured using a plate luminometer (BMG Labtech, FLUOstar Optima, Cary, NC). Data were analyzed by plotting the relative light units (RLU) per second.

In vivo Bioluminescence Imaging

Mice were weighed to calculate the volume of substrate according to the dose of 4 mg/kg of body weight and anesthetized. The calculated volume of the 5 mg/ml of stock substrate solution was mixed with 100 µl of PBS and injected via retro-orbital route [31]. *In vivo* bioluminescence images were acquired immediately over a period of 5 min using a Xenogen IVIS® Lumina II (Caliper Life Sciences) equipped with a cooled couple-charged device (CCD) camera (PerkinElmer Co., Alameda CA). Signal intensity was quantified using the camera control program, Living Image software version 4, and shown as photons/second/cm^2/steridian (p/s/cm^2/sr).

Cell Sorting, Lineage Analyses, and Transgene Expression

Twelve-weeks post-transplantation of human CD34$^+$ cells in primary recipient NSG mice, bone marrow cells were flushed from the bones of the hind limb with sterile PBS. Red blood cells were hemolyzed with ammonium chloride buffer. Cells were then labeled with fluorescein isothiocyanate (FITC) conjugated anti human CD45 and allophyocyanine (APC) conjugated anti mouse CD45 antibodies, and the percentage of human CD45-positive cells was calculated. For sorting of lineage specific cells, the bone marrow cells were labeled with FITC-conjugated anti human CD71 for erythroid, phycoerythrin (PE)-conjugated anti human CD19 for B cells, and APC-conjugated anti-human CD11b for monocytes and neutrophils. All antibodies were from BD Biosciences (San Jose, CA). Each lineage-specific cells were sorted using BD Aria TMIIu Fluorescence-Activated Cell Sorter (BD Biosciences). For determining Gluc activity in the sorted cell populations, $\sim4\times10^4$ cells from each lineage were suspended in 100 ml PBS. Five ml of the cell mixtures were used for the *in vitro* Gluc activity assay as described above.

Secondary Transplantation

Twelve-weeks post-primary transplantation, the whole bone marrow cells from a mouse transplanted with human CD34$^+$ cells transduced with DM-scAAV6-B19p6-Gluc vectors were isolated as described above. Approximately 2×10^6 bone marrow cells were transplanted into NSG mice ($n=4$) via retro-orbital injection following irradiation with 250 cGy. Mice were maintained on 0.2 mg/ml enrofloxacin in drinking water (Bayer Healthcare, KS). Six-weeks post secondary transplantation, mice were subjected to whole-body bioluminescence imaging *in vivo* as described above.

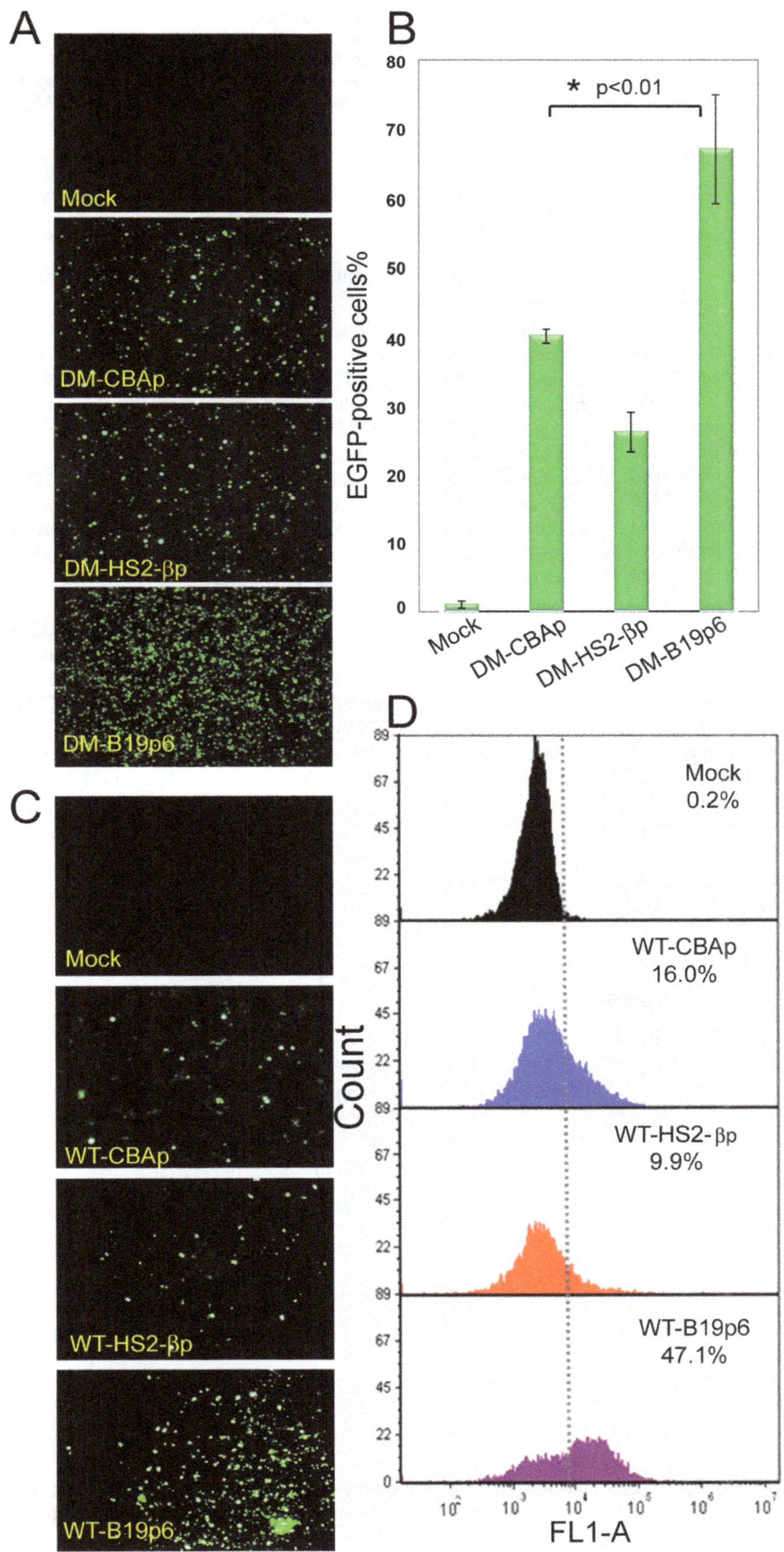
A
Mock
DM-CBAp
DM-HS2-βp
DM-B19p6
B
* p<0.01
EGFP-positive cells%
80
70
60
50
40
30
20
10
0
Mock
DM-CBAp
DM-HS2-βp
DM-B19p6
C
Mock
WT-CBAp
WT-HS2-βp
WT-B19p6
D
Mock
0.2%
WT-CBAp
16.0%
WT-HS2-βp
9.9%
WT-B19p6
47.1%
Count
FL1-A

Figure 2. Transcriptional potential of CBAp, HS2-βp, and B19p6 promoters in human hematopoietic cells. Approximately 1×10^4 cells were either infected with DM scAAV6 vectors (K562 cells) or WT scAAV6 vectors (human CD34⁺ cells) expressing the EGFP gene under the control of the three different promoters at 5×10^3 vgs/cell (K562 cells) or 2×10^4 vgs/cell (human $CD34^+$ cells), respectively. Transgene expression in K562 cells (Panels A and B) and human $CD34^+$ cells (Panels C and D) was determined 72 hrs post-infection by fluorescence microscopy and quantitated by the flow cytometry as described above. The original image magnifications were 100× (Panel A) and 200× (Panel B). *DM-scB19p6-EGFP vs. DM-scAAV6-HS2-βp-EGFP vectors, $p<0.01$.

Results

Transduction Efficiency of Single- and Double-tyrosine Mutant scAAV6 Serotype Vectors in Human Hematopoietic Cells *in vitro*

We recently identified AAV6 as the most efficient serotype in transducing primary human HSCs, and that site-directed mutagenesis of specific surface-exposed tyrosine residues (Y705 and Y731) further increased the transduction efficiency of these vectors. Since we have previously reported that the transduction efficiency of AAV2 and AAV3 serotype vectors could be further improved by combining the single tyrosine-mutations, we wished to evaluate the transduction efficiency of the Y705F+Y731F double-mutant (DM) scAAV6 vectors. Both human erythroleukemia K562 cells, and primary human $CD34^+$ cells were either mock-infected, or infected with WT, or single (Y705F)-, or DM (Y705+731F) scAAV6 vectors. K562 cells were infected with 5×10^3 vgs/cell, and human $CD34^+$ cells were infected with 2×10^4 vgs/cell. Transgene expression was determined by fluorescence microscopy and quantified by flow cytometry. These results are shown in Figure 1. As can be seen, the transduction efficiency of DM scAAV-CBAp-enhanced green fluorescent protein (EGFP) vectors was significantly higher than that of either WT or single-mutant scAAV6 vectors, both in K562 cells (Panels A and B) and in $CD34^+$ cells (Panels C and D). The percentage of EGFP-positive cells increased from 24.0±4.0% to 46.0±6.1% in K562 cells, and from 16.0±2.0% to 73.7%±5.1% in $CD34^+$ cells.

Transcriptional Potential of CBAp, HS2-βbp, and B19p6 Promoters

With the ultimate objective of developing recombinant AAVs vectors for the potential gene therapy of human hemoglobinopathies, we next evaluated the transcriptional potential of the following two erythroid cell-specific promoters: HS2-βp, and the B19p6. The ubiquitous CBAp was used as an appropriate control. scAAV6 vectors containing the EGFP gene under the control of the three promoters were used to infect primary human $CD34^+$ cells under identical conditions, and transgene expression was evaluated 72 hrs post-infection. These results are shown in Figure 2. In K562 cells (Panels A and B), the EGFP expression level from DM-scAAV6-B19p6-EGFP vectors was ~67.0±7.9%, which is significantly higher that from DM-scAAV6-CBAp-EGFP vectors (~40.0±1.0%), and from DM-scAAV6-HS2-βbp-EGFP vectors (~26.1±2.9%). Similarly, in human $CD34^+$ cells (Panels C and D), whereas little transgene expression occurred in mock-infected cells, ~16% of cells transduced with scAAV6-CBAp-EGFP vectors were EGFP-positive. Transgene expression from scAAV6-HS2-βbp-EGFP occurred in ~10% of cells, whereas ~47% of cells transduced with scAAV6-B19p6-EGFP vectors were EGFP-positive.

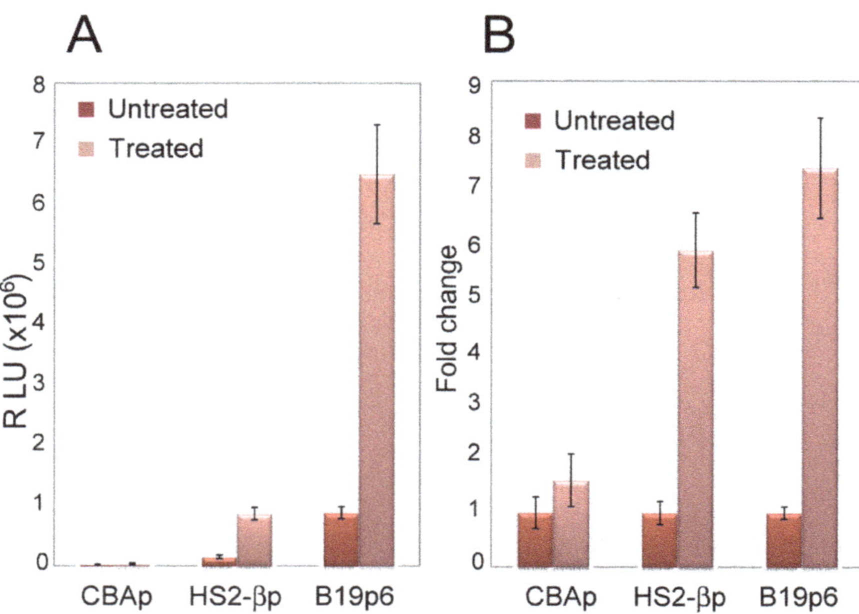

Figure 3. Transcriptional potential of CBAp, HS2-βp and B19p6 promoters in human erythroleukemia cells following erythroid differentiation. Equivalent numbers of mock-treated, or Epo-induced erythroid-differentiated K562 cells were infected with 5×10^3 vgs/cell of scAAV6-Gluc vectors, and transgene expression was determined 18 hrs post-infection (A). Fold changes in transgene expression from the three promoters were calculated from untreated vs. Epo-treated groups (B).

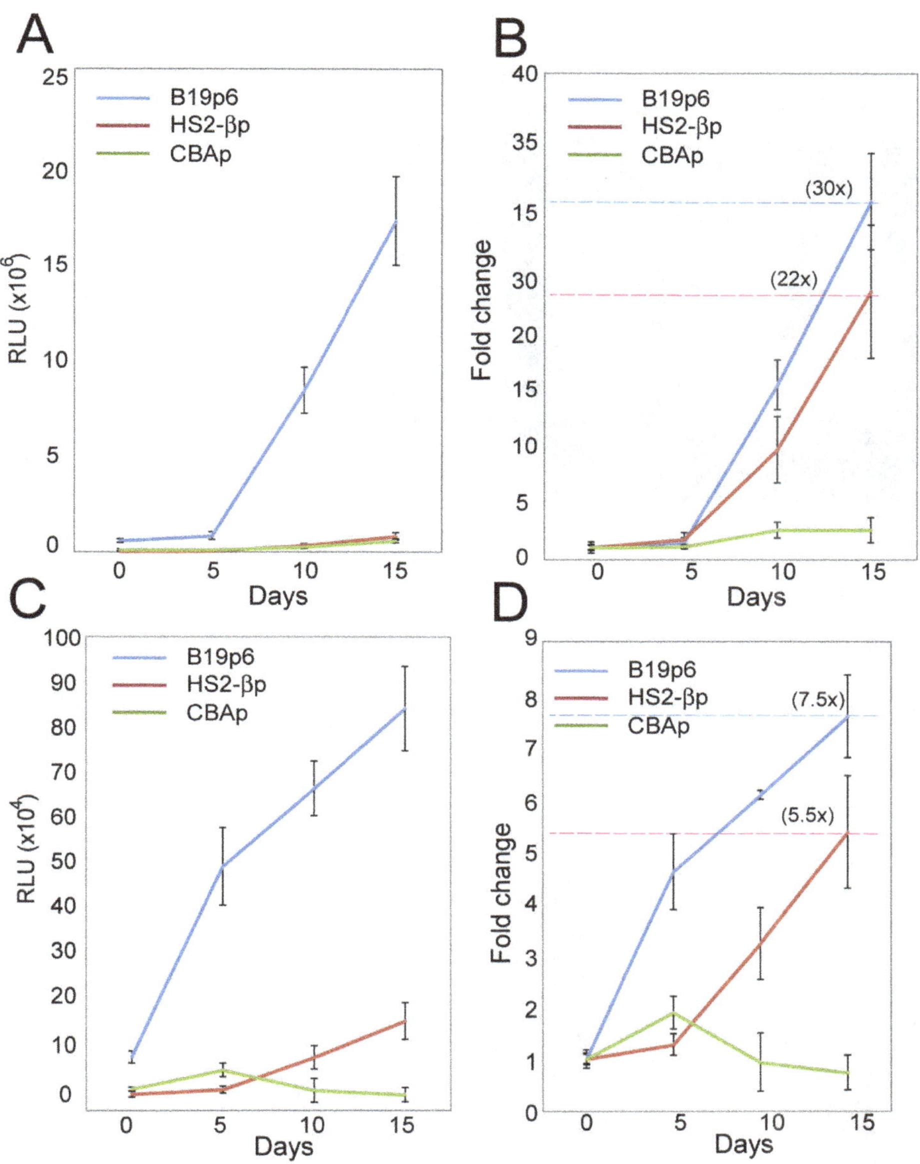

Figure 4. Transcriptional potential of CBAp, HS2-βp and B19p6 promoters in primary human CD34⁺ and CD36⁺ human cells following erythroid differentiation. Approximately 1.5×10^4 $CD34^+$ cells, and $\sim2\times10^4$ primary human $CD36^+$ erythroid progenitor cells were cultured with or without Epo (3 U/ml) for various indicated times, and infected with 1×10^4 vgs/cell scAAV6-Gluc vectors under identical conditions. Transgene expression levels were determined at 18 hrs post-infection at each time-point. Gluc activity at various time-points was normalized to the group without Epo-induction, and the normalized absolute values are shown as average ± standard deviation from triplicates for $CD34^+$ cells (Panel A), and for $CD36^+$ cells (Panel C). Fold changes in transgene expression following erythroid-differentiation were calculated by dividing the normalized Gluc activities by the initial activity on Day 0 (Panels B and D).

Transgene Expression from the CBAp, HS2-βbp, and B19p6 Promoters following Erythroid Differentiation *in vitro*

Since HS2-βp and B19p6 are erythroid cell-specific promoters, we wished to examine whether transgene expression from these promoters could be further increased following erythroid differentiation of K562 cells. K562 cells were cultured for 4 days in the presence or absence of the 3 U/ml of erythropoietin (Epo), and equivalent numbers of cells were either mock-infected, or infected with 5×10^3 vgs/cell of Y705+731F DM-scAAV6 vectors expressing the Gluc reporter gene under the control of the CBAp, HS2-βp, or the B19p6 promoters as described in Materials and Methods. Gluc activity was determined 18 hrs post-infection. As can be seen in Figure 3, transgene expression from B19p6 promoter in untreated K562 cells was significantly higher than that from CBAp and HS2-βp promoters (Panel A). The extent of transgene expression from both HS2-βp and B19p6 increased up to 7-fold following Epo-induced differentiation, whereas no significant change was observed from the CBAp, with or without Epo-induced differentiation (Panel B). Similar results were observed with butyrate- or HU-induced erythroid differentiation of K562 cells (data not shown). However, since HU has been shown to increase the transduction efficiency of AAV vectors [33],

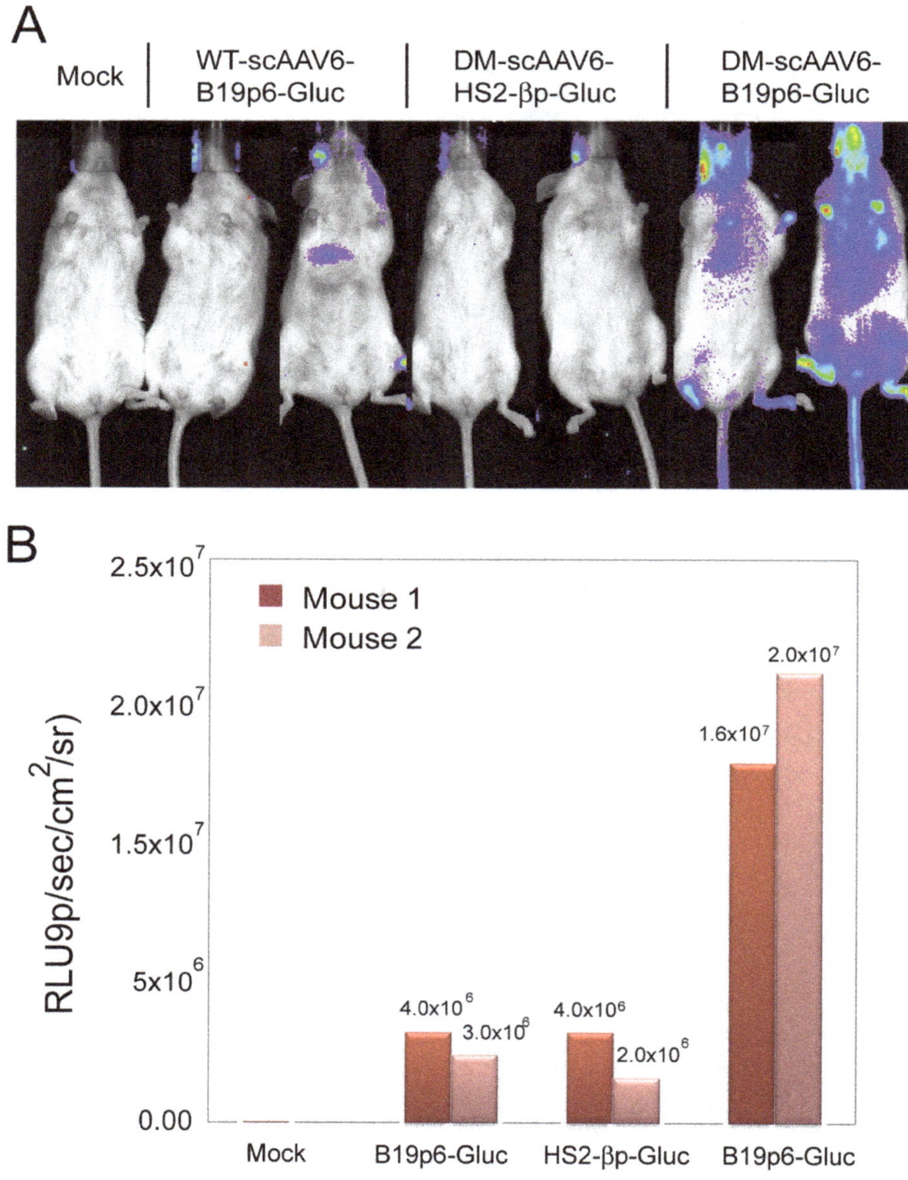

Figure 5. Bioluminescence imaging of mice transplanted with human CD34⁺ cell *in vivo*. NSG mice transplanted with mock-infected, or various indicated scAAV6 vector-infected primary human $CD34^+$ cells was acquired by a Xenogen IVIS® Imaging System 6-weeks post-transplantation. Images of representative animals from each group are shown (Panel A). The luminescence signal intensity was quantified as photons/second/cm^2/steridian (p/s/cm^2/sr) using the Living Image® software (Panel B).

and butyrate has been reported to be related to activation of p38 MAP kinase [34], which also affects AAV transduction [35], the observed increase in transgene expression may not solely be credited to erythroid differentiation.

Epo is also commonly used to induce erythroid differentiation in $CD34^+$ cells [29]. In the current study, $CD34^+$ cells were cultured for various indicated days in the presence or absence of Epo, and equivalent numbers of cells were either mock-infected, or infected with 1×10^4 vgs/cell of Y705+731F DM-scAAV6-Gluc vectors. Gluc activity was determined 18 hrs post-infection at each time-point. These results are shown in Figure 4 (Panels A and B). As is evident, transgene expression from both HS2-βp and B19p6 kept increasing until the end of the experiments, whereas expression from the CBAp remained unaffected, the extent of transgene expression from the HS2-βp and the B19p6 promoters increased up to 22-fold and 30-fold, respectively, 15 days post-erythroid differentiation. Similar results were obtained with primary human $CD36^+$ erythroid progenitor cells (Figure 4, Panels C and D). The extent of transgene expression from the HS2-βp and the B19p6 promoters increased up to 5.5-fold and 7.5-fold, respectively, 12 days post-erythroid differentiation.

Transgene Expression from the HS2-βp and B19p6 Promoters in a Xenograft Murine Model *in vivo*

Transgene expression from the HS2-βp and the B19p6 promoter was also evaluated in an immuno-deficient xenograft mouse model *in vivo*. Female non-obese diabetic [36] severe

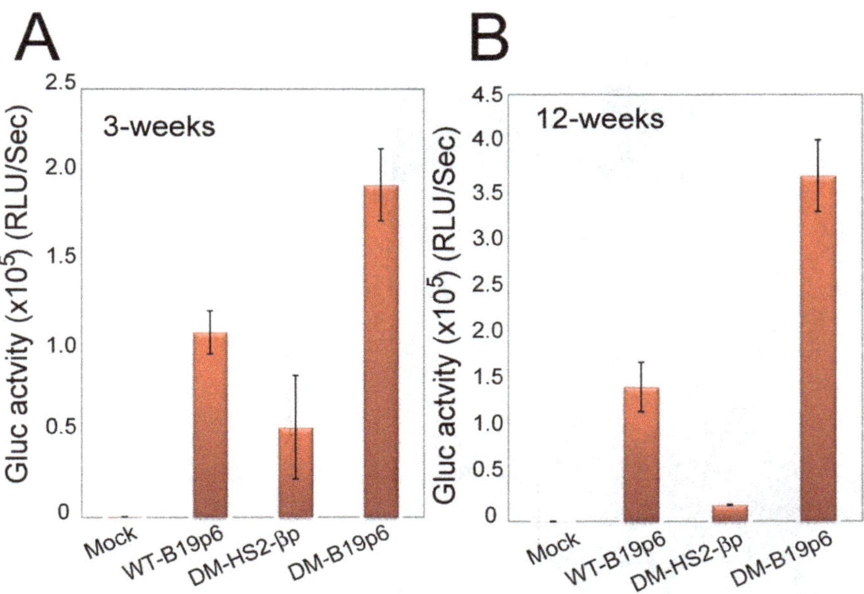

Figure 6. Relative levels of transgene expression from HS2-βp and B19p6 promoters in primary human CD34$^+$ cells following xenotransplantation in NSG mice. Approximately 1×10^6 primary human CD34$^+$ cells were either mock-infected, or infected with 2×10^4 vgs/cell of WT-scAAV6-B19p6-Gluc, Y705+731F DM-scAAV6-HS2-βbp-Gluc, or Y705+731F DM-scAAV6-B19p6-Gluc vectors under identical conditions, and engrafted into NSG mice as described under Materials and Methods. Gluc activity was measured 3 weeks (Panel A) and 12-weeks (Panel B) post-engraftment in peripheral blood using a luminometer. Total relative light units (RLU) per second were calculated, and results are presented as mean ± s.d., with $P<0.001$ as calculated by student's t-test.

combined immune-deficient (SCID), gamma (NSG) mice have been reported to be a good xenotransplantation model for assaying human cell engraftment [37]. In our present study, $\sim 1 \times 10^6$ primary human CD34$^+$ cells were either mock-infected, or infected by WT or Y705+731F DM-scAAV6 vectors expressing Gluc under the control of HS2-βp or the B19p6 promoters, respectively.

Whole-body bioluminescence images (Figure 5, Panel A), acquired as detailed in Materials and Methods at 6 weeks post-implantation, corroborated that whereas no transgene expression occurred in mice transplanted with mock-infected human CD34$^+$

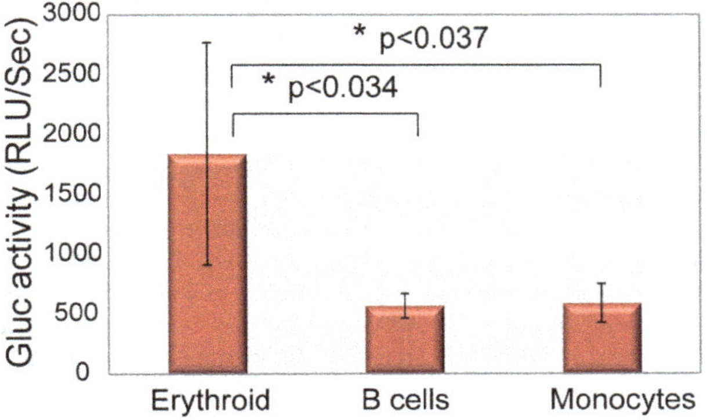

Figure 7. Transgene expression in various human hematopoietic lineages 12-weeks post-transplantation of human CD34$^+$ cells in primary recipient NSG mice. Bone marrow cells were harvested and human lineage-specific cells were sorted and Gluc activity in the sorted cell populations, was determined as described above. $*p<0.034$ (erythroid vs. B cells) and $*p<0.037$ (erythroid vs. monocytes).

cells, expression from the B19p6 promoter in Y705+731F DM-scAAV6 vectors was up to 5-fold higher than that from the B19p6 promoter in WT scAAV6 vectors, or from the HS2-βbp promoter in Y705+731F DM-scAAV6 vectors (Figure 5, Panel B).

Since Gluc is secreted and it has very high tissue absorption, human CD34$^+$ cell engraftment in NSG mice and transgene expression levels were monitored *in vivo* both by Gluc activity in peripheral blood (3 weeks and 12 weeks post-transplantation). As can be seen in Figure 6A, Gluc expression from the B19p6 promoter in the WT scAAV6 vectors was >2-fold higher than that from the HS2-βp promoter in the Y705+731F double-mutant scAAV6 vectors, and expression from the B19p6 promoter in the Y705+731F double-mutant scAAV6 vectors was ~4-fold higher than that from the HS2-βbp promoter in Y705+731F double-mutant scAAV6 vectors in peripheral blood in NSG mice 3 weeks post-transplantation (Panel A). The extent of transgene expression was further increased from the B19p6 promoter 12 weeks post-transplantation (Panel B).

In order to evaluate whether the observed transgene expression from the B19p6 promoter was restricted to human erythroid progenitor cells, whole bone marrow cells were harvested from primary recipient mice 12 weeks post-transplantation. Anti-human antibodies were used to sort for erythroid, B cells, and monocytes using lineage-specific antibodies as described under Materials and Methods. Gluc activity in the sorted cell populations was determined as described above. These results, shown in Figure 7, suggest that transgene expression from the B19p6 promoter is largely restricted to human erythroid progenitor cells.

To further evaluate whether long-term repopulating human stem cells were transduced, whole bone marrow cells from a mouse transplanted with human CD34$^+$ cells transduced with DM-scAAV6-B19p6-Gluc vectors were isolated 12-weeks post-transplantation, and transplanted into secondary recipient mice (n = 4). Whole-body bioluminescence imaging *in vivo* was per-

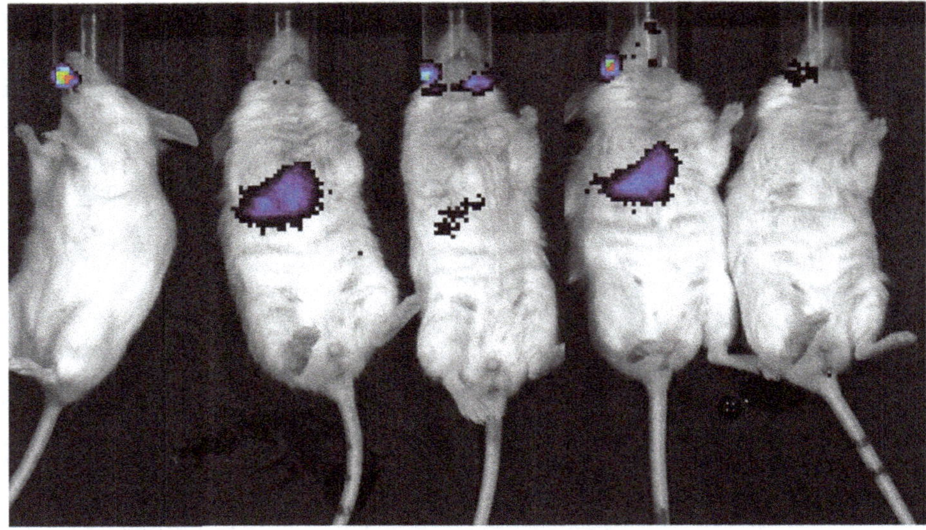

Figure 8. Bioluminescence imaging of mice following secondary transplantation. Whole bone marrow cells from NSG mice transplanted with mock-infected, or DM scAAV6-B19p6-Gluc vector-infected primary human CD34$^+$ cells were harvested 12-weeks post-primary transplantation, and transplanted into secondary recipient mice. Six-weeks post secondary transplantation, mice were subjected to whole-body bioluminescence imaging *in vivo* as described above.

formed 6-weeks post-secondary transplantation as described above. As can be seen in Figure 8, transgene expression was observed in each animal, albeit at low levels, due to $<1\%$ engraftment of human cells (data not shown). These results, nonetheless, document that DM scAAV6 vectors are capable of transducing long-term repopulating human stem cells.

Discussion

An ideal gene therapy vector for the potential gene therapy of b-thalassemia and sickle cell disease would be one with which high-efficiency transduction of primitive human HSCs could be achieved, and following erythroid differentiation, robust levels of expression of the transduced human b-globin gene could be obtained. The development of lentiviral vectors by a number of investigators has indeed achieved these objectives [38–45], but their long-term safety still remains an open question [1]. We and others have described the development of the first generation of recombinant AAV2 vectors for the potential gene therapy of b-thalassemia and sickle cell disease [4–8], but in retrospect, it has become clear that the use of the WT AAV2 capsid, and the single-stranded nature of the vector genome, were major obstacles to achieving therapeutic levels of the human b-globin gene [6,8,46–48]. In addition, the use of murine models of these diseases was not predictive of the potential efficacy of a number of alternative serotypes of AAV vectors [27,28].

Based on more recent studies by us and others [12–14], in which AAV6 was identified to be the most efficient serotype for transducing human HSCs, and our observation that B19p6 is more robust than HS2-βp for mediating erythroid lineage-restricted expression [27], we reasoned that combining these features might lead to the development of an ideal vector for the potential gene therapy of β-thalassemia and sickle cell disease, especially since the safety and efficacy of AAV vectors have now been established unequivocally in a number of Phase I/II clinical trials in humans [49–53]. Indeed, the Y705+731F double-mutant scAAV6 vectors containing the B19p6, described here, were determined to be the most efficient in transducing primary human CD34$^+$ cells, and mediating erythroid lineage-restricted transgene expression, both *in vitro* and *in vivo*. It is also possible that the transduction efficiency of these vectors can be augmented further, based on our recent observations that site-directed mutagenesis of specific surface-exposed serine and threonine residues improves the transduction efficiency of AAV2 serotype vectors [35], and most of these residues are highly conserved in all AAV serotypes.

The basic underlying molecular mechanism of increased transduction efficiency of the Y705+731F double-mutant scAAV6 vectors in human CD34$^+$ cells is not readily apparent. Based on our recent studies with tyrosine-mutant AAV2 and AAV3 serotype vectors [15,17], we favor the hypothesis that improved intracellular trafficking and/or nuclear transport lead to the observed effect. However, the alternative hypothesis that a more efficient cellular receptor-mediated viral vector entry also play a role, cannot be ruled out since the extent of transgene expression from the B19p6 promoter in human CD36$^+$ erythroid progenitor cells was ~20-fold lower than the more primitive CD34$^+$ HSCs (compare Figures 4 A, B and Figure 4 C, D). Thus, additional studies are warranted to address these issues, as well as to identify the authentic receptor for AAV6 for human HSCs, since in a recent report, EGFR was recently identified to be the cellular receptor for AAV6 [54], and Denard *et al.* [55] reported that galectin 3-binding protein in human sera agglutinates AAV6 vectors, which resulted in decreased transduction efficiency of these vectors. In our studies, pre-treatment of CD34$^+$ cells with EGF had no effect on the transduction efficacy of AAV6 vectors, and K562 cells, which are known to lack expression of EGFR [56], could be efficiently transduced by AAV6 vectors, which was inhibited by FBS (data not shown).

Although erythroid lineage-restricted transgene expression from the B19p6 promoter in primary human HSCs *in vitro* has previously been reported [26], those studies were carried out with the first generation single-stranded AAV2 serotype vectors, which were clearly sub-optimal. We subsequently utilized scAAV1 and scAAV7 serotype vectors, and corroborated the erythroid cell-specificity of the B19p6 promoter *in vivo* [27,28], those studies were carried out in murine HSCs, which were clearly not predictive for human HSCs. In the present studies, we documented sustained transgene expression in human HSCs, both in primary as well as in secondary transplant recipient mice. However, because of less than 1% engraftment of human cells in secondary transplant recipients, we were unable to document stable integration of the AAV proviral genomes. In this context, it is important to emphasize that the general conclusion that AAV genomes do not integrate, has largely been derived from previously published studies, all of which were carried out with post-mitotic cells and tissues, such as liver, muscle, brain, and retina, in which the AAV genomes remain episomal, although integration in liver has been reported by several investigators [57–60]. In our previously published studies with primary murine HSCs, stable integration of the AAV proviral genomes has been documented in both primary as well as secondary transplant recipient mice [7,27,28,61,62], and in a more recently published collaborative study, we have also documented long-term transduction and multi-lineage engraftment of human HSCs in a mouse xenograft model [63]. Thus, our working hypothesis has been that unlike in post-mitotic cells, AAV vectors do integrate in HSCs. The fact that in a recent report by Weltner *et al.* [64], all 4 reprogramming genes were shown to be integrated following AAV vector-mediated generation of induced pluripotent stem (iPS) cells, provides further support to our hypothesis.

The development of the optimized scAAV6-B19p6 vectors described here, with which high-efficiency transduction of human HSCs, and erythroid lineage-restricted expression can be achieved *in vivo*, and the possibility that the transduction efficiency of these vectors can be further augmented by introducing additional mutations in surface-exposed specific serine and threonine residues, similar to those described for AAV2 [35,65], bodes well for the eventual use of these vectors in the potential gene therapy of human hemoglobinopathies in general, and b-thalassemia and sickle cell disease in particular.

Acknowledgments

We thank Drs. Philippe Leboulch, R. Jude Samulski, and Xiao Xiao for their kind gifts of recombinant plasmids. We also thank Drs. Kenneth I. Berns and Sergei Zolotukhin for a critical review of this manuscript.

Author Contributions

Conceived and designed the experiments: LS XL GRJ MCY MT AS. Performed the experiments: LS XL GRJ YW GVA CL LZ. Analyzed the data: LS XL GRJ GVA CL LZ GG MCY MT AS. Contributed reagents/materials/analysis tools: LZ GG CL. Wrote the paper: LS XL GRJ MCY AS.

References

1. Cavazzana-Calvo M, Payen E, Negre O, Wang G, Hehir K, et al. (2010) Transfusion independence and HMGA2 activation after gene therapy of human beta-thalassaemia. Nature 467: 318–322.
2. Mueller C, Flotte TR (2008) Clinical gene therapy using recombinant adeno-associated virus vectors. Gene Ther 15: 858–863.
3. Mingozzi F, High KA (2011) Therapeutic in vivo gene transfer for genetic disease using AAV: progress and challenges. Nat Rev Genet 12: 341–355.
4. Walsh CE, Liu JM, Xiao X, Young NS, Nienhuis AW, et al. (1992) Regulated high level expression of a human gamma-globin gene introduced into erythroid cells by an adeno-associated virus vector. Proc Natl Acad Sci U S A 89: 7257–7261.
5. Miller JL, Walsh CE, Ney PA, Samulski RJ, Nienhuis AW (1993) Single-copy transduction and expression of human gamma-globin in K562 erythroleukemia cells using recombinant adeno-associated virus vectors: the effect of mutations in NF-E2 and GATA-1 binding motifs within the hypersensitivity site 2 enhancer. Blood 82: 1900–1906.
6. Zhou SZ, Li Q, Stamatoyannopoulos G, Srivastava A (1996) Adeno-associated virus 2-mediated transduction and erythroid cell-specific expression of a human beta-globin gene. Gene Ther 3: 223–229.
7. Ponnazhagan S, Yoder MC, Srivastava A (1997) Adeno-associated virus type 2-mediated transduction of murine hematopoietic cells with long-term repopulating ability and sustained expression of a human globin gene in vivo. J Virol 71: 3098–3104.
8. Tan M, Qing K, Zhou S, Yoder MC, Srivastava A (2001) Adeno-associated virus 2-mediated transduction and erythroid lineage-restricted long-term expression of the human beta-globin gene in hematopoietic cells from homozygous beta-thalassemic mice. Mol Ther 3: 940–946.
9. Gao G, Vandenberghe LH, Alvira MR, Lu Y, Calcedo R, et al. (2004) Clades of Adeno-associated viruses are widely disseminated in human tissues. J Virol 78: 6381–6388.
10. Gao GP, Alvira MR, Wang L, Calcedo R, Johnston J, et al. (2002) Novel adeno-associated viruses from rhesus monkeys as vectors for human gene therapy. Proc Natl Acad Sci U S A 99: 11854–11859.
11. Gao G, Alvira MR, Somanathan S, Lu Y, Vandenberghe LH, et al. (2003) Adeno-associated viruses undergo substantial evolution in primates during natural infections. Proc Natl Acad Sci U S A 100: 6081–6086.
12. Schuhmann NK, Pozzoli O, Sallach J, Huber A, Avitabile D, et al. (2010) Gene transfer into human cord blood-derived CD34(+) cells by adeno-associated viral vectors. Exp Hematol 38: 707–717.
13. Veldwijk MR, Sellner L, Stiefelhagen M, Kleinschmidt JA, Laufs S, et al. (2010) Pseudotyped recombinant adeno-associated viral vectors mediate efficient gene transfer into primary human CD34(+) peripheral blood progenitor cells. Cytotherapy 12: 107–112.
14. Song L, Kauss MA, Kopin E, Chandra M, Ul-Hasan T, et al. (2013). Optimizing the transduction efficiency of human hematopoietic stem cells using capsid-modified AAV6 vectors in vitro and in a xenograft mouse model in vivo. Cytotherapy, in press.
15. Zhong L, Li B, Mah CS, Govindasamy L, Agbandje-McKenna M, et al. (2008) Next generation of adeno-associated virus 2 vectors: point mutations in tyrosines lead to high-efficiency transduction at lower doses. Proc Natl Acad Sci U S A 105: 7827–7832.
16. Kauss MA, Smith LJ, Zhong L, Srivastava A, Wong KK Jr, et al. (2010) Enhanced long-term transduction and multilineage engraftment of human hematopoietic stem cells transduced with tyrosine-modified recombinant adeno-associated virus serotype 2. Hum Gene Ther 21: 1129–1136.
17. Cheng B, Ling C, Dai Y, Lu Y, Glushakova LG, et al. (2012) Development of optimized AAV3 serotype vectors: mechanism of high-efficiency transduction of human liver cancer cells. Gene Ther. 19: 375–384,
18. Qiao C, Zhang W, Yuan Z, Shin JH, Li J, et al. (2010) Adeno-associated virus serotype 6 capsid tyrosine-to-phenylalanine mutations improve gene transfer to skeletal muscle. Hum Gene Ther 21: 1343–1348.
19. Ussher JE, Taylor JA (2010) Optimized transduction of human monocyte-derived dendritic cells by recombinant adeno-associated virus serotype 6. Hum Gene Ther 21: 1675–1686.
20. Dalkara D, Byrne LC, Lee T, Hoffmann NV, Schaffer DV, et al. (2012) Enhanced gene delivery to the neonatal retina through systemic administration of tyrosine-mutated AAV9. Gene Therapy 19: 176–181.
21. Tuan D, Kong S, Hu K (1992) Transcription of the hypersensitive site HS2 enhancer in erythroid cells. Proc Natl Acad Sci U S A 89: 11219–11223.
22. Pawliuk R, Bachelot T, Raftopoulos H, Kalberer C, Humphries RK, et al. (1998) Retroviral vectors aimed at the gene therapy of human beta-globin gene disorders. Ann N Y Acad Sci 850: 151–162.
23. Shade RO, Blundell MC, Cotmore SF, Tattersall P, Astell CR (1986) Nucleotide sequence and genome organization of human parvovirus B19 isolated from the serum of a child during aplastic crisis. J Virol 58: 921–936.
24. Ponnazhagan S, Woody MJ, Wang XS, Zhou SZ, Srivastava A (1995) Transcriptional transactivation of of parvovirus B19 promoters in in non-permissive cells by adenovirus type 2. J Virol 69: 8096–8101.
25. Wang XS, Yoder MC, Zhou SZ, Srivastava A (1995) Parvovirus B19 promoter at map unit 6 confers autonomous replication competence and erythroid specificity to adeno-associated virus 2 in primary human hematopoietic progenitor cells. Proc Natl Acad Sci U S A 92: 12416–12420.
26. Kurpad C, Mukherjee P, Wang XS, Ponnazhagan S, Li L, et al. (1999) Adeno-associated virus 2-mediated transduction and erythroid lineage-restricted expression from parvovirus B19p6 promoter in primary human hematopoietic progenitor cells. J Hematother Stem Cell Res 8: 585–592.

27. Maina N, Han Z, Li X, Hu Z, Zhong L, et al. (2008) Recombinant self-complementary adeno-associated virus serotype vector-mediated hematopoietic stem cell transduction and lineage-restricted, long-term transgene expression in a murine serial bone marrow transplantation model. Hum Gene Ther 19: 376–383.
28. Maina N, Zhong L, Li X, Zhao W, Han Z, et al. (2008) Optimization of recombinant adeno-associated viral vectors for human beta-globin gene transfer and transgene expression. Hum Gene Ther 19: 365–375.
29. Myklebust JH, Smeland EB, Josefsen D, Sioud M (2000) Protein kinase C-alpha isoform is involved in erythropoietin-induced erythroid differentiation of CD34(+) progenitor cells from human bone marrow. Blood 95: 510–518.
30. Notta F, Doulatov S, Dick JE (2010) Engraftment of human hematopoietic stem cells is more efficient in female NOD/SCID/IL-2Rgc-null recipients. Blood 115: 3704–3707.
31. Tannous BA (2009) Gaussia luciferase reporter assay for monitoring biological processes in culture and in vivo. Nat Protoc 4: 582–591.
32. Wurdinger T, Badr C, Pike L, de Kleine R, Weissleder R, et al. (2008) A secreted luciferase for ex vivo monitoring of in vivo processes. Nat Methods 5: 171–173.
33. Yakobson B, Koch T, Winocour E (1987) Replication of adeno-associated virus in synchronized cells without the addition of a helper virus. J Virol 61: 972–981.
34. Witt O, Sand K, Pekrun A (2000) Butyrate-induced erythroid differentiation of human K562 leukemia cells involves inhibition of ERK and activation of p38 MAP kinase pathways. Blood 95: 2391–2396.
35. Aslanidi GV, Rivers AE, Ortiz L, Govindasamy L, Ling C, et al. (2012) High-efficiency transduction of human monocyte-derived dendritic cells by capsid-modified recombinant AAV2 vectors. Vaccine 30: 3908–3917.
36. Miyachi T, Adachi M, Hinoda Y, Imai K (1999) Butyrate augments interferon-alpha-induced S phase accumulation and persistent tyrosine phosphorylation of cdc2 in K562 cells. Br J Cancer 79: 1018–1024.
37. McDermott SP, Eppert K, Lechman ER, Doedens M, Dick JE (2010) Comparison of human cord blood engraftment between immunocompromised mouse strains. Blood 116: 193–200.
38. May C, Rivella S, Callegari J, Heller G, Gaensler KM, et al. (2000) Therapeutic haemoglobin synthesis in beta-thalassaemic mice expressing lentivirus-encoded human beta-globin. Nature 406: 82–86.
39. Pawliuk R, Westerman KA, Fabry ME, Payen E, Tighe R, et al. (2001) Correction of sickle cell disease in transgenic mouse models by gene therapy. Science 294: 2368–2371.
40. Imren S, Payen E, Westerman KA, Pawliuk R, Fabry ME, et al. (2002) Permanent and panerythroid correction of murine beta thalassemia by multiple lentiviral integration in hematopoietic stem cells. Proc Natl Acad Sci U S A 99: 14380–14385.
41. Wilber A, Hargrove PW, Kim YS, Riberdy JM, Sankaran VG, et al. (2011) Therapeutic levels of fetal hemoglobin in erythroid progeny of beta-thalassemic CD34+ cells after lentiviral vector-mediated gene transfer. Blood 117: 2817–2826.
42. Levasseur DN, Ryan TM, Pawlik KM, Townes TM (2003) Correction of a mouse model of sickle cell disease: lentiviral/antisickling beta-globin gene transduction of unmobilized, purified hematopoietic stem cells. Blood 102: 4312–4319.
43. Oh IH, Fabry ME, Humphries RK, Pawliuk R, Leboulch P, et al. (2004) Expression of an anti-sickling beta-globin in human erythroblasts derived from retrovirally transduced primitive normal and sickle cell disease hematopoietic cells. Exp Hematol 32: 461–469.
44. Imren S, Fabry ME, Westerman KA, Pawliuk R, Tang P, et al. (2004) High-level beta-globin expression and preferred intragenic integration after lentiviral transduction of human cord blood stem cells. J Clin Invest 114: 953–962.
45. Puthenveetil G, Scholes J, Carbonell D, Qureshi N, Xia P, et al. (2004) Successful correction of the human beta-thalassemia major phenotype using a lentiviral vector. Blood. 104: 3445–3453.
46. Fisher KJ, Gao GP, Weitzman MD, DeMatteo R, Burda JF, et al. (1996) Transduction with recombinant adeno-associated virus for gene therapy is limited by leading-strand synthesis. J Virol 70: 520–532.
47. Ferrari FK, Samulski T, Shenk T, Samulski RJ (1996) Second-strand synthesis is a rate-limiting step for efficient transduction by recombinant adeno-associated virus vectors. J Virol 70: 3227–3234.
48. Ponnazhagan S, Mukherjee P, Wang XS, Qing K, Kube DM, et al. (1997) Adeno-associated virus type 2-mediated transduction in primary human bone marrow-derived CD34+ hematopoietic progenitor cells: donor variation and correlation of transgene expression with cellular differentiation. J Virol 71: 8262–8267.
49. Bainbridge JW, Smith AJ, Barker SS, Robbie S, Henderson R, et al. (2008) Effect of gene therapy on visual function in Leber's congenital amaurosis. N Engl J Med 358: 2231–2239.
50. Maguire AM, Simonelli F, Pierce EA, Pugh EN Jr, Mingozzi F, et al. (2008) Safety and efficacy of gene transfer for Leber's congenital amaurosis. N Engl J Med 358: 2240–2248.
51. Cideciyan AV, Aleman TS, Boye SL, Schwartz SB, Kaushal S, et al. (2008) Human gene therapy for RPE65 isomerase deficiency activates the retinoid cycle of vision but with slow rod kinetics. Proc Natl Acad Sci U S A 105: 15112–15117.
52. Hauswirth WW, Aleman TS, Kaushal S, Cideciyan AV, Schwartz SB, et al. (2008) Treatment of leber congenital amaurosis due to RPE65 mutations by ocular subretinal injection of adeno-associated virus gene vector: short-term results of a phase I trial. Hum Gene Ther 19: 979–990.
53. Nathwani AC, Tuddenham EG, Rangarajan S, Rosales C, McIntosh J, et al. (2011) Adenovirus-associated virus vector-mediated gene transfer in hemophilia B. N Engl J Med 365: 2357–2365.
54. Weller ML, Amornphimoltham P, Schmidt M, Wilson PA, Gutkind JS, et al. (2010) Epidermal growth factor receptor is a co-receptor for adeno-associated virus serotype 6. Nat Med 16: 662–664.
55. Denard J, Beley C, Kotin R, Lai-Kuen R, Blot S, et al. (2012) Human galectin 3 binding protein interacts with recombinant adeno-associated virus type 6. J Virol 86: 6620–6631.
56. Allen H, Hsuan J, Clark S, Maziarz R, Waterfield MD, et al. (1990) Expression of epidermal-growth-factor receptor in the K562 cell line by transfection. Altered receptor biochemistry. Biochem J 271: 785–790.
57. Nakai H, Iwaki Y, Kay MA, Couto LB (1999). Isolation of recombinant adeno-associated virus vector-cellular DNA junctions from mouse liver. J Virol. 73: 5438–5447.
58. Song S, Lu Y, Choi YK, Han Y, Tang Q, et al. (2004) DNA-dependent PK inhibits adeno-associated virus DNA integration. Proc Natl Acad Sci USA. 101: 2112–2116.
59. Donsante A, Miller DG, Li Y, Vogler C, Brunt EM, et al. (2007). AAV vector integration sites in mouse hepatocellular carcinoma. Science. 317: 477.
60. Li H, Malani N, Hamilton SR, Schlachterman A, Bussadori G, et al. (2011). Assessing the potential for AAV vector genotoxicity in a murine model. Blood. 117: 3311–3319.
61. Zhong L, Li W, Li Y, Zhao W, Wu J, et al. (2006). Evaluation of primitive murine hematopoietic stem and progenitor cell transduction *in vitro* and *in vivo* by recombinant adeno-associated virus vector serotypes 1 through 5. Hum Gene Therapy. 17: 321–333.
62. Han Z, Zhong L, Maina N, Hu Z, Li X, et al. (2008). Stable integration of recombinant adeno-associated virus vector genomes after transduction of murine hematopoietic stem cells. Hum Gene Therapy. 19: 267–278.
63. Kauss MA, Smith LJ, Zhong L, Srivastava A, Wong KK Jr, et al. (2010). Enhanced long-term transduction and multilineage engraftment of human hematopoietic stem cells transduced with tyrosine-modified recombinant adeno-associated virus 2. Hum Gene Therapy. 21: 1129–1136.
64. Weltner J, Anisimov A, Alitalo K, Otonkoski T, Trokovic R (2012). Induced pluripotent stem cell clones reprogrammed via recombinant adeno-associated virus-mediated transduction contain integrated vector sequences. J Virol. 86: 4463–4467.
65. Aslanidi GV, Rivers AE, Ortiz L, Song L, Ling C, et al. (2013). Optimization of the capsid of recombinant adeno-associated virus 2 (AAV2) vectors: The final threshold? PLoS One, in press.

21

An *In Vitro* and *In Vivo* Evaluation of a Reporter Gene/ Probe System hERL/^{18}F-FES

Chunxia Qin[1], Xiaoli Lan[1]*, Jiang He[2], Xiaotian Xia[1], Yueli Tian[1], Zhijun Pei[1], Hui Yuan[1], Yongxue Zhang[1]

1 Department of Nuclear Medicine, Union Hospital, Tongji Medical College, Huazhong University of Science and Technology, Wuhan, China, **2** Department of Radiology and Medical Imaging, University of Virginia, School of Medicine, Charlottesville, Virginia, United States of America

Abstract

Purpose: To evaluate the feasibility of a reporter gene/probe system, namely the human estrogen receptor ligand binding domain (hERL)/16α-[^{18}F] fluoro-17β-estradiol (^{18}F-FES), for monitoring gene and cell therapy.

Methods: The recombinant adenovirus vector Ad5-hERL-IRES-VEGF (Ad-EIV), carrying a reporter gene (hERL) and a therapeutic gene (vascular endothelial growth factor, VEGF165) through an internal ribosome entry site (IRES), was constructed. After transfection of Ad-EIV into bone marrow mesenchymal stem cells (Ad-EIV-MSCs), hERL and VEGF165 mRNA and protein expressions were identified using Real-Time qRT-PCR and immunofluorescence. The uptake of ^{18}F-FES was measured in both Ad-EIV-MSCs and nontransfected MSCs after different incubation time. Micro-PET/CT images were obtained at 1 day after injection of Ad-EIV-MSCs into the left foreleg of the rat. The right foreleg was injected with nontransfected MSCs, which served as self-control.

Results: After transfection with Ad-EIV, the mRNA and protein expression of hERL and VEGF165 were successfully detected in MSCs, and correlated well with each other ($R^2 = 0.9840$, $P < 0.05$). This indicated the reporter gene could reflect the therapeutic gene indirectly. Ad-EIV-MSCs uptake of ^{18}F-FES increased with incubation time with a peak value of 9.13%±0.33% at 150 min, which was significantly higher than that of the control group. A far higher level of radioactivity could be seen in the left foreleg on the micro-PET/CT image than in the opposite foreleg.

Conclusion: These preliminary *in vitro* and *in vivo* studies confirmed that hERL/^{18}F-FES might be used as a novel reporter gene/probe system for monitoring gene and cell therapy. This imaging platform may have broad applications for basic research and clinical studies.

Editor: Rudolf Kirchmair, Medical University Innsbruck, Austria

Funding: This study was supported by the National Nature Science Foundation of China (Grant Numbers: 30970853, 81071200 and 30830041), the China Postdoctoral Science Foundation (2005037194), and Hubei Province Science Fund for Distinguished Young Scholars (2010CDA094). The funders' websites are http://www.nsfc.gov.cn/Portal0/default152.htm for the National Nature Science Foundation of China, http://210.79.234.200/V1/Manage/Login.aspx for the China Postdoctoral Science Foundation, and http://www.hbstd.gov.cn/jh/default.jsp for Hubei Province Science Fund for Distinguished Young Scholars. The funders had no role in study design, data collection and analysis, decision to publish, or preparation of the manuscript.

Competing Interests: The authors have declared that no competing interests exist.

* E-mail: LXL730724@hotmail.com

Introduction

Gene and cell therapy holds great promise as a potential treatment for various diseases, especially for ischemic disease and cancer research [1]. However, some problems such as a lack of tracing cells and monitoring gene expression after treatment exist. Currently, PET reporter gene/probe systems are the prevalent molecular imaging strategy for monitoring therapeutic cell and gene expression in terms of magnitude, location and duration, wherein the therapeutic gene is co-expressed together with the reporter gene which enables indirect external monitoring expression of the therapeutic gene [2,3,4].

There are two kinds of reporter genes commonly used for radionuclide imaging. One is herpes simplex virus type 1 thymidine kinase (HSV1-tk). The other is based on a membrane associated receptor or transporter, such as the dopamine 2 receptor, somatostatin receptor and sodium iodide symporter (NIS) [5,6,7]. However, both kinds of reporter genes come with shortcomings. HSV1-tk is also known as "suicide gene", its application is limited due to the toxic effects of the expression products on normal cells [8]; Membrane associated receptor or transporter may cause a series of physical problems related to the cellular signal transduction [9]. Thus exploration and development of a novel reporter gene imaging system that is safe and effective was an important component of this study. An ideal reporter gene system used for radionuclide imaging should have the following features. First, the reporter gene should be non-toxic, non-immunogenic, non-secretary, small in size, and have no endogenous protein present in the target region. Second, the tracer should be safe for use in humans and be able to combine with the reporting protein effectively after permeating the cell membrane, preferably the blood brain barrier when the tracer is used to study some brain diseases [10].

In the present study, we developed a reporter gene imaging system that uses the human estrogen receptor ligand-binding domain (hERL) as the reporter gene and 16α-[^{18}F]-fluoro-17β-estradiol (^{18}F-FES) as the radio-ligand. As a reporter gene, hERL has many advantages. First, it is a fragment of the estrogen receptor and has no transcriptional role in estrogen gene regulation due to lack of N-terminal region, avoiding unnecessary physiological role and keeping the feature of estrogen specifically. Second, hERL is a human protein, meaning that it is not or is only minimally immunogenic. In addition, there is very low endogenous expression of estrogen receptor except for the uterus, ovaries and mammary glands. Thus hERL can be used as an exogenous gene and introduced into target cells or tissues without endogenous protein interference. Estrogen receptor is a member of the nuclear hormone family of intracellular receptors [11]. Since estrogen is a steroidal hormone, it can pass through the phospholipid membranes of the cell [12,13]. When estrogen enters the nucleus, it binds to the estrogen receptor. So estrogen or its analogues, which can recognize and specifically bind to ERL, were selected as the reporter probes to monitor the reporter gene. At present, many radionuclides, such as $^{125/131/123}$I, ^{18}F and ^{99m}Tc, can be used to label estrogen or its derivatives [14,15]. 16α-[^{18}F]fluoro-17β-estradiol (^{18}F-FES) is a well-established positron emission tomography (PET) tracer with a known labeling procedure, and as a small lipophilic molecule, it has a well-characterized biodistribution and high blood–brain barrier permeability [16,17,18,19,20]. ^{18}F-FES can get internalized into ER expressing cells and bind with ER, then accumulates and traps in the targeted cells. It has already been clinically used for the diagnosis of breast cancer and gynecological carcinomas of the pelvic cavity [21,22]. All of these characteristics make ^{18}F-FES perfect for reporter gene imaging.

In relation to reporter gene imaging, researches mainly focused on cancer, while cell/gene therapy with great potential in many other diseases is rarely involved. Bone mesenchymal stem cells (MSCs) account for a small population of cells in bone marrow. They constitute a non-hematopoietic component with the capacity to differentiate into a variety of cell lineages, including adipocytes, osteocytes, chondrocytes, cardiomyocytes, neuro progenitors, and stromal cells [23]. In addition, MSCs can be readily isolated and expanded in vitro. So MSCs are considered to be a promising platform for cell and gene therapy for a variety of diseases, including tissue/organ damage, inflammation and cancer [24]. In the past decade much progress has been made in the development of gene therapy. Vascular endothelial growth factor (VEGF) is a potent angiogenic cytokine and has been delivered as a recombinant protein, using plasmids or viral gene constructs to encourage blood vessel formation in ischemic tissues [25,26]. In the present study, MSCs and VEGF165 were used as the therapeutic cell and gene; hERL/^{18}F-FES was used as the reporter gene/probe system to monitor the expression of the therapeutic gene and stem cell indirectly in vivo. The aim of our study was to evaluate the feasibility of a new reporter gene/probe system, hERL/^{18}F-FES, for monitoring gene and cell therapy, and to provide a theoretical basis for in vivo imaging using animal models of ischemic heart disease.

Materials and Methods

Gene Transfer Vector

Recombinant adenoviruses vector Ad5-hERL-IRES-VEGF (Ad-EIV), carrying a reporter gene (hERL) and a therapeutic gene (VEGF165) through an internal ribosome entry site (IRES), was constructed and purified in Vector Gene Technology (Beijing, China). The hERL and VEGF genes in the recombinant vectors were identified using the polymerase chain reaction (PCR). The viral titer of Ad5-hERL-IRES-VEGF was 1×10^9 TU/ml as determined using the 50% Tissue Culture Infective Dose (TCID50) method.

Rat Bone Mesenchymal Stem Cell Isolation and Culture

All protocols involving animals were conducted according to the standards of international regulations. Sprague-Dawley rats aged 6–8 weeks and weighing 100–150 g were obtained from the Experimental Animal Center of Tongji Medical College, Huazhong University of Science and Technology (Wuhan, China). They were euthanized with an overdose of chloral hydrate solution. MSCs were harvested and cultured as described previously [27,28]. Briefly, both tibias and femurs were dissected free, the ends of the bones were then cut and the bone marrow was extracted and rinsed in 10 mL of Dulbecco's modified Eagle's medium/Ham's F-12 nutrient mixture (DMEM/F12; Hyclone, Beijing, China) with a syringe. Cells were then washed twice with culture medium (DMEM/F12 containing 15% fetal bovine serum) and planted in 75 cm^2 flasks. They were incubated at 37 °C in a humidified atmosphere containing 5% carbon dioxide (CO_2). After 3 days, non-adherent cells were removed by replacing the medium and adherent cells further cultured in culture medium for 4 supplementary days. Cells were trypsinized at 80%–90% confluence using 0.25% trypsin solution, and cell viability was checked using the trypan blue dye exclusion test and replated to fresh flasks.

MSC phenotype was considered positive for CD44 and CD90, and negative for CD34 and CD45 [29]. In order to characterize the phenotype of MSCs, immunocytochemical analyses were performed with CD34 and CD44 antibodies. MSCs at passage three were fixed in 4% paraformaldehyde for 30 min, and then permeabilized with 0.1% Triton X-100 for 15 min. After the cells were washed with phosphate-buffered saline (PBS), they were incubated overnight with primary mouse antibodies directed against either the rat CD34 (ready for use, Maixin, China) or CD44 (1:200, Zhongshan, China) surface antigens at 4 °C. Mouse IgG was added instead of primary antibodies as an isotype control. Cells were then washed with PBS followed by incubation with a secondary antibody (ChemMateTMEnVision+/HRP) for 45 min at room temperature. The signals were visualized using diaminobenzidine substrate and counterstained using hematoxylin. In addition, for further confirmation, the proportion of CD45− and CD90+ cells was analyzed using flow cytometry. Cells at passage three were used. After trypsinization, 2×10^5 cells were resuspended in 300 μL of PBS and incubated with antibodies directed against either the CD45 (Anti-Rat CD45.2 FITC; eBioscience) or the CD90 (Anti-Mouse/Rat CD90.1 [Thy-1.1] PE; eBioscience) antigens for 30 min. The cells were then washed with PBS, fixed in CellFix (eBioscience) and analyzed using flow cytometry. Data were generated using the CELLQUEST software. Isotype control antibody containing mouse IgG1 FITC and IgG2 PE was used as a control.

In Vitro Viral Infections

MSCs between passages three and ten were transfected with various Ad-EIV viral titers (multiplicity of infection (MOI) = 0, 25, 50, 75 or 100) according to the aim of the experiment. Take a 6-well-plate and MOI = 100 as an example. About 5×10^5 MSCs per well were incubated with 1×10^7 TU of adenoviral (10 μl) diluted in 1 ml of Opti-MEM medium without fetal calf serum (FCS) at 37 °C for 4 h, and then the viral supernatant was removed and replaced with culture medium. The adenovirus-infected cells were called Ad-EIV-MSCs and were used after 48 h of infection. MSCs incubated with Opti-MEM at the same volume served as the control, but without virus transfection.

Real-Time qRT-PCR

The transcription levels of ER and VEGF genes were quantified by real-time reverse transcription (RT)-PCR. Total RNA was isolated from cells using TRIzol® reagent (Invitrogen, Carlsbad, CA, USA) and cDNA was then synthesized from total RNA using SuperScript™ II Reverse Transcriptase according to the manufacturer's protocols (Invitrogen). Real-time RT-PCR using synthesized cDNA as a template was performed with three pairs of PCR primers (Table 1) and a SYBR green mix (Thunderbird SYBR qPCR Mix; Toyobo, Osaka, Japan). The reaction was done in triplicate. Glyceraldehyde phosphate dehydrogenase (GAPDH) was used as an internal control gene. Relative gene expression of ER and VEGF were analyzed using comparative threshold circle (C_T) method, which means the amplification fold change of ER or VEGF relative to GAPDH in the transfected cells compared with the control nontransfected cells.

Immunofluorescence Assay for hERL and VEGF165 Expression

MSCs were transfected with Ad-VIE (MOI = 100) for 48 h. Cells were then fixed with 4% paraformaldehyde and permeabilized with 0.1% Triton X-100 for 15 min. Primary antibodies, monoclonal antibodies to ERα (Santa Cruz, USA) at a dilution of 1:200 and VEGF (Beyotime, China) at a dilution of 1:200, were added to the cells and incubated overnight at 4 °C. After washing with PBS for three times, cells were incubated with CY3-conjugated goat anti-mouse or rabbit antibody (1:50) for 45 min. The cells were then washed with PBS and incubated with hochest33258 for 10 min. All fluorescent staining was visualized using a fluorescence microscope. Rabbit IgG was added instead of primary antibodies as an isotype control.

Radiolabelling of Estradiol

^{18}F-FES was prepared using a conventional ^{18}F-FDG module and established procedures were used according to the published references [30,31,32]. Fluorine-18 was produced by the ^{18}O (p,n) ^{18}F reaction on ^{18}O-enriched water as target material. The necessary precursor, 3-O-methoxymethyl-16, 17-O-sulfuryl-16-epiestriol (MMSE) was purchased from Huayi Isotopes Co. (Changshu, China). Briefly, the total procedure of ^{18}F-FES preparation consisted of three steps as follows: (a) fluorination, (b) hydrolysis, and (c) high performance liquid chromatography (HPLC) purification of the final product. The yield of ^{18}F-FES was 50.0±2.35%, and the radiochemical purity was 96.1±0.3% (n = 4).

Table 1. Primers used for qRT-PCR analysis

Gene		Primer sequence	Length (bp)
Human VEGF165	Forward	5'-ATGACGAGGGCCTGGAGTGT-3'	227
	Reverse	5'- ACATTTACACGTCTGCGGATCT-3'	
Human ER	Forward	5'-GAAGTGCAAGAACGTGGTG-3'	149
	Reverse	5'-AATGCGATGAAGTAGAGCC-3'	
Rat GAPDH	Forward	5'-CGCTAACATCAAATGGGGTG-3'	201
	Reverse	5'-TTGCTGACAATCTTGAGGGAG-3'	

Cellular Uptake of ^{18}F-FES

ER activity was evaluated by measuring the cellular uptake of ^{18}F-FES. For this purpose, Ad-EIV-MSCs (MOI = 100) and control nontransfected MSCs in 24-well plates were incubated at 37 °C with 200 μL of ^{18}F-FES (2 μCi/mL) for 30, 60, 90, 120 and 150 min. At the end of the incubation period, the radioactive medium was collected from each well, followed by rinsing three times with PBS. The medium and rinses were combined into a tube for the purpose of counting of extra cellular radioactivity. Subsequently, the cells were lysed with 1 N sodium hydroxide solution and the wells were rinsed three times with PBS. Both cell lysate and rinses were collected into an additional tube for counting of intracellular radioactivity. Radioactivity was measured using a gamma counter and corrected for decay. Triplicate samples were performed for all uptake studies. The uptake rate was calculated according to the following formula: Uptake Rate (%) = $\text{Count}_{\text{intracellular}}/(\text{Count}_{\text{extra cellular}}+\text{Count}_{\text{intracellular}})\times 100\%$.

In Vivo Micro-PET/CT Imaging

To assess the feasibility of the reporter gene/probe system hERL/^{18}F-FES for monitoring gene and cell therapy in vivo, micro-PET/CT were performed in rats. Four rats were prepared for imaging. For each rat, $3-5\times10^6$ Ad-EIV-MSCs (MOI = 100) suspended in 100 μL of PBS were injected intramuscularly into left foreleg, and nontransfected MSCs with same number were injected into the opposite foreleg served as a self-control. Positron emission tomography (PET) imaging was performed on a micro-PET/CT scanner (Siemens Inc, Germany) at 1 day after MSCs injection. The injected dose of ^{18}F-FES was 200–300 μCi per animal. Images were obtained at 1 h after intravenous tail vein injection of ^{18}F-FES. During imaging, the animals were maintained under 10% chloral hydrate anesthesia (0.3 mL/100 g), and placed in prone position on the bed of the scanner. Two bed positions were acquired.

The images were reconstructed and identical regions of interest (ROIs) were drawn on bilateral foreleg areas of rat images. The counts per pixel per minute were converted to tracer activity (Bq/mL) using a calibration constant obtained from scanning a cylindrical phantom. The ROI counts per mL per min were converted to counts per gram per min (assuming a tissue density of 1 g/mL), and divided by the injected dose to obtain an image ROI-derived tissue uptake index expressed as percent injected dose per gram of tissue (% ID/g).

Statistical Analysis

Data are expressed as mean ± SD. Group comparisons were performed using a two-tailed Student t test or one-way ANOVA where appropriate. P values less than 0.05 were considered statistically significant.

Results

Mesenchymal Stem Cell Culture and Identification

Most of the cells collected from bone marrow rinses by centrifuge were mononuclear MSCs. The primary cells were circular and began to stick after 24 h, and the morphology of cells changed to spindle or short rod-like in 3–4 days. About 1 week later, the cells formed colonies and were arranged like radial or concentric circles. They grew to 80%–90% confluence on days 7–10 after initial plating and had a definition of passage 0. Cells between passages three and ten were maintained in a spindle-shaped and fibroblast-like form and were used for experiments. Immuno-cytochemistry and flow cytometry showed most of the cells were positive for CD44 and CD90 but negative for CD34 and

CD45 (Fig. 1). The osteogenic differentiation and adipogenic differentiation capacity of MSCs have been confirmed by our group previously [33]. These MSCs immunophenotype profiles agreed well with previously reported expression patterns of surface antigens using rMSCs [28].

Strong Correlations between Reporter and Therapeutic Genes Indicated by qRT-PCR and Immunofluorescence

The results of qRT-PCR showed an obvious mRNA expression of hERL and VEGF165 in Ad-EIV-MSCs, while the control nontransfected MSCs revealed low hERL and VEGF165 mRNA expression (Fig. 2 A). Over the range of viral titers tested, a high correlation ($R^2 = 0.9840$, $P<0.05$) existed between the expressions of the two linked genes (Fig. 2 B). Figure 3 shows an immunofluorescence image that exhibited protein expression of hERL and VEGF165. From the PCR and immunofluorescence results, the mRNA and protein expression of VEGF165 was stronger than that of hERL. These results demonstrated successful transduction of the reporter and therapeutic gene at the same time, and the reporter gene could reflect the therapeutic gene indirectly.

Cellular Uptake of ^{18}F-FES

Figure 4 demonstrated a time-dependent increase in the accumulation of ^{18}F-FES in both the Ad-EIV-MSCs (MOI = 100) and control nontransfected MSCs, and the highest uptake rate occurred at 150 min, with the peak values of 9.13%±0.33% (n = 3) and 4.27%±0.27% (n = 3), respectively. The results obtained from the control group showed a remarkable difference compared with Ad-EIV-MSCs at each time point (t = 10.574–40.260, $P<0.01$), which supported the specificity of ^{18}F-FES for hERL.

In Vivo Micro-PET/CT Imaging

Much higher radioactivity could be seen in the left foreleg where Ad-EIV-MSCs were injected than that in the opposite foreleg, which served as self-control (Fig. 5). Identical ROIs were drawn on the left and right forelegs, and the uptake values were 0.46±0.11% ID/g and 0.11±0.03% ID/g (n = 4), respectively ($P<0.05$).

Discussion

In order to evaluate the success of stem cell transplantation and to monitor the expression of therapeutic genes in living individuals, development of noninvasive imaging modalities capable of identifying the location, magnitude and duration of cellular survival and fate is required [27]. One of best techniques available is radionuclide reporter gene imaging, which enables accurate non-invasive monitoring of therapeutic genes and cells, quantitatively and repeatedly.

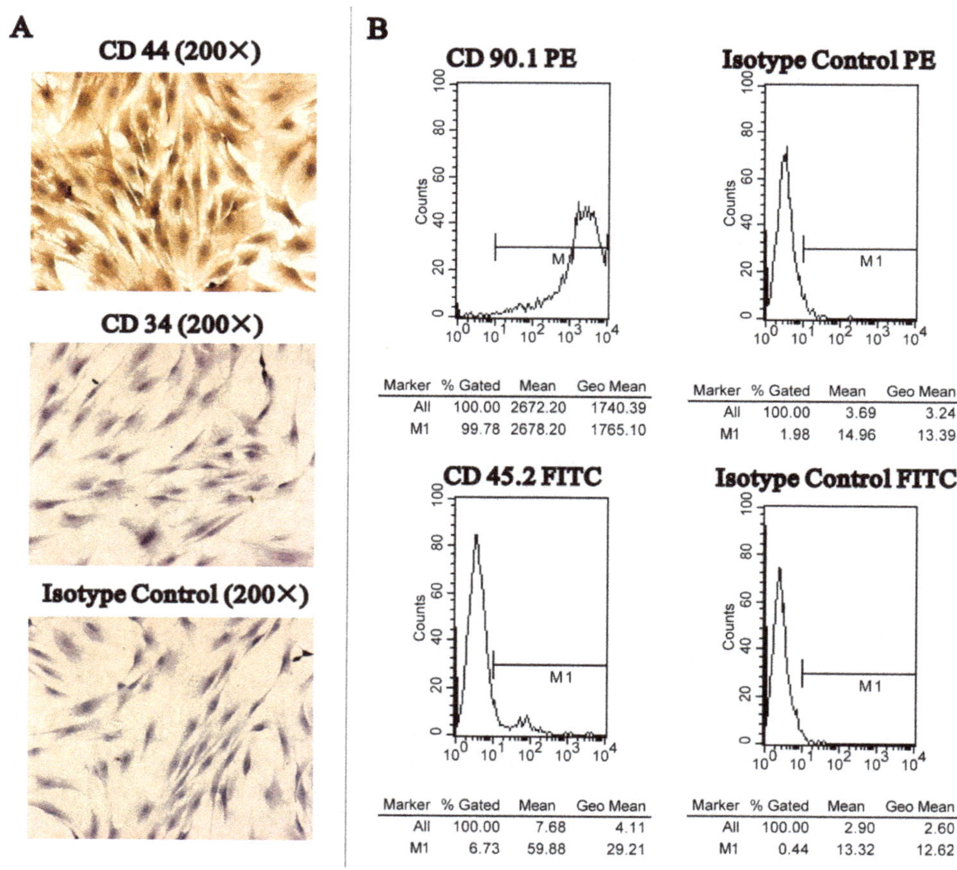

Figure 1. Detection of surface markers of MSCs. A. Immunocytochemistry results showed that MSCs were positive for CD44 (upper), and negative for CD34 (middle) and isotype control (lower). B. Flow cytometry analysis of MSCs. Almost the entire tested MSCs showed positive for CD90 (left upper), and negative for CD45 (left lower), isotype control Ig G2 PE (right upper) and isotype control Ig G1 FITC (right lower).

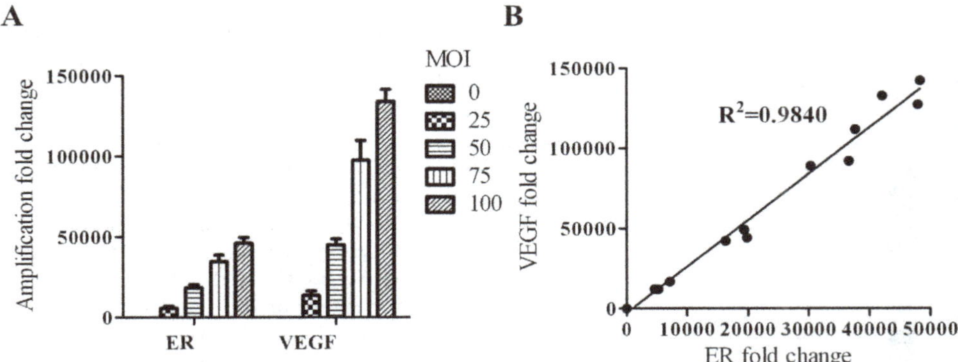

Figure 2. hERL and VEGF165 expression in MSCs detected by qRT-PCR. A revealed the relative expression of hERL and VEGF165 increased with adenovirus titer. Very low expression of both genes was seen in the control nontransfected group (MOI = 0), and VEGF165 gene expression showed stronger than that of the hERL gene. B presented the high correlation of the expression of hERL and VEGF165 ($R^2 = 0.9840$).

Recently, investigators have developed a reporter gene PET tracer system, hERL/^{18}F-FES, for monitoring gene therapy noninvasively [2,10,34]. Plasmid or adenovirus was used as the carrier of the reporter gene; human thymidine phosphorylase was used as a therapeutic gene and uptake of [^{3}H] estradiol demonstrated specific uptake in infected cells. In the present study, MSCs were used as the platform for gene therapy and recombinant adenovirus Ad5-hERL-IRES-VEGF was used as the vector. The aim was to evaluate the feasibility of a new reporter gene/probe system hERL/^{18}F-FES for monitoring gene and cell therapy; the ultimate goal is to monitor MSCs and VEGF165 gene therapy in vivo. This is the first report on the novel reporter gene system hERL/^{18}F-FES being used for monitoring cell/gene therapy in vivo. We demonstrated its feasibility from our primary in vitro and in vivo results, which may provide a good foundation for further study.

In order to achieve gene therapy, a carrier or 'vector' is required to deliver the therapeutic genetic material into the special target cells. Different gene delivery systems with various favorable characteristics have been developed. Adenovirus is still the preferred gene delivery vector owing to its high efficiency [2,35,36]. This is especially true in humans where high levels of short-term gene expression, such as for therapeutic angiogenesis, are required. Compared with other cell types considered for cardiomyopathy, MSCs appear to possess unique properties that may allow for convenient and highly effective cell therapy. MSCs

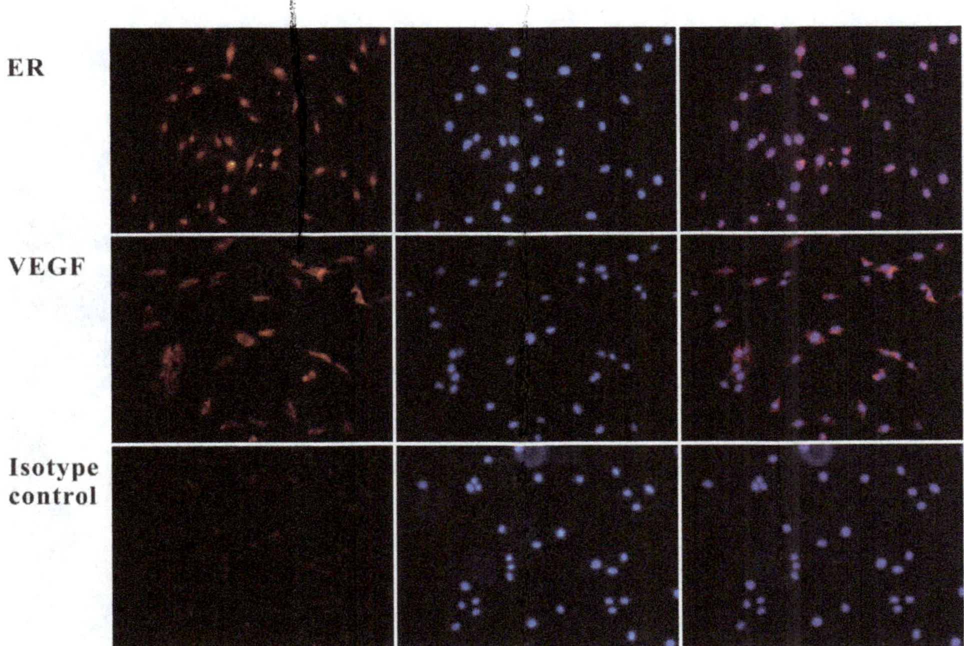

Figure 3. Immunofluorescence results for hERL and VEGF165 expression in Ad-EIV-MSCs (200×). The upper row showed an intense/ moderate immunoreactive signal in the peri-nuclear/nuclear regions, which suggested the expression of the estrogen receptor-α subtype. The image on the left was the positive expression of ER, and the middle one was the nucleus staining under the same field of vision. The image on the right was the overlay image, which showed the sub-cellular localization of ER clearly. The middle row showed an intense immune-reactive signal of VEGF165, which was detected in the cytoplasm. The order of the image was same as the upper row. The third row was the isotype control result.

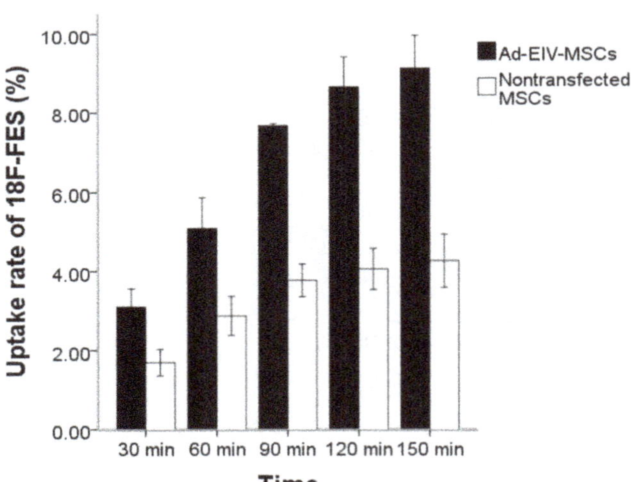

Figure 4. Time-dependent cellular uptake experiment. Data are means and standard deviations from three independent experiments.

can be used allogenetically and delivered systemically, and can differentiate into many cell types in the proper microenvironments. Furthermore, MSCs can be readily transduced by a variety of vectors and maintain transgene expression after in vivo differentiation [27].

In the initial in vitro studies, our data showed that the reporter gene hERL and the therapeutic gene VEGF165 were successfully transfected into MSCs through the recombinant adenoviruses vector Ad5-hERL-IRES-VEGF. These two genes co-expressed and correlated well with each other. These findings indicated that the adenovirus was a good vector with high transfect efficiency and provide a theoretical basis for animal research in vivo. In the cellular uptake experiment, uptake rates of ^{18}F-FES in Ad-VIE-MSCs at all time points were much higher than those of nontransfected MSCs. However, a small but detectable rise in uptake was also seen in the nontransfected MSCs. It may be related to the non-specific uptake or conglutination of ^{18}F-FES, and this non-specific uptake increased over time. Moreover, nontransfected MSCs perhaps have a very low expression of ER.

In the primary in vivo study, we injected virus infected MSCs into rat foreleg muscle and used micro-PET/CT imaging for evaluation. After intravenous injection, ^{18}F-FES has been shown to distribute rapidly in the whole body, including the brain. It is also washed out rapidly, with the exception of ER-expressing tissue and tissues such as the liver, kidney, bladder and intestines, for these organs are the primary organs involved in ^{18}F-FES metabolism and excretion [16,37]. Positive accumulation of ^{18}F-FES localized in the left foreleg was observed. The region of high ^{18}F-FES uptake indicated hERL expression. Some bone uptakes were observed, which indicates either defluorination of ^{18}F-FES in vivo or ^{18}F- impurity presenting in the probe. The biodistribution of ^{18}F-FES observed using micro-PET imaging in the present study was similar to that reported in previous studies [38,39].

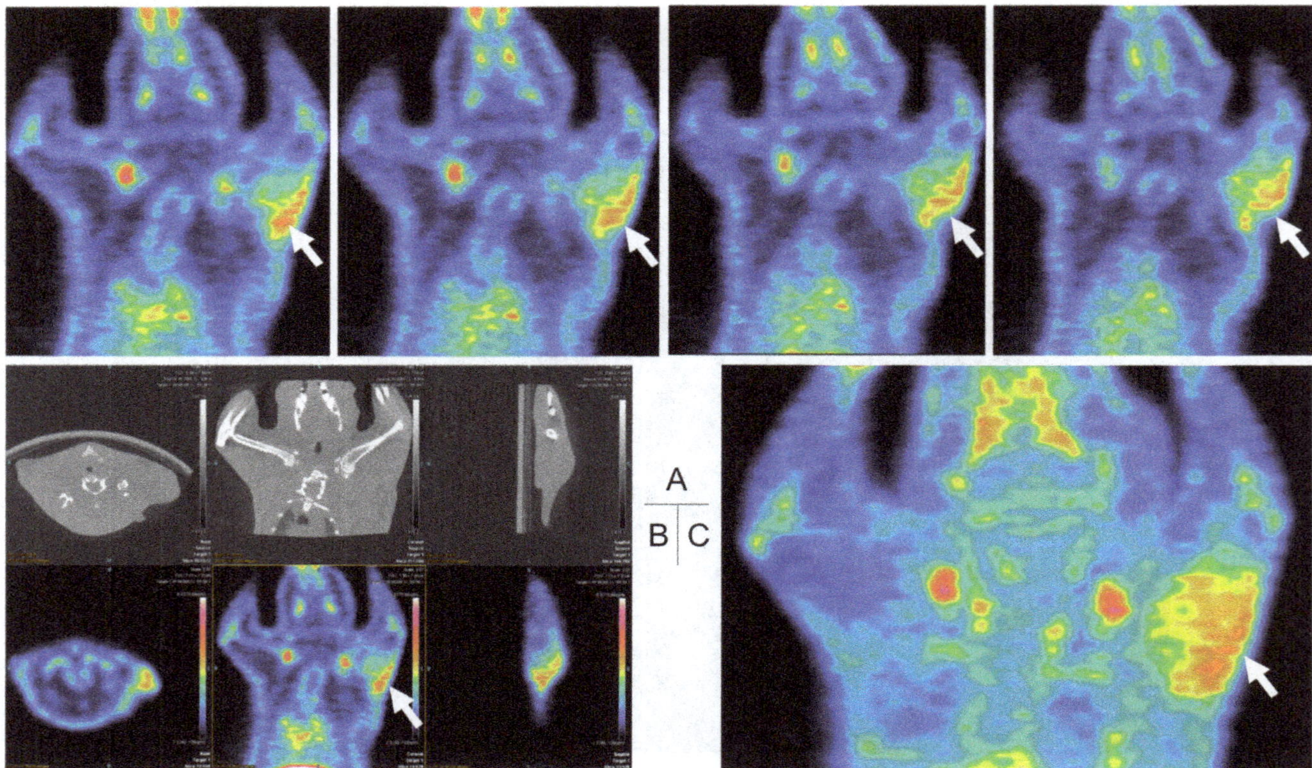

Figure 5. Micro-PET/CT images of a representative animal. ^{18}F-FES PET/CT scan was performed to detect hERL expression in the left forearm of rat. Intense ^{18}F-FES uptake (arrows) was observed at the left forearm, while no uptake of ^{18}F-FES at the contralateral forearm. (A. Coronal slices of an animal's PET imaging; B. The transverse, coronal and sagittal images of CT (upper) and PET (lower) images; C. Image of maximum intensity projection.).

The advantage of our study was that the PET probe ^{18}F-FES is a radiopharmaceutical already being used for human studies, which can access a wide range of tissues, including the brain. In addition, because the reporter hERL gene lacks a DNA binding domain it can no longer work as a transcription factor, and has no physiological function. Thus, it's possible to obtain images of the therapeutic gene and stem cells through the reporter gene indirectly. All of these features could facilitate easier translation of our system from the bench to bedside.

Our study had some limitations that should be acknowledged. First, our recombinant adenovirus did not contain the fluorescence (GFP or RFP) gene, so we could not observe transfection efficiency using the fluorescence microscopy which is very convenient. Second, our current study lacked a radio-ligand receptor binding assay. Unlabeled estradiol should have been used to block the estrogen receptor and test non-specific binding. A competitive binding assay is also needed.

Although further studies, such as those involving a receptor binding assay and in vivo animal models are still needed, the positive in vitro results and proof-of-concept in vivo images obtained in our study using a rat muscle model indicated that our new reporter gene/reporter probe system is potentially applicable for monitoring gene/cell therapy.

Conclusion

In summary, our study demonstrated that Ad5-hERL-IRES-VEGF was a good vector for the reporter gene hERL and the therapy gene VEGF165. Cultured MSCs infected by Ad-EIV expressed therapeutic and reporter genes simultaneously, and accumulated the radioligand ^{18}F-FES specifically. Successful micro-PET/CT imaging of the rat left foreleg injected with Ad-EIV-MSCs demonstrated the efficacy of utilizing hERL as reporter gene, and ^{18}F-FES as PET probe for monitoring gene and cell therapy in vivo. These findings demonstrated that hERL/^{18}F-FES is feasible for monitoring gene/cell therapy and provided sufficient evidence to warrant further studies.

Acknowledgments

Thanks are offered to Dr. Biao Li and Dr. Sheng Liang at Ruijin Hospital, Shanghai Jiaotong University, for their kind help in preparing ^{18}F-FES and performing micro-PET/CT imaging.

Author Contributions

Conceived and designed the experiments: XL JH YZ. Performed the experiments: CQ XL XX YT ZP HY. Analyzed the data: CQ XL. Contributed reagents/materials/analysis tools: CQ XL. Wrote the paper: CQ XL.

References

1. Bonaros N, Bernecker O, Ott H, Schlechta B, Kocher AA (2005) Cell- and gene therapy for ischemic heart disease. Minerva Cardioangiol 53: 265–273.
2. Lohith TG, Furukawa T, Mori T, Kobayashi M, Fujibayashi Y (2008) Basic evaluation of FES-hERL PET tracer-reporter gene system for in vivo monitoring of adenoviral-mediated gene therapy. Mol Imaging Biol 10: 245–252.
3. Lan X, Yin X, Wang R, Liu Y, Zhang Y (2009) Comparative study of cellular kinetics of reporter probe [(131)I]FIAU in neonatal cardiac myocytes after transfer of HSV1-tk reporter gene with two vectors. Nucl Med Biol 36: 207–213.
4. Hu J, Zhang Y, Sun X, Li D, Li C, et al. (2011) A novel technique for the preparation of (125)I-5-trimethylstannyl-1-(2-deoxy-2-fluoro-beta-D-arabino-furanosyl) urail and its biodistribution pattern in Kunming mice. J Huazhong Univ Sci Technolog Med Sci 31: 693–695.
5. Zhang H, Moroz MA, Serganova I, Ku T, Huang R, et al. (2011) Imaging expression of the human somatostatin receptor subtype-2 reporter gene with 68Ga-DOTATOC. J Nucl Med 52: 123–131.
6. Gambhir SS, Barrio JR, Herschman HR, Phelps ME (1999) Assays for noninvasive imaging of reporter gene expression. Nucl Med Biol 26: 481–490.
7. Blasberg RG, Gelovani J (2002) Molecular-genetic imaging: a nuclear medicine-based perspective. Mol Imaging 1: 280–300.
8. Freeman SM, Ramesh R, Marrogi AJ (1997) Immune system in suicide-gene therapy. Lancet 349: 2–3.
9. Likar Y, Dobrenkov K, Olszewska M, Vider E, Shenker L, et al. (2008) A new acycloguanosine-specific supermutant of herpes simplex virus type 1 thymidine kinase suitable for PET imaging and suicide gene therapy for potential use in patients treated with pyrimidine-based cytotoxic drugs. J Nucl Med 49: 713–720.
10. Takamatsu S, Furukawa T, Mori T, Yonekura Y, Fujibayashi Y (2005) Noninvasive imaging of transplanted living functional cells transfected with a reporter estrogen receptor gene. Nucl Med Biol 32: 821–829.
11. Kumar V, Green S, Stack G, Berry M, Jin JR, et al. (1987) Functional domains of the human estrogen receptor. Cell 51: 941–951.
12. Evans RM (1988) The steroid and thyroid hormone receptor superfamily. Science 240: 889–895.
13. Beato M, Herrlich P, Schutz G (1995) Steroid hormone receptors: many actors in search of a plot. Cell 83: 851–857.
14. Takahashi N, Yang DJ, Kohanim S, Oh CS, Yu DF, et al. (2007) Targeted functional imaging of estrogen receptors with 99mTc-GAP-EDL. Eur J Nucl Med Mol Imaging 34: 354–362.
15. Melo e Silva MC, Patrcio L, Gano L, Sa e Melo ML, Inohae E, et al. (2001) Synthesis and biological evaluation of two new radiolabelled estrogens: [125I](E)-3-methoxy-17alpha-iodovinylestra-1,3,5(10),6-tetraen-17beta-ol and [125I](Z)-3-methoxy-17α-iodovinylestra-1,3,5(10),6-tetraen-17β-ol. Appl Radiat Isot 54: 227–239.
16. Kiesewetter DO, Kilbourn MR, Landvatter SW, Heiman DF, Katzenellenbogen JA, et al. (1984) Preparation of four fluorine- 18-labeled estrogens and their selective uptakes in target tissues of immature rats. J Nucl Med 25: 1212–1221.
17. Romer J, Fuchtner F, Steinbach J, Kasch H (2001) Automated synthesis of 16alpha-[18F]fluoroestradiol-3,17beta-disulphamate. Appl Radiat Isot 55: 631–639.
18. Mathias CJ, Welch MJ, Katzenellenbogen JA, Brodack JW, Kilbourn MR, et al. (1987) Characterization of the uptake of 16 alpha-([18F]fluoro)-17 beta-estradiol in DMBA-induced mammary tumors. Int J Rad Appl Instrum B 14: 15–25.
19. Mankoff DA, Peterson LM, Tewson TJ, Link JM, Gralow JR, et al. (2001) [18F]fluoroestradiol radiation dosimetry in human PET studies. J Nucl Med 42: 679–684.
20. Sasaki M, Fukumura T, Kuwabara Y, Yoshida T, Nakagawa M, et al. (2000) Biodistribution and breast tumor uptake of 16alpha-[18F]-fluoro-17beta-estradiol in rat. Ann Nucl Med 14: 127–130.
21. McGuire AH, Dehdashti F, Siegel BA, Lyss AP, Brodack JW, et al. (1991) Positron tomographic assessment of 16 alpha-[18F] fluoro-17 beta-estradiol uptake in metastatic breast carcinoma. J Nucl Med 32: 1526–1531.
22. Kumar P, Mercer J, Doerkson C, Tonkin K, McEwan AJ (2007) Clinical production, stability studies and PET imaging with 16-alpha-[18F]fluoroestra-diol ([18F]FES) in ER positive breast cancer patients. J Pharm Pharm Sci 10: 256s–265s.
23. Pittenger MF, Mackay AM, Beck SC, Jaiswal RK, Douglas R, et al. (1999) Multilineage potential of adult human mesenchymal stem cells. Science 284: 143–147.
24. Ozawa K, Sato K, Oh I, Ozaki K, Uchibori R, et al. (2008) Cell and gene therapy using mesenchymal stem cells (MSCs). J Autoimmun 30: 121–127.
25. Modarai B, Humphries J, Burnand KG, Gossage JA, Waltham M, et al. (2008) Adenovirus-mediated VEGF gene therapy enhances venous thrombus recanalization and resolution. Arterioscler Thromb Vasc Biol 28: 1753–1759.
26. Kalil RA, Salles FB, Giusti, II, Rodrigues CG, Han SW, et al. (2010) VEGF gene therapy for angiogenesis in refractory angina: phase I/II clinical trial. Rev Bras Cir Cardiovasc 25: 311–321.
27. Roelants V, Labar D, de Meester C, Havaux X, Tabilio A, et al. (2008) Comparison between adenoviral and retroviral vectors for the transduction of the thymidine kinase PET reporter gene in rat mesenchymal stem cells. J Nucl Med 49: 1836–1844.
28. Javazon EH, Colter DC, Schwarz EJ, Prockop DJ (2001) Rat marrow stromal cells are more sensitive to plating density and expand more rapidly from single-cell-derived colonies than human marrow stromal cells. Stem Cells 19: 219–225.
29. Mansilla E, Marin GH, Drago H, Sturla F, Salas E, et al. (2006) Bloodstream cells phenotypically identical to human mesenchymal bone marrow stem cells circulate in large amounts under the influence of acute large skin damage: new evidence for their use in regenerative medicine. Transplant Proc 38: 967–969.
30. Oh SJ, Chi DY, Mosdzianowski C, Kil HS, Ryu JS, et al. (2007) The automatic production of 16alpha-[18F]fluoroestradiol using a conventional [18F]FDG module with a disposable cassette system. Appl Radiat Isot 65: 676–681.
31. Romer J, Fuchtner F, Steinbach J, Johannsen B (1999) Automated production of 16alpha-[18F]fluoroestradiol for breast cancer imaging. Nucl Med Biol 26: 473–479.
32. Mori T, Kasamatsu S, Mosdzianowski C, Welch MJ, Yonekura Y, et al. (2006) Automatic synthesis of 16 alpha-[(18)F]fluoro-17beta-estradiol using a cassette-type [(18)F]fluorodeoxyglucose synthesizer. Nucl Med Biol 33: 281–286.

33. Hu S, Cao W, Lan X, He Y, Lang J, et al. (2011) Comparison of rNIS and hNIS as reporter genes for noninvasive imaging of bone mesenchymal stem cells transplanted into infarcted rat myocardium. Mol Imaging 10: 227–237.
34. Furukawa T, Lohith TG, Takamatsu S, Mori T, Tanaka T, et al. (2006) Potential of the FES-hERL PET reporter gene system–basic evaluation for gene therapy monitoring. Nucl Med Biol 33: 145–151.
35. Stewart DJ, Hilton JD, Arnold JM, Gregoire J, Rivard A, et al. (2006) Angiogenic gene therapy in patients with nonrevascularizable ischemic heart disease: a phase 2 randomized, controlled trial of AdVEGF(121) (AdVEGF121) versus maximum medical treatment. Gene Ther 13: 1503–1511.
36. Wong GK, Chiu AT (2011) Gene therapy, gene targeting and induced pluripotent stem cells: applications in monogenic disease treatment. Biotechnol Adv 29: 1–10.
37. Mankoff DA, Tewson TJ, Eary JF (1997) Analysis of blood clearance and labeled metabolites for the estrogen receptor tracer [F-18]-16 alpha-fluoroestradiol (FES). Nucl Med Biol 24: 341–348.
38. Benard F, Ahmed N, Beauregard JM, Rousseau J, Aliaga A, et al. (2008) [18F]Fluorinated estradiol derivatives for oestrogen receptor imaging: impact of substituents, formulation and specific activity on the biodistribution in breast tumour-bearing mice. Eur J Nucl Med Mol Imaging 35: 1473–1479.
39. Seimbille Y, Rousseau J, Benard F, Morin C, Ali H, et al. (2002) 18F-labeled difluoroestradiols: preparation and preclinical evaluation as estrogen receptor-binding radiopharmaceuticals. Steroids 67: 765–775.

Hybrid Sequencing Approach Applied to Human Fecal Metagenomic Clone Libraries Revealed Clones with Potential Biotechnological Applications

Mária Džunková[1,2], Giuseppe D'Auria[1,2]*, David Pérez-Villarroya[1], Andrés Moya[1,2]

1 Joint Unit of Research in Genomics and Health, Centre for Public Health Research (CSISP) - Cavanilles Institute for Biodiversity and Evolutionary Biology, University of Valencia, Valencia, Spain, **2** CIBER en Epidemiología y Salud Pública (CIBEResp), Madrid, Spain

Abstract

Natural environments represent an incredible source of microbial genetic diversity. Discovery of novel biomolecules involves biotechnological methods that often require the design and implementation of biochemical assays to screen clone libraries. However, when an assay is applied to thousands of clones, one may eventually end up with very few positive clones which, in most of the cases, have to be "domesticated" for downstream characterization and application, and this makes screening both laborious and expensive. The negative clones, which are not considered by the selected assay, may also have biotechnological potential; however, unfortunately they would remain unexplored. Knowledge of the clone sequences provides important clues about potential biotechnological application of the clones in the library; however, the sequencing of clones one-by-one would be very time-consuming and expensive. In this study, we characterized the first metagenomic clone library from the feces of a healthy human volunteer, using a method based on 454 pyrosequencing coupled with a clone-by-clone Sanger end-sequencing. Instead of whole individual clone sequencing, we sequenced 358 clones in a pool. The medium-large insert (7–15 kb) cloning strategy allowed us to assemble these clones correctly, and to assign the clone ends to maintain the link between the position of a living clone in the library and the annotated contig from the 454 assembly. Finally, we found several open reading frames (ORFs) with previously described potential medical application. The proposed approach allows planning *ad-hoc* biochemical assays for the clones of interest, and the appropriate sub-cloning strategy for gene expression in suitable vectors/hosts.

Editor: Jonathan H. Badger, J. Craig Venter Institute, United States of America

Funding: This work was funded by grant CP09/00049 Miguel Servet, Instituto de Salud Carlos III, Spain to GD; by projects SAF2009-13032-C02-01 from the Spanish Ministry for Science and Innovation (MCINN), FU2008-04501-E from Spanish Ministry for Science and Innovation (MCINN) in the frame of ERA-Net PathoGenoMics and Prometeo/2009/092 from Conselleria D'Educació Generalitat Valenciana, Spain, to AM. MD is recipient of a fellowship from Spanish Ministry of Education FPU2010. The funders had no role in study design, data collection and analysis, decision to publish, or preparation of the manuscript.

Competing Interests: The authors have declared that no competing interests exist.

* E-mail: dauria_giu@gva.es

Introduction

Since the late nineties, metagenomic-based methodologies have been applied to decipher the composition and gene content of bacterial communities in the environment, as well as to detect novel biomolecules for subsequent functional screening [1,2]. The majority of anti-microbial or anti-cancer drugs have a natural origin [3] and the most disparate environments (sea water, extreme environments, soil) have been studied by metagenomic approaches [4–6]. Such studies have led to the discovery of many novel biocatalysts such as lipases or esterases [7–10], cellulases [11,12], chitinases [13], DNA polymerases [14], proteases [15], and a wide range of antibiotics [16]. Symbiotic metagenomes are also promising when it comes to seeking molecules with medical applications given their connection to the healthy status of hosts [17]. Despite this fact, to date no metagenomic library from human symbiotic ecosystems has been screened for novel biomolecules.

Several strategies can be followed to discover new bacterial products in metagenomic samples [18]. One of them is the construction of clone libraries. Small-insert libraries (plasmid vectors) are employed to identify bioproducts encoded by a single gene or a small operon. Large-insert libraries (cosmid vectors or bacterial artificial chromosomes) can be used to isolate larger gene clusters, which could encode for complete pathways [1,4]. One of the possible screening methods is functional-based screening, in which a given metagenomic library is tested against a wide spectra of screening assays, aiming to identify clones possessing interesting features. Sequence-based screening involves the selection of positive clones for a PCR reaction specifically designed for a gene of interest. A third possible method is substrate-induced gene-expression screening (SIGEX), which has been successfully applied to select clones whose expression is induced by a given substrate [19]. However, in spite of the efforts to screen for natural bioproducts, both discovery rate and application have dramatically declined [20].

In all the above-mentioned methods, an assay designed to discover a single novel biomolecule must be applied to the whole clone library (often containing thousands of clones), finally giving only a few positive clones (if any), which makes the screening process very inefficient. However, the clones that are negative for that specific assay could also contain sequences with an interesting biotechnological potential; however, unfortunately in this case they would remain unexplored.

Prior knowledge of clone sequences can help researchers to design the appropriate screening assays and, thus, to increase the biotechnological application potential of the library (novel biomolecule per clone library rate). However, sequencing clones one-by-one using any type of sequencing platform would be very time-consuming and expensive.

Here, we propose a hybrid sequencing approach based on 454 pyrosequencing coupled with a clone-by-clone Sanger end-sequencing. This technique allows genetic information to be gathered from individual clones in a short time and with reduced sequencing costs. Instead of whole individual clone sequencing, we sequenced the clones in a pool and the medium-large insert (7–15 kb) cloning strategy allowed us to assemble these 358 sequenced clones correctly and assign them the correct Sanger reads of clone ends. Thus, the clone-end sequences maintain the link between the living clones and the annotated contigs from 454 assemblies, and so serve to locate the clone of interest in the clone library. The retrieved data facilitate planning consecutive biochemical assays for a given clone of interest. Moreover, the choice of the easy-handling plasmid vector enables an appropriate sub-cloning strategy to be designed for gene expression in suitable vectors/hosts. This article reports the characterization of the first metagenomic clone library from the fecal sample of a healthy human volunteer.

Materials and Methods

Isolation of Bacterial Cells from a Fecal Sample and DNA Extraction

The study was approved by the Ethics and Research Committee of the Centre for Public Health Research (CSISP) of Valencia, Spain. The volunteer involved in this study provided a written informed consent. One ml of fresh feces from the healthy volunteer was resuspended in 3 ml of salt solution (0.9% NaCl) by vortexing and then centrifuged at 2000 rpm for 2 min. The supernatant was transferred to a 15 ml tube. Microbial cells were purified as previously described [21]. Bacterial DNA was extracted by the Ausubel protocol (1992) including lysozyme, SDS and CTAB treatment, phenol-chloroform purification and isopropanol-ammonium acetate precipitation [21,22].

Preparation of the Clone Library

Seven µg of extracted bacterial DNA was digested with EcoRI enzyme (Roche, ref.: 10703737001) at 37°C for 2 hours and then resolved on 0.5% TAE agarose gel at 15 V for 16 hours. DNA fragments measuring between 7 and 15 Kb were cut out from the gel without exposure to UV light. DNA elution was performed in the Elutrap device (Whatman, ref.: 10447700) running at 150 V for 3 hours. Amicon 50 K columns (Millipore, ref.: UFC503024) were used for sample concentration and for the exchange of the electrophoresis buffer into water. Fragments shorter than 1.5 Kb were completely removed to allow ligation of longer ones by adding 100 µl of Agencourt Ampure Xp magnetic beads (Beckman Coulter, ref.: 082A63881) to the DNA sample, diluted in 200 µl 10 mM Tris-HCl. DNA was bound to the magnetic beads on a magnetic particle concentrator (Invitrogen, ref.: 123-21D) and purified by 70% ethanol. Size selected DNA was finally resuspended in 20 µl 10 mM Tris-HCl.

Two µl of sample DNA was ligated to EcoRI pBluescript (Agilent, ref.: 212250) with Takara DNA ligation kit (Takara, ref.: 6024) at 16°C overnight. The ligation reaction was transformed into One Shot TOP10 electrocompetent cells (Invitrogen) at 1800 Volts (Electroporator 2510, Eppendorf). Transformed cells were incubated in 1 ml of SOC medium at 37°C for 1.5 hours and then spread on LB agar plates containing ampicillin (100 µg/ml), XGAL (50 µg/ml), and IPTG (1 mM) and incubated at 37°C overnight.

Sequencing of Clones

White colonies were picked and placed separately in 1 ml of LB with 100 µg/ml ampicillin into 96 well plate and left to grow overnight at 37°C. Plasmid minipreps were performed using 100 µl of solution 1 (50 mM sucrose, 25 mM TrisHCl pH 8, 10 mM EDTA), 200 µl of solution 2 (0.2% NaOH, 1% SDS) and 150 µl of solution 3 (3 M potassium acetate, 2 M acetic acid, pH 4.8). Plasmid DNA was resuspended in 30 µl of water. Twenty ng of each of the 358 clones were pooled together.

The shotgun library was prepared from 1 µg of the pooled sample according to manufacturer instructions (Roche, Rapid Library Preparation Method Manual GS FLX+ Series XL+, May 2011). The sample was then sequenced on 1/8 of PicoTiterPlate by GS FLX+ system. Sequencing depth has been calculated in order to reach coverage of about 10×, distributed among the 358 clones.

Plasmid DNA obtained by miniprep from each clone (about 60 ng) was sequenced separately by the Sanger method on DNA ABI 3730 (Applied Biosystems) using M13 forward or M13 reverse primers.

Assembly and Annotation

In order to remove vector sequences (2961 bp), Smalt 0.5.8. tool (Wellcome Trust Sanger Institute, http://www.sanger.ac.uk/resources/software/smalt/) was used and plasmid sequences coordinates were employed in the following assembly step to avoid unnecessary vector assembly. Pyrosequencing reads were assembled by MIRA3 applying typical *de-novo* genome 454 assembly parameters [23].

Aiming to a correct mapping of clone ends, vector sequences present in Sanger reads were cut out. Sanger reads were then mapped on 454 assembly by Staden package v 4.11.2 and the resulting contigs were revised manually [24].

For protein annotation, contigs longer than 1000 bp were selected. ORFs (open reading frames) were identified by Glimmer 3 [25] and annotated by KAAS - KEGG Automatic Annotation Server, KEGG BRITE [26,27]. Annotated ORFs were further enriched by InterProScan Sequence Search [28,29]. The InterPro database makes use of different scanning tools and integrates predictive models or signatures from diverse source repositories: BlastProDom [30], Coil [31], FPrintScan [32], Gene3D [33], HAMAP [34], HMMPanther [35], HMMPfam [36], HMMPIR [37], HMMSmart [38], HMMTigr [39], PatternScan and ProfileScan [40], Seg [28,29], SignalPHMM [41], Superfamily [42], TMHMM [43]. InterPro combines individual strengths of these different annotation sources and provides comprehensive information about protein families, domains and functional sites. Protein names resulting from InterProScan Sequence Search were submitted to the Brenda database to obtain a general overview of possible protein application [44].

A figure with the flow chart of the proposed approach is shown in Figure S1.

Accession Numbers

Sequences were deposited in EMBL-EBI Sequence Read Archive (SRA) with study number ERP001596 (http://www.ebi.ac.uk/ena/data/view/ERP001596).

Results and Discussion

Sequencing Results and Assembly

In total, 57,469 out of 87,898 reads were assembled into 473 contigs, with an average coverage of 14.67X, while N50 contig size was 8,241. The largest contig measured 23,504 bp. Twelve clones containing only the vector (false positives with no insert) were excluded from the analysis.

The hybrid assembly revealed that 57 contigs correctly matched more than one Sanger sequence, showing a probable partial digestion or that inserts can proceed from different original microbial genetic rearrangement. Only six Sanger sequences could not be mapped to 454 contigs.

The assembly results show that on using the strategy of cloning the medium-large inserts (7–15 kb) into plasmids, there is no need for additional paired-end 454 sequencing; moreover, the coverage for correct assembling was sufficient. The sequence length of the pBluescript plasmid (2961 bp) is lower than the length of commercially available fosmid of BAC vectors (8–17 kb), which reduces the number of reads containing vector sequences.

General Overview on Annotated ORFs

Out of 473 contigs, 316 were larger than 1000 bp and used for the analysis. Glimmer3 identified 1790 ORFs. The average length of ORFs was 249 amino acids, while the shortest and the longest ones were 38 and 2381 amino acids, respectively. HMMPfam annotated 742 different proteins in our assembly and Seg scanning application identified 1,859 matches (see Table 1). The complete table of ORF annotation by all annotation tools of InterProScan Sequence Search is shown in Table S1.

Figure 1 shows the distribution of KEGG annotation by protein families. The annotated enzymes corresponded to 121 different KEGG metabolic pathways. It is noteworthy that we found almost complete metabolic pathways of valine, leucine and isoleucine biosynthesis (see Figure S2).

Annotated ORFs with Reported Industrial Applications

The clone library derived from the fecal sample of a healthy volunteer provided genetic information of several clones containing enzymes with previously known applications. Figure 2 shows a description of some clones of interest and a summary is given in Table 2.

Clone 2H2 (Figure 2, panel a) contained arginine deiminase (ADI). This enzyme has also been found in bacteria, archaea (*Pseudomonas*, *Mycoplasma*, *Halobacterium*, *Lactobacillus*, *Lactococcus* [45]) and some eukaryotes, but not in mammalian cells which synthesize arginine from citrulline. Arginine auxotrophic cancer cells lack active citrulline to arginine recycling pathway and, therefore, an arginine-degrading enzyme may eradicate them effectively [46]. ADI has been tested successfully as an anti-tumoral drug for the treatment of arginine-auxotrophic tumors, hepatocellular carcinoma and melanoma [47]. ADI also improves liver function in patients with chronic hepatitis C virus (HCV) infection and selectively inhibits HCV replication *in vitro* [48]. Moreover, ADI could also be employed in the treatment of nitric oxide synthase-related neuronal diseases, which was demonstrated in a co-culture of neurons and microglia [49].

Clone 2C1 (Figure 2, panel b) contained a gene annotated as uridine kinase (uridine-cytidine kinase, HMMPanther annotation) or as uracil phosphoribosyltransferase (HMMPfam and KAAS KEGG annotations). A proposed gene therapy is based on the strategy that a non-mammalian gene encoding a certain enzyme is transduced in tumor cells and its expression catalyses the activation of a pro-drug to a cytotoxin that induces tumor cell death [50]. A cytosine deaminase-uracil phosphoribosyltransferase fusion gene has been used in clinical gene therapy trials to improve strong chemotherapeutic agents, in which 5-fluorouracil is catalyzed by cellular enzymes to fluoronucleotides, subsequently inhibiting DNA or RNA synthesis [51–53]. Uridine kinase and uracil phosphoribosyltransferase are enzymes catalyzing the formation of uridine 5′-monophosphate from uridine and adenine

Table 1. InterProScan annotation overview.

Annotation tool	Total number of matches	Total number of unique protein names
BlastProDom	26	18
Coil	190	1
FPrintScan	732	107
Gene3D	1312	226
HAMAP	112	95
HMMPanther	1017	165
HMMPfam	1526	742
HMMPIR	93	74
HMMSmart	318	109
HMMTigr	341	257
PatternScan	257	140
ProfileScan	384	129
Seg	1859	1
SignalPHMM	394	1
superfamily	1188	226
TMHMM	1535	1

Total number of matches and total number of unique protein names assigned by different annotation tools provided by InterProScan. This table summarizes Table S1, which contains the whole list of protein matches in our assembly. The number of matches is higher than the number of unique protein names because one type of protein could be found in several contigs or one ORF could contain several matches to the same protein.

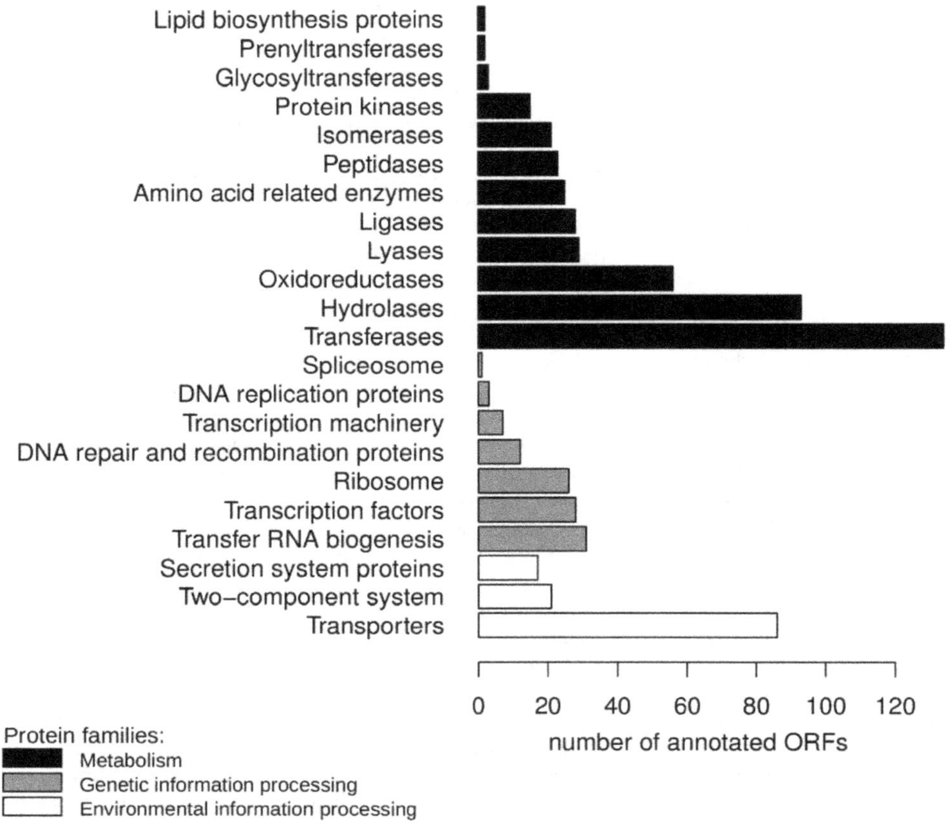

Figure 1. KEGG categories distribution. Distribution of KEGG categories identified among ORFs.

5′-triphosphate and from uracil and phosphoribosyl-α-l-pyrophosphate in the pyrimidine salvage pathway, respectively [54]. Uracil phosphoribosyltransferase was also successfully applied in the treatment of hepatitis C virus (HCV) infection where ribavirin (1-b-D-ribofuranosyl-1, 2, 4-triazole), a synthetic nucleoside analog, is currently used in combination with interferon-α or peginterferon-α [55]. In HCV infection, because the vast majority of replication occurs in hepatocytes, selective delivery of ribavirin into those liver cells would be desirable to enhance antiviral activity and also avoid systemic side effects. In 2008, VirovicJukic showed that human uridine-kytidine kinase-1 recognizes ribavirin and phosphorylates it [56]. Introducing a phosphate group in ribavirin facilitates the preparation of a novel protein conjugate of ribavirin, which has the potential for targeted delivery to specific cell types.

Another enzyme of interest is choloylglycine hydrolase (bile salt hydrolase) found in contig 2B3 (Figure 2, panel c). Choloylglycine hydrolase is present in many bacterial species inhabiting the human gut, and has been found to have cholesterol lowering effects [57].

We found alginate lyase in contig HK3UA (Figure 2, Panel d). Alkawash (2006) demonstrated in an *in vitro* biofilm system that co-administration of antibiotics with alginate lyase from *Bacillus circulans* might benefit cystic fibrosis patients by increasing the efficacy of antibiotic in the respiratory tract [58]. Once mucoid (alginate-producing) strains of *Pseudomonas aeruginosa* have become established in the patient's respiratory tracts, they can rarely be eliminated by antibiotic treatment alone. Alginate lyase was also found to have application in plant culture techniques *in vitro*. It has been applied successfully for the extraction of protoplasts for food research and regeneration of a variety of algal species, including brown algae, and serves as an alternative for various mechanical and chemical methods [59].

Clones Related to Potential Applications Treating Human Enzyme Deficiencies

Several studies indicate an association between common neurodevelopmental disorders and gut microbiota. The microbial colonization process triggers signaling mechanisms that can influence central nervous system development and might be linked to autism [60,61]. In the clone library, we found enzymes with a homolog in humans, whose deficiency has been described to lead to neurological diseases. These clones should be investigated in greater depth to explain the interactions between gut microbiota and the human central nervous system.

It is known that bacteria can mediate gene transfer, which has led to the utilization of various bacterial strains in gene therapy [62–65]. Several publications demonstrate the considerable potential of using genetically modified lactic acid bacteria to deliver therapeutic peptides and proteins to the mucosa [66]. Greater knowledge of the interactions between humans and their gut bacteria may open up new hypothetical therapeutic approaches based on gene therapy for neurological diseases. For example, we found an ORF in contig 7H8 (Figure 2, panel e) annotated as spermine synthase (HMMPfam) or spermidine synthase (KAAS KEGG). Spermidine synthase converts putrescine into spermidine, and spermine synthase converts spermidine into spermine [67]. Spermine deficiency in human causes

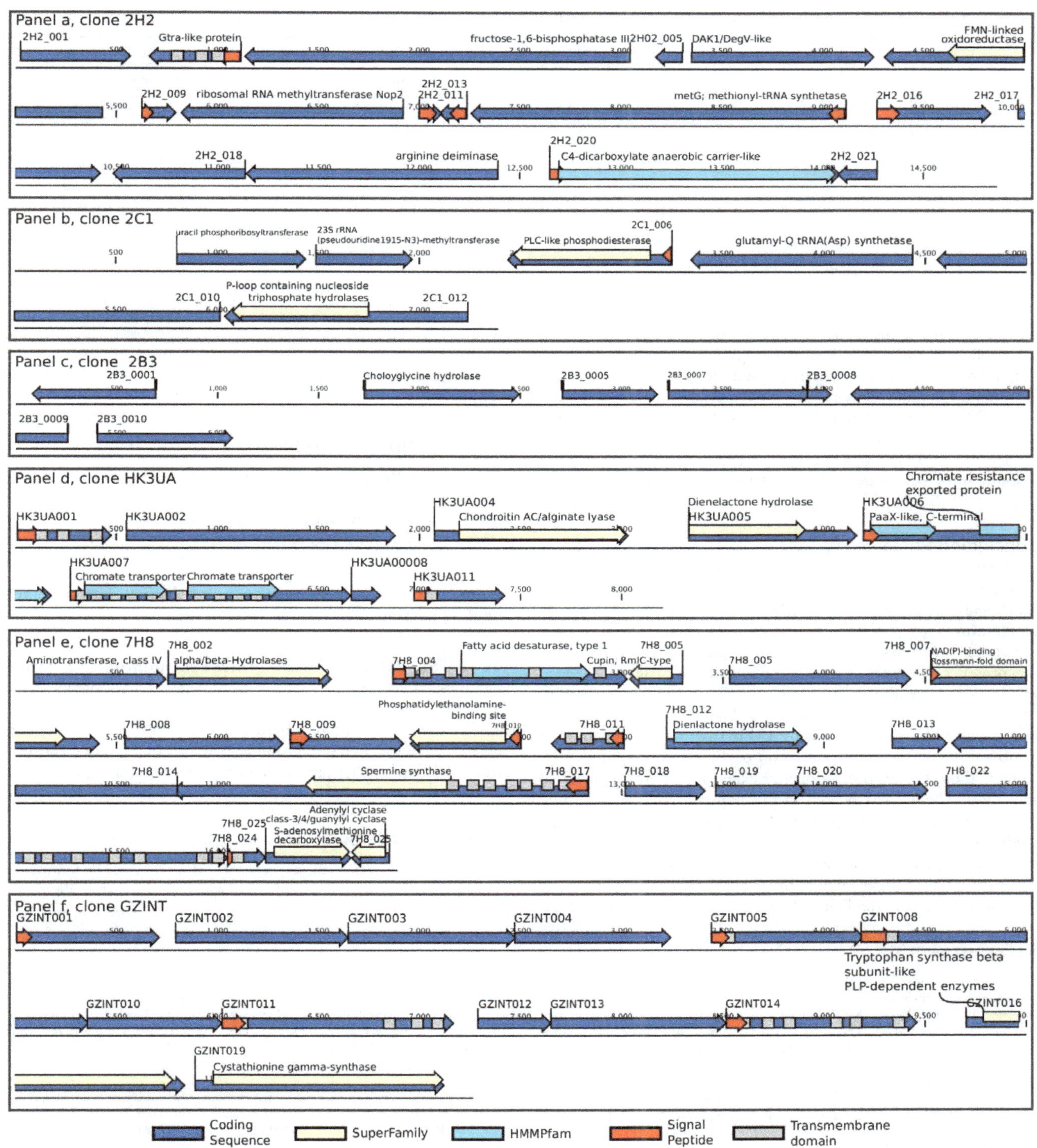

Figure 2. Annotated ORFs with reported industrial applications. Figure describes ORFs annotation of selected clones of interest. Annotation colors describe the kind of annotation (see legend). Every panel describes a different clone (see results section text for detailed descriptions).

the Snyder-Robinson syndrome, an X-linked mental retardation disorder [68]. Wang (2004) suggested that attempts to increase spermine by dietary manipulation, drug treatment or gene therapy may be successful in preventing the Snyder-Robinson syndrome [69].

Cystathionine β-synthase (CBS) is a vitamin B6-dependent trans-sulfuration enzyme needed to synthesize cysteine from methionine. A CBS deficiency causes homocystinuria, a rare autosomal recessive disease, characterized by mental retardation, psychiatric disturbances, skeletal abnormalities, and vascular

Table 2. ORFs with potential industrial or medical applications.

Protein name	Contig ID	ORF number	Contig length
Arginine deiminase	2H2	19	14.867 bp
Uracil phosphoribosyl transferase/Uridine kinase	2C1	1	7.390 bp
Choloylglycine hydrolase	2B3	4	6.393 bp
Alginate lyase	HK3UA	4	8.204 bp
Spermine synthase	7H8	17	16.889 bp
Cystathionine synthase	GZINT	16 and 19	12.265 bp

Columns describe ORF annotations, contig identifiers and ORFs identifier.

disorders [70]. Only around half of the patients with CBS deficiency respond to pyridoxine therapy [71]; thus, gene therapy might be an alternative for those that do not respond to this treatment. Oh and collaborators (2004) used three kinds of human CBS cDNA to construct vectors for gene therapy, demonstrating positive effects on homocystinuria affected mice [72]. In our clone library, the ORF 16 of contig GZINT was annotated as cystathionine β-synthase and ORF 19 as cystathionine γ-synthase (Figure 2, panel f).

Concluding Remarks

Metagenomics of the human microbiome can provide genetic information about the DNA of bacteria inhabiting human-related ecological niches, adapted to physiological conditions such as temperature, pH, redox potential, etc. The assembly and annotation of clones produced from a library of this kind reveal the presence of several proteins for which industrial or medical applications have already been reported. They can also be used to study proteins of unknown function. The screening of a clone library with inserts of 7–15 Kb by 454 pyrosequencing enabled us to obtain the annotation information of the genes present in each clone without the need of prior and expensive *ad hoc* biochemical screening. The approach used in this paper started by analyzing 358 clones and ended up with 316 assembled and annotated contigs. The proposed method is perfectly scalable enabling work to tackle larger clone libraries, proportionally increasing sequencing efforts. This strategy enables the link to be maintained between the information and the living clones, providing annotation of the whole library; thus, particular clones of interest can undergo further testing by the most appropriate biochemical assay and/or sub-cloning for appropriate selection of vectors and/or host, if required.

Supporting Information

Figure S1 Protocol flow chart. The figure summarizes the protocols applied to construct the clone library, pyrosequencing of pooled clones, individual clone Sanger end sequencing, contigs/clone-ends matching and annotations.

Figure S2 Valine biosynthesis pathway. Green frames indicate enzymes found in the library.

Table S1 Whole library InterPro annotation table. Columns describe: ORF name bounded to the original clone name in the library; amino acid length; InterPro inquired database; database match; match description; ORF match start position; ORF match end position; match p-value; date of search; InterPro match code; protein name; protein description.

Author Contributions

Conceived and designed the experiments: MD GD AM. Performed the experiments: MD DPV. Analyzed the data: MD GD. Wrote the paper: MD GD AM.

References

1. Simon C, Daniel R (2011) Metagenomic analyses: past and future trends. Applied and environmental microbiology 77: 1153–1161.
2. Stein JL, Marsh TL, Wu KY, Shizuya H, DeLong EF (1996) Characterization of uncultivated prokaryotes: isolation and analysis of a 40-kilobase-pair genome fragment from a planktonic marine archaeon. Journal of bacteriology 178: 591–599.
3. Harvey a (2000) Strategies for discovering drugs from previously unexplored natural products. Drug discovery today 5: 294–300.
4. Daniel R (2005) The metagenomics of soil. Nature reviews Microbiology 3: 470–478.
5. DeLong EF (2005) Microbial community genomics in the ocean. Nature reviews Microbiology 3: 459–469.
6. Rhee J-K, Ahn D-G, Kim Y-G, Oh J-W (2005) New Thermophilic and Thermostable Esterase with Sequence Similarity to the Hormone-Sensitive Lipase Family, Cloned from a Metagenomic Library. Applied and Environmental Microbiology 71: 817–825.
7. Cieśliński H, Białkowskaa A, Tkaczuk K, Długołecka A, Kur J, et al. (2009) Identification and molecular modeling of a novel lipase from an Antarctic soil metagenomic library. Polish journal of microbiology/Polskie Towarzystwo Mikrobiologów = The Polish Society of Microbiologists 58: 199–204.
8. Elend C, Schmeisser C, Leggewie C, Babiak P, Carballeira JD, et al. (2006) Isolation and biochemical characterization of two novel metagenome-derived esterases. Applied and environmental microbiology 72: 3637–3645.
9. Heath C, Hu XP, Cary SC, Cowan D (2009) Identification of a novel alkaliphilic esterase active at low temperatures by screening a metagenomic library from antarctic desert soil. Applied and environmental microbiology 75: 4657–4659.
10. Henne A, Schmitz RA, Bömeke M, Gottschalk G, Daniel R (2000) Screening of environmental DNA libraries for the presence of genes conferring lipolytic activity on Escherichia coli. Applied and environmental microbiology 66: 3113–3116.
11. Duan C-J, Xian L, Zhao G-C, Feng Y, Pang H, et al. (2009) Isolation and partial characterization of novel genes encoding acidic cellulases from metagenomes of buffalo rumens. Journal of applied microbiology 107: 245–256.
12. Healy FG, Ray RM, Aldrich HC, Wilkie AC, Ingram LO, et al. (1995) Direct isolation of functional genes encoding cellulases from the microbial consortia in a thermophilic, anaerobic digester maintained on lignocellulose. Applied microbiology and biotechnology 43: 667–674.
13. Hjort K, Bergström M, Adesina MF, Jansson JK, Smalla K, et al. (2010) Chitinase genes revealed and compared in bacterial isolates, DNA extracts and a metagenomic library from a phytopathogen-suppressive soil. FEMS microbiology ecology 71: 197–207.
14. Simon C, Herath J, Rockstroh S, Daniel R (2009) Rapid identification of genes encoding DNA polymerases by function-based screening of metagenomic libraries derived from glacial ice. Applied and environmental microbiology 75: 2964–2968.
15. Waschkowitz T, Rockstroh S, Daniel R (2009) Isolation and characterization of metalloproteases with a novel domain structure by construction and screening of

metagenomic libraries. Applied and environmental microbiology 75: 2506–2516.
16. Riesenfeld CS, Goodman RM, Handelsman J (2004) Uncultured soil bacteria are a reservoir of new antibiotic resistance genes. Environmental microbiology 6: 981–989.
17. Brady SF, Simmons L, Kim JH, Schmidt EW (2009) Metagenomic approaches to natural products from free-living and symbiotic organisms. Natural product reports 26: 1488–1503.
18. Strohl W (2000) The role of natural products in a modern drug discovery program. Drug discovery today 5: 39–41.
19. Simon C, Daniel R (2009) Achievements and new knowledge unraveled by metagenomic approaches. Applied microbiology and biotechnology 85: 265–276.
20. Yun J, Ryu S (2005) Screening for novel enzymes from metagenome and SIGEX, as a way to improve it. Microbial cell factories 4: 8.
21. Peris-Bondia F, Latorre A, Artacho A, Moya A, D'Auria G (2011) The active human gut microbiota differs from the total microbiota. PloS one 6: e22448.
22. Ausubel FM, Brent R, Kinston R, Moore D, Seidman JG, et al. (1992) Current protocol in molecular biology. Current protocols in molecular biology: 211–245.
23. Chevreux B, Wetter T, Suhai S (1999) Genome Sequence Assembly Using Trace Signals and Additional Sequence Information. Hannover, Germany. 45–56.
24. Staden R, Beal KF, Bonfield JK (2000) The Staden package, 1998. Methods in molecular biology (Clifton, NJ) 132: 115–130.
25. Delcher AL, Harmon D, Kasif S, White O, Salzberg SL (1999) Improved microbial gene identification with GLIMMER. Nucleic acids research 27: 4636–4641.
26. Kanehisa M, Goto S, Sato Y, Furumichi M, Tanabe M (2011) KEGG for integration and interpretation of large-scale molecular data sets. Nucleic Acids Research 40: D109–D114.
27. Moriya Y, Itoh M, Okuda S, Yoshizawa AC, Kanehisa M (2007) KAAS: an automatic genome annotation and pathway reconstruction server. Nucleic acids research 35: W182–185.
28. Quevillon E, Silventoinen V, Pillai S, Harte N, Mulder N, et al. (2005) InterProScan: protein domains identifier. Nucleic Acids Res 33: W116–120.
29. Hunter S, Jones P, Mitchell A, Apweiler R, Attwood T, et al. (2012) InterPro in 2011: new developments in the family and domain prediction database. Nucleic Acids Research 40: D306–D312.
30. Corpet F (2000) ProDom and ProDom-CG: tools for protein domain analysis and whole genome comparisons. Nucleic Acids Research 28: 267–269.
31. Lupas A, Van Dyke M, Stock J (1991) Predicting coiled coils from protein sequences. Science 252: 1162–1164.
32. Scordis P, Flower DR, Attwood TK (1999) FingerPRINTScan: intelligent searching of the PRINTS motif database. Bioinformatics 15: 799–806.
33. Pearl F, Todd A, Sillitoe I, Dibley M, Redfern O, et al. (2005) The CATH Domain Structure Database and related resources Gene3D and DHS provide comprehensive domain family information for genome analysis. Nucleic acids research 33: D247–251.
34. Lima T, Auchincloss AH, Coudert E, Keller G, Michoud K, et al. (2009) HAMAP: a database of completely sequenced microbial proteome sets and manually curated microbial protein families in UniProtKB/Swiss-Prot. Nucleic acids research 37: D471–478.
35. Mi H, Lazareva-Ulitsky B, Loo R, Kejariwal A, Vandergriff J, et al. (2005) The PANTHER database of protein families, subfamilies, functions and pathways. Nucleic acids research 33: D284–288.
36. Bateman A, Birney E, Durbin R, Eddy SR, Howe KL, et al. (2000) The Pfam protein families database. Nucleic acids research 28: 263–266.
37. Wu CH, Yeh L-SL, Huang H, Arminski L, Castro-Alvear J, et al. (2003) The Protein Information Resource. Nucleic acids research 31: 345–347.
38. Letunic I, Doerks T, Bork P (2012) SMART 7: recent updates to the protein domain annotation resource. Nucleic acids research 40: D302–305.
39. Haft DH, Selengut JD, White O (2003) The TIGRFAMs database of protein families. Nucleic acids research 31: 371–373.
40. Hulo N, Bairoch A, Bulliard V, Cerutti L, De Castro E, et al. (2006) The PROSITE database. Nucleic acids research 34: D227–230.
41. Nielsen H, Engelbrecht J, Brunak S, von Heijne G (1997) Identification of prokaryotic and eukaryotic signal peptides and prediction of their cleavage sites. Protein engineering 10: 1–6.
42. Gough J, Karplus K, Hughey R, Chothia C (2001) Assignment of homology to genome sequences using a library of hidden Markov models that represent all proteins of known structure. Journal of molecular biology 313: 903–919.
43. Krogh A, Larsson B, von Heijne G, Sonnhammer EL (2001) Predicting transmembrane protein topology with a hidden Markov model: application to complete genomes. Journal of molecular biology 305: 567–580.
44. Scheer M, Grote A, Chang A, Schomburg I, Munaretto C, et al. (2011) BRENDA, the enzyme information system in 2011. Nucleic acids research 39: D670–676.
45. Ni Y, Schwaneberg U, Sun Z-H (2008) Arginine deiminase, a potential anti-tumor drug. Cancer letters 261: 1–11.
46. Takaku H, Matsumoto M, Misawa S, Miyazaki K (1995) Anti-tumor activity of arginine deiminase from Mycoplasma argini and its growth-inhibitory mechanism. Japanese journal of cancer research Gann 86: 840–846.
47. Ensor CM, Holtsberg FW, Bomalaski JS, Clark MA (2002) Pegylated arginine deiminase (ADI-SS PEG20,000 mw) inhibits human melanomas and hepatocellular carcinomas in vitro and in vivo. Cancer research 62: 5443–5450.
48. Izzo F, Montella M, Orlando AP, Nasti G, Beneduce G, et al. (2007) Pegylated arginine deiminase lowers hepatitis C viral titers and inhibits nitric oxide synthesis. Journal of Gastroenterology and Hepatology 22: 86–91.
49. Yu H-H, Wu F-LL, Lin S-E, Shen L-J (2008) Recombinant arginine deiminase reduces inducible nitric oxide synthase iNOS-mediated neurotoxicity in a coculture of neurons and microglia. Journal of Neuroscience Research 86: 2963–2972.
50. Greco O, Dachs GU (2001) Gene directed enzyme/prodrug therapy of cancer: historical appraisal and future prospectives. Journal of Cellular Physiology 187: 22–36.
51. Crystal RG, Hirschowitz E, Lieberman M, Daly J, Kazam E, et al. (1997) Phase I study of direct administration of a replication deficient adenovirus vector containing the E. coli cytosine deaminase gene to metastatic colon carcinoma of the liver in association with the oral administration of the pro-drug 5-fluorocytosine. Human gene therapy 8: 985–1001.
52. Daher GC, Harris BE, Diasio RB (1990) Metabolism of pyrimidine analogues and their nucleosides. Pharmacology therapeutics 48: 189–222.
53. Pandha HS, Martin LA, Rigg A, Hurst HC, Stamp GW, et al. (1999) Genetic prodrug activation therapy for breast cancer: A phase I clinical trial of erbB-2-directed suicide gene expression. Journal of clinical oncology : official journal of the American Society of Clinical Oncology 17: 2180–2189.
54. Islam MR, Kim H, Kang S-W, Kim J-S, Jeong Y-M, et al. (2007) Functional characterization of a gene encoding a dual domain for uridine kinase and uracil phosphoribosyltransferase in Arabidopsis thaliana. Plant molecular biology 63: 465–477.
55. McHutchison JG, Gordon SC, Schiff ER, Shiffman ML, Lee WM, et al. (1998) Interferon Alfa-2b Alone or in Combination with Ribavirin as Initial Treatment for Chronic Hepatitis C. New England Journal of Medicine 339: 1485–1492.
56. Virovic Jukic L, Duvnjak M, Wu CH, Wu GY (2008) Human uridine-cytidine kinase phosphorylation of ribavirin: a convenient method for activation of ribavirin for conjugation to proteins. Journal of biomedical science 15: 205–213.
57. Pereira DIA, Gibson GR (2002) Effects of consumption of probiotics and prebiotics on serum lipid levels in humans. Critical Reviews in Biochemistry and Molecular Biology 37: 259–281.
58. Alkawash MA, Soothill JS, Schiller NL (2006) Alginate lyase enhances antibiotic killing of mucoid Pseudomonas aeruginosa in biofilms. APMIS acta pathologica microbiologica et immunologica Scandinavica 114: 131–138.
59. Wong TY, Preston LA, Schiller NL (2000) ALGINATE LYASE: review of major sources and enzyme characteristics, structure-function analysis, biological roles, and applications. Annual Review of Microbiology 54: 289–340.
60. Finegold SM, Dowd SE, Gontcharova V, Liu C, Henley KE, et al. (2010) Pyrosequencing study of fecal microflora of autistic and control children. Anaerobe 16: 444–453.
61. Heijtz RD, Wang S, Anuar F, Qian Y, Björkholm B, et al. (2011) Normal gut microbiota modulates brain development and behavior. Proceedings of the National Academy of Sciences of the United States of America 108: 3047–3052.
62. Niethammer AG, Xiang R, Becker JC, Wodrich H, Pertl U, et al. (2002) A DNA vaccine against VEGF receptor 2 prevents effective angiogenesis and inhibits tumor growth. Nature medicine 8: 1369–1375.
63. Sizemore DR, Branstrom AA, Sadoff JC (1995) Attenuated Shigella as a DNA delivery vehicle for DNA-mediated immunization. Science 270: 299–302.
64. Steidler L, Hans W, Schotte L, Neirynck S, Obermeier F, et al. (2000) Treatment of murine colitis by Lactococcus lactis secreting interleukin-10. Science 289: 1352–1355.
65. Vassaux G, Nitcheu J, Jezzard S, Lemoine NR (2006) Bacterial gene therapy strategies. The Journal of pathology 208: 290–298.
66. Wells J (2011) Mucosal vaccination and therapy with genetically modified lactic acid bacteria. Annual review of food science and technology 2: 423–445.
67. Coffino P (2001) Regulation of cellular polyamines by antizyme. Nature Reviews Molecular Cell Biology 2: 188–194.
68. Cason AL, Ikeguchi Y, Skinner C, Wood TC, Holden KR, et al. (2003) X-linked spermine synthase gene (SMS) defect: the first polyamine deficiency syndrome. European journal of human genetics EJHG 11: 937–944.
69. Wang X, Ikeguchi Y, McCloskey DE, Nelson P, Pegg AE (2004) Spermine synthesis is required for normal viability, growth, and fertility in the mouse. The Journal of Biological Chemistry 279: 51370–51375.
70. Mudd SH, Finkelstein JD, Irreverre F, Laster L (1964) HOMOCYSTINURIA: AN ENZYMATIC DEFECT. Science 143: 1443–1445.
71. Mudd SH, Edwards WA, Loeb PM, Brown MS, Laster L (1970) Homocystinuria due to cystathionine synthase deficiency: the effect of pyridoxine. Journal of Clinical Investigation 49: 1762–1773.
72. Oh H-J, Park E-S, Kruger W, Jung S-C, Lee J-S (2004) 181. Human CBS (Cystathionine β-Synthase) Gene Transfer Mediated by Recombinant Adeno-Associated Virus Vector. Molecular Therapy 9: S69–S70.

23

Novel Therapeutic Approaches for Various Cancer Types using a Modified Sleeping Beauty-based Gene Delivery System

In-Sun Hong[1,2]⁹, Hwa-Yong Lee[1,2]⁹, Hyun-Pyo Kim[3]*

1 Adult Stem cell Research Center, Seoul National University, Seoul, Republic of Korea, **2** Department of Veterinary Public Health, Laboratory of Stem Cell and Tumor Biology, Seoul National University, Seoul, Republic of Korea, **3** Department of Biomedical Science, Jungwon University, Chungbuk, Korea

Abstract

Successful gene therapy largely depends on the selective introduction of therapeutic genes into the appropriate target cancer cells. One of the most effective and promising approaches for targeting tumor tissue during gene delivery is the use of viral vectors, which allow for high efficiency gene delivery. However, the use of viral vectors is not without risks and safety concerns, such as toxicities, a host immune response towards the viral antigens or potential viral recombination into the host's chromosome; these risks limit the clinical application of viral vectors. The Sleeping Beauty (SB) transposon-based system is an attractive, non-viral alternative to viral delivery systems. SB may be less immunogenic than the viral vector system due to its lack of viral sequences. The SB-based gene delivery system can stably integrate into the host cell genome to produce the therapeutic gene product over the lifetime of a cell. However, when compared to viral vectors, the non-viral SB-based gene delivery system still has limited therapeutic efficacy due to the lack of long-lasting gene expression potential and tumor cell specific gene transfer ability. These limitations could be overcome by modifying the SB system through the introduction of the hTERT promoter and the SV40 enhancer. In this study, a modified SB delivery system, under control of the hTERT promoter in conjunction with the SV40 enhancer, was able to successfully transfer the suicide gene (HSV-TK) into multiple types of cancer cells. The modified SB transfected cancer cells exhibited a significantly increased cancer cell specific death rate. These data suggest that our modified SB-based gene delivery system can be used as a safe and efficient tool for cancer cell specific therapeutic gene transfer and stable long-term expression.

Editor: Eduard Ayuso, University of Nantes, France

Funding: This study was supported by a grant (Project Code No.,Z-1541745-2012-13-09) from Animal and Plant Quarantine Agency, Ministry of Agriculture, Food and Rural Affairs. The funders had no role in study design, data collection and analysis, decision to publish, or preparation of the manuscript.

Competing Interests: The authors have declared that no competing interests exist.

* E-mail: khpsss@jwu.ac.kr

⁹ These authors contributed equally to this work.

Introduction

Gene-directed enzyme prodrug therapy (GDEPT) is one of the promising alternatives to conventional chemotherapy; GDEPT minimizes systemic toxicities through the introduction of catalytic enzymes that convert low- or non-toxic prodrugs into toxic metabolites in tumor cells [1]. This therapeutic system comprises of inactive low- or non-toxic prodrugs and a gene encoding an enzyme [2]. After genetically modifying the tumor cells to express such enzymes and the systemic administration of the prodrug, the prodrug is locally converted by the enzyme into toxic metabolites, leading to the selective killing of the tumor cells. Because the toxic metabolite is only produced and released in the local tumor site where the gene is delivered, resulting in a greatly reduced circulating concentration of the free toxic drug, this therapeutic system is called local chemotherapy. There are several genes encoding prodrug-activating enzymes. Among them, the most common gene is Herpes Simplex Virus-1 Thymidine Kinase (HSV-TK), a well characterized suicide gene that can be isolated from the Herpes simplex virus or *E. coli* [3,4]. HSV-TK converts the systemically administered prodrug gancyclovir (GCV) into a toxic metabolite that kills cancer cells [5]. This combination method has been successfully applied to many clinical areas, such as gene therapy for cancer treatment [6] and graft-versus-host disease (GVHD) [7].

Successful GDEPT largely depends on the selective introduction of the suicide gene into the appropriate target cancer cells. One of the most effective and promising approaches for gene delivery into the target tumor tissue is the use of viral vectors, which allow for high efficiency gene transfer [8,9]. However, these vectors currently have risks and safety concerns, such as toxicities, host immune responses towards the viral antigens or potential viral recombination into the host's chromosomes, which limit their clinical application [10]. Another problem with the use of viral vectors for gene therapy is that viral vector preparation is laborious and expensive [11,12] Therefore, a better alternative may be to develop a gene delivery method that would direct therapeutic agents to appropriate sites and constitutively express therapeutic genes within or near the tumor site without these limitations.

The transposon-based system is an attractive, non-viral alternative to the viral delivery systems. Transposons are discrete segments of DNA that have the inherent ability to move from site to site and can replicate themselves within the genome using the host cell's organelles and other machinery. However, when compared to viral vectors, transposons are not infectious, and their activities are therefore confined to intracellular compartments with specific functions. In invertebrates, several different types of endogenous transposons have been extensively used, such as the Tc1 mariner-like element in *Caenorhabditis elegans* and the P element in *Drosophila* [13,14]. Unfortunately, no such active and endogenous transposons are available in vertebrates due to the accumulated mutations within the transposon sequence [15]. One approach to overcome this problem in vertebrates was the molecular reconstruction of a genetically active vertebrate Tc1/ mariner-type transposable element called Sleeping Beauty (SB) from the ancient "dead" transposon fossils found in fish genomes [16]. SB shows efficient transpositional activity in mouse embryonic stem (ES) cells [17], mouse somatic tissue [18], and mouse germ line [19]. In addition, SB has shown tremendous success as an efficient gene delivery vehicle in mouse models of human disease [20–23]. In previous studies, song et al. found that SB transposon mediate suicide gene expression in hepatocellular carcinoma causing apoptosis [24] and telomerase gene transfer to protect against chemicals (t-BH, CCl4, or d-GalN)- induced acute cellular injury [25].

However, when compared to viral vectors, the non-viral SB based gene delivery system still has limited therapeutic efficacy due to the lack of long-lasting gene expression and cancer cell specific gene transfer ability. The hTERT gene is frequently reactivated in approximately 90% of immortalized human cells and cancer cells of various origins [26–28]. hTERT promoter has been extensively used in targeted cancer gene therapy [29–31]. Additionally, the SV40 enhancer has been extensively used to improve the activity of promoters to promote long-lasting gene expression [32]. Thus, to increase the promoter strength while maintaining tissue specificity, we used a recombinant SV40 enhancer containing a tumor-specific hTERT promoter [33]. While song et al. have reported an association between modified SB and suppression of tumor growth [24], their study have been confined to those of single hepatocellular carcinoma cell line (Hep3B) in which univeral antitumor effects in various cancer cell types are lacking. Similarly, although tumor suppressive effects of modified SB have been suggested, these effects are confirmed by a single in vitro assay (ATP cell viability assay) in which a more comprehensive profile of the antitumor effects of modified SB is still lacking [24]. Therefore, in the present study, the modified SB-based gene delivery system was used to transfer the suicide gene (HSV-TK) into multiple types of cancer cells, including H358 (lung cancer), H1299 (lung cancer), PC3 (prostate cancer), DU145 (prostate cancer), and OVCAR3 (ovarian cancer) cells with various experimental approaches including TUNEL assay, cell viability assay, FACS analysis, and in vivo experiment. These data suggest that modified SB-based gene delivery system can be used as a safe and efficient tool for cancer cell specific therapeutic gene transfer and stable long-term expression.

Materials and Methods

Cell culture

Human normal fibroblast, WI-38 and IMR-90 cells were maintained in DMEM (GIBCO BRL, Germany) supplemented with 10% fatal calf serum (FCS) (HyClone, Logan, USA), penicillin (50 units/ml), and streptomycin (50 ug/ml) in the presence of 5% CO_2. H358 (lung cancer), H1299 (lung cancer), PC3 (prostate cancer), DU145 (prostate cancer), and OVCAR3 (ovarian cancer) were grown in RPMI1640 supplemented with 10% FCS, penicillin (50 units/ml), and streptomycin (50 ug/ml) in 5% CO2. All cell lines were obtained from Korea Cell Line Bank (Seoul, Korea).

Animal experiments

Lung cancer cells (H358), prostate cancer cell line (DU-145), and ovarian cancer cells (OVCAR3) were harvested by trypsinization, and 1×10^5 viable cells (as determined by trypan blue exclusion) in a total volume of 200 µl were injected subcutaneously into 6- to 10-week-old, NOD/SCID mice. Two days following tumor seeding, animals were intravenously injected via tail veins with 100 mg/kg gancyclovir (GCV) along with either 25 µg of empty plasmid (pT. hTp. Con) or modified SB system (pT.hTp.HSV-tk.Con). Mice were sacrificed 28 days after tumor injection, and the effect of modified SB system on tumor growth was evaluated by measuring tumor size. To minimize suffering, all surgical procedure was performed under sodium pentobarbital anesthesia. Animal experiments were approved by the ethics committee for Animal Experiments of Jungwon University (Permit Number: 2013-0610).

RT-PCR analysis

Total RNA was isolated from each cells using the Absolutely RNA Microprep kit (Stratagene, La Jolla, USA) according to the manufacturer's protocol and treated with DNase I to prevent genomic DNA contamination. cDNA synthesis was performed with 1 ug of RNA using the SuperScript III reverse transcriptase (Invitrogen, Calsbad, USA) with Oligo(dT) primer (Promega, Madison, USA) to a final volume of 20 ul. 1 ul aliquots of cDNA were used to amplify the cDNA in 20 ul of total reaction. PCR conditions for amplification were: 94°C for 5 min; 30 cycles at 94°C for 1 min, at 55°C for 1 min, and at 72°C for 90 sec; and finally, 72°C for 10 min). hTR cDNA was amplified with hTR specific primer set (5′-tttgtctaaccctaactgagaagg-3′ as forward and 5′-tgtgagccgagtcctgggtgcacg-3′ as reverse). hTERT cDNA was amplified with forward primer (5′-cggaagagtctggagcaa-3′) and reverse primer (5′-ggatgaagcggagtctgga-3′). Differences in expression from each sample were normalized to the GAPDH (forward 5′-aacgagcggttccgatgccctgag-3′; reverse 5′-tgtcgccttcaccgttccagt t-3′). The PCR products were separated by 2% agarose gel electrophoresis containing 0.5 µg/ml of ethidium bromide.

Construction of plasmids

Plasmids for the Sleeping Beauty-transposon system, pCMV-SB and pCMV-mSB (a transposase having a missense mutation in its C-terminal Asp-Asp-Glu motif) were kindly provided by Dr. Joonseok Song (University of Pittsburgh) [25]. To construct the transposon plasmid, pGL3-hT-Con and pGL3-hT-TK-Con plasmids were cut with KpnI and BamHI restriction enzymes. A luciferase and the HSV-TK gene were ligated with pT-MCS vector, which gave rise to pT.hTp.Con and pT.hTp.HSV-tk.Con vectors respectively (Fig. 1). The hTERT promoter and the SV40 enhancer region were amplified by PCR using Ex Taq DNA polymerase (Takara, Shiga, Japan) and subcloned into the pGL3-hT-Con vector. The hTERT promoter forward (5′-accaggtagtggattcgcgggcacaga-3′) and reverse (5′-agatctagggcttcccacgtgcgcag-3′) primers, and the SV40E forward (5′-gcattcgatggagcgg-3′) and reverse (5′-ggatccgctgtggaatg-3′) primers were used. PCR was performed for 35 cycles at 94°C for 1 min, at 60°C for 1 min, and at 72°C for 1 min.

Luciferase assay

Luciferase assays were carried out using Luciferase Assay System (Promega, Madison, USA) and AutoLumat LB953

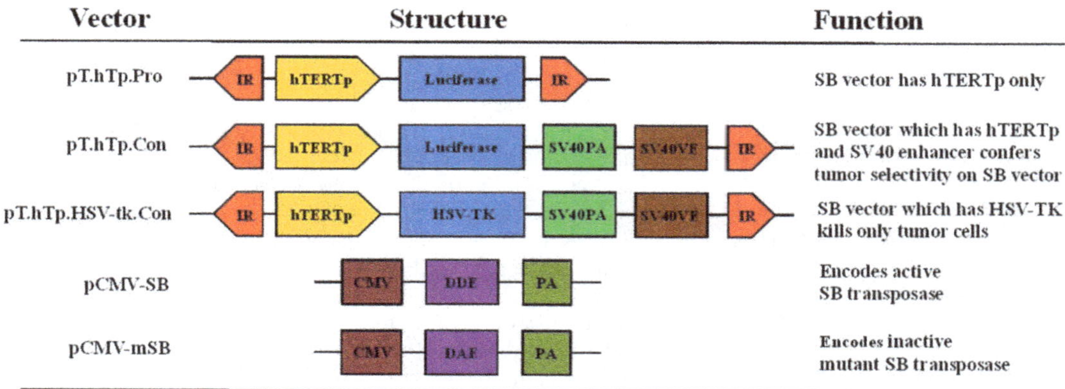

Figure 1. Schematic representation of the Sleeping Beauty transposon including the hTERT promoter and SV40 enhancer used in our studies. To construct the transposon plasmid, the pGL3-hT-Con and pGL3-hT-TK-Con plasmids were cut with KpnI and BamHI; the ends of the luciferase cassette and the HSV-TK cassette were filled in using DNA polymerase I and blunt end ligated into the pT-MCS vector, resulting in the pT.hTp.Con and pT.hTp.HSV-tk.Con vectors, respectively. The pT.hTp.nori.Con plasmid was constructed from the pTnori plasmid through the insertion of the human telomerase promoter (hTERTp) and the SV40 enhancer. The SV40 promoter was replaced with hTERTp by digesting the pTnori plasmid with SexAI and BglII. The SV40 enhancer was inserted between the BsmI and BamHI sites of pTnori. The hTERT promoter and the SV40 enhancer region were amplified by PCR from the pGL3-hT-Con vector using Ex-Taq polymerase.

luminometer (Berthold, Wildbad, Germany) according to the manufacturer's protocols. In brief, 3×10^4 cells seeded in a 16-mm tissue culture dish were transfected with 1 ug of luciferase reporter plasmids and 0.25 ug of pSV-β-galactosidase control plasmid vector. Cell lysates were prepared 48 hours after transfection by adding 100 ul of reporter lysis buffer and their luciferase activities were measured. The pGL3-Promoter plasmid containing SV40 promoter was used as a positive control. The luciferase activity of the pGL3-Promoter plasmid in each cell line was considered to be 1, and the relative luciferase activity was calculated. All luciferase assays were performed in triplicate.

Plasmid transfection with GCV treatment in vitro

Cancer and normal cells (10^5 cells per dish) were plated in 35-mm culture dishes prior to transfection, and they were transfected with pCMV-SB or pCMV-mSB plasmid with pT.hTp.HSV-TK.Con plasmid using Lipofectamine 2000 transfection reagent (Invitrogen, Carlsbad, USA). After incubation at 37°C for 3 days, 2 ml of media containing various concentrations of Ganciclovir (GCV; InvivoGen, San Diego, USA) were added to the cells. All of the data shown in this report were obtained from at least three independent experiments.

TUNEL assay

DNA strand breaks in apoptotic cells were measured by the TUNEL assay using the In-situ Detection Kit (Roche Molecular Biochemicals, Germany). Samples were fixed with 4% paraformaldehyde in PBS for 15 min and incubated in a 0.1% ice-cold Triton X-100 solution for permeabilization for 10 min according to the manufacturer's instructions. Cell were then washed 3 times with PBS and reacted with 50 μl of the TUNEL reaction mixture at 37°C for 60 min in a dark, humidified chamber. Cells were washed three times in PBS. Under fluorescence microscopy, the number of TUNEL-positive cells was counted.

Apoptosis assay

The apoptotic rates in normal and cancer cells were measured by an Annexin V-FITC Kit (Invitrogen, Carlsbad, USA). Briefly, the pT.hTp.HSV-TK.Con and pCMV-SB transfected cells were treated with GCV (50 ug/ml, 3 hr at 37°C) after 10 days of transfection. Cells were harvested and rinsed with a 1× annexin-binding buffer and then resuspended with 100 ul of a 1× annexin-binding buffer. After adding 5 ul of FITC annexin V and 1 ul of propidium iodide (PI; 100 ug/ml), cells were incubated at room temperature for 15 minutes in the dark. The proportion of viable cells were analyzed by FACScalibur flow cytometer (Becton Dickinson, San Jose, CA) and quantified by Flowjo software (Tree Star Inc., Ashland, USA).

Cytotoxicity assay

A number of 5×10^3 pT.hTp.HSV-TK.Con and pCMV-SB transfected cells were inoculated into 96-well plate. The plate was then incubated at 37°C and 5% CO2 for 24 hours. GCV was added at the concentration level of 10, 30, 50 ug/ml in triplicate for each concentration level. The cells were then incubated for 3 hours and were added with MTT, where the cells were cultured for another 4 hours. Supernatant was then removed and DMSO was added to dissolve the MTT formazan crystals. OD value at 570 nm was detected by a microplate reader. Cell survival rate was calculated by: survival rate (%) = A/B×100 (A: OD value of pT.hTp.HSV-TK.Con and pCMV-SB transfected cells; B: OD value of pT.hTp.Con and pCMV-SB). All experiments were performed in triplicate. Survival curve was generated with mean viabilities of each cell lines as ordinate axis and the concentrations of GCV as abscissa axis

Statistical analysis

Each set of experiments was performed in duplicate or triplicate. Results from each experiment replicate were presented as the mean ± SD. Data were assessed by one-way analysis of variance (ANOVA) and significant results were further assessed by Tukey's multiple comparison tests. Statistical significance was defined at a P level of <0.05.

Results

hTERT is a promising target for the SB-mediated gene therapy

Successful gene therapy largely depends on the selective expression of a suicide gene in appropriate target cancer cells, but not in the normal surrounding cells. The human telomerase reverse transcriptase (hTERT) gene, which encodes the catalytic subunit of telomerase, is highly expressed in embryonic stem cells and is progressively down-regulated during differentiation, resulting in complete silencing in fully differentiated somatic cells. hTERT is frequently reactivated in approximately 90% of immortalized human cells and cancer cells of various origins [26–28]. Therefore, it can be a promising target for gene therapy in a variety of tumor types. First, we examined the expression profiles of the human telomerase RNA components (hTR) and hTERT using RT-PCR in fibroblasts and various cancer cell lines. hTR was constitutively expressed in both the fibroblasts and the cancer cell lines, which were consistent with previous observations [34]. The expression of hTERT was detected in all cancer cells, including two lung cancer cell lines (H358 and H1299), two prostate cancer cell lines (PC3 and DU145), and an ovarian cancer cell line (OVCAR3), but it was not detected in the two fibroblast cell lines (WI-38 and IMR-90) (Fig. 2). Therefore, expression of hTERT appeared to be tightly connected to tumor development, and hTERT could be a promising target for the SB-mediated gene therapy of the various cancer types.

Tumor specific activation of the hTERT promoter by the SV40 enhancer

Because the normal or natural promoter was not strong enough to induce efficient expression of the therapeutic genes in certain tumor cells, a powerful tumor-specific promoter is essential to achieve successful long-lasting therapeutic gene expression. The Simian virus 40 (SV40) enhancer has been extensively used to improve the activity of promoters [32] and the 3 poly(A) tail is important for the stability and translation mRNA [35]. Thus, to increase the promoter strength while maintaining tissue specificity, we constructed a recombinant hTERT promoter that contained the SV40 enhancer and SV40 PolyA (Simian virus 40 PolyA, also called PolyA). The SV40 enhancer sequence was amplified and inserted into the multiple clone site (MCS) downstream of the hTERT promoter. The transcription activity following transfection with the pT-hTp-Con plasmid (with SV40 enhancer and SV40 PolyA) or the pT-hTp-Pro plasmid (without SV40 enhancer and SV40 PolyA) was detected and compared in the normal and cancer cell lines, and the effect of the SV40 enhancer on the activity of the tumor specific hTERT promoter was evaluated. As shown in Fig. 3, the pT-hTp-Con plasmid, which contains the SV40 enhancer and SV40 PolyA, showed a significant increase in transcript activity in the telomerase positive cancer cell lines, whereas there was no change in the two normal fibroblast cell lines. These results showed that the hTERT promoter exhibited relatively high transcriptional activities in most of the tumor cell lines while exhibiting little activity in the normal fibroblast cell lines, and the SV40 enhancer and SV40 PolyA significantly increased the activity of the hTERT promoter exclusively in the cancer cell lines.

Long-term sustainability of the modified SB delivery system in various types of cancer cells

Successful gene therapy depends on the long-term sustainability of therapeutic gene expression to cure or slow down the progression of cancer development. Therefore, we next examined whether the SB delivery system modified with the hTERT promoter and the SV40 enhancer sustained long-lasting thera-

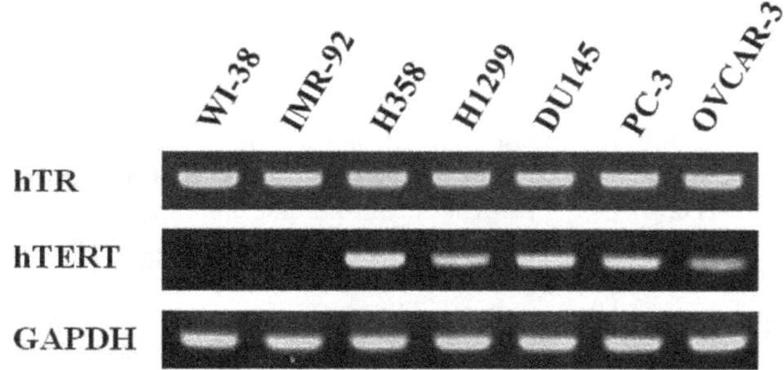

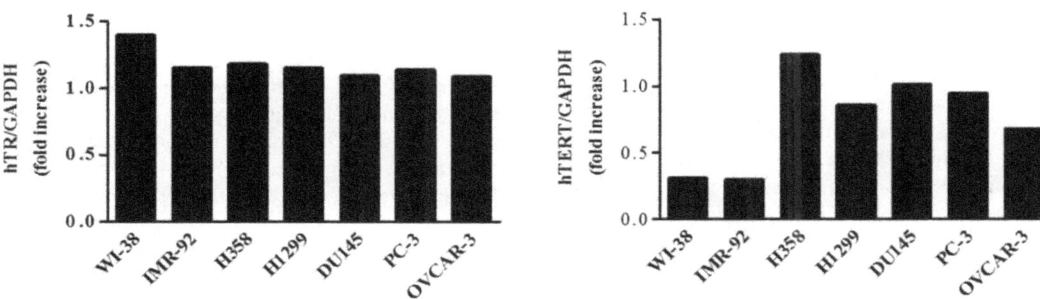

Figure 2. Comparison of the hTR and hTERT expression profiles of multiple cancer cell lines and normal fibroblasts. hTR and hTERT expression levels in various cancer cell lines and normal fibroblasts were determined using RT-PCR. Total RNA was amplified using hTR and hTERT specific primers (top and middle, respectively). GAPDH expression was used as an internal control for the normalization of hTR and hTERT expression. hTR was constitutively expressed in both the fibroblasts and the cancer cell lines. The expression of hTERT was detected in all cancer cells, whereas it was not detected in the two fibroblast cell lines. Lung cancer cell lines (H358 and H1299); prostate cancer cell lines (PC3 and DU145); ovarian cancer cell line (OVCAR3); fibroblast cell lines (WI-38 and IMR-90).

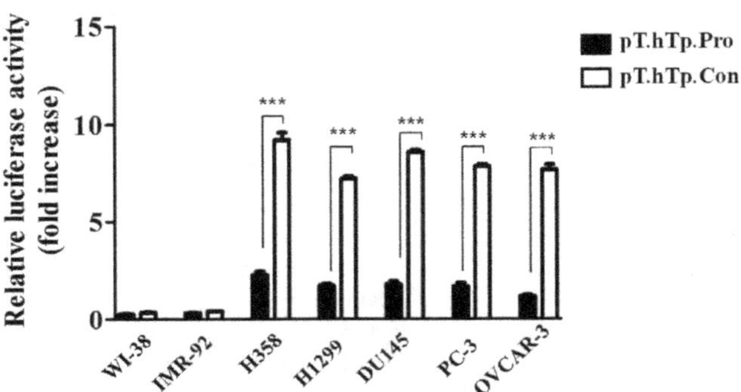

Figure 3. Comparison of the hTERT-mediated transcriptional activity of various cancer cell lines and normal fibroblasts with or without the SV40 enhancer and SV40 PolyA. Following the transfection of either the pT-hTp-Con plasmid (with SV40 enhancer and SV40 PolyA) or the pT-hTp-Pro plasmid (without SV40 enhancer and SV40 PolyA), the luciferase activity was detected and compared in normal and cancer cell lines. In telomerase positive cancer cell lines, the SV40 enhancer and SV40 PolyA activated the hTERT gene promoter by at least 7-fold compared to the hTERT gene promoter activity without these sequences. Relative luciferase activity was standardized to the transfection of the control pGL3-promotor plasmid. Lung cancer cell lines (H358 and H1299); prostate cancer cell lines (PC3 and DU145); ovarian cancer cell line (OVCAR3); fibroblast cell lines (WI-38 and IMR-90). The results are shown as the mean ± SD from three independent experiments. * $P<0.05$, ** $P<0.01$, and *** $P<0.001$.

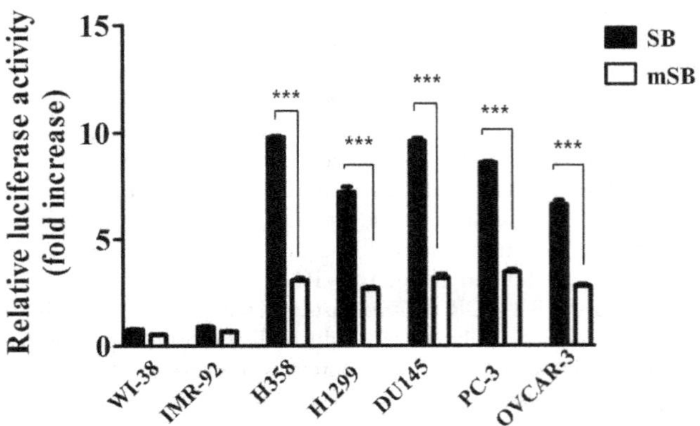

Figure 4. Long-lasting hTERT-mediated transcriptional activity in various types of cancer cells. Luciferase assays were used to determine the promoter activities of the luciferase expressing plasmid pT-hTp-Con following co-transfection with either the active helper plasmid (pCMV-SB) or the inactive helper plasmid (pCMV-mSB) in H358, H1299, PC3, DU145, OVCAR3, WI-38, and IMR-90 cells. All cancer cell lines that contained the SB-based gene delivery system, under the control of the hTERT promoter and the SV40 enhancer, sustained relatively higher levels of long-term luciferase activity than the normal fibroblasts 10 days after transfection. Relative luciferase activity was standardized to the transfection of the control pGL3-promotor plasmid. Lung cancer cell lines (H358 and H1299); prostate cancer cell lines (PC3 and DU145); ovarian cancer cell line (OVCAR3); fibroblast cell lines (WI-38 and IMR-90). The results are shown as the mean ± SD from three independent experiments. * $P<0.05$, ** $P<0.01$, and *** $P<0.001$.

peutic gene expression in various types of cancer cell lines. Because the transposase-producing helper plasmid is essential for the insertion of SB into the host genomes, we co-transfected normal fibroblast and cancer cell lines with a luciferase expressing version of the pT-hTp-Con plasmid along with either the active helper plasmid (pCMV-SB) or the inactive helper plasmid (pCMV-mSB). All cancer cell lines sustained relatively higher levels of long-term luciferase activity using the SB delivery system under control of the hTERT promoter and the SV40 enhancer compared to the normal fibroblasts; there was no change in the two normal fibroblast cell lines 10 days after transfection (Fig. 4). These findings suggest that the modified SB delivery system is a promising way to enhance the therapeutic efficiency when long-term expression of the therapeutic products is required.

Modified SB delivery system increases tumor cell specific cytotoxicity

Successful cancer treatment using gene therapy largely depends on the specific delivery of the therapeutic product into the appropriate target cancer cells. Gene-directed enzyme prodrug therapy (GDEPT) is a promising alternative to conventional chemotherapy; GDEPT minimizes the systemic toxicities of conventional chemotherapy drugs by introducing catalytic enzymes into tumor cells; these enzymes then convert low- or non-toxic prodrugs into toxic metabolites [1]. After genetically modifying the tumor cells to express the catalytic enzymes, systemic administration of the prodrug, which is locally converted by the enzyme into cytotoxic metabolites, leads to the selective killing of tumor cells. To determine the tumor cell specific toxic effect of our SB-based gene delivery system, cancer cells and normal fibroblasts were co-transfected with the modified SB system (pT.hTp.HSV-tk.Con) along with the active helper plasmid (pCMV-SB) following the administration of 50 µg/mL gancyclovir (GCV). We then performed TUNEL assays on cells 10 days after transfection to identify the apoptotic cells, which are characterized by the presence of densely stained circular bodies that represent the fragmented DNA of apoptotic cells. As shown in Fig. 5, the TUNEL assays demonstrated that the modified SB transfected cancer cells showed a significantly increased death rate compared to the normal fibroblasts in the presence of 50 µg/mL GCV. To further confirm this tumor specific cell death by the SB-based gene delivery system, a cell viability assay was used to evaluate the cancer cell specific cytotoxicity in the normal fibroblasts and cancer cell lines treated with GCV in a dose-dependent manner. GCV alone had negligible effect on the cell viability (Fig. 6A), whereas transfection of the modified SB (pT.hTp.HSV-tk.Con) system following administration of GCV significantly decreased cancer cell viability in a dose-dependent manner (Fig. 6B). Additionally, cell death was also determined by flow cytometry to identify cells that were stained with both Annexin V/FITC and propidium iodide (PI). The data from the TUNEL and cell viability assays were consistent with our flow cytometry results (Fig. 7). These results suggest that our SB-based gene delivery system mediated tumor cell specific therapeutic gene delivery, which in turn induced tumor-specific apoptosis. Our in vitro data suggested that the modified SB transfected cancer cells showed a significantly increased death rate compared to the normal fibroblasts. Therefore, we next investigated whether tumor growth could be suppressed by modified SB delivery system in vivo. In some experimental groups, tumor growth was successfully suppressed by modified SB delivery system, while the other groups did not show an apparent anti-tumor effect (Fig. 8).

Discussion

Many commonly used chemotherapy drugs lack tumor specificity, and the doses required to reach therapeutic levels in the tumor are often toxic to the surrounding normal tissues. Therefore, prodrug-activating systems that include suicide gene

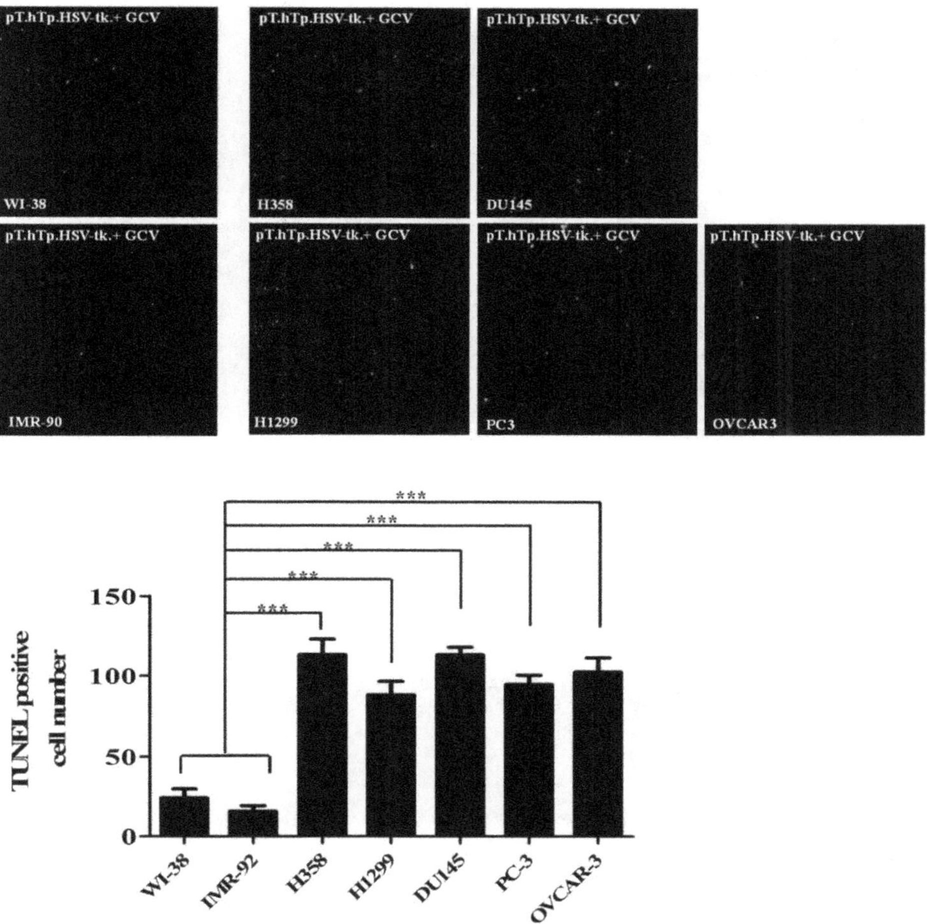

Figure 5. Cancer cell specific effect of the SB-based gene delivery system with the hTERT promoter. The levels of cell apoptosis were assessed using the TUNEL assay after transfection of the SB system (pT.hTp.HSV-tk.Con with active helper plasmid) and following administration of 50 μg/mL GCV at 3 day post-transfection. TUNEL-positive cells were characterized by densely stained circular bodies that represent the fragmented DNA of apoptotic cells. SB transfected cancer cells showed a significantly increased number of TUNEL-positive cells compared to normal fibroblasts in the presence of 50 μg/mL GCV. Lung cancer cell lines (H358 and H1299); prostate cancer cell lines (PC3 and DU145); ovarian cancer cell line (OVCAR3); fibroblast cell lines (WI-38 and IMR-90). The results are shown as the mean ± SD from three independent experiments. * $P<0.05$, ** $P<0.01$, and *** $P<0.001$.

therapy are promising alternatives to conventional chemotherapy; these systems minimize the systemic toxicities of conventional chemotherapy drugs. For clinical application, the suicide genes need to satisfy the following criteria: a) these genes must be either not expressed or present at extremely low levels in the host; and b) the gene must have a high catalytic activity to achieve a sufficient level of the toxic metabolite in the tumors [36]. Ideally, tumor-targeted prodrugs must meet the following criteria: a) the prodrug must be less toxic or non-toxic prior to activation (cleavage) by the suicide gene product; b) the prodrug must have a selective binding affinity for the transfected suicide gene product; and c) an active metabolite of the prodrug must have an extended half-life so that the treatment dose can be reduced [36].

Of the suicide gene/prodrug therapy systems, by far the combination of HSV-TK and GCV is the most frequently used in cancer gene therapy. The HSV-TK gene is transfected into the tumor cells to convert the systemically administered non-toxic prodrug GCV into a toxic metabolite [37]. HSV-TK catalyzes GCV into monophosphorylated GCV (GCV-MP), which is then converted into the toxic triphosphate form of GCV (deoxythymidine triphosphate). This triphosphate metabolite is an analog of purine; incorporation of this analog during DNA synthesis inhibits DNA polymerase, leading to the observed toxicity [38]. Therefore, this combination method has been successfully applied to many clinical areas, such as gene therapy for cancer treatment [6], as an efficient tool for controlling graft-versus-host disease (GVHD) [7], and as positron emission tomography (PET) reporter probes [39]. However, this combination system is not effective enough to eradicate malignant tumors due to the poor transfection efficiency of the HSV-TK gene, resulting in significantly lower expression levels of the gene product *in vitro* and *in vivo* [40]; poor expression of the HSV-TK gene requires that higher doses GCV are used during treatment. High doses of GCV appear to be associated with hematologic toxicities, such as leucopenia and thrombocytopenia, renal toxicity, and other adverse side effects [41]. These disadvantages have greatly limited the clinical application of the HSV-TK/GCV system. However, it is generally thought that these limitations are associated with the poor transfection efficiency of the gene delivery systems used in these experiments

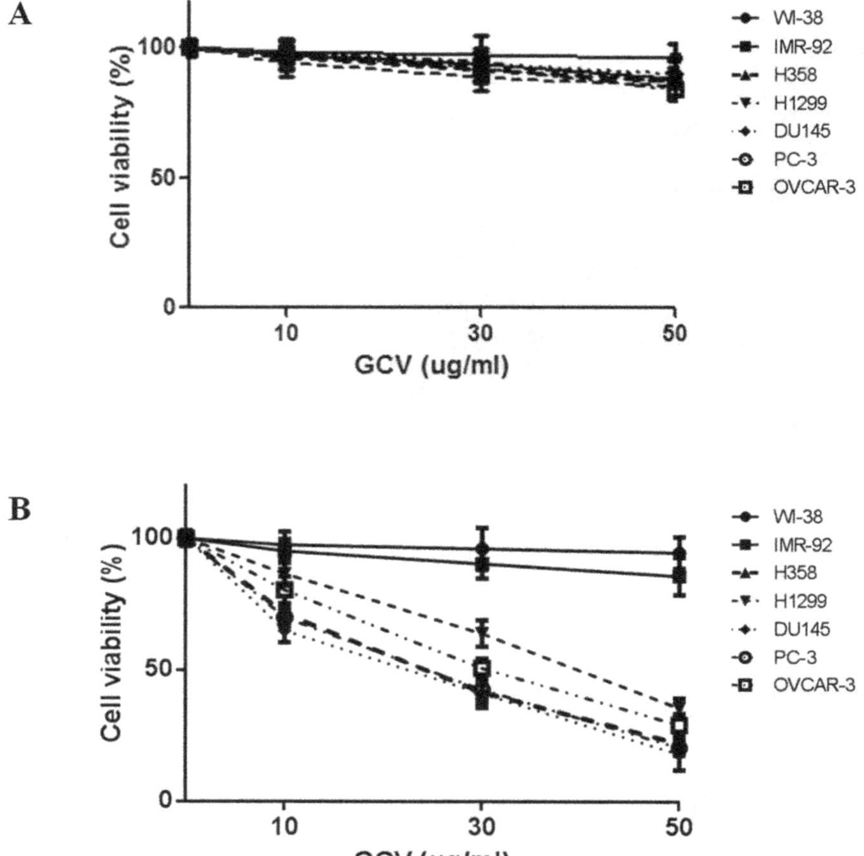

Figure 6. Cancer cell specific effect of the SB-based gene delivery system with the hTERT promoter on cell viability. Cell viability was assessed using the MTT with or without transfection of the SB system (pT.hTp.HSV-tk.Con with active helper plasmid) following administration of 10, 30, or 50 µg/mL GCV at 3 day post-transfection. GCV alone had negligible effect on effect on the cell viability (A), whereas transfection of the SB system (pT.hTp.HSV-tk.Con with active helper plasmid) following administration of GCV significantly decreased the cancer cell viability in a dose-dependent manner (B). Lung cancer cell lines (H358 and H1299); prostate cancer cell lines (PC3 and DU145); ovarian cancer cell line (OVCAR3); fibroblast cell lines (WI-38 and IMR-90). The results are shown as the mean ± SD from three independent experiments. * $P<0.05$, ** $P<0.01$, and *** $P<0.001$.

rather than a failure of the combination gene therapy using HSV-TK and GCV [42].

Several studies have focused on increasing the transfection efficiency and the expression level of the HSV-TK gene to improve the therapeutic potential of the HSV-TK/GCV combination system. Many transfection methods have been attempted to improve the transfection efficiency, but most of the observed effects did not meet the clinical requirements, such as safe, non-immunogenic, easy to produce, target specific, and long-lasting expression in tumor cells. The SB transposon-based system is an attractive, non-viral alternative to the previously used viral delivery systems. SB may be less immunogenic than viral vector systems due to lack of viral sequences [43]. The SB-based gene delivery system can stably integrate into the host cell's genome to produce the suicide gene product over the cell's lifetime [44]. SB-mediated transposition has been shown to occur in a variety of cell culture systems including zebrafish [45], mouse embryo [46], mouse lung and liver [47–49], and human primary blood lymphocytes [50]. However, when compared to the viral vectors, the non-viral SB-based gene delivery system had limited therapeutic efficacy due to the lack of long-lasting gene expression and tumor cell specific gene transfer ability. This limitation can be overcome through the addition of the hTERT promoter and the SV40 enhancer to the SB transposon. hTERT, the catalytic subunit of telomerase, is highly expressed in embryonic stem cells, is progressively down-regulated during differentiation, and is silenced in fully differentiated somatic cells. hTERT is frequently reactivated in approximately 90% of immortalized human cells and cancer cells of various origins [26–28]. Moreover, its powerful promoter is essential to achieve long-term stable expression of a therapeutic gene. The SV40 enhancer has been extensively used to improve the activity of promoters [32]. Thus, to increase the promoter strength while maintaining tissue specificity, we constructed a recombinant SV40 enhancer containing the tumor-specific hTERT promoter.

Our in vitro data suggested that the modified SB transfected cancer cells showed a significantly increased death rate compared to the normal fibroblasts. Therefore, we next investigated whether tumor growth could be suppressed by modified SB delivery system in vivo. In some experimental groups, tumor growth was successfully suppressed by modified SB delivery system, while the other groups did not show an apparent anti-tumor effect (Fig. 8). These in vivo variations among the experimental subjects possibly due to the following: 1) the lower in vivo transfection

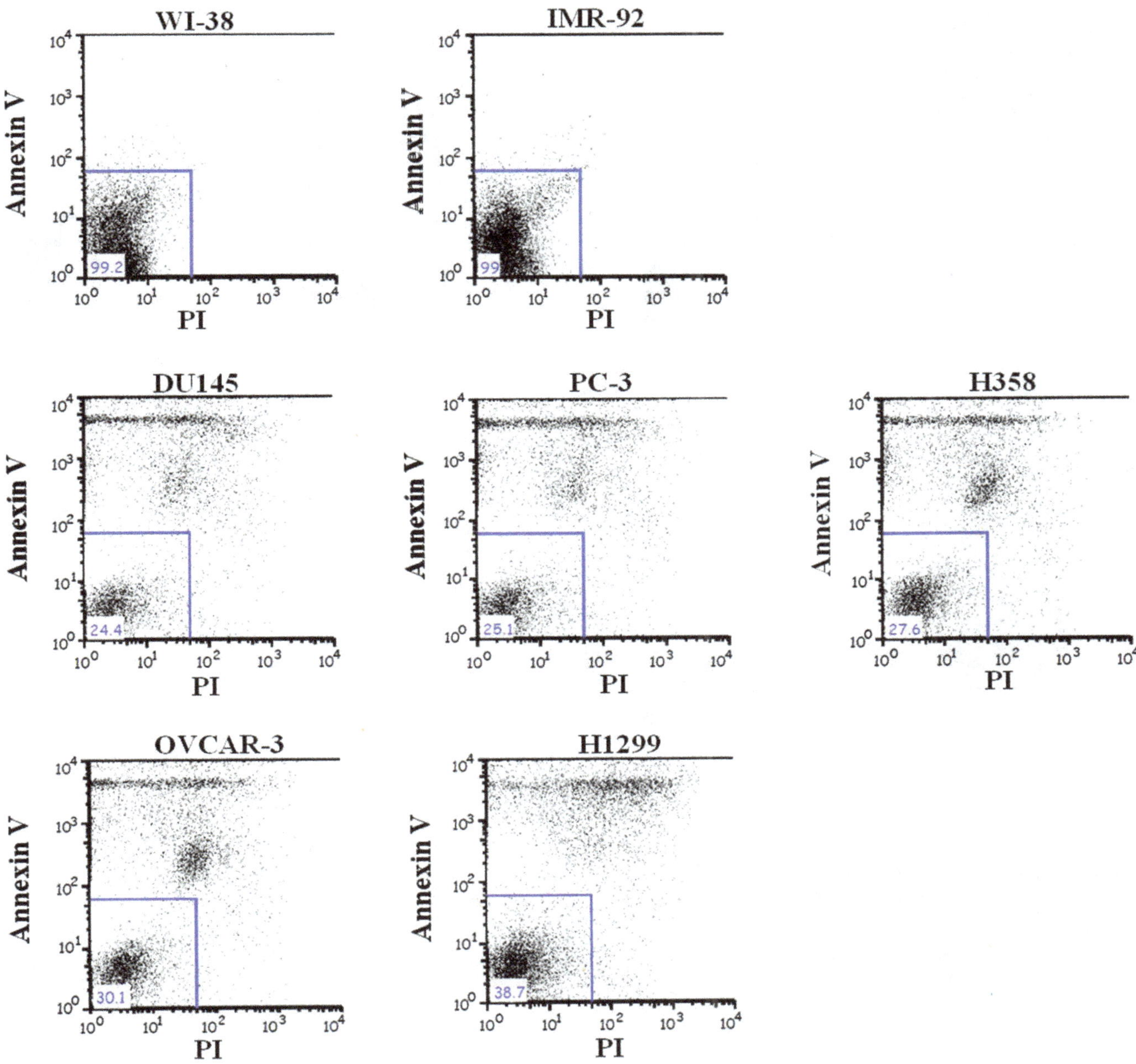

Figure 7. Flow cytometry analysis of the SB-based gene delivery system with the hTERT promoter on cancer cell apoptosis. Cancer cell lines and normal fibroblasts were transfected with the SB system (pT.hTp.HSV-tk.Con with active helper plasmid). Cells were then challenged with 50 µg/mL GCV, followed by Annexin V-FITC/PI staining and FACS analysis at 3 day post-transfection. Lung cancer cell lines (H358 and H1299); prostate cancer cell lines (PC3 and DU145); ovarian cancer cell line (OVCAR3); fibroblast cell lines (WI-38 and IMR-90).

efficiency of SB plasmid can be related directly to the lower anti-tumor effect of modified SB delivery system in vivo; 2) One of the critical parameters for a successful expression of systemic administration of plasmid DNA is the volume of DNA solution administered. Previous study demonstrated that plasmid delivery to rodent by the tail vein is effective as long as the volume of injected DNA solution is adjusted to 7–8% of body weight [51]; 3) rapid injection (less than 10 s) is also critical parameters for gene delivery with highest level of gene expression [51].

In this study, the SB-based delivery system, under the control of the hTERT promoter with the SV40 enhancer, was used to achieve successful target specific transfer of the HSV-TK gene into multiple types of cancer. Our SB-based system induced HSV-TK gene expression exclusively in cancer cells due to the cancer cell specific hTERT promoter activity, and therefore only the cancer cells were susceptible to the administration of the GCV prodrug. In the presence of GCV, the SB transfected cancer cells showed a significantly increased death rate compared to the normal fibroblasts. The viability of the SB transfected cancer cells was significantly lower than that of the normal fibroblasts following GCV treatment; this result was dose-dependent. These data suggest that our modified SB-based gene delivery system can be used as a safe and efficient tool for stable HSV-TK gene transfer and long-term expression. However, several critical questions still

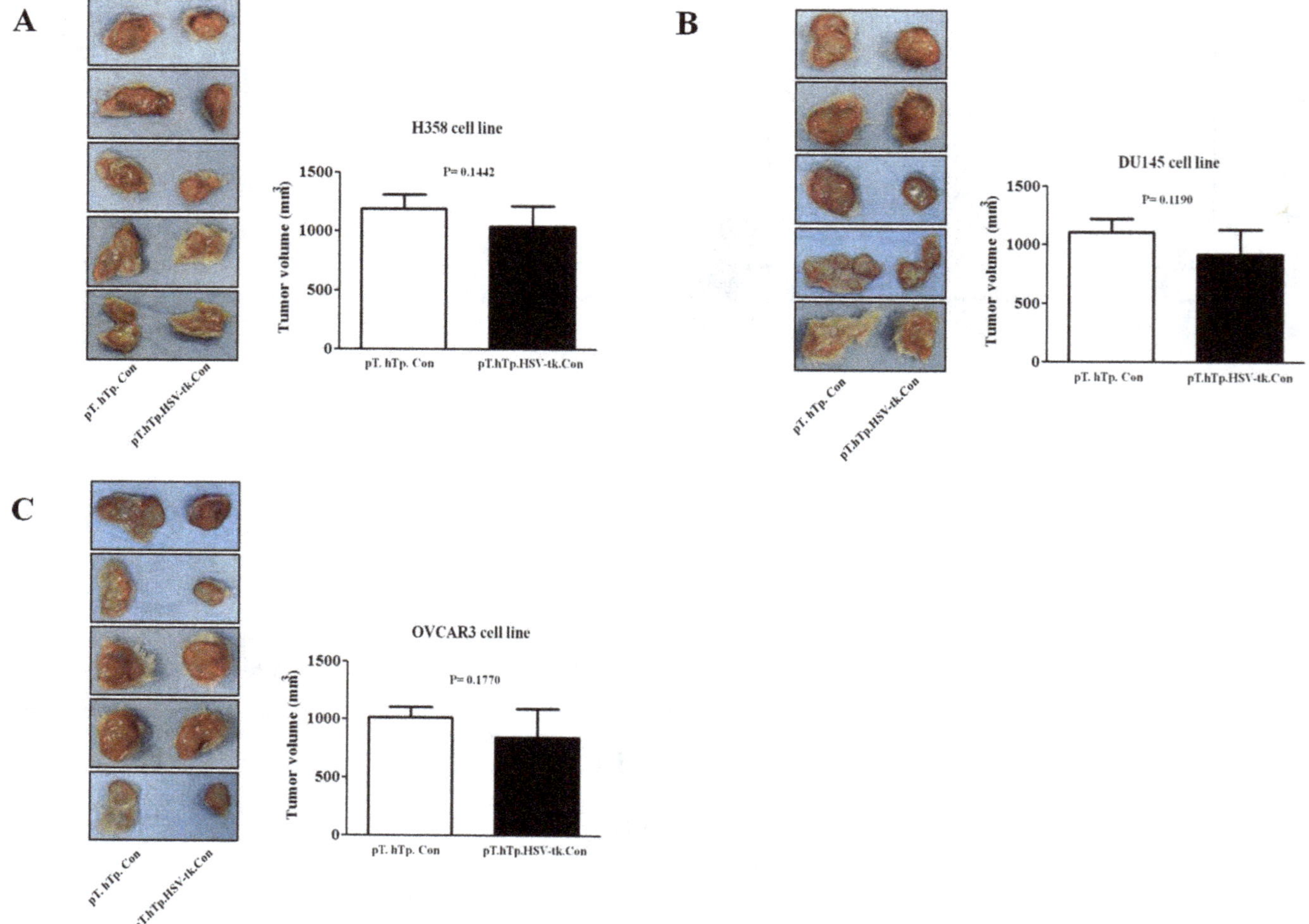

Figure 8. The effect of modified SB system on the tumor growth in vivo. Lung cancer cells (H358) (A), prostate cancer cell line (DU-145) (B), and ovarian cancer cells (OVCAR3) (C) were harvested by trypsinization, and 1×10^5 viable cells (as determined by trypan blue exclusion) in a total volume of 200 µl were injected subcutaneously. Two days following tumor seeding, animals were intravenously injected via tail veins with 100 mg/kg gancyclovir (GCV) along with either co-transfection of the empty plasmid (pT. hTp. Con) with the active helper plasmid (pCMV-SB) or co-transfection of the SB system (pT.hTp.HSV-tk.Con) with the active helper plasmid (pCMV-SB). Mice were sacrificed 28 days after tumor injection, and the effect of modified SB system on tumor growth was evaluated by measuring tumor size.

need to be answered before a clinical trial of SB mediated therapeutic gene delivery can commence. First, it is still possible that SB functions as an insertion mutagen that disrupts the structure of the host gene where it resides, resulting in tumor formation. Second, SB and its associated carriers, such as PEI, can instigate an inflammatory response. Finally, our understanding of the interactions between SB and intracellular molecules is still rudimentary.

Author Contributions

Conceived and designed the experiments: HPK. Performed the experiments: ISH HYL HPK. Analyzed the data: ISH HYL HPK. Wrote the paper: ISH HYL HPK.

References

1. Both GW (2009) Gene-directed enzyme prodrug therapy for cancer: a glimpse into the future? Discov Med 8: 97–103.
2. Rainov NG, Dobberstein KU, Sena-Esteves M, Herrlinger U, Kramm CM, et al. (1998) New prodrug activation gene therapy for cancer using cytochrome P450 4B1 and 2-aminoanthracene/4-ipomeanol. Hum Gene Ther 9: 1261–1273.
3. Miller AD (1992) Human gene therapy comes of age. Nature 357: 455–460.
4. Black ME, Newcomb TG, Wilson HM, Loeb LA (1996) Creation of drug-specific herpes simplex virus type 1 thymidine kinase mutants for gene therapy. Proc Natl Acad Sci U S A 93: 3525–3529.
5. Elion GB, Furman PA, Fyfe JA, de Miranda P, Beauchamp L, et al. (1977) Selectivity of action of an antiherpetic agent, 9-(2-hydroxyethoxymethyl) guanine. Proc Natl Acad Sci U S A 74: 5716–5720.
6. Sterman DH, Recio A, Vachani A, Sun J, Cheung L, et al. (2005) Long-term follow-up of patients with malignant pleural mesothelioma receiving high-dose adenovirus herpes simplex thymidine kinase/ganciclovir suicide gene therapy. Clin Cancer Res 11: 7444–7453.
7. Ciceri F, Bonini C, Gallo-Stampino C, Bordignon C (2005) Modulation of GvHD by suicide-gene transduced donor T lymphocytes: clinical applications in mismatched transplantation. Cytotherapy 7: 144–149.
8. Davidson BL, Stein CS, Heth JA, Martins I, Kotin RM, et al. (2000) Recombinant adeno-associated virus type 2, 4, and 5 vectors: transduction of

variant cell types and regions in the mammalian central nervous system. Proc Natl Acad Sci U S A 97: 3428–3432.

9. Fischer A, Hacein-Bey-Abina S, Lagresle C, Garrigue A, Cavazana-Calvo M (2005) [Gene therapy of severe combined immunodeficiency disease: proof of principle of efficiency and safety issues. Gene therapy, primary immunodeficiencies, retrovirus, lentivirus, genome]. Bull Acad Natl Med 189: 779–785; discussion 786–778.
10. Nair V (2008) Retrovirus-induced oncogenesis and safety of retroviral vectors. Curr Opin Mol Ther 10: 431–438.
11. Grimm D, Kleinschmidt JA (1999) Progress in adeno-associated virus type 2 vector production: promises and prospects for clinical use. Hum Gene Ther 10: 2445–2450.
12. Pan RY, Xiao X, Chen SL, Li J, Lin LC, et al. (1999) Disease-inducible transgene expression from a recombinant adeno-associated virus vector in a rat arthritis model. J Virol 73: 3410–3417.
13. Cooley L, Kelley R, Spradling A (1988) Insertional mutagenesis of the Drosophila genome with single P elements. Science 239: 1121–1128.
14. Plasterk RH (1996) The Tc1/mariner transposon family. Curr Top Microbiol Immunol 204: 125–143.
15. Lohe AR, Moriyama EN, Lidholm DA, Hartl DL (1995) Horizontal transmission, vertical inactivation, and stochastic loss of mariner-like transposable elements. Mol Biol Evol 12: 62–72.
16. Ivics Z, Hackett PB, Plasterk RH, Izsvak Z (1997) Molecular reconstruction of Sleeping Beauty, a Tc1-like transposon from fish, and its transposition in human cells. Cell 91: 501–510.
17. Luo G, Ivics Z, Izsvak Z, Bradley A (1998) Chromosomal transposition of a Tc1/mariner-like element in mouse embryonic stem cells. Proc Natl Acad Sci U S A 95: 10769–10773.
18. Yant SR, Meuse L, Chiu W, Ivics Z, Izsvak Z, et al. (2000) Somatic integration and long-term transgene expression in normal and haemophilic mice using a DNA transposon system. Nat Genet 25: 35–41.
19. Fischer SE, Wienholds E, Plasterk RH (2001) Regulated transposition of a fish transposon in the mouse germ line. Proc Natl Acad Sci U S A 98: 6759–6764.
20. Izsvak Z, Ivics Z (2004) Sleeping beauty transposition: biology and applications for molecular therapy. Mol Ther 9: 147–156.
21. Montini E, Held PK, Noll M, Morcinek N, Al-Dhalimy M, et al. (2002) In vivo correction of murine tyrosinemia type I by DNA-mediated transposition. Mol Ther 6: 759–769.
22. Ortiz-Urda S, Lin Q, Yant SR, Keene D, Kay MA, et al. (2003) Sustainable correction of junctional epidermolysis bullosa via transposon-mediated nonviral gene transfer. Gene Ther 10: 1099–1104.
23. Yant SR, Ehrhardt A, Mikkelsen JG, Meuse L, Pham T, et al. (2002) Transposition from a gutless adeno-transposon vector stabilizes transgene expression in vivo. Nat Biotechnol 20: 999–1005.
24. Song J, Kim C, Ochoa ER (2009) Sleeping Beauty-mediated suicide gene therapy of hepatocellular carcinoma. Biosci Biotechnol Biochem 73: 165–168.
25. Song JS, Murase N, Demetris AJ, Michalopoulos GK, Ochoa ER (2007) Protection from acute cellular injury using Sleeping Beauty mediated telomerase gene transfer. Biochem Biophys Res Commun 363: 253–256.
26. Wright WE, Piatyszek MA, Rainey WE, Byrd W, Shay JW (1996) Telomerase activity in human germline and embryonic tissues and cells. Dev Genet 18: 173–179.
27. Avilion AA, Piatyszek MA, Gupta J, Shay JW, Bacchetti S, et al. (1996) Human telomerase RNA and telomerase activity in immortal cell lines and tumor tissues. Cancer Res 56: 645–650.
28. Shay JW, Bacchetti S (1997) A survey of telomerase activity in human cancer. Eur J Cancer 33: 787–791.
29. Bilsland AE, Fletcher-Monaghan A, Keith WN (2005) Properties of a telomerase-specific Cre/Lox switch for transcriptionally targeted cancer gene therapy. Neoplasia 7: 1020–1029.
30. Plumb JA, Bilsland A, Kakani R, Zhao J, Glasspool RM, et al. (2001) Telomerase-specific suicide gene therapy vectors expressing bacterial nitroreductase sensitize human cancer cells to the pro-drug CB1954. Oncogene 20: 7797–7803.
31. Abdul-Ghani R, Ohana P, Matouk I, Ayesh S, Ayesh B, et al. (2000) Use of transcriptional regulatory sequences of telomerase (hTER and hTERT) for selective killing of cancer cells. Mol Ther 2: 539–544.
32. Li S, MacLaughlin FC, Fewell JG, Gondo M, Wang J, et al. (2001) Muscle-specific enhancement of gene expression by incorporation of SV40 enhancer in the expression plasmid. Gene Ther 8: 494–497.
33. Song JS (2004) Activity of the human telomerase catalytic subunit (hTERT) gene promoter could be increased by the SV40 enhancer. Biosci Biotechnol Biochem 68: 1634–1639.
34. Yi X, Tesmer VM, Savre-Train I, Shay JW, Wright WE (1999) Both transcriptional and posttranscriptional mechanisms regulate human telomerase template RNA levels. Mol Cell Biol 19: 3989–3997.
35. Guhaniyogi J, Brewer G (2001) Regulation of mRNA stability in mammalian cells. Gene 265: 11–23.
36. Singh Y, Palombo M, Sinko PJ (2008) Recent trends in targeted anticancer prodrug and conjugate design. Curr Med Chem 15: 1802–1826.
37. Hedley D, Ogilvie L, Springer C (2007) Carboxypeptidase-G2-based gene-directed enzyme-prodrug therapy: a new weapon in the GDEPT armoury. Nat Rev Cancer 7: 870–879.
38. Matthews T, Boehme R (1988) Antiviral activity and mechanism of action of ganciclovir. Rev Infect Dis 10 Suppl 3: S490–494.
39. Ponomarev V, Doubrovin M, Serganova I, Vider J, Shavrin A, et al. (2004) A novel triple-modality reporter gene for whole-body fluorescent, bioluminescent, and nuclear noninvasive imaging. Eur J Nucl Med Mol Imaging 31: 740–751.
40. Rainov NG (2000) A phase III clinical evaluation of herpes simplex virus type 1 thymidine kinase and ganciclovir gene therapy as an adjuvant to surgical resection and radiation in adults with previously untreated glioblastoma multiforme. Hum Gene Ther 11: 2389–2401.
41. Winston DJ, Wirin D, Shaked A, Busuttil RW (1995) Randomised comparison of ganciclovir and high-dose acyclovir for long-term cytomegalovirus prophylaxis in liver-transplant recipients. Lancet 346: 69–74.
42. Portsmouth D, Hlavaty J, Renner M (2007) Suicide genes for cancer therapy. Mol Aspects Med 28: 4–41.
43. Ding S, Wu X, Li G, Han M, Zhuang Y, et al. (2005) Efficient transposition of the piggyBac (PB) transposon in mammalian cells and mice. Cell 122: 473–483.
44. Ivics Z, Izsvak Z (2006) Transposons for gene therapy! Curr Gene Ther 6: 593–607.
45. Balciunas D, Ekker SC (2005) Trapping fish genes with transposons. Zebrafish 1: 335–341.
46. Dupuy AJ, Akagi K, Largaespada DA, Copeland NG, Jenkins NA (2005) Mammalian mutagenesis using a highly mobile somatic Sleeping Beauty transposon system. Nature 436: 221–226.
47. Belur LR, Frandsen JL, Dupuy AJ, Ingbar DH, Largaespada DA, et al. (2003) Gene insertion and long-term expression in lung mediated by the Sleeping Beauty transposon system. Mol Ther 8: 501–507.
48. Aronovich EL, Bell JB, Khan SA, Belur LR, Gunther R, et al. (2009) Systemic correction of storage disease in MPS I NOD/SCID mice using the sleeping beauty transposon system. Mol Ther 17: 1136–1144.
49. Kren BT, Unger GM, Sjeklocha L, Trossen AA, Korman V, et al. (2009) Nanocapsule-delivered Sleeping Beauty mediates therapeutic Factor VIII expression in liver sinusoidal endothelial cells of hemophilia A mice. J Clin Invest 119: 2086–2099.
50. Huang X, Guo H, Kang J, Choi S, Zhou TC, et al. (2008) Sleeping Beauty transposon-mediated engineering of human primary T cells for therapy of CD19+ lymphoid malignancies. Mol Ther 16: 580–589.
51. Zhou T, Kamimura K, Zhang G, Liu D (2010) Intracellular gene transfer in rats by tail vein injection of plasmid DNA. AAPS J 12: 692–698.

Permissions

All chapters in this book were first published in PLOS ONE, by The Public Library of Science; hereby published with permission under the Creative Commons Attribution License or equivalent. Every chapter published in this book has been scrutinized by our experts. Their significance has been extensively debated. The topics covered herein carry significant findings which will fuel the growth of the discipline. They may even be implemented as practical applications or may be referred to as a beginning point for another development.

The contributors of this book come from diverse backgrounds, making this book a truly international effort. This book will bring forth new frontiers with its revolutionizing research information and detailed analysis of the nascent developments around the world.

We would like to thank all the contributing authors for lending their expertise to make the book truly unique. They have played a crucial role in the development of this book. Without their invaluable contributions this book wouldn't have been possible. They have made vital efforts to compile up to date information on the varied aspects of this subject to make this book a valuable addition to the collection of many professionals and students.

This book was conceptualized with the vision of imparting up-to-date information and advanced data in this field. To ensure the same, a matchless editorial board was set up. Every individual on the board went through rigorous rounds of assessment to prove their worth. After which they invested a large part of their time researching and compiling the most relevant data for our readers.

The editorial board has been involved in producing this book since its inception. They have spent rigorous hours researching and exploring the diverse topics which have resulted in the successful publishing of this book. They have passed on their knowledge of decades through this book. To expedite this challenging task, the publisher supported the team at every step. A small team of assistant editors was also appointed to further simplify the editing procedure and attain best results for the readers.

Apart from the editorial board, the designing team has also invested a significant amount of their time in understanding the subject and creating the most relevant covers. They scrutinized every image to scout for the most suitable representation of the subject and create an appropriate cover for the book.

The publishing team has been an ardent support to the editorial, designing and production team. Their endless efforts to recruit the best for this project, has resulted in the accomplishment of this book. They are a veteran in the field of academics and their pool of knowledge is as vast as their experience in printing. Their expertise and guidance has proved useful at every step. Their uncompromising quality standards have made this book an exceptional effort. Their encouragement from time to time has been an inspiration for everyone.

The publisher and the editorial board hope that this book will prove to be a valuable piece of knowledge for researchers, students, practitioners and scholars across the globe.

List of Contributors

Rui Guo, M Zhang, Yun Xi, Shuo Shi, Ying Miao and Biao Li
Department of Nuclear Medicine, Rui Jin Hospital, School of medicine, Shanghai JiaoTong University, Shanghai, China

Yufei Ma and Sheng Liang
Department of Nuclear Medicine, Xin Hua Hospital, School of medicine, Shanghai JiaoTong University, Shanghai, China

Wen-Tao Deng, Jie Li, Song Mao, Sanford L. Boye, Li Liu, Vince A. Chiodo, Xuan Liu, Wei Shi and Ye Tao and William W. Hauswirth
Department of Ophthalmology, College of Medicine, University of Florida, Gainesville, Florida, United States of America

Ji-jing Pang and Xufeng Dai
Department of Ophthalmology, College of Medicine, University of Florida, Gainesville, Florida, United States of America
Eye Hospital, School of Optometry and Ophthalmology, Wenzhou Medical College, Wenzhou, China

Bo Lei and Keqing Zhang
Chongqing Key Laboratory of Ophthalmology, Ophthalmology, The First Affiliated Hospital of Chongqing Medical University, Chongqing, China

Drew Everhart and Yumiko Umino
Ophthalmology, SUNY Upstate Medical University, Syracuse, New York, United States of America,

Bo Chang
The Jackson Laboratory, Bar Harbor, Maine, United States of America

Sunilima Sinha, Ashish Tandon, Rangan Gupta, Jonathan C. K. Tovey and Ajay Sharma
Harry S. Truman Veterans Memorial Hospital, Columbia, Missouri, United States of America
Mason Eye Institute, School of Medicine, University of Missouri, Columbia, Missouri, United States of America

Rajiv R. Mohan
Harry S. Truman Veterans Memorial Hospital, Columbia, Missouri, United States of America
Mason Eye Institute, School of Medicine, University of Missouri, Columbia, Missouri, United States of America
College of Veterinary Medicine, University of Missouri, Columbia, Missouri, United States of America

Lichun Tian
Zhongshan Ophthalmic Center, Sun Yat-sen University, Guangzhou, People's Republic of China
The First Affiliated Hospital of Chongqing Medical University, Chongqing Key Laboratory of Ophthalmology and Chongqing Eye Institute, Chongqing, People's Republic of China

Peizeng Yang, Bo Lei, Ju Shao, Chaokui Wang, Qin Xiang, Lin Wei and Zhougui Peng
The First Affiliated Hospital of Chongqing Medical University, Chongqing Key Laboratory of Ophthalmology and Chongqing Eye Institute, Chongqing, People's Republic of China

Aize Kijlstra
Eye Research Institute Maastricht, Department of Ophthalmology, University Hospital Maastricht, Maastricht, The Netherlands

Hideto Chono, Naoki Saito, Hiroshi Tsuda, Junichi Mineno and Ikunoshin Kato
Center for Cell and Gene Therapy, Takara Bio Inc, Otsu, Shiga, Japan

Hiroaki Shibata, Naohide Ageyama, Keiji Terao and Yasuhiro Yasutomi
Tsukuba Primate Research Center, National Institute of Biomedical Innovation, Tsukuba, Ibaraki, Japan

Lauren E. Woodard, Annahita Keravala, W. Edward Jung, Orly L. Wapinski and Michele P. Calos
Department of Genetics, Stanford University School of Medicine, Stanford, California, United States of America

Qiwei Yang and Dean W. Felsher
Division of Oncology, Department of Medicine, Stanford University School of Medicine, Stanford, California, United States of America

Hsiao-Hsuan Tsai and Tae Heung Kang
Department of Pathology, Johns Hopkins Medical Institutions, Baltimore, Maryland, United States of America

Chien-Fu Hung
Department of Pathology, Johns Hopkins Medical Institutions, Baltimore, Maryland, United States of America

Department of Oncology, Johns Hopkins Medical Institutions, Baltimore, Maryland, United States of America

Richard R. Roden
Department of Pathology, Johns Hopkins Medical Institutions, Baltimore, Maryland, United States of America
Department of Oncology, Johns Hopkins Medical Institutions, Baltimore, Maryland, United States of America
Department of Obstetrics and Gynecology, Johns Hopkins Medical Institutions, Baltimore, Maryland, United States of America

T.-C. Wu
Department of Pathology, Johns Hopkins Medical Institutions, Baltimore, Maryland, United States of America
Department of Oncology, Johns Hopkins Medical Institutions, Baltimore, Maryland, United States of America
Department of Obstetrics and Gynecology, Johns Hopkins Medical Institutions, Baltimore, Maryland, United States of America
Department of Molecular Microbiology and Immunology, Johns Hopkins Medical Institutions, Baltimore, Maryland, United States of America

An Jen Chiang
Department of Pathology, Johns Hopkins Medical Institutions, Baltimore, Maryland, United States of America
Department of Obstetrics and Gynecology, Kaohsiung Veterans General Hospital, Kaohsiung, Taiwan
Division of Obstetrics and Gynecology, National Yang-Ming University School of Medicine, Taipei, Taiwan,
Department of Biological Sciences, National Sun Yat-Sen University, Kaohsiung, Taiwan

Martin G. Pomper
Department of Radiology, Johns Hopkins School of Medicine, Baltimore, Maryland, United States of America

Marianthi Karali, Anna Manfredi, Agostina Puppo, Elena Marrocco, Annagiusi Gargiulo, Mariacarmela Allocca and Enrico Maria Surace
Telethon Institute of Genetics and Medicine (TIGEM), Naples, Italy

Alberto Auricchio
Telethon Institute of Genetics and Medicine (TIGEM), Naples, Italy
Medical Genetics, Department of Pediatrics, University of Naples Federico II, Naples, Italy

Sandro Banfi
Telethon Institute of Genetics and Medicine (TIGEM), Naples, Italy
Medical Genetics, Department of General Pathology, Second University of Naples, Naples, Italy

Francesca Simonelli
Telethon Institute of Genetics and Medicine (TIGEM), Naples, Italy
Department of Ophthalmology, Second University of Naples, Naples, Italy

Massimo Giunti and Maria Laura Bacci
Department of Veterinary Medical Science (DSMVET), University of Bologna, Bologna, Italy,

Michele Della Corte and Settimio Rossi
Department of Ophthalmology, Second University of Naples, Naples, Italy

Swathi Balaji, Louis Le, Alice Leung, Mounira Habli and Helen N. Jones
Center for Molecular Fetal Therapy, Division of Pediatric, General, Thoracic and Fetal Surgery, Cincinnati Children's Hospital Medical Center and The University of Cincinnati College of Medicine, Cincinnati, Ohio, United States of America

Sundeep G. Keswani, Foong-Yen Lim and Timothy M. Crombleholme
Center for Molecular Fetal Therapy, Division of Pediatric, General, Thoracic and Fetal Surgery, Cincinnati Children's Hospital Medical Center and The University of Cincinnati College of Medicine, Cincinnati, Ohio, United States of America
The Children's Institute for Surgical Science, The Children's Hospital of Philadelphia, Philadelphia, Pennsylvania, United States of America

Anna B. Katz
The Children's Institute for Surgical Science, The Children's Hospital of Philadelphia, Philadelphia, Pennsylvania, United States of America

James M. Wilson
Gene Therapy Program, Department of Pathology and Laboratory Medicine, University of Pennsylvania School of Medicine, Philadelphia, Pennsylvania, United States of America

Jörn A. Lohmeyer, Daniel F. Müller and Hans-Günther Machens
Department of Plastic Surgery and Hand Surgery, Faculty of Medicine, University Hospital Rechts der Isar, Technische Universität München, Munich, Germany

Ziyang Zhang
Department of Plastic Surgery and Hand Surgery, Faculty of Medicine, University Hospital Rechts der Isar, Technische Universität München, Munich, Germany
Department of Plastic Surgery and Hand Surgery, University of Lübeck, Lübeck, Germany

José-Tomás Egaña
Department of Plastic Surgery and Hand Surgery, Faculty of Medicine, University Hospital Rechts der Isar, Technische Universität München, Munich, Germany
Facultad de Ciencias, Center for Genome Regulation, Universidad de Chile, Santiago, Chile

Alex Slobodianski, Astrid Arnold and Jessica Nehlsen
Department of Plastic Surgery and Hand Surgery, University of Lübeck, Lübeck, Germany

Wulf D. Ito
Cardiovascular Center Oberallgaeu, Academic Teaching Hospital, University of Ulm, Immenstadt, Germany

Shaoxiang Weng
Department of Cardiovascular Diseases, School of Medicine, Sir Run Run Shaw Hospital, Zhejiang University, Hangzhou, China
Experimental Angiology, Medical Department II, University Hospital Lübeck, Lübeck, Germany

Natalie Lund
Experimental Angiology, Medical Department II, University Hospital Lübeck, Lübeck, Germany

Jihong Liu
Department of Urology, Tongji Hospital, Huazhong University of Science and Technology, Wuhan, China
David M. Markusic, Dirk R. de Waart and Jurgen Seppen Academic Medical Center, Tytgat Institute for Liver and Intestinal Research, Amsterdam, The Netherlands

Priscila O. e Giuseppe, Nadia H. Martins, Andreia N. Meza, Camila R. os Santos, Humberto and Mario T. Murakami
Laboratório Nacional de Biociências (LNBio), Centro Nacional de Pesquisa em Energia e Materiais, Campinas, São Paulo, Brazil

D'Muniz Pereira
Instituto de Física de São Carlos, Grupo de Cristalografia, Universidade de São Paulo, São Carlos, São Paulo, Brazil

Yufang Zuo, Jiangxue Wu, Shiping Yang, Haijiao Yan, Li Tan, Xiangqi Meng, Xiaofang Ying, Ranyi Liu and Tiebang Kang
State Key Laboratory of Oncology in South China, Cancer Center, Sun Yat-Sen University, Guangzhou, People's Republic of China

Wenlin Huang
State Key Laboratory of Oncology in South China, Cancer Center, Sun Yat-Sen University, Guangzhou, People's Republic of China
Institute of Microbiology, Chinese Academy of Science, Beijing, People's Republic of China

Zumin Xu
State Key Laboratory of Oncology in South China, Cancer Center, Sun Yat-Sen University, Guangzhou, People's Republic of China
Department of Radiation Oncology, Cancer Center, Sun Yat-Sen University, Guangzhou, People's Republic of China

Jinglun Xue and Jinzhong Chen
State Key Laboratory of Genetic Engineering, Institute of Genetics, School of Life Science, Fudan University, Shanghai, China

Xiaoyan Dong
State Key Laboratory of Genetic Engineering, Institute of Genetics, School of Life Science, Fudan University, Shanghai, China
Beijing FivePlus Molecular Medicine Institute, Beijing, China

Zheyue Dong, Wei Shen and Gang Zheng
Beijing FivePlus Molecular Medicine Institute, Beijing, China

Wenhong Tian, Gang Wang, Xiaobing Wu and Yue Wang
State Key Laboratory for Molecular Virology and Genetic Engineering, National Institute for Viral Disease Control and Prevention, Chinese Center for Disease Control and Prevention, Beijing, China

Eduardo Gallatti Yasumura, Roberta Sessa Stilhano, Vívian Yochiko Samoto, Priscila Keiko Matsumoto, Leonardo Pinto de Carvalho, Valderez Bastos Valero Lapchik and Sang Won Han
Research Center for Gene Therapy, Department of Biophysics, Universidade Federal de São Paulo, São Paulo, São Paulo, Brazil

Erick L. Ayuni, Marie Noelle Giraud, Alexander Kadner, Thierry Caus, Thierry P. Carrel and Hendrik T. Tevaearai
Department of Cardiovascular Surgery, University Hospital of Berne, Berne, Switzerland

Amiq Gazdhar and Ralph A. Schmid
Division of General Thoracic Surgery, University Hospital of Berne, Berne, Switzerland

Mathias Gugger
Department of Pathology, University of Berne, Berne, Switzerland,

Marco Cecchini
Department of Urology, University Hospital of Berne, Berne, Switzerland

Johanna P. Laakkonen, Tatjana Engler, Florian Kreppel and Stefan Kochanek
Department of Gene Therapy, University of Ulm, Ulm, Germany

Ignacio A. Romero and Babette Weksler
Inserm, U1016, Cochin Institute, Paris, France

Pierre- Olivier Couraud
Inserm, U1016, Cochin Institute, Paris, France
CNRS, UMR8104, Paris, France
University Paris Descartes, Paris, France

Huading Lu, Yuhu Dai, Lulu Lv and Huiqing Zhao
Department of Orthopedics, Third Affiliated Hospital of Sun Yat-sen University, Guangzhou, P.R.China

Yuji Kashiwakura, Jun Mimuro, Seiji Madoiwa, Akira Ishiwata, Atsushi Yasumoto, Asuka Sakata, Tsukasa Ohmori and Yoichi Sakata
Research Division of Cell and Molecular Medicine, Center for Molecular Medicine, Jichi Medical University, Shimotsuke, Tochigi-ken, Japan

Akira Onishi, Daiichiro Fuchimoto, Shunichi Suzuki, Misae Suzuki and Shoichiro Sembon
Transgenic Animal Research Center, National Institute of Agrobiological Sciences, Tsukuba, Ibaraki-ken, Japan

Masaki Iwamoto
Transgenic Animal Research Center, National Institute of Agrobiological Sciences, Tsukuba, Ibaraki-ken, Japan
Advanced Technology Development Team, Prime Tech Ltd., Tsuchiura, Ibaraki-ken, Japan

Michiko Hashimoto and Satoko Yazaki
Advanced Technology Development Team, Prime Tech Ltd.,Tsuchiura, Ibaraki-ken, Japan

Mengqun Tan
Experimental Hematology Laboratory, Department of Physiology, School of Basic Medical Sciences, Central South University, Changsha, China
Shenzhen Institute of Xiangya Biomedicine, Shenzhen, China

Liujiang Song
Experimental Hematology Laboratory, Department of Physiology, School of Basic Medical Sciences, Central South University, Changsha, China
Shenzhen Institute of Xiangya Biomedicine, Shenzhen, China
Division of Cellular and Molecular Therapy, Department of Pediatrics, University of Florida College of Medicine, Gainesville, Florida, United States of America
Powell Gene Therapy Center, University of Florida College of Medicine, Gainesville, Florida, United States of America
Genetics Institute, University of Florida College of Medicine, Gainesville, Florida, United States of America

Yuan Wang
Department of Traditional Chinese Medicine, Changhai Hospital, Second Military Medical University, Shanghai, China
Shanghai University of Traditional Chinese Medicine, Shanghai, China

Chunxia Qin, Xiaoli Lan, Xiaotian Xia, Yueli Tian, Zhijun Pei, Hui Yuan and Yongxue Zhang
Department of Nuclear Medicine, Union Hospital, Tongji Medical College, Huazhong University of Science and Technology, Wuhan, China

Jiang He
Department of Radiology and Medical Imaging, University of Virginia, School of Medicine, Charlottesville, Virginia, United States of America

David Pérez-Villarroya
Joint Unit of Research in Genomics and Health, Centre for Public Health Research (CSISP) - Cavanilles Institute for Biodiversity and Evolutionary Biology, University of Valencia, Valencia, Spain

Mária Džunková, Giuseppe D'Auria and Andrés Moya
Joint Unit of Research in Genomics and Health, Centre for Public Health Research (CSISP) - Cavanilles Institute for Biodiversity and Evolutionary Biology, University of Valencia, Valencia, Spain
CIBER en Epidemiología y Salud Pública (CIBEResp), Madrid, Spain

In-Sun Hong and Hwa-Yong Lee
Adult Stem cell Research Center, Seoul National University, Seoul, Republic of Korea
Department of Veterinary Public Health, Laboratory of Stem Cell and Tumor Biology, Seoul National University, Seoul, Republic of Korea

Hyun-Pyo Kim
Department of Biomedical Science, Jungwon University, Chungbuk, Korea

Index